The

A I D S

Dictionary

OTHER BOOKS BY SARAH BARBARA WATSTEIN

AIDS and Women: A Sourcebook

End-User Searching in Libraries

Formal Planning in College Libraries

On Account of Sex, 1987–1992

On Account of Sex: An Annotated Bibliography on the Status of Women in Librarianship, 1982–1987

The

A I D S

Dictionary

Sarah Barbara Watstein, M.L.S., M.P.A.

With

Karen Chandler, M.D.

Facts On File, Inc.

The AIDS Dictionary

Facts On File, Inc.
11 Penn Plaza
New York NY 10001

Library of Congress Cataloging-in-Publication Data

Watstein, Sarah.
The AIDS dictionary / Sarah Watstein.
p.   cm
Includes bibliographical references and index.
ISBN 0-8160-3149-5(hc) ISBN 0-8160-3754-X (pb) (alk. paper)
1.   AIDS (Disease)—Dictionaries.   I. Title.
RC607.A26W383   1997
616.97′92′003—dc21   97-8114

Facts On File books are available at special discounts when purchased in bulk quantities for businesses, associations, institutions, or sales promotions. Please call our Special Sales Department in New York at 212/967-8800 or 800/322-8755.

You can find Facts On File on the World Wide Web at
http://www.factsonfile.com

The AIDS Dictionary is a reference work intended to help readers become better informed about HIV, AIDS, and related subjects. It is not a complete, exhaustive, or up-to-the-minute compilation, a medical text, a scientific work, or a diagnostic manual or guide to practical treatment, and should not be consulted as such. Under no circumstances can the use of this book be an adequate substitute for examination, diagnosis, and treatment by a physician or other trained medical practitioner in a properly equipped facility. The authors and publisher disclaim any liability arising directly or indirectly from any such use of this book. *All matters regarding health and health care require medical consultation and supervision.*

Text design by Cathy Rincon and Hermitage Publishing Services
Cover design by Nora Wertz

Printed in the United States of America

VB Hermitage 10 9 8 7 6 5 4 3 2 1

This books is printed on acid-free paper.

Contents

For Pam, especially;
for those friends who believe with me that knowledge = power;
and for those we have all loved and lost.
— S.B.W.

ACKNOWLEDGMENTS

To thank everyone who contributed to the conception, writing, and publication of *The AIDS Dictionary* would take several pages, but several special acknowledgments must be made. My colleagues at Virginia Commonwealth University supplied me with plenty of encouragement and support. Over the years this project has been evolving, the people with whom I worked as a volunteer—in New York City at the Gay Men's Health Crisis, in Richmond at the Richmond AIDS Ministry and the Richmond Organization for Sexual Minority Youth—were also encouraging, and eager to share their considerable knowledge. I gratefully thank them all.

This project would never have existed without the technical expertise of Wendy Helmer. Her commitment to this project, and her unwavering support for me personally, were a great help. Thanks also to Caroline Sutton, formerly of Facts On File, for her belief in this book, and finally, to my editors Drew Silver and Eleanora von Dehsen for their willingness to take on this project and for their detailed attention over the years despite already overfull schedules.

—S.B.W.

INTRODUCTION

Imagine a world without HIV/AIDS. A world beyond the virus and the dread of disease; without other fears we have gotten all too used to: fear of the public's attitude toward those infected; fear of the stigma, prudery, bigotry, and hypocrisy that give the epidemic fertile ground to grow in. A world in which policymakers no longer have to fight for funding of AIDS research and patient care; in which health care professionals no longer have to fight to stop discrimination against AIDS patients; in which communities are no longer torn asunder by rage and grief. A world in which AIDS activists no longer have to fight to disseminate information freely. Is this our future? We'd like to imagine it is.

Today, infection with human immunodeficiency virus (HIV), the virus that causes the acquired immunodeficiency syndrome (AIDS), remains one of the country's and the world's greatest health challenges. Despite some good news in the past few years, AIDS remains both a devastating illness and a major public health crisis in both the developed and the developing world. As science has learned more about it, and discovered ways to restrain it temporarily, its character has changed, as have the statistics of the epidemic. But it is still unpredictable, still a congeries of symptoms for which there is neither a cure nor a vaccine. We still don't have even a rough estimate of its incubation period. We have barely glimpsed its face, much less found a way to stop it.

AIDS has been in the public consciousness since 1981, and has been the subject of countless books and articles. There is an enormous scientific and medical literature, a growing academic literature of cultural and social analysis and criticism, and reference books for general and specialized audiences. In the trade market there is a growing *literary* literature of AIDS—novelists, poets, short story writers, dramatists, journalists, and editors continue to be moved by the pandemic and to address it in their work. Surprisingly, however, there hasn't been a really comprehensive, easy-to-use source of basic information for laypeople. This book grew out of an awareness of this gap in the literature and the authors' commitment to making a difference for the better in the lives of both those infected with, and those affected by, the virus.

Discussions of HIV and AIDS involve many complex, ever-changing issues in a variety of subject areas. Today, in the second decade of the pandemic, most would concur that the vocabulary of HIV and AIDS is growing rapidly as we learn more and more about them. The purpose of *The AIDS Dictionary* is to help readers become better informed by acquainting them with key terms and phrases that populate the HIV/AIDS lexicon. A secondary purpose is to fill the need for a reference source on HIV and AIDS in both academic and public libraries. Every effort has been made to ensure that the information in this work is accurate and up to date, but HIV/AIDS is a field that is vast and rapidly changing, and it is not possible to guarantee that there are no errors. Readers seeking definitive answers will not find them in this or any other book on this subject.

The AIDS Dictionary consists of more than 3,000 entries, most short and all free of moralizing, stigmatizing, and euphemism. In addition to the basic biological and medical aspects of the disease, it addresses many of the financial, legal, and even political and social ramifications of the pandemic. Appendixes provide a statistical snapshot of the pandemic and a list of HIV/AIDS abbreviations, as well as selected resources available by phone or on the Internet for researchers, medical practitioners, and persons with HIV/AIDS.

The authors hope that you find *The AIDS Dicitionary* a useful reference tool and welcome comments and suggestions on any aspect of this work. Please send comments to: The Authors, *The AIDS Dictionary*, c/o Facts On File, 11 Penn Plaza, New York, NY 10001–2006.

—Sarah Barbara Watstein
Karen Chandler, M.D.

The

A I D S

Dictionary

abacavir A new NUCLEOSIDE ANALOG heading for FOOD AND DRUG ADMINISTRATION approval by mid-1998. Clinical trials show that in NAIVE patients, abacavir has a profound potency, similar to a PROTEASE INHIBITOR. However, all is not so well when treatment-experienced patients are examined. Preliminary resistance analysis shows that the likelihood of failing to respond to abacavir increased according to the number of mutations on the REVERSE TRANSCRIPTASE of an individual's HIV, regardless of whether those mutations specifically reduced sensitivity to the new drug. HIV with four or more reverse transcripase mutations had little or no susceptibility to abacavir. The intricacies of abacavir resistance have yet to be fully delineated, but as of this writing it is to be feared that abacavir will not work so well in people who have already taken nucleoside analogs. A second concern about abacavir is its life-threatening allergic reactions. Glaxo Wellcome, the drug's manufacturer, has acknowledged that patients with a rash and initial systemic symptoms should not restart abacavir. Anaphylactic reactions have been seen in a small percentage of patients.

abdomen Area of the body between the thorax (chest) and the pelvis. Contains vital organs such as the stomach, lower part of the esophagus, small and large intestines, liver, gallbladder, spleen, pancreas, and bladder and reproductive organs.

abortion Induced premature termination of pregnancy; almost always done before the fetus reaches the stage of viability (ability to live outside the womb). The legal threshold of viability differs from state to state but is usually 20 to 24 weeks. Some premature NEONATES younger than 24 weeks or weighing less than 500 grams are viable. Symptoms commonly experienced during abortion include uterine contractions, uterine hemorrhage (sometimes including tissue), dilation of the CERVIX, and ejection of fetal material. Abortion done at the request of the mother is called *elective* abortion, in contrast to therapeutic abortions, done when the mental or physical health of the mother would be endangered by continued pregnancy or when the fetus is known to have, in standard medical parlance, "a condition incompatible with life." Abortions may be induced by drugs, by suction, by scraping the lining of the uterus, by injection of a sterile hypertonic solution into the amniotic cavity, or by surgery. Premature terminations of pregnancy that occur spontaneously are called *miscarriages*.

abscess Pus-filled cavity in any part of the body that occurs as a result of disintegration or displacement of tissue. A serious complication of PELVIC INFLAMMATORY DISEASE.

abstinence Going without or refraining voluntarily, particularly from indulgence in food, alcoholic beverages, or sexual activity (some people include masturbation in this definition, others do not). Sexual abstinence is an option people have exercised for a variety of reasons ranging from moral or religious conviction to fear of pregnancy or disease. Some people, including some religious orders, practice celibacy, or permanent abstinence from all sexual activity (historically, the term *celibacy* has also been used to mean simply the state of being unmarried). Some couples practice abstinence as a means of contraception: In "natural" family planning, periodic abstinence is practiced during the fertile period of the woman's menstrual cycle.

Sexual abstinence is one means of avoiding AIDS and other SEXUALLY TRANSMITTED DISEASEs. Some people opt never to have sex with anyone before or outside of permanent, exclusive sexual relationships, rather than renounce sex entirely; but for society generally, as history and everyday observation show, abstinence has not been found to be a practical or effective means of preventing infection. Today, emphasis is placed on changing sexual behavior and reducing the risk of infection through sexual contact. The positive aspects of SAFE SEX are stressed instead of emphasizing the negative aspects of UNSAFE SEX.

accelerated approval The abbreviated regulatory process under which the U.S. FOOD AND DRUG ADMINISTRATION (FDA) grants conditional marketing approval for a new drug based on early clinical testing data. Accelerated approval allows pharmaceutical manufacturers to bring to market as quickly as possible drugs for the treatment of serious or life-threatening diseases such as HIV/AIDS, and is based on relatively short-term evidence of laboratory "markers" of effectiveness (see SURROGATE MARKERS). The agency requires that drug makers provide more substantial proof of effectiveness after drugs are on the market, according to the more stringent traditional criteria, including adequate information on definitive endpoints such as disease progression and mortality rates. It could withdraw approval if such evidence is not forthcoming. Some AIDS activists have questioned the wisdom of recent accelerated drug approvals, such as that of 3TC. They concur that the drugs need to be made available as quickly as possible, but question that we will ever find out how best to use them. These activists would like to see the FDA require more stringent testing after approval.

access to injection equipment   See NEEDLE ACCESS.

access to legal services   Part of the American ideal is that everyone has the right to legal services when they are necessary. Nonetheless, people with HIV have sometimes been denied this right. There are several reasons for this. First, in terms of its scope, incidence, transmissibility, and the challenges it poses to society as a whole, HIV is unlike other illnesses with which our modern society has dealt. Second, because of its unique characteristics, the degree of ignorance about the disease remains high, and the degree of fear even higher. The legal system, after all, is run by people who are subject to the same ignorance and fear as everyone else. Additionally, persons with HIV disease have special problems that they bring to the legal system. And the system may indeed be really trying to provide such persons with an equal opportunity at fairness by giving them a helping hand in order to equalize their chance at justice with the chance enjoyed by persons not infected with HIV. In general, the courts have been slow in recognizing these special problems, for instance, protecting the privacy of people with AIDS (PWAs), weighed against the need to protect the public from transmission of HIV; balancing risks to the defendant and the public in determining the sentence for a PWA convicted of a crime; dealing with the fears of court personnel about courtroom contact with PWAs; and introducing new aspects of old issues of discrimination in employment, housing, public accommodations and schools.

The American Bar Association's (ABA) Policy on AIDS was adopted in August 1989. It sets forth four principles. First, the judiciary and the organized bar should encourage attorneys and judges to become knowledgeable about HIV and its related legal issues and should provide appropriate education and training in these areas. Second, the judiciary and the organized bar should support the allocation of additional private and public resources, including the further development of pro bono activities, for the delivery of legal services to individuals affected by HIV. Third, attorneys should not refuse to represent clients or limit or modify their representation of clients because of the clients' known or perceived HIV status. Fourth, judicial or administrative proceedings involving participants known or perceived to be HIV-infected should be conducted in the same fashion as any other such proceedings. Extraordinary safety or security precautions should not be undertaken based solely upon the participants' known or perceived HIV status.

access to medical care   The degree of ease with which the consumer can secure health services. Along with AVAILABIL-ITY, access is a key criterion used to measure the adequacy of a health care system. Access, especially early in the course of their illness, is a particularly important issue for those infected with HIV, who require a broad array of services at all times. Early access to drugs and therapies for the treatment of HIV infection includes access to promising treatments before full marketing approval. Historically, within the context of HIV/AIDS, pharmaceutical companies and government agencies alike have been unenthusiastic if not hostile towards early treatment access.

accessory cells   LYMPHOID cells predominantly of the MONOCYTE and MACROPHAGE lineage that cooperate with T and B LYMPHOCYTEs in the formation of ANTIBODIES and in other IMMUNE RESPONSEs.

accessory molecules   Membrane GLYCOPROTEINs of the Ig superfamily on certain T cell surfaces, additional to the T cell receptors themselves, regulating adhesion between T cell and ANTIGEN-PRESENTING CELLs (APCs).

acemannan   An anti-HIV drug (trade name Carrisyn). Acemannan, a complex carbohydrate extracted from the aloe vera plant, has been shown to have a broad spectrum of action against viruses that infect warm-blooded animals and HIV IN VITRO. Additionally, the drug has been shown to stimulate host immunity. This property places acemannan in a new class of substances known as BIOLOGICAL RESPONSE MODIFIERs (BRMs). The acemannan molecule is absorbed intact into the bloodstream where it accumulates in MACROPHAGEs, multipurpose white blood cells vital to IMMUNE SYSTEM function. After absorbing acemannan, the macrophages increase their production of vital immunologic protein substances, called CYTOKINEs. These include INTERLEUKIN-1 and TUMOR NECROSIS FACTOR. These substances function to elicit the cascade of host immune defenses, including escalated production of natural KILLER CELLs vital to the body's ability to fight off so-called OPPORTUNISTIC INFECTIONs. See ALOE VERA.

acetaminophen   A synthetic drug with antipyretic (antifever) and ANALGESIC actions similar to aspirin. It does not have the anti-inflammatory or antirheumatic actions of aspirin. It is available without a prescription. As a prescription medicine, it is used in combination with stronger pain relievers for the treatment of moderate-to-severe pain. It is also used in a number of cold and flu products in combination with ANTIHISTAMINEs, decongestants, and sleeping medications. Acetaminophen is available in many forms and doses, under many trade names.

achlorhydria   The absence of free hydrochloric acid in the gastric juices, a result of atrophy of the gastric mucous membrane. Also called gastric anacidity. May be associated with CARCINOMA, gastric ulcer, pernicious anemia, ADRENAL INSUFFICIENCY, or chronic gastritis.

acid-fast   Resistant to decolorization with acidified organic solvents after staining with a dye. This property is used as the basis of a test for identifying acid-fast bacilli (AFB) such as MYCOBACTERIUM TUBERCULOSIS and other MYCOBACTERIA.

acid-fast bacillus   See ACID-FAST.

acidophilus   Bacteria that help maintain or restore a supportive bacterial environment in an intestinal tract affected by disease and ANTIBIOTICs. *Acidophilus* also may be useful in preventing CANDIDIASIS (thrush) in the throat, mouth, and vagina. Most HIV-positive people have some form of digestive imbalance at some time. Daily *acidophilus* supplementation is suggested to prevent or mitigate such problems. Among the benefits of *acidophilus* are production of significant amounts of folic acid, vitamin B12 and other B-complex vitamins, reduction of intestinal gas and diarrhea and increased production of lactase, leading to improved digestion of dairy products. *Acidophilus* is found in yogurt and is available in capsule form in health food stores.

ACIDS   See ACQUIRED COMMUNITY IMMUNE DEFICIENCY SYNDROME.

acquired community immune deficiency syndrome (ACIDS)   An early name for what is now called ACQUIRED IMMUNODEFICIENCY SYNDROME (AIDS).

acquired immune deficiency syndrome   An early name for what is now called ACQUIRED IMMUNODEFICIENCY SYNDROME (AIDS).

acquired immunodeficiency syndrome (AIDS)   An infectious disease characterized by failure of the IMMUNE SYSTEM and believed to be caused by the HUMAN IMMUNODEFICIENCY VIRUS (HIV), one of a large group of IMMUNODEFICIENCY viruses (IVs) widespread among primates and other mammals. The now universal acronym was first used by the Centers for Disease Control and Prevention (CDC) of the U.S. Public Health Service in the fall of 1982.

AIDS and HIV are not the same thing. AIDS is best understood as the latest stage of the illness resulting from infection with the HIV virus, characterized by the appearance of difficult-to-treat OPPORTUNISTIC INFECTIONS and malignancies which profoundly decreased immunity is unable to control. See SYNDROME; AIDS-DEFINING DIAGNOSIS.

ACT-UP   See AIDS COALITION TO UNLEASH POWER; ACTIVISM.

ACTG   See AIDS CLINICAL TRIALS GROUPs.

activated lymphocytes   LYMPHOCYTEs that have been stimulated by specific ANTIGEN or nonspecific MITOGEN.

activated macrophages   Mature MACROPHAGEs IN A Metabolic state caused by various stimuli, especially PHAGOCYTOSIS or LYMPHOKINE activity.

active immunity   Resistance to a disease resulting from the production of ANTIBODIES in a person who has been inoculated with an ANTIGEN. See also PASSIVE IMMUNITY.

activism   The practice of direct action or involvement as a means of achieving political or other social or civic goals. In recent decades, activism has emerged as an effective way for those without great financial resources or political clout to participate in public debate over issues as diverse as institutionalized racism, class bias, reproductive rights, sexism, heterosexism, ableism.

AIDS activism is a way to respond collectively and constructively to the epidemic in all of its enormity and complexity, keeping it alive as an urgent public issue. It serves many specific purposes. Perhaps most importantly, AIDS activism empowers persons with HIV/AIDS by helping them organize around, and even figure out what their issues are. For both individuals and groups, it provides a means to fight discrimination and to overcome, or begin to overcome, a history of powerlessness. It provides a constant challenge to government agencies, social service providers, the medical establishment, the media and the public.

On the HIV/AIDS issue, letter writing, postcard campaigns, leafletting, conducting safe-sex "tupperware" parties for adults, setting up information tables outside high schools, creating videotapes, questioning public officials and, for gays and lesbians, forcing colleagues and families to confront an issue they may have preferred to evade by "coming out," are all forms of activism. ACT-UP (AIDS COALITION TO UNLEASH POWER), formed in 1987 in New York by a group outraged at the government's mismanagement of the AIDS crisis, was one of the earliest and still probably the best known AIDS activist group.

Significantly, although AIDS activism has not decreased, in recent years there have been far fewer of the kind of attention-getting acts that deliberately disrupt some public function or ceremony. The reason is that earlier efforts have succeeded in putting AIDS on the public agenda. AIDS activists are now consulted by the CDC and other agencies on health policy, to the benefit of the public. Although many have taken issue with some of the tactics employed by organized activist groups in their early years, most would agree that they have served a good purpose.

activity   The ability in a drug, to control or inhibit a PATHOGEN. Activity may be determined in the laboratory and differs from EFFICACY, which is the ability of a treatment to alter the course of clinical disease.

ACTU   See AIDS CLINICAL TRIALS GROUPs.

acupressure   Based on the principles of ACUPUNCTURE, this ancient Chinese technique involves the use of finger pressure, rather than needles, on specific "chi" points on the body to relieve tension and stress, as well as menstrual pain, cramps, arthritis, headaches, and eyestrain. Acupressure is also said to prevent and combat colds, improve muscle tone, boost energy levels, and be generally useful in preventive health care.

Acupressure, like acupuncture, is intended to relieve muscular tension, increasing the flow of blood—and therefore of oxygen and nutrients—to tissues throughout the body. This helps promote physical calmness and mental alertness, and aids in healing by removing waste products. Many researchers now believe that acupuncture and acupressure trigger the release of ENDORPHINS, neurochemicals that relieve pain. Both techniques have been used with some success to provide relief to people with HIV and AIDS.

acupuncture   A Chinese medical therapy in which needles are used to press "chi," or energy, points on the surface of the body. Traditional Chinese medical theory holds that energy imbalance is the cause of all illness. Acupuncture seeks to diagnose such an imbalance before a detectable physiological impairment occurs. Acupuncturists focus on helping patients balance the chi energy within and between the five major organ systems: the heart, lungs, liver, spleen, and kidneys. To restore health, an acupuncturist uses long, very thin needles as "antennas" to direct chi to organs or functions of the body. The needles can also be used to drain chi where it is excessive, and to decrease or increase moisture and heat. The acupuncturist does this by selecting points along the body's fourteen "meridians" that affect the functioning of specific organs and puncturing and stimulating tissue at these locations. The needles penetrate to just below the epidermis and do not draw blood or cause discomfort. Sometimes heat is used, along with massage or electrical impulses.

The World Health Organization (WHO) currently recognizes more than forty medical problems, ranging from allergies to arthritis and AIDS, that can be helped by acupuncture treatment. Acupuncture has become a respectable therapy in American hospitals in the last twenty years, and is used to reduce pain in patients with sore throats, sickle-cell anemia, dysmenorrhea, aftereffects of dental surgery, hysterectomies, chronic back disorders, migraine headaches and other ailments. It has been used successfully to induce cessation of smoking and to treat alcoholism and opiate addiction. Acupuncture has also been used to reduce pain in patients undergoing cancer chemotherapy and, of course, HIV/AIDS and related opportunistic infections and diseases.

In most states of the United States, acupuncturists must be medical doctors and have certification from the National Commission of Acupuncturists. However, some states do not regulate the practice at all. It is advisable to check a practitioner's credentials before a visit.

An acupuncturist generally uses a history and physical examination of the patient in making a diagnosis. In addition to asking questions, he focuses his attention on the character of the pulse and the appearance of the tongue. Sophisticated biological testing is not employed. The goal of the history and the physical is to assess the balance of yin and yang in the patient, and to guide the acupuncturist in selecting the correct chi points for a particular condition. Several treatments may be required over a period of weeks or months. The goal of therapy is to correct deficiencies or excesses of chi, thus restoring health. See also ACUPRESSURE.

acute   In medicine, this term describes intense short-term symptoms or illnesses that either resolve or evolve into long-lasting chronic disease manifestation.

acute aseptic meningitis   See MENINGITIS.

acute encephalopathy   See ENCEPHALOPATHY.

acute HIV exanthem   A severe skin eruption or rash that manifests itself as a result of HUMAN IMMUNODEFICIENCY VIRUS.

acute HIV infection   See HIV INFECTION.

acute phase proteins   SERUM PROTEINs whose levels increase during infection or inflammatory reactions. See INFLAMMATION.

acute phase reactions   Increases in certain PLASMA PROTEINs in response to almost any disease process that causes tissue damage. The blood sedimentation rate is influenced by these increases, as is the synthesis of C-reactive protein. The reaction is induced by INTERLEUKIN-1, INTERLEUKIN-6, and TUMOR NECROSIS FACTOR. This factor is important in prompting the body defenses against MICROORGANISMs.

acute PID   See PELVIC INFLAMMATORY DISEASE (PID).

acute salpingitis   See PELVIC INFLAMMATORY DISEASE; SALPINGITIS.

acyclovir   A NUCLEOSIDE ANALOG like AZT, acyclovir is an ANTIMICROBIAL and ANTIVIRAL drug approved for use against HERPES SIMPLEX I (fever blisters, cold sores), herpes simplex II (genital herpes), HERPES ZOSTER (shingles), CYTOMEGALOVIRUS and EPSTEIN-BARR VIRUS. Acyclovir is sometimes used as an adjunct to AZT, although the effectiveness of the combination is the subject of controversy (both drugs are manufactured by Glaxo Wellcome). It has been suggested that high doses of acyclovir may strengthen the REVERSE TRANSCRIPTASE INHIBITORs, and that it may improve health by suppressing herpes or other opportunistic viral infections, but neither hypothesis has been proven. Either one, if confirmed, could represent a strategy for buttressing weak anti-HIV medications by improving the body's overall microbial environment. Side effects include arthralgias, diarrhea, headache, nausea, vomiting, and dizziness. Psychosis may be seen at high doses. Topical administration (ointment) may cause burning and stinging; skin may became hypersensitive with subsequent use. In combination with ZIDOVUDINE, severe drowsiness and lethargy may occur, but an increase in antiretroviral activity has been seen. Combined use with probenecid increases the half-life of acyclovir by decreasing its excretion. Increased antiviral activity has been seen in combination with ALPHA-INTERFERON *in vitro*. Combination with nephrotoxic drugs increases the risk of nephrotoxicity. High IV doses in combination with other bone marrow suppressant agents (i.e., high-dose trimethoprim/sulfamethoxazole) may induce blood dyscrasias.

To date, acyclovir's effect on HIV levels, has not been established, nor has its anti-AIDS mechanism been definitively elucidated. It remains to be seen whether acyclovir is useful in cases of HIV with no evidence of herpes simplex infection. How best to use acyclovir, the proper dosages, and the duration of its benefit are open questions.

Acyclovir is available for oral (considered most effective), intravenous, and topical administration. It is marketed under the trade name Zovirax.

ADA   See AMERICANS WITH DISABILITIES ACT.

ADAP   See AIDS DRUG ASSISTANCE PROGRAMS.

adaptation   1. Adjustment of an organism to a change in internal or external conditions or circumstances. 2. In ophthalmology, adjustment of the eye to various intensities of light, accomplished by changing the size of the pupil and through chemical changes inside the eye. 3. In psychology, a change in quality, intensity, or distinctness of sensation occurring after continuous stimulation of constant intensity. 4. In dentistry, the proper fitting of dentures or orthodontic bands to the teeth, or closeness of a filling to walls of a cavity.

adaptive immunity   A series or complex of host defenses characterized by extreme specificity and memory mediated by ANTIBODY or T CELLs. See IMMUNITY.

ADC   See AIDS DEMENTIA COMPLEX.

ADCC   See ANTIBODY-DEPENDENT CELL-MEDIATED CYTO-TOXICITY.

adefovir   Another new antiviral heading for FOOD AND DRUG ADMINISTRATION consideration by the middle of 1998. Gilead Sciences' adefovir is a NUCLEOSIDE ANALOG with a twist, or actually a tail. Adefovir, the oral prodrug version of PMEA, comes with a phosphate group attached, the first of three that cells add to nucleosides to energize them before they can be strung together to form new DNA or RNA. By skipping the first of these activation steps, which can be a real bottleneck, adefovir in theory is more readily available within cells to attack HIV than the standard nucleoside analogs (technically adefovir is a nucleotide analog). Its intracellular stability is also higher than the nucleoside drugs'. To date little information has been released about adefovir's activity. Adefovir's main purpose probably is to contribute a little extra HIV suppression and hence more durability to a combination regimen that is already achieving a substantial response in the individual. Two advantages to adefovir are that resistance mutations are rare during treatment and that it accumulates within cells. This latter advantage can also be a disadvantage when those cells start to feel the adverse effects of the drug, which is just as inherently toxic as the nucleoside analogs. For starters, adefovir reduces cellular levels of L-carnitine, a natural substance necessary for converting lipids to energy within cells, and patients taking the drug must also take L-carnitine supplements. Particularly sensitive to adefovir are the kidney cells; to protect this organ those on adefovir must have their kidney function checked each month, via lab tests for serum creatinine and protein in the urine. Brand name Preveon.

addiction   Although there is disagreement among authorities as to how inclusive this designation should be, addiction is generally recognized to be a state of intense dependence upon a substance that chemically alters the functioning of the central nervous system, characterized by uncontrollable use of the substance, tolerance for its pleasure-giving effects, and manifestations of withdrawal symptoms when it is withheld. These features constitute physical dependence—a state of physical incorporation of the substance into the fundamental biochemistry of the brain. Habitual repeated behaviors such as overeating, reading, and television-watching are sometimes loosely referred to as addictions, but the term is properly used to indicate physiological need to experience the effects on the central nervous system of the addictive substance.

In regard to alcohol and drugs, addiction is distinguished from other noncompulsive ways of use such as *experimental* (trying a drink or a drug to see what it does); *social* or *recreational* (using a drink or a drug to enhance an activity or an event); *situational* (using a drink or a drug for a specific temporary pharmacological effect, such as relaxation of tension); and *intensified* (daily use without signs of compulsion).

The life of addicts is one of compulsion. Seven stages of addictive behavior have been noted. First, use of the addictive substance so that the user loses awareness of the amount and frequency of use. Second, the effects of the substance become unpredictable. Third, use becomes indiscriminate, and the user is no longer careful about the circumstances in which he or she uses it. Fourth, the user exhibits fear of abstinence and acts to secure or protect his supply; he feels better simply by having the substance in his possession. Fifth, the user develops a peer support group of fellow users and may reject nonusers. Sixth, where circumstances (such as the illegal status of some addictive substances) encourage them, the user develops self-protective, often pathological behaviors, including lying, stealing, and cheating, and may also engage in trafficking. Finally, the user develops the destructive physical and psychological effects of the prolonged use at toxic levels of the addictive substance—most commonly alcohol, tobacco, or a narcotic drug.

Addison's disease   A disease resulting from a disorder of the adrenal glands, resulting in deficiency or lack of secretion of adrenocortical HORMONEs. It may be a result of TUBERCULOSIS or autoimmune-induced adrenal disease. Its symptons include occasional discoloration of the skin and mucous membranes, irregular patches of vitiligo (depigmentation of the skin), black freckles over head and neck, fever, tumors, HEMORRHAGIC NECROSIS, weakness, FATIGUE, HYPOTENSION, NAUSEA, vomiting, ANOREXIA, weight loss, and sometimes HYPOGLYCEMIA. If not treated, it is usually fatal. See also ADRENAL FUNCTION and ADRENAL INSUFFICIENCY.

adenine arabinoside   See VIDARABINE.

adenopathy   Swelling or enlargement of the LYMPH NODEs.

adenovirus   One of a group of closely related VIRUSEs that can cause infections of the upper respiratory tract. These viruses have also appeared in latent infections in some people. Many types of adenoviruses have been isolated and designated by number. In addition to human adenoviruses there are also animal types. Adenoviruses may induce malignancy.

adherence   In medicine, following or adhering to a prescribed therapeutic regimen.

adhesion   The binding, or "sticking" of migratory LEUKO-CYTEs to endothelial or structural cells by the interaction of complementary adhesion PROTEINs.

adjustment disorder   A maladaptive reaction to an identifiable psychological or social stress that occurs within three months of the onset of the stressful situation. The reaction is characterized by impairment of function or symptoms in excess of the norm for that stress. The symptoms may be expected to remit either when the stress ceases, or a new, more functional adaptation is achieved.

adjuvant   Assisting. In medicine, a drug added to a therapy to increase the effectiveness of the treatment. In immunology, one of a variety of substances, including inorganic gels such as alum, aluminum hydroxide, and aluminum phosphate, that increase antigenic response (see ANTIGEN). A compound capable of potentiating an immune response.

administration   In medicine, the introduction of a drug or chemical into the body.

administration, route of   The method—INTRAVENOUS, oral or topical—of introducing a drug or chemical into the body.

administrative law judge (ALJ)   An outside, impartial officer appointed to hear disputes and render decisions regarding the administrative determinations of many state and federal government agencies. An applicant who has been turned down for benefits in a SOCIAL SECURITY ADMINISTRATION (SSA) program, for instance, may request an ALJ hearing.

adolescence   The period in which full sexual development occurs, between the onset of puberty and sexual maturity. It is characterized by physical growth, the appearance of secondary sexual characteristics, intense and wildly changeable emotions and strong sexual urges (sometimes known as "raging hormones").
   This development is a gradual process and its timing varies among individuals. It is defined by the National Library of Medicine as ranging from ages 13 to 18, but other institutions and disciplines hold that it ranges as broadly as from ages 11 to 25.

adoption   The assumption of complete parental responsibility for children by persons who are not the natural parents. Formal adoption is an exhaustive legal procedure.

adrenal function   The action performed by the ADRENAL GLAND.

adrenal gland   One of two ENDOCRINE GLANDs located on the top of the kidneys; each consists of an adrenal cortex, which secretes cortisol and aldosterone, and an adrenal medulla, which secretes epinephrine and norepinephrine

adrenal insufficiency   Abnormally low or decreased production of adrenal corticoid hormone by the ADRENAL GLAND. ADDISON'S DISEASE is the result.

adult day services   Day-long social service and care programs for incapacitated adults, on the model of senior citizens' or children's day care programs. Sponsored by the Department of Veterans Affairs (formerly the Veterans Administration [VA]).

adult respiratory distress syndrome (ARDS)   A form of restrictive lung disease caused by increased permeability of the pulmonary capillaries or the alveolar EPITHELIUM, characterized by the presence of an abnormally large amount of fluid in the tissue. The condition often develops after severe infection, trauma, or systemic illness. It has approximately a 50-percent fatality rate.

adult services   Social services such as counseling, home chore aid, meals-on-wheels, discharge planning, program placement, drug abuse treatment, and so on, provided to adult welfare recipients as well as to some moderate-income aged and disabled people.

adverse event   In medicine, a toxic reaction to therapy.

Advil   See IBUPROFEN.

advocacy   In regard to social services and health care, action taken on behalf of individuals by themselves or others to ensure appropriate access to and availability of such services.

aerosol   In medicine, the action by which a drug, such as PENTAMIDINE, is turned into a fine spray or mist by a nebulizer for administration by inhaling. See ADMINISTRATION, ROUTE OF.

aerosol pentamidine   See PENTAMIDINE: AEROSOL.

AETC   See AIDS EDUCATION AND TRAINING CENTERS (AETC) PROGRAM.

AFB isolation   A specific type of hospital isolation for persons with acute MYCOBACTERIUM TUBERCULOSIS. Its purpose is to prevent the spread of infection during the infectious phase of the disease. See ACID-FAST.

AFDC   See AID TO FAMILIES WITH DEPENDENT CHILDREN.

AFDC foster care   FOSTER CARE for children who originated in families receiving benefits under the AID TO FAMILIES WITH DEPENDENT CHILDREN (AFDC) program. It includes MEDICAID coverage of the children.

affective   Pertaining to feelings, emotions, or mental states.

affective disorder   Any disorder of affect, that is, of the feelings or emotions, characterized by mood swings and depression. It is not caused by, but may accompany, other physical or mental disorders. Affective disorders are common in HIV/AIDS patients.

African swine fever   A viral disease caused by an IMMUN-ODEFICIENCY-distinct agent, first isolated in Africa. It has also been found in Brazil, Cuba, the Dominican Republic, Haiti, and western Europe. Early in the AIDS epidemic it was suspected to be the causative agent of the acquired immunodeficiency syndrome.

age   In psychology, the stage of development reached by an individual, as expressed in terms of the chronological age of an average individual at a comparable stage of development or accomplishment.

agent   Something that causes a biological, chemical, or physical effect. BACTERIA that cause a disease are agents of that disease; medicine administered to treat a DISEASE or illness is a therapeutic agent.

AHG   See FACTOR VIII.

A.I.D.   See ARTIFICIAL INSEMINATION by donor.

aid and attendance   A term used by the DEPARTMENT OF VETERANS AFFAIRS (VA) to designate the home chore aid a disabled veteran pensioner must purchase because he or she is too incapacitated for daily living activities and for which he or she is therefore eligible for a higher pension income.

Aid to Families with Dependent Children (AFDC)   One of a number of federal welfare programs that provides temporary financial assistance to needy families with dependent children. The principal agency designated to carry out welfare, the Department of Health and Human Service's Administration for Children and Families' (ACF) Office of Family Assistance (OFA) saw its mission transformed by the Personal Responsibility and Work Opportunity Reconciliation Act of 1996. This law was designed to "end welfare as we know it," in the words of both President Bill Clinton and the Republicans in Congress. See TEMPORARY ASSISTANCE FOR NEEDY FAMILIES (TANF).

Aid to the Permanently and Totally Disabled (APTD)   A federal-state welfare program for poor disabled persons. It was replaced by the federal SUPPLEMENTAL SECURITY INCOME (SSI) program in 1974, but the term is still used in some states to refer to STATE SUPPLEMENTARY PAYMENT (SSP) programs.

AIDS   See ACQUIRED IMMUNODEFICIENCY SYNDROME.

AIDS advocacy organization   See COMMUNITY-BASED ORGANIZATION.

AIDS and cultural analysis   See CULTURAL ANALYSIS AND AIDS.

AIDS and cultural discourse   See CULTURAL ANALYSIS AND AIDS; AIDS DISCOURSE.

AIDS-associated retrovirus (ARV)   Isolates of the retrovirus that causes AIDS. See HUMAN IMMUNODEFICIENCY VIRUS (HIV).

AIDS-associated virus (AAV)   An early name for HUMAN IMMUNODEFICIENCY VIRUS (HIV).

AIDS buyers' club   Any of a network of outlets that provide access to alternative treatments, often on a cost-plus basis. Typically a nonprofit organization set up by persons with HIV or AIDS, a buyers club helps its members buy nutritional and other products, especially those not readily available elsewhere, at wholesale prices. Buyers' clubs also protect their members by making more sophisticated product selection and purchasing decisions than individuals would be likely to do on their own and negotiating better prices. They often have products independently tested, helping members avoid shoddy products.

Clubs also share information and negotiate as a unit when necessary, so they provide the power of a national network, one entirely dedicated to serving the interests of HIV positive people and finding the best treatments available. Buyers' clubs serve an important quality control function in the marketplace.

Their importance also goes beyond their role in the market. They often serve as treatment-oriented support groups. Members share information not only about products but about physicians, clinics, and therapies, including all kinds of conventional, experimental, or alternative treatments. These grassroots groups fill the gap left by major AIDS support organizations that have usually refused to allow their support group to focus on treatment information.

In practice, buyers' clubs vary widely. Some of the smaller ones skip the considerable paperwork of incorporating as a nonprofit, so technically they are for-profit businesses even if they do not actually make money. Some clubs will ship products; others are not set up to do that. Some need to collect money in advance before placing orders; others have stock on hand. Clubs are located throughout the United States, and in foreign countries as well.

AIDS case definition   As with any disease, a consistent definition was developed for AIDS so that the CENTERS FOR DISEASE CONTROL AND PREVENTION (CDC) could track the spread of AIDS and implement strategies to prevent the transmission of infection. Devised in 1987, the CDC AIDS definition describes a case of AIDS according to a narrow list of criteria and specifically according to whether an individual has experienced one or more of a number of infections and cancers, known as "indicator" diseases. These cases, and only these cases, are included in the CDC's surveillance reports of AIDS diagnoses and fatalities. Based on the CDC's experience (in the early and mid-1980s) with people with HIV, at the time predominantly gay men, the AIDS case definition systematically excluded women, injection drug users, low-income people, and other populations. These people with AIDS were, in turn, unable to be officially diagnosed as having AIDS. While the way in which the CDC defines AIDS may seem remote from the daily lives of people with HIV, it does, in fact, have a profound impact on their access to health care and benefits. For example, many entitlement programs determine an individual's eligibility for benefits according to whether or not s/he has CDC-defined AIDS. In addition, as a second example, federal and state funds are often allocated on the basis of the CDC-defined AIDS cases reported. What is at issue therefore is, when does an HIV infection become AIDS and when does AIDS become disabling.

In 1992, bowing to increasing public pressure from patients, health professionals, activists, and others, federal officials proposed an expanded definition of AIDS that included a laboratory test of immune function and added three illnesses (invasive cancer of the cervix, pulmonary tuberculosis, and two or more episodes of bacterial pneumonia) to 23 other complicating ailments listed in the 1987 definition. The proposed definition also included any adult infected with HIV who has 200 or fewer CD4 cells per cubic milliliter of blood, or about one-fifth the normal level. No such measurement was part of the original definition. The expansion of the AIDS definition to include the gynecological symptoms and diseases of women with HIV paved the way for research and treatment for women-specific infections. The new definition went into effect in 1993, and resulted, as was predicted, in a significant increase in the number of AIDS cases. The change did not have a significant impact on insurance and other benefits because Social Security Administration officials do not rely on the CDC definition in determining disability.

AIDS Clinical Trials Group (ACTG)

Also known as AIDS Clinical Trials Unit (ACTU). A nationwide, multicenter clinical trials network that tests new drugs and treatment strategies for adults and children infected with HIV that is sponsored and administered by the National Institute of Allergy and Infectious Diseases (NIAID). The ACTG was established by NIAID in 1987 and remains the largest network of its kind in the world. The specific goals of the ACTG are threefold: to evaluate innovative therapeutic strategies and interventions to control HIV infection and its complications; to facilitate rapid translation of basic research into clinical research and practice; and to provide a flexible resource for state-of-the-art, multidisciplinary clinical trials that address the goals and objectives of NIAID's therapeutics research agenda. NIAID contracts with institutions such as hospitals, academic medical centers, and so forth to perform the actual drug trials through a grant process, with a principal investigator controlling the trial.

The ACTG is an outgrowth of NIAID's first major programs for the evaluation of potential treatments for people with AIDS, which began in the summer of 1986. The original 36 AIDS Clinical Trials Units included two sites that enrolled children with AIDS. Additional pediatric sites were added between 1988 and 1989, and again in 1992. After a competitive renewal in 1992, the ACTG grew to include 35 adult and 22 pediatric AIDS Clinical Trial Units, in addition to a statistical and data analysis center and an operations office. More than 35,000 adults and 6,000 children and adolescents have enrolled in ACTG clinical trials ranging from early single-site safety studies to large-scale, multicenter efficacy trials.

In 1993, NIAID conducted a comprehensive evaluation of the ACTG to assess its mission, scientific agenda, and future direction, as well as the group's organizational structure and efficiency. This review was carried out by an exter-

nal scientific review panel that evaluated the ACTG's scientific plans, and NIAID staff working group that assessed organizational and managerial issues. Both review groups recommended that the leadership of the ACTG be strengthened, giving it increased authority and accountability for development and management of its scientific program. The reviewers also recommended that the ACTG place greater emphasis on pathogenesis-based clinical research. These recommendations and others, including the separation of the Adult ACTG from the Pediatric ACTG, were incorporated into a Request for Applications for the competitive renewal of Adult ACTG, published in August 1994. Three types of applications were solicited: one for prospective AIDS Clinical Trials Units, one for a Coordinating and Operations Center, and another for a Statistical and Data Management Center. Two separate committees were convened to review the three types of applications. Applications recommended for further consideration went through a second level of external peer review by the National Advisory Allergy and Infectious Diseases Council, before a final decision was made on the sites that would be funded. Among the criteria considered in the review process were the scientific and technical merit of the applications, the qualifications of key personnel, experience in multicenter HIV/AIDS clinical research, adequacy of plans for inclusion of women and minorities, and a demonstrated ability to accrue a certain number of patients each year.

Today, the ACTGs remain the largest network of their kind in the world. A consortium of academically affiliated clinicians responsible for conducting a large portion of clinical research of AIDS in the United States constitutes the backbone of the ACTGs. Medical centers throughout the United States that conduct clinical trials of drugs for treating people with HIV infection are also members of the consortium. Specifically, the drugs are for treating opportunistic infections or tumors as well as HIV itself, and for stimulating the immune system. ACTGs are funded federally through the National Institutes of Heath.

ACTG trials have been the source of most of the information currently available on how best to treat people with HIV infection and related diseases. ACTG research also has defined the standard preventive therapies and treatments for many opportunistic infections. When a drug is given ACTG status it means that a specific protocol and a series of sites were chosen to carry out government-funded clinical trials of the drug in order to study the drug's effect in people living with HIV/AIDS.

AIDS Coalition to Unleash Power (ACT-UP)

An AIDS activist organization founded in 1987 in New York City. Composed mainly of young gays and lesbians with a desire to be politically active, ACT-UP quickly became the strongest and best known organization of its kind. In its heyday, ACT-UP had to move its weekly New York meeting from a small community center in Greenwich Village to a more commodious auditorium at the Cooper Union. There, at what was then the epicenter of AIDS activism, as many as 700 people would show up, pumping each other full of a take-no-prisoners fervor and plotting brash demonstrations that would halt traffic, heckle politicians, and guarantee prominent coverage on the evening news. From interrupting trading at the New York Stock Exchange to disrupting a sermon by Cardinal O'Connor inside St. Patrick's Cathedral, its nervy tactics became a staple of television news. Its leaflets and logos formed a sort of visual iconography in many cities, including New York, where it used to be difficult to use an automated teller machine without seeing a decal bearing a pink triangle and the caveat "silence=death," or to walk a few blocks without seeing a rendering of a bloody handprint. Indeed, in its heyday in New York just about every possible target was zapped, and many of those demonstrations made the newspapers and the television news.

Several big moments in ACT-UP's history merit mention. In March 1987, at ACT-UP's first demonstration, 17 members were arrested on Wall Street as 250 protested drug company profiteering and other issues. In April 1989 four ACT-UP members were arrested after barricading themselves inside a Burroughs Wellcome office in North Carolina to protest the high cost of AZT. In September 1989 seven ACT-UP members interrupted trading on the New York Stock Exchange floor. In December 1989 some 4,500 people converged on St. Patrick's Cathedral in New York City to protest church opposition to safer-sex education and legal abortion. A total of 111 people were arrested, including 43 inside for disrupting a sermon by Cardinal O'Connor. In October 1992, while the AIDS quilt was on display in Washington, ACT-UP mourners broke through police lines and threw ashes of people who had died of AIDS on the White House lawn.

ACT-UP served a variety of purposes, not the least of which was to train a whole generation of activists in a range of social-change work and advocacy. ACT-UP demanded increased financing for medical research and accelerated drug development; today, much of this has come to pass. In March 1987, when ACT-UP held its inaugural demonstration on Wall Street, the annual budget allotted by the National Institutes of Health for AIDS research was about $290 million and AZT was the only antiviral AIDS drug that was approved by the FOOD AND DRUG ADMINISTRATION. As of March 1997, the annual research budget was an estimated $1.5 billion and there were ten approved ANTIVIRAL drugs, including four PROTEASE INHIBITORs, which seem by far to be the most effective medications to date. Moreover, the time from initial development of a drug to its availability to patients has been cut from about seven or eight years to less than three. ACT-UP was a compelling force behind these changes. Above all, ACT-UP irrefutably accomplished its bedrock goal: to make Americans pay some attention to AIDS. It did this with unmitigated gall and undeniable panache that in New York, San Francisco, Los Angeles, and many other cities, turned ACT-UP into the coolest club to which homosexuals could belong. And it did this while surviving on donations and the sale of T-shirts and artwork.

Today, ACT-UP is a shadow of its former self. This reflects, in part, the deaths of many of its leaders, the infighting that fractured the group, the seemingly inevitable mellowing of any radical movement, and the degree to which the armies that amassed to battle AIDS traveled a spectrum of grief from anger to acceptance. It also is because ACT-UP's energy did not so much dissipate as dis-

perse, with members marching off in different, more specialized directions and with an array of other AIDS-related organizations spun off from or inspired by it. Most interestingly, and perhaps most significantly, it also reflects the extent to which the protesters once clamoring at the dining room door have gained a place at the table.

See ACTIVISM.

AIDS-defining diagnosis   See AIDS CASE DEFINITION.

AIDS-defining illness   One of a number of serious illnesses that occurs in HIV-positive individuals and contributes to a diagnosis of AIDS. See ACQUIRED IMMUNODEFICIENCY SYNDROME; AIDS CASE DEFINITION.

AIDS dementia   See AIDS DEMENTIA COMPLEX.

AIDS dementia complex (ADC)   Dementia is the deterioration or loss of intellectual capacity, including memory, judgment, and ability to concentrate. AIDS dementia complex is the dementia that appears to result from HIV infection of the brain or an inflammatory reaction to such an infection. It is also known as HIV ENCEPHALITIS, HIV ENCEPHALOPATHY, MULTIFOCAL GIANT-CELL ENCEPHALITIS, and SUBACUTE ENCEPHALITIS.

AIDS dementia is relatively common in the late stages of HIV infection. It may represent a complex of several disease processes involving inflammatory immune system CYTOKINEs and OXIDATIVE STRESS as well as HIV itself. Symptoms include apathy, decreased concentration and memory, and slowness of thought and motor movements. ADC is usually progressive. Some 30 percent of people with AIDS experience minor cognitive impairment, while 20 percent have a serious deficit, affecting their ability to function in social or occupational settings.

Standard treatment of ADC consists of high-dose regimens of AZIDOTHYMIDINE (AZT). Administration of DIDEOXYINOSINE (ddI) is another potential treatment, but ddI's poor penetration of the blood-brain barrier may affect efficacy. Another possibility is AZT plus DIDEOXYCYTIDINE (ddC). NIMODIPINE (a CALCIUM CHANNEL BLOCKER), PENTOXIFYLLINE (a reputed antagonist of TUMOR NECROSIS FACTOR), and PEPTIDE T (a synthetic peptide that mimics the cell binding site on HIV's surface protein GP120) are among the drugs that might improve neurologic functions without affecting HIV replication. In patients with psychomotor slowing, use of psychostimulants may be helpful. Agitation and mania can be treated with neuroleptics (drugs that produce symptoms resembling those of diseases of the nervous system) or lithium, starting at low doses.

AIDS discourse   The complex of formal speech and writing that examines what HIV and AIDS have been made to mean socially and culturally, both in the lives of the people and communities coping with AIDS and HIV infection, and in society as a whole; the totality of informed discussion about AIDS. See CULTURAL ANALYSIS AND AIDS.

AIDS drug assistance programs (ADAPs)   ADAPs are the most heavily utilized AIDS programs in the nation, with, as of early 1996, more than 50,000 people enrolled. The federally funded ADAP system began in 1987 as a way of providing free AIDS drugs to low- or moderate-income people not covered by Medicaid or third-party insurance. Since 1990, ADAPs have been funded under the RYAN WHITE CARE ACT, the main source of federal funds for AIDS care. Each state administers its own ADAP, so eligibility criteria and formularies (the list of covered drugs) vary from state to state. Today many of the states' ADAPs are running out of money. The funding shortfall has led AIDS organizations to press for more funds at the state and federal levels, but no solution is in sight. Increased caseloads and drug usage, higher drug costs, and more expensive combination therapies coupled with stagnant financial resources have placed ADAPs across the country in jeopardy.

ADAPs' woes underscore a frightening reality of the American health care system. More and more people with HIV who rely on government health care or MANAGED-CARE plans may find that newer and more expensive drugs remain unreimbursed. Breakthrough drugs, like PROTEASE INHIBITORs, that have a major life-prolonging potential for people with HIV may be available only to the very few who have jobs that offer top-of-line insurance coverage.

AIDS education and training centers   See AIDS EDUCATION AND TRAINING CENTERS (AETC) PROGRAM.

AIDS Education and Training Centers (AETC) Program
The National AIDS Education and Training Centers Program was established in 1987 to increase the number of health care providers who are effectively educated and motivated to counsel, diagnose, treat, and manage individuals with HIV infection and to assist in the prevention of high-risk behaviors that may lead to infection. The program conducts targeted, multidisciplinary HIV education and training programs for health care providers through a network of 15 regional centers. Information dissemination efforts emphasize electronic communication and include cosponsorship of the quarterly national HIV Clinical Conference Call series.

The program began with four AETCs that focused on educating providers about the epidemiology of AIDS and how to identify groups at increased risk of infection. By 1991, in response to the growth of the epidemic, the program had increased the number of regional AETCs to cover all 50 states, the Virgin Islands, and Puerto Rico. Clinical training of primary care providers (physicians, nurses, dentists) became the primary focus, with a secondary emphasis on training providers in mental health and allied fields. Most resources have been concentrated on areas of high HIV incidence.

Allocation of program resources and scheduling of activities are based on a comprehensive local, state and regional needs assessment. The toll free National HIV/AIDS ETC Clinical Telephone Consultation Service (800-933-3413) is especially helpful to providers less experienced with HIV care or those practicing in rural areas.

AIDS enteropathy   Any intestinal disease appearing in a person with AIDS.

AIDS orphan   A child or youth who has lost parents, foster and adoptive parents, grandparents, siblings, friends, neighbors, or other crucial caregivers to the AIDS epidemic. AIDS orphans generally do not have the disease themselves and are not viewed as patients by the medical community. Often unable to share their family secrets and losses, they are often invisible to service communities, schools, churches, and courts. Few professionals seem to be helping to plan for their futures, or even recognize that they exist. CONFIDENTIALITY and disclosure, custody and placement, benefits programs, and bereavement are some of the issues these children and youth face. An additional challenge these children and youth face is that the general public is not well educated about the issue.

Children and youth whose lives are touched by the HIV/AIDS epidemic confront not one epidemic but two: as the disease spreads, so does the epidemic of indifference to the children's and youths' plight. The indifference arises in part from ignorance. Breaking society's silence about these children who must struggle to survive AIDS in their families is one means of arresting the epidemic of indifference. It is noted that there are numerous national organizations that provide useful information to HIV-affected children and youth and their families.

AIDS prodrome   Any sign or symptom indicative of the onset of AIDS.

AIDS-related complex (ARC)   A health condition in which some of the signs and symptoms of HIV infection (stages 1 to 5) have appeared, but none of the opportunistic infections associated with AIDS. At the onset of the epidemic the term designated the condition of HIV-infected individuals not diagnosed with AIDS but with compromised immune systems and decreased T-CELL COUNTs. The term is no longer officially recognized by the CDC.

AIDS-related condition   A serious stage of HIV infection characterized by opportunistic infections other than those clearly associated with AIDS. In effect, a variety of AIDS.

AIDS-related virus (ARV)   A strain of HUMAN IMMUNODEFICIENCY VIRUS (HIV) found in HOMOSEXUAL men in 1984 in Atlanta, Georgia. This was one of the names given the virus responsible for AIDS early in the epidemic, before the terminology was standardized.

AIDS service organization (ASO)   Generally, a nongovernmental nonprofit group that provides services such as medical care, counseling, legal and housing assistance, and access to food banks to those infected with HIV.

The first was the Gay Men's Health Crisis, created in New York in 1981 by the playwright Larry Kramer and others. Today, ASOs are the principal institutional vehicles of volunteer, community-based AIDS prevention and care efforts.

Though they may operate at a local, regional or national level, most of these organizations are quite small, staffed and supported by a remarkable variety of activists, from gay men and lesbians, social and health care workers, ministers' wives, injection drug users, alcoholics in recovery, and friends and family members of people with AIDS.

ASOs have for years been central to society's response to AIDS, but the future is unclear as the epidemic spreads to new populations, as charismatic leaders burn out or die, and as societal needs outstrip volunteer efforts and modest financial resources.

AIDS Treatment Evaluation Units (ATEU)   Original name of the AIDS CLINICAL TRIALS GROUP, established by the National Institute of Allergy and Infectious Diseases in 1986 to test new AIDS-related drugs.

AIDS virus   In medical literature, HIV, the virus responsible for AIDS, is called by various other names dating from early in the AIDS epidermic. Though it continues to be debated, the basic terminology has been fairly well standardized.

AIDSLINE   A National Library of Medicine (NLM) database that contains citations to AIDS-related literature. The citations are derived from various NLM databases, including Cancerlit, Health Planning and Administration, and Medline.

AIDSphobia   A term coined to denote an unrealistic fear and dread of the acquired immunodeficiency syndrome and of those afflicted with it.

AIDSspeak   A vernacular created by public health officials, politicians, and AIDS activists to discuss issues related to the pandemic. Among its characteristics is the use of nonjudgmental language.

airborne transmission   Process by which an infectious AGENT passes through the air from a CARRIER to others in the form of tiny inhalant droplets. Typically the process begins with a sneeze or a cough.

AL-721   An immune stimulant believed to inhibit the replication of the HIV virus, AL-721 was, prior to the marketing of AZT, the unofficial, "underground" treatment of choice for people with AIDS. This inexpensive egg-based compound was developed in 1979 at Israel's Weitzmann Institute of Science to remove cholesterol from cell walls. Use of AL-721 was discarded after a single, tiny, loosely-controlled clinical trial at St. Luke's-Roosevelt Hospital in New York. Most research on AL-721 has been done outside of the United States.

alanine aminotransaminase (ALT)   A LIVER ENZYME that plays a role in PROTEIN metabolism. Elevated SERUM levels of ALT are a sign of liver damage from disease or drugs. ALT is also known as SGPT (serum glutamic pyruvic transaminase).

albendazole   A broad-spectrum antihelmintic (i.e., drug used to treat a range of species of helminths [parasitic worms]. Several studies have found that it is active against MICROSPORIDIOSIS, a form of extreme diarrhea caused by two intestinal protozoa species that are increasingly recognized in people with AIDS.

alcoholism   ADDICTION to alcoholic beverages. A primary chronic disease with genetic, psychosocial, and environmental factors influencing its development and manifestations. A progressive disease, alcoholism can cause physical, psychological, and social harm and can be fatal.

alkaline phosphatase   An ENZYME produced in the liver as well as in bone and other tissues. Elevated SERUM levels of the enzyme are indicative of LIVER disease, bile duct obstruction in particular.

allergen   A protein or HAPTEN that induces the formation of anaphylactic antibodies and may precipitate an IMMUNE RESPONSE; a substance that causes an ALLERGIC REACTION. Among common allergens are inhalants (dusts, pollens, fungi, smoke, perfumes, odors of plastics); foods (wheat, eggs, milk, chocolate, strawberries); drugs (aspirin, antibiotics, serums); infectious agents (bacteria, viruses, fungi, animal parasites) and contactants (chemicals, animals, plants, metals).

allergic dermatitis   See ATOPIC DERMATITIS.

allergic eczema   See ATOPIC DERMATITIS.

allergic reaction   Physiological response triggered by an ALLERGEN. See ALLERGY.

allergy   A hypersensitivity to an ALLERGEN (an environmental HAPTEN or ANTIGEN), resulting in tissue inflammation, fever, organ dysfunction, and other physiological manifestations. The most common allergic reactions are on the skin and in the respiratory and GASTROINTESTINAL TRACTS.

allogeneic (allogenic)   Having a different genetic constitution. The term is often used to refer to intraspecific (within a species) genetic variations.

aloe vera   A species of the genus *Aloe*, a member of the lily family. There are at least 120 known species of aloe, many of which have been used as botanical medicines. The sap and rind portions of the aloe vera leaf contain analgesics, anti-inflammatory compounds, minerals, and beneficial fatty acids. Aloe vera is widely known as a skin moisturizer and healing agent, especially in treating cuts, burns, insect stings, bruises, acne, poison ivy, welts, ulcerated skin lesions, eczema, and sunburns. It has also been used to treat stomach disorders, ulcers, and many colon-related disorders, including colitis. Aloe juice may be used to treat food allergies, varicose veins, skin cancer, and arthritis as well. Aloe vera may help stop the spread of some viruses, such as HERPES SIMPLEX I and II, VARICELLA ZOSTER VIRUS, pseudorabies virus, and the influenza virus.

alpha-interferon (IFN-A)   Alpha interferon is a natural protein secreted by immune cells in response to viral infection. A manufactured version of IFN-A is approved to treat KAPOSI'S SARCOMA, hepatitis B, and hepatitis C. Alpha-interferon has been shown to be effective in preventing replication of the human immunodeficiency virus IN VITRO (in the laboratory). Its TOXICITY significantly limits its use IN VIVO (in the living body).

A current study under the auspices of the National Institute of Allergy and Infectious Diseases is investigating whether low-dose oral alpha interferon (LDOAI) therapy is effective in reducing the symptoms of AIDS. The use of LDOAI in the United States has been controversial, in part because the data about its effectiveness are conflicting and in part because LDOAI products are sometimes used to the exclusion of other therapies of proven value. Large multicenter randomized placebo-controlled trials have shown that LDOAI provides no benefit in fighting HIV, the virus that causes AIDS, or in improving the immune system of those infected. Nonetheless, LDOAI products have been used in the United States, particularly in African-American communities, based on reports that these agents have beneficial effects on HIV-related symptoms, weight loss, and the severity of opportunistic infections associated with HIV infection.

alprazolam   A triazolo-benzodiazepine antianxiety agent. It is sold under the trade name Xanax.

ALT   See ALANINE AMINOTRANSAMINASE.

altered mental state   A changed functional state of mind—as manifested in behavior, appearance, speech, memory, judgment, and responsiveness to stimuli of all kinds—that is markedly different from an individual's norm.

alternative health care   See ALTERNATIVE TREATMENT.

alternative insemination   See ARTIFICIAL INSEMINATION.

alternative delivery system (ADS)   A term coined to describe a variety of health care forms other than the traditional fee-for-service model, such as health maintenance organizations (HMOs) and preferred provider organizations (PPOs).

alternative medicine   Approaches to medical diagnosis and therapy that have been developed outside the established standards, practices, and institutional sites of conventional medical science. Included are a great number of theories and "systems," including therapeutic NUTRITION, CHIROPRACTIC, HOMEOPATHY, structural, energetic therapies and MIND-BODY THERAPIES; traditional non-Western ethnomedicinal systems such as CHINESE MEDICINE and AYURVEDA, which combine botanical medicine with other applications; other uses of botanical substances; and various treatments that simply have not been accepted by the medical establishment. This is not to say that, were these methods subjected to scientific study, all of them would be found to be ineffective. Alternative medicine has been variously called "natural," "complementary" (the preferred term in Europe), and numerous other terms referring to elements of a particular modality or tradition. "Alternative medicine" is not equivalent to "HOLISTIC medicine," a more narrow term.

Traditional ethnomedicinal systems are typically holistic, meaning that they aim to treat the whole person rather than

a specific disease or symptom and that they therefore address not only the physical patient but also the mind and spirit. It is typically assumed that each individual possesses an innate healing capacity (an "immune system" in the broadest sense), and the goal of such treatment generally is to reinforce this, restoring strength and "balance" to weakened systems with a variety of natural modalities: foods, herbs and other botanicals, "body work," detoxification, and so on, tailored as much as possible for the individual. The use of alternative therapies for AIDS grew out of this same eclectic mix.

alternative therapy   See ALTERNATIVE TREATMENT.

alternative treatment   Generally, therapy with procedures or agents that are not approved by the Food and Drug Administration (FDA) or other certifying authority. Alternative medical treatments have been used by a significant proportion of people with HIV, often to complement approved treatments. Some alternative treatments have been investigated in laboratory settings and observational studies, and a few have undergone clinical trials; others are being used without having undergone any studies. Alternative treatments are available for a variety of conditions, including weakened immune system, stress, drug abuse, mental disorders, common health problems, pregnancy, childbirth and infant care, dental care, eye, ear, nose and throat disorders, cancer and heart disorders, and aging. Alternative medicine combines many different Eastern and Western medical specialties: AYURVEDA medicine, CHINESE MEDICINE, ACUPUNCTURE and ACUPRESSURE, NUTRITION, exercise, NATUROPATHIC MEDICINE, HOMEOPATHY, botanical medicine, CHIROPRACTIC, and MASSAGE. Although all these methods have been lumped together in the generic category "alternative health care," they differ substantially from each other in philosophy, modality, cost, and other important ways. Although often touted as nontoxic, some herbs or nutritional supplements can have significant toxicities if used in sufficient quantities. Additionally, just as there is no universal language, so no single medical system or tradition—Eastern or Western, ancient or modern, scientific or unscientific—can provide the magic lantern that reveals all the mysteries of the human body. All alternative treatments share one similarity—very little is known about their activity in the human body and their usefulness in treating AIDS, even those that seem beneficial.

In 1992, for the first time in the then eight-year history of the International Conference on AIDS, alternative and traditional indigenous medicines had a prominent place. Politically, that year marked a change in the course of the conference toward greater attention to alternative or traditional treatments, in addition to mainstream pharmaceutical industry drugs. Many physicians and researchers believe that as time passes and the limitations of Western medicine become more defined, it is increasingly important for there to be cooperation among different medical traditions.

In 1993, partly as a response to the growing popularity of alternative medicine in the United States, President Clinton signed into law on June 14, 1993, the National Institutes of Health Revitalization Act, now known as Public Law 103–43.

In the law, Congress permanently established the Office of Alternative Medicine (OAM) within the Office of the Director of National Institutes of Health. The purpose of the OAM is "to facilitate the evaluation of alternative medical modalities, including acupuncture and Oriental medicine, homeopathic medicine and physical manipulation therapies."

Some members of the AIDS community dismiss all alternative treatments, regardless of evidence demonstrating efficacy, and others defend all alternative treatments, regardless of evidence demonstrating lack of efficacy or toxicity. The reality seems to be that some alternative treatments may be effective, some are clearly ineffective, and most are in some degree toxic. The chief difficulty with using alternative treatments is a lack of empirical data. In the absence of the usual university, government, or corporate sponsorship of scientific research into them, there is no infrastructure that systematically addresses the potential benefits and risks of alternative treatments.

Since toxicity studies on most alternative treatments have not been conducted, it must be assumed that they may be toxic. There is no legal or regulatory mandate to disclose negative side effects. It must be kept in mind that profit is as big a motive for the marketers of "alternative" medicines as it is for the conventional pharmaceutical industry.

Access is also an issue with regard to alternative approaches to AIDS treatment. Alternative medicine, with its roots in traditional ethnomedicine, has the reputation of being a "new age" phenomenon, of interest mainly to the affluent middle class. This is due to its fringe status, which means that insurance and entitlement programs do not cover it, rather than to any lack of interest on the part of lower-income people. Increasing the availability of potentially useful treatments is directly related to their gaining wider acceptance among the medical and insurance industries.

Among the most common alternative agents are plants and plant extracts, derived from natural products or medicinal herbs. These are used for their possible antiviral properties and antibacterial and antifungal activity in the treatment of opportunistic infections. They include acemannan, astragalus, bitter melon, blue-green algae, burdock, garlic extract, glycyrrhizin, hypericin, iscador, maitake mushroom, mulberry roots and seeds, pine cone extracts, red marine algae, shiitake mushrooms, Siberian ginseng, traditional medicinal herbs, trichosanthin, and woundwaret.

Nutritional supplements are used in an attempt to restore natural levels of nutrients, to enhance resistance to opportunistic infections, and, when taken in high doses, to treat various HIV/AIDS-related conditions. Vitamins, minerals, and other substances in this category include BETA-CAROTENE, calcium, FOLIC ACID, iron, vitamins B_6 and B_{12}, VITAMIN C, vitamin E, ACIDOPHILUS, colostrum, COENZYME Q10, L-lysine, N-ACETYLCYSTEINE, and SELENIUM.

Dietary management is used to maintain or improve general health. Special regimes, such as those eliminating refined sugar or yeast to prevent or treat fungal infections, can be used as prophylaxis or treatment.

Physical techniques are used to treat certain conditions, relieve physical symptoms, and improve comfort and the quality of life. They can be combined with other therapies without fear of interactions with medication. Treatments include acupuncture, chiropractic manipulation, hydrotherapy, and massage.

Spiritual and psychological approaches seek to provide a holistic balance to complement other treatment strategies for HIV/AIDS. Although benefits are highly individual and subjective, they can contribute to an overall state of health. Treatments include hypnotherapy, meditation, psychotherapy, spiritual healing, stress reduction, and visualization.

Other treatments include ASPIRIN, colonics, dehydroepiandrosterone (DHEA) DNCB (dinitrichlorobenzene), ozone therapy (super oxygenation), passive immunotherapy, shark cartilage powder, shark liver oil, snake venom, and thymus extracts.

alveolar proteinosis See PULMONARY ALVEOLAR PROTEINOSIS.

alveolus (pl. alveoli) Any small, saclike cavity in the body, such as an air cell of the lung or an erosion or ulcer in the gastric mucous membrane. Also, the socket of a tooth.

Alzheimer's disease A chronic, organic mental disorder; a form of presenile dementia due to atrophy of the frontal and occipital lobes of the brain. Onset is usually between age 40 and 60. Its effects include progressive irreversible loss of memory, deterioration of intellectual functions, apathy, speech and gait disturbance, and disorientation. Its course may take from a few months to four or five years to progress to complete loss of intellectual function.

AmBisome See AMPHOTERICIN B.

ambulatory care Care treatment provided to ambulatory (mobile, not hospitalized) patients.

Amcil See AMPICILLIN.

ameba See AMOEBA.

amebiasis A parasitic intestinal infection caused by tiny unicellular microorganisms called AMOEBAs, especially *Entamoeba histolytica*. Many patients remain asymptomatic, but the disease is generally characterized by dysentery with diarrhea, weakness, prostration, nausea, vomiting, and pain. One serious complication is amebic hepatitis.

amebic dysentery Infection with *Entamoeba histolytica*. Also called hepatic AMEBIASIS.

amebic hepatitis Amebic abscess of the liver caused by infection with *Entamoeba histolytica*.

amenorrhea Absence or suppression of menstruation. Amenorrhea is normal before puberty, after menopause, and during pregnancy and lactation. Primary amenorrhea is the failure of the menstruation cycle to begin at puberty; this may result from a congenital defect in the reproductive organs. The term usually refers to a condition caused by reasons other than these. Secondary amenorrhea is the suspension of menstruation after it has been established at puberty, and may result from an illness, a change of environment, or irradiation or removal of the uterus or ovaries. It is also associated with certain metabolic disorders (obesity, malnutrition, diabetes) and certain systemic diseases (SYPHILIS, TUBERCULOSIS, nephritis). Amenorrhea may also result from emotional causes (excitement, anorexia nervosa), pituitary disorders (hormonal imbalance of estrogen, progesterone, or FOLLICLE-STIMULATING HORMONE), or eating disorders (OBESITY, ANOREXIA).

America Responds to AIDS   An AIDS education campaign launched in 1988 by the Centers for Disease Control and Prevention (CDC) to promote public awareness.

American Association of Blood Banks   Association comprising blood banks and individuals that promotes blood banking, operates a clearinghouse for the exchange of blood and credits for blood, conducts educational and training programs, and supports and sponsors research.

Americans with Disabilities Act (ADA)   Signed into law on July 26, 1990, by President Bush, this legislation guarantees equal opportunity for, and prohibits discrimination against, persons with disabilities regarding employment, public accommodation (essentially every type of business and service provider), transportation, state and local government and services, and telecommunications.

In the ADA the term *disability* describes a broad range of conditions often inappropriately taken into account by employers and businesses. The ADA definition of disability is not the same as that used to establish eligibility for benefit programs under other legislation. The ADA prohibits discrimination against all people with disabilities, specifically including people with HIV disease, defined to include everything from asymptomatic HIV infection to full AIDS. The ADA also protects from discrimination people who are perceived as having or somehow carrying HIV disease. These could include friends, family members, lovers, caretakers of people with AIDS PWAs, or volunteers serving the PWA community.

Under the ADA, an employer may not refuse to hire someone simply because she has HIV disease, nor may it fire someone or refuse to a promote him simply because he has HIV disease. In other words, an employer may not discriminate against an otherwise qualified person with HIV disease. To be qualified, an individual must be able to perform all the essential functions of a job, despite his or her HIV. This includes being well enough to get to work on a regular basis and to perform the job adequately. Under the ADA, an employer must make "reasonable accommodations" for persons with disabilities. This means that the employer has a responsibility to make changes in a job that will help the person perform the job adequately. This could include establishing flexible work schedules and allowing a person time off for medical treatment. An employee, however, must request such accommodation. Furthermore, under the ADA, an employer only has to make "reasonable" accommodations that will not impose an "undue hardship" on it. If an employer shows that it would be a significant difficulty or expense to make a certain accommodation, it does not have to make it.

The ADA treats the testing issue as well. An employer may not require that an employee take an HIV-ANTIBODY TEST unless the employer proves that the test results are necessary for the employee's performance on the job. The act does allow the HIV-antibody test to be included in a general physical examination if one is required after a conditional offer of employment is made to a job applicant. But the test may not be selectively administered in a discriminatory manner, and the employer may not withdraw the conditional offer of employment unless the test results indicate that the applicant is no longer qualified for the job.

The ADA does not apply to the federal government, but a very similar statute, the REHABILITATION ACT OF 1973, does apply to the executive branch. The ADA also does not mention housing because there is already a federal law, the FAIR HOUSING ACT (as amended by Congress in 1989), that prohibits discrimination against people with disabilities (including HIV disease) in the sale and rental of private housing.

Beyond employment issues, the ADA further prohibits discrimination based on disability in "public accommodations." In the ADA, that term covers not only its traditional meaning—hotels, restaurants, theaters, convention centers, and such, but virtually every type of business or service provider in the country, including doctors, dentists, pharmacists, and even lawyers. These public accommodations may not discriminate in the delivery of goods or services against a person because of that person's HIV disease or because the person is regarded as having HIV disease or associates with persons with HIV disease.

The employment portion of the ADA (Title I) is enforced by the Equal Employment Opportunities Commission (EEOC). The public accommodation provision of the ADA (Title III) can be enforced by filing a lawsuit in court or, in some instances, by filing a complaint with the Department of Justice, which is empowered to undertake an investigation and compliance review. The public entity portion of the ADA (Title II) is enforced by the Department of Justice.

amikacin   An ANTIMICROBIAL, AMINOGLYCOSIDE ANTIBIOTIC, amikacin is indicated for MYCOBACTERIUM AVIUM COMPLEX (MAC) and multidrug-resistant MYCOBACTERIUM TUBERCULOSIS. Side effects include NEPHROTOXICITY and OTOTOXICITY. Amikacin should not be used with other nephrotoxic drugs such as AMPHOTERICIN B, vancomycin, loop diuretics and other aminoglycosides, or with other ototoxic drugs. Amikacin may potentiate the effects of neuromuscular blockers. It is sold under the trade name Amikin.

amino acid   Any of twenty nitrogen-containing acids that are the building blocks for proteins and required for human growth. Occurring freely within organisms, amino acids contain an amine group and a carboxyl group.

amino acid therapy   A questionable form of AIDS therapy available outside the United States, especially in Mexico. Results to date have not proven to be long-term.

aminoglycoside   One of a number of ANTIBIOTICS derived or synthesized from species of *Streptomyces* bacteria.

aminosalicylic acid   An antituberculosis drug believed to delay development of bacterial resistance. Its effectiveness is greatly enhanced when used in combination with STREPTO-MYCIN and ISONIAZID (INH).

amitriptyline   A tricyclic antidepressant. Although the Food and Drug Administration (FDA) has not approved such use, it is sometimes given to HIV-infected people to reduce the pain associated with peripheral neuropathy, a condition characterized by numbness, tingling or pain in the feet, legs, arms, or hands. It is thought to work by increasing the concentrations of neurotransmitters called serotonin and norepinephrine in the brain.

This class of antidepressants is usually taken over a long period of time; amitriptyline should not be taken by people who have HIV dementia or AIDS dementia complex because it may cause acute delirium. Additionally, most antidepressants increase the risk of seizures in people susceptible to them. Because seizures are not uncommon in HIV disease, people who are infected with the virus should be cautious about taking all antidepressants, including those in the tricyclic class.

Amitriptyline is available in tablet and injectable form. The most common side effects include sleepiness, blurred vision, disorientation, confusion, hallucinations, muscle spasms, seizures, dry mouth, constipation, difficult urination, worsening glaucoma, and sensitivity to bright light or sunlight.

amniotic fluid   The transparent, almost colorless liquid contained in the inner membrane (amnion) that holds a suspended fetus. It protects the fetus from physical impact, insulates against temperature variations and prevents the fetus from adhering to the amnion and the amnion from adhering to the fetus. Amniotic fluid is continually absorbed and replenished; about one third of the water in the amniotic fluid is replaced each hour.

amoeba (pl. amoebae)   A one-celled, microscopic protozoan organism, found in soil and water, that may infect humans, causing AMEBIASIS. It sends out fingerlike projections of protoplasm (pseudopodia) that enable it to move about and through which it obtains nourishment. The pseudopodia also keep the shape of the amoeba in constant flux. Amoebae reproduce by binary fission, with the nucleus dividing by mitosis.

amoebiasis   See AMEBIASIS.

amoebic dysentery   See AMEBIC DYSENTERY.

amoebic hepatitis   See AMEBIC HEPATITIS.

amoxicillin   An antibiotic drug; semisynthetic derivative of ampicillin effective against a broad spectrum of gram-positive and gram-negative bacteria. In people with HIV, amoxicillin is used specifically to treat bacterial inflammation of the sinuses (sinusitis), diarrhea caused by salmonella, and vaginal ulcers (chancroid) caused by *Haemophilus ducreyi*. Amoxicillin works by interfering with a susceptible bacteria's ability to build cell walls. It is converted by the body into AMPICILLIN. The primary difference between the two is that amoxicillin is resistant to acid in the stomach, which means that more of the active drug gets into the intestines where it is absorbed.

Amoxicillin is generally well tolerated. The most common side effects are minor and include rashes, heartburn, nausea, vomiting or diarrhea. These side effects are likely to occur in people who are allergic to penicillin or have a history of allergy, asthma, or hay fever. Rarely, some people taking amoxicillin experience agitation, anxiety, insomnia, dizziness, confusion or behavioral changes.

In recent years, bacteria have become more resistant to amoxicillin and other penicillin-type antibiotics. Resistance may occur more frequently in the HIV-positive population because of their widespread use of such drugs. In cases of resistance additional antibiotics that kill bacteria by a different mechanism are often needed. Trade names for amoxicillin include Amoxil, Moxicillin, Wymax, and Augmentin. Augmentin is amoxicillin plus clavulante.

Amoxil   See AMOXICILLIN.

amphetamine   One of a group of organic compounds that act as CENTRAL NERVOUS SYSTEM stimulants. Sometimes referred to as speed, amphetamines if abused may lead to psychological dependence, producing symptoms ranging from restlessness to psychosis in severe cases. The preparation most commonly used is the sulfate, marketed in tablet and capsule form.

amphotericin B   An antibiotic. Amphotericin B (trade name Fungizone) is the standard treatment for many infections caused by fungi, including those that affect people infected with HIV: CANDIDA, CRYPTOCOCCUS, HISTOPLASMA, coccidiodes, and ASPERGILLUS. People with HIV are routinely given amphotericin B for initial treatment of severe cryptococcosis, histoplasmosis, aspergillosis, blastomycosis, and COCCIDIOIDOMYCOSIS. Amphotericin B, which in the United States is currently given only intravenously, is highly effective. (An oral form is available in Europe and is being tested in the United States.) Unfortunately, it is also one of the most toxic antibodies known. Amphotericin B is metabolized slowly and can be found in urine up to seven weeks after treatment. The drug works by attacking the cell walls of the fungi. Because human and fungal cell walls contain similar compounds, amphotericin B's side effects may be a result of the drug attacking human cells as well.

The most important side effects include kidney damage, anemia, disturbances in the balance of electrolytes, nausea and vomiting, headache, fever and chills, altered blood pressure, changes in appetite, and phlebitis or inflammation of the vein into which the drug is injected. These reactions are usually most severe with the first few doses and usually diminish with subsequent treatment. The serious kidney toxicities caused by amphotericin B are most evident when treatment lasts six to ten weeks or longer. Many of these side effects can be reduced in severity or eliminated by stopping the drug, by continuing the drug in a lower dose or by taking other medications at the same time that will counteract them. Medications that affect kidney functions, such as AMINOGLYCOSIDE antibiotics, FOSCARNET, and PENTAMIDINE, should be prescribed to patients on amphotericin with extreme caution.

Because of amphotericin B's toxicity, other drugs, like KETOCONAZOLE and FLUCONAZOLE, are preferred in situations in which they are considered likely to be as effective or nearly as effective. One potentially more effective and safer alternative to standard amphotericin may be liposomal amphotericins. In these "high-tech" versions of the drug, amphotericin is encapsulated in tiny fat globules known as liposomes. LIPOSOMAL AMPHOTERICIN must be administered through intravenous infusion like the standard drug, but it is hypothesized that the LIPOSOMEs may be preferentially absorbed at the sites of infection, thereby avoiding most of amphotericin's side effects and potentially extending the length of time amphotericin therapy can be tolerated.

ampicillin   A semisynthetic penicillin, this broad-spectrum antibiotic is effective against various gram-negative and gram-positive bacteria. Predominantly used in the treatment of urinary system and urinary tract infections, it is also used to treat prolonged bronchial infections. Trade names include AMCILL, OMNIPEN, POLYCILLIN, and Principen.

ampicillin sodium   Monosodium salt of ampicillin. Trade names include omnipen-N, polycillin-N, and Principen-N.

amplification   Multiplication of a virus either through the body of an individual host or through a population of hosts. Extreme amplification is the multiplication of a virus everywhere in a host, partly transforming the host into a virus. Host here refers to an organism supporting a parasite in or on its body and to its own detriment.

ampligen   A non-nucleoside drug found in the late 1980s to be ineffective against AIDS. Previously it had been thought to have the activity of both an antiviral and an immunomodulator.

amprenavir   A PROTEASE INHIBITOR now under development, amprenavir represents Glaxo Wellcome's adaptation of the basic, highly potent and HIV-specific SAQUINAVIR structure to achieve greater availability in the body. The Vertex Pharmaceuticals scientists who originally created amprenavir (before it was sold to Galxo) went several steps beyond nelfinavir, arriving at a molecule that is yet more compact and looks even less like a peptide (a short protein-like sequence of amino acids). Amprenavir has similar efficacy to other protease inhibitors, but it is better tolerated and dosing is only twice a day. The extent that amprenavir can be used in real life against HIV resistant to other protease inhibitors remains to be determined.

amyl nitrite   A fluorocarbon that, inhaled, dilates the blood vessels, producing a temporary "rush" or "high." Used to treat angina and asthma, it has become popular for enhancing sexual experience. Known as "POPPERS."

amyl nitrite inhalant   See ISOBUTYL NITRITE INHALERS.

amylase   A starch-splitting enzyme secreted by the salivary glands and the pancreas to aid digestion of food. An increase in amylase serum levels may indicate pancreatitis, a possible life-threatening consequence of ddI.

anabolic steroids   Anabolic steroids are testosterone derivatives designed to increase strength and muscle mass. Testosterone performs these functions in the body, but its masculinizing effects make it an inappropriate therapy for men who already have normal testosterone levels, or for women. The synthetic anabolic steroids, such as nandrolone, oxandrolone, methandrostenolone and oxymetholone, were designed to be less masculinizing than testosterone and are often used to treat men with AIDS. These men often have low testicular function or testosterone deficiencies caused by HIV suppression of normal endocrine-gland function or by drugs (like KETOCONAZOLE) used to treat opportunistic infections. These deficiencies are associated with weakness and loss of lean tissue mass.

Weight loss is a common symptom in people with HIV. It can be caused by opportunistic infections that interfere with the ability to absorb nutrients. Oral problems such as thrush or dry mouth may contribute to decreased food intake. Weight loss can also be caused by a poorly understood condition called HIV-related wasting, where lean muscle mass is lost even when a person is eating properly.

Oral and injectable testosterone have long been available to treat testosterone deficiencies. The oral form is metabolized by the liver and can cause serious liver toxicities, so it is infrequently used. Injectable forms of the drugs are used more commonly, but they cause transient high levels of the drug in the blood, which may increase the risk of side effects.

Anabolic steroids have the advantage of being dramatically cheaper than most therapies being studied for AIDS-related wasting. The ability of anabolic steroids to increase muscle mass and break down fat in healthy, exercising people is well-documented and doctors can legally prescribe therapeutic doses. Despite the numerous anecdotal reports of steroid use in people with AIDS-related wasting, its long-term safety and efficacy has yet to be established in controlled studies. Additionally, for treatment of HIV-related weight loss, anabolic steroids are only effective for men with abnormally low testosterone levels. Consequently, before initiating treatment, physicians usually measure their patients' testosterone levels. For maximum effect against wasting, both adequate nutrition and exercise should be combined with anabolic steroid therapy. The drugs make cells ready to build tissue, but they have little effect without the proper building blocks (especially protein) and exercise. Use of steroids by people with no urgent medical reason for it, however, is considered extremely dangerous. Aside from undesirable potential side effects such as (in women) hirsutism, masculinization and clitoral hypertrophy, such use affects immune system functioning and has been associated with muscular deterioration and brain cancer.

anal eroticism   Finding sexual enjoyment in the stimulation of one's own or a partner's anus.

anal intercourse Sexual intercourse involving the insertion of one partner's penis into the other's anus. The man who inserts his penis into the anus of his partner is performing *insertive* or *active* anal intercourse. The partner is experiencing *passive* anal intercourse.

Anal intercourse without a condom with an infected partner carries a high risk for HIV infection and other sexually transmitted diseases (STDs) because it often causes small tears in the rectal tissue and other internal injuries, through which infected semen can enter the bloodstream. Generally speaking, a condom does not offer quite the same protection in anal intercourse as in vaginal intercourse. Because the anus is usually tighter than the vagina, the condom may slip or break more easily. Additionally, it is not yet clear whether spermicides containing NONOXYNOL-9 can be safely used inside the rectum. Nonetheless a lubricant containing nonoxynol-9 can further reduce the risk. The same condom should not be used for both anal and vaginal intercourse.

anal-oral sex See ANILINGUS.

anal sex See ANAL EROTICISM; ANAL INTERCOURSE.

analgesic A compound that reduces or relieves pain without reducing consciousness. Tylenol, ASPIRIN, and the OPIATES are examples of analgesic drugs.

anaphylactic shock See ANAPHYLAXIS.

anaphylaxis A systemic allergic reaction (also called anaphylactic shock) of immediate hypersensitivity to a drug or other antigen that results in life-threatening respiratory distress usually accompanied by shock and collapse of blood vessels. Symptoms include acute respiratory distress; hypotension; edema; rash; tachycardia; pale, cool skin; convulsions; and cyanosis. If untreated, unconsciousness and death may be the outcome. Edema can be life threatening if the larynx is involved, since air flow is obstructed with even minimal swelling.

Anaphylaxis occurs in nearly all vertebrates. It results from sensitization of tissue-fixed mast cells by cytotropic antibodies following exposure to an ANTIGEN.

anemia A condition in which the hemoglobin content of the blood (carried in the red blood cells), is less than that required to meet the oxygen demands of the body, producing fatigue and other symptoms. The condition may be caused by too few red blood cells, too little hemoglobin, or both. Because variables such as lifestyle, location, age, and sex can influence red cell and hemoglobin concentrations, it is not possible to state that anemia exists when the hemoglobin is less than a specific value. If the onset of anemia is slow, the body may adjust so well that there will be no functional impairment even though the hemoglobin may be less than 6 gm/100 ml of blood. Symptoms, in addition to fatigue, include pallor of skin, fingernail beds, and mucous membranes; weakness; vertigo; headache; sore tongue; drowsiness; general malaise; dyspnea; tachycardia; palpitation; angina pectoris; gastrointestinal disturbances; amenorrhea; loss of libido; slight fever.

Anemia is not a disease; it may be a symptom of various diseases or of malnutrition. When the reduction of red blood cells, responsible for delivering oxygen to all parts of the body, is severe, the result is fatigue. Anemia can be triggered by HIV infection, an opportunistic infection, or by several of the drugs commonly taken by people with AIDS. Drugs often responsible include trimethoprim-sulfamethoxazole, other sulfa drugs, PENTAMIDINE, AMPHOTERICIN B, and AZT. When anemia is severe, it can be corrected with transfusions. When drugs are responsible, the drugs can be reduced in dose or discontinued.

anergic See ANERGY.

anergy The lack of reaction to ANTIGENs; a state of impaired or absent CELL-MEDIATED IMMUNITY, diagnosable through administration of a common skin test. Used of T-CELLS, the term refers specifically to the lack of response to a normally stimulatory MHC-PEPTIDE complex on an ANTIGEN-PRESENTING CELL.

angiogenesis The formation of new blood vessels. Tumors and KAPOSI'S SARCOMA lesions stimulate angiogenesis to supply themselves with blood.

angular cheilitis See PERLECHE.

angular cheilosis See PERLECHE.

angular stomatis See PERLECHE.

anilinctus See ANILINGUS.

anilingus Sexual activity involving contact between the mouth and the anus; anal-oral sex. Also called anilinctus.

animal models Drug trials done in animals prior to human studies. For example, tests of various substances in standardized genetic strains of mice or the tests of HIV VACCINE in CHIMPANZEES.

anogenital wart Raised skin in the anal or genital region occurring as a response to infection with PAPILLOMA virus.

anomanual intercourse Sexual contact involving placing a hand in a partner's anus. After insertion the hand is made into a fist and a thrusting motion is made.

anonymous testing Persons who decide to get tested for HIV may want to do so anonymously. Centers for such testing have been established in many cities. The standard procedure is to assign a testee an i.d. number before testing, so that the testing agency never knows his or her personal identity. Test results are identified only by the number and cannot be traced. No name or other identification is required, taken, or reported. Anonymous testing differs from confidential testing, in which a testee's doctor and others in his or her office know the test results, which become part of the testee's private medical record.

Locations of anonymous testing centers are available through any AIDS hot line or local public health service. Tests are often free of charge.

anorectal disease   A PATHOLOGICAL condition of the anus and rectum, or the area joining the two, which is manifested by a characteristic set of clinical signs and symptoms.

anorexia   Lack or loss of appetite for food (sometimes known as inappetence). This is common in the onset of fevers and systemic illnesses, certain psychiatric illnesses, depression, and malaise, and in disorders of the alimentary tracts, especially the stomach. It also is a common result of alcoholic excesses and drug addiction. Many drugs and medical procedures have the undesired side effect of causing malaise with concurrent anorexia.

Because anorexia is a common HIV disease–related complication, a patient's appetite is a key piece of clinical information; causes of inappetence may include undiagnosed or untreated opportunistic infections. Many drugs used against HIV have side effects that include nausea and anorexia. As the number of medications given to an HIV/AIDS patient grows, the impact on his or her overall well-being, including nutritional status, must continually be reassessed. Small, frequent meals and calorically dense foods and beverages are often recommended; shared meals and changes in eating place are encouraged, and NUTRITIONAL SUPPLEMENTS are frequently indicated. In many cases, patients learn to prepare their own high calorie/high nutrient drinks, significantly reducing their cost.

Anorexia is a symptom or side effect of a serious health problem. *Anorexia nervosa*, often referred to simply as anorexia, is a serious (psychological) disorder in itself, the pathological absence or *suppression* of appetite. Unlike the anorexia suffered by so many patients with HIV/AIDS, cancer and other illnesses, anorexia nervosa is not associated with the presence of any physical illness.

anoscope   A long narrow tube with lenses at both ends, used to examine the rectal walls closely.

Antabuse   See DISULFIRAM.

antenatal   Occurring before birth.

antenatal diagnosis   A determination of the health and genetic status of a fetus. Methods include amniocentesis, chorionic villus sampling, cell culture, biochemical methods, nonstress testing, oxytocin challenge test, biophysical profile, amnioscopy, amniography, and ultrasound. See PARENTAL TESTING.

antepartum care   See PRENATAL CARE.

anthrax   An acute infectious bacterial disease caused by *Bacillus anthacis*. It generally attacks cattle, goats, horses, or sheep but may be passed on to humans through contact with infected animals, their discharges, or contaminated animal products. Failure to properly treat anthrax may be fatal. Also called CHARBON, MILZBRAND, and SPLENIC FEVER.

anthroposophic medicine   Medicine practiced according to anthroposophy, an occult spiritual system developed by the social philosopher and mystic Rudolf Steiner (1861–1925). Anthroposophic medicine attempts to take into account the spiritual as well as the physical components of illness. A treatment regime may include herbal and homeopathic medicines as well as special dietary practices, art therapy, movement therapy, massage and specially prepared baths.

anti-anxiety drugs   An umbrella term for a number of compounds (also called anxiolytic drugs), including the BENZODIAZEPINE drugs and the muscle relaxant MEPROBAMATE, that are used for reducing anxiety. They are sometimes referred to as minor TRANQUILIZERS.

antibacterial   Destructive of the growth of BACTERIA; any agent that has such an effect.

antibiosis   An antagonistic process or relationship between living organisms, specifically MICROORGANISMS. This natural destructiveness, or antibiotic activity, is the basis for the effectiveness of ANTIBIOTIC drugs.

antibiotic   Pertaining to ANTIBIOSIS, the natural destructiveness of some microorganisms against others; any of a class of drugs that exploits this phenomenon to fight microbial infections.

Antibiotics are made from natural substances and incorporate specific living microorganisms (in relatively weak solution) that kill or inhibit the growth of those causing infection. Effective antibiotic drugs have been developed for use against most BACTERIA, fungi (see FUNGUS), PARASITEs and VIRUSes that cause infection in humans. Some of the antibiotics most frequently given to the HIV-infected include TRIMETHOPRIM-SULFAMETHOXAZOLE (TMF-SMX) and other sulfa drugs, PENTAMIDINE, KETOCONAZOLE, AMPHOTERICIN B, PYRIMETHAMINE, GANCICLOVIR, ACYCLOVIR, PENICILLIN, ERYTHROMYCIN, NYSTATIN, CLOTRIMAZOLE, and AZT.

In recent years it has become clear that antibiotics have been overused. The consequence is that the infectious organisms they once destroyed have evolved strains resistant to them. See DRUG RESISTANCE.

antibiotic resistance   See DRUG RESISTANCE.

antibiotic therapy   See ANTIBIOTIC.

antibody   A chemical substance developed by the immune system to fight an infectious agent found in the body. Specifically, antibodies are members of a class of proteins known as immunoglobulins, which are produced and secreted by B-lymphocytes in response to the presence of specific antigens. For most antigens, the B-lymphocytes take one or two weeks to produce antibodies; for HIV the time required may be months. Immunoglobulins can be found in the blood or secretory fluids. Although antibodies share many properties, each one is highly specific. Once a specific antibody is formed in response to a specific antigen, the cell has a "memory" of this event. This "memory" usually renders the person immune to the specific substance or microorganism in the future.

The presence of antibodies may be linked to vaccination, previous infection, perinatal transfer of bodily fluids between mother and fetus, or unknown exposure. The body also possesses natural antibodies that react without apparent contact with a specific antigen. Antibodies neutralize toxins and interact with other components of the immune system to eliminate infectious microorganisms for the body. In AIDS, these antibodies are usually not effective in neutralizing infection.

At the dawning of the AIDS epidemic, scientists had a very simplistic view of the immune system: antibodies, antibodies, and more antibodies. Now they are finding that the human immune system is much more complicated than they previously imagined. Most people are familiar with antibodies and believe that they provide protection against the opportunistic infections in AIDS. It is now known that production of antibodies enables viral and other microbial pathogens to flourish because it does not destroy the infected cells that are the source of infection, but only temporarily controls cell-free or cell-surface infectious microbes. The other arm of the immune system, cell-mediated immunity, is critical in controlling and clearing the infectious agents that cause opportunistic diseases in AIDS. See also CELL-MEDIATED IMMUNITY or CELLULAR IMMUNITY.

antibody-dependent cell-mediated cytotoxicity   A form of LYMPHOCYTE-MEDIATED cytotoxicity in which an effector cell kills an antibody-coated target cell, presumably by recognition of the Fc region of the cell-bound antibody through an FC RECEPTOR present on the EFFECTOR lymphocyte.

antibody-dependent cellular cytotoxicity   Direct killing of an infected cell by antibody-coated lymphocytes.

antibody envy   An accusation sometimes leveled at HIV-negative individuals who seek to express or explore the damage the AIDS epidemic has done to those not infected. The expression of an opinion, or even a simple assertion of fact or statement of an issue, may enrage some who are HIV-positive or have an AIDS-related illness, as if the HIV-negative had no right to speak publicly. When they do they may be accused of "robbing" resources from the "truly needy." Such accusations serve to divide and discourage those who wish to help, and to minimize and discount the severity of the impact of the epidemic in the lives of those who are HIV-negative and in the community as a whole.

antibody-negative   Not having been infected with a particular ANTIGEN, such as HIV, at any time and therefore not having developed antibodies to it; a blood test result showing this to be the case. See ANTIBODY; ANTIBODY-POSITIVE; ANTIBODY TESTING.

antibody-positive   Having been infected with a particular ANTIGEN, such as HIV, at some time, and developed antibodies to it; a blood test result showing this condition to exist. See ANTIBODY; ANTIBODY-NEGATIVE; ANTIBODY TESTING.

antibody testing   A clinical procedure used to determine the presence of an ANTIBODY in the blood. In the case of HIV, because it takes some time after infection for antibodies to develop, the tests currently in use are not foolproof. Experts disagree about the time it takes, but most people infected with HIV develop antibodies within six months. The chance of testing error is minuscule but not nonexistent. The preliminary test currently in use for HIV antibodies, the ENZYME-LINKED IMMUNOABSORBENT ASSAY (ELISA), is designed to err in the direction of a positive reading. Such a result must be confirmed with a second test, usually the WESTERN BLOT test. See ANTIBODY; ANTIBODY-NEGATIVE; ANTIBODY-POSITIVE.

antibody therapy   The use of antibodies to treat patients with IMMUNODEFICIENCY. This is done by using PARENTERAL IMMUNE GLOBULIN.

anticoagulant   A substance that delays or counteracts blood clotting (coagulation).

anticonvulsant   Preventing or relieving convulsions; a drug that does so.

antidepressant   Tending to relieve depression; a drug that relieves depression and similar mood disorders by influencing neurotransmitters in the brain. There are three types of antidepressants: bicyclic, tricyclic, and tetracyclic. Probably the best-known, and most used, antidepressant is the bicyclic fluoxetine (trade name Prozac). Tricyclic antidepressants inhibit the reuptake of 5-HT and norepinephrine. Popular tricyclic antidepressants include amitriptyline (Elavil, Endep), imipramine (Janimine, Tofranil), and nortriptyline (Aventyl, Pamelor). Other antidepressants include bupropion (Wellbutrin), fluvoxamine (Luvox), nefazodone (Serzone), paroxetine (Paxil), tranzodone (Desyrel), and the MONOAMINE OXIDASE INHIBITORS (MAOIs). MAOIs block the absorption of amines such as dopamine, adrenalin, and noradrenalin, allowing these stimulants to accumulate at the synapses in the brain. Popular MAOIs include phenelzine (Nardil) and tranylcypromine (Parnate). The selective serotonin reuptake inhibitors (SSRIs) act by blocking the reuptake of serotonin, resulting in a higher concentration of serotonin in the synapses, increasing activity at the serotonin receptor sites. Sertraline (Zoloft) is a popular SSRI.

antidiarrheal   Tending to prevent or suppress diarrhoea; a substance used to prevent or treat diarrhea.

antidiuretic hormone   See VASOPRESSIN.

antifungal   Acting against FUNGUS; any agent that kills or inhibits the growth or reproduction of fungi or is used to treat fungal infections.

antigen   A foreign substance, usually a protein, that stimulates an immune response. Autoantigens are antigens on the body's own cells. Antigens on all other cells are called foreign antigens. Antigens include proteins, toxins, or other substance or microorganism that the body's immune system recognizes as foreign and attempts to destroy. Specific substances called antigen receptors are found on the surfaces of both B LYMPHOCYTES and T LYMPHOCYTES. These antigen receptors make possible the reaction of B and T lymphocytes to antigens. Without the antigen receptors, the lymphocytes cannot respond to the presence of antigens and no immune response can take place.

antigen-binding site   The part of an immunoglobulin that binds an antigen.

antigen-presenting cell (APC)   A cell that processes a protein antigen by fragmenting it into peptides that are presented on the cell surface in concert with class II major histocompatibility molecules for interaction with the appropriate T-CELL RECEPTOR. B cells, T cells, DENDRITIC CELLS, and MACROPHAGES can perform this function.

antigen processing   The conversion of an antigen by proteolysis into a form in which it can be recognized by lymphocytes.

antigen processing cell (APC)   A cell, such as a MACROPHAGE or DENDRITIC CELL, that digests foreign bodies and exhibits the resulting antigen on its surface in an effort to find and activate the CD4 T-HELPER CELLS responsive to that antigen.

antigen test   A test that looks directly for the presence of a virus in the body rather than for antibodies to that virus. An antigen test for AIDS looks for HIV.

antigenic shift   Changes over time in the surface antigens of certain viruses, caused by genetic mutations.

antigenicity   The condition of being able to produce an IMMUNE RESPONSE to an ANTIBODY.

antihemophilic factor   Blood coagulation FACTOR VIII. It is available commercially under the trade names Antihemophilic Globulin, Hemofil, Hemofil F, and Profilate.

antihemophilic factor A   See FACTOR VIII.

antihistamine   Any of various drugs that counteract histamine in the body; often used to relieve the symptoms of allergic reactions and colds.

anti-infective   Acting against infection; a drug designed to do so. Many such drugs, including ANTIVIRALs, ANTIBACTERIALs, ANTIFUNGALs, and ANTIPROTOZOALs, are used widely in AIDS treatment to prevent the onset of opportunistic infections. The use of most of these drugs, even in short-term treatment of acute illness, has been shown to have a negative impact on cell-mediated immune functions by decreasing lymphocyte populations and impairing T-cell function. Long-term use of unlikely combinations of drugs has not, to date, been evaluated for possible synergies that may result in profound immunosuppression. Conceivably, these side effects could prove to be lethal to an already immune-compromised individual.

Weakening of the immune system has also been found to occur in antiviral regimes targeting primary HIV infection itself. The development of resistance to and immunosuppression caused by AZT is now understood to be a consequence of widespread antiviral therapy.

anti-inflammatory   A substance that counteracts or suppresses inflammation. There are two types of anti-inflammatory drugs: STEROIDS, such as cortisone, and NONSTEROIDS, such as aspirin.

antimanic drugs   Agents that prevent or arrest mania, a mental disorder characterized by irrational excitement and hyperactivity, which sometimes appears in people with AIDS.

antimicrobial   An agent that destroys or prevents the growth of microorganisms such as bacteria, fungus, or parasites.

antimoniotungstate   A drug found to be poisonous to the blood when tested for possible use in treating infection with HIV. The drug was developed in the 1970s as a potential treatment for CREUTZFELD-JAKOB disease. It acts by inhibiting REVERSE TRANSCRIPTASE.

antineoplastic   Preventing the development, growth, or spread of malignant cells; an agent that has such effect.

antioxidant   A substance that may prevent FREE RADICALs (chemicals with free electrons, or oxidants) from causing cell damage. VITAMINS A, C, and E are antioxidants.

antioxidant therapy   Treatment with ANTIOXIDANTS, substances that tend to reduce damage caused by the presence of oxidants in the blood.

"Renegade" oxygen atoms, known as FREE RADICALs or singlet oxygen, have been shown to damage the cellular component of the immune system. Many people living with immune deficiencies therefore attempt to reduce such damage by supplementing their diets with antioxidant nutrients and vitamins. This is a part of an approach to illness known as orthomolecular medicine. Antioxidants have been used to reduce stress, to treat Alzheimer's and cancer, for lens functioning, macular degeneration, and to reduce heart disease.

Oxygen free radicals are produced by several unavoidable factors in our environment. Toxins, highly processed foods, large amounts of saturated fats in our diets, and, significantly, stress, can cause oxygen in the blood to degenerate from its stable and useful form. Antioxidant therapies seek to remedy deficiencies caused by these factors, decrease damage to the immune system and, speculatively, slow down the aging process. Orthomolecular therapeutic agents include BETA-CAROTENE (a nontoxic form of VITAMIN A that can be stored in the body); COENZYME Q 10 (a nutrient used in Japan as an anti-cancer agent); GERMANIUM (a fossilized plant product used widely in Japan as a cancer preventative); GLUTHATHIONE peroxidase (a complement to superoxide); SUPEROXIDE DISMUTASE (one of the basic building blocks of the body's antioxidant response, usually extracted from wheat or barley sprouts); VITAMIN C (probably the most widely used orthomolecular therapeutic agent, and also the most controversial); and vitamin E and SELENIUM (two minerals that must be combined to function optimally, essential to cell and tissue repair). In addition to supplementing their diets with antioxidant nutrients and vitamins, many people chose to add antioxidant foods to their diets; yams, butternut and winter squash, pumpkin, carrots, spinach, broccoli, iceberg lettuce, endive, kale, tomatoes, cantaloupe, apricots, mango, and papaya are good sources of antioxidants.

antiprotozoal   Tending to kill or inhibit the multiplication of single-celled microorganisms called PROTOZOA; a drug that has such an effect.

antipsychotic   Tending to alleviate the symptoms of psychotic disorders; any drug that has such an effect. Major tranquilizers, including especially phenothiazine derivatives such as chlorpromazine (trade name Largactil) and thioridazine, are used primarily in the treatment of schizophrenia and other disorders involving psychotic symptoms. Lithium compounds are used primarily in the treatment of bipolar (manic-depressive) disorder. Psychosis is a common manifestation in the late stages of AIDS.

antiretroviral   Active against RETROVIRUSes; a drug that has such activity. Antiretroviral drugs reduce the replication rate of retroviruses such as HIV and are widely used in the treatment of HIV-infected persons. The first antiretroviral drug approved by the FOOD AND DRUG ADMINISTRATION was AZIDOTHYMIDINE. The most commonly used are ZIDOVUDINE (AZT), DIDANOSINE (ddI), and ZALCITABINE (ddC).

Antiretroviral therapy can reduce the risk of death in asymptomatic patients with intermediate-stage HIV disease. Moreover, research has shown that ddI alone, ddI in combination with AZT, and ddc in combination with AZT are all superior to AZT alone in preventing serious consequences of HIV infection, including CD4+ T-CELL decline, whether or not there has been previous treatment with AZT.

Today, preferred regimens generally include two or three drugs, based on the patient's condition. Often, the three-drug combination includes a PROTEASE INHIBITOR. MONOTHERAPY, almost invariably with ddI, is a reasonable alternative for patients who refuse a heavier regimen or show intolerance for AZT. To date, there is little data to support rational decisions about whether to employ antiretroviral therapy. Often, a combination of symptoms and SURROGATE MARKERS (CD4 and viral load) is considered. CD4 and VIRAL LOAD values considered to indicate such treatment vary widely among physicians. Some rely on algorithms to determine when to start. Patients' lifestyles, preferences, and ability to comply are also taken into account. In the absence of sufficient information, some physicians are relying on their own and others' clinical experience to guide them in the development of new treatment modalities.

Decisions to stop or switch therapies most often involve toxicity and adverse events. Others are based on combinations of symptoms and surrogate markers, patients' requests, and poor compliance. Many physicians discontinue antiretroviral regimens when the side effects are judged to exceed the potential benefits. This is fairly common in very

advanced illness, when the need to treat CMV and MAI and to prevent PCP is more urgent than antiretroviral therapy. Others stop when no further benefit is demonstrated or there's more benefit from PROPHYLAXIS alone.

The waning effectiveness that has been seen in antiretroviral therapy over time is generally attributed to the emergence of drug-resistant strains of HIV (see DRUG RESISTANCE). Many researchers hope that combination therapy will increase the time necessary for resistant strains of virus to emerge. In the meantime, it has been shown that dual-resistance HIV that can replicate in the presence of both AZT and 3TC is indeed possible, and that dual-resistant virus can be detected one year after the addition of AZT to the regimen of symptomatic HIV-infected individuals undergoing 3TC monotherapy. This acquisition of dual-resistant virus may in part account for the return of viral load to pretreatment levels in those treated at first with 3TC monotherapy and then AZT/3TC combination therapy, although this does not always mean that the combination will lose its antiviral effect. And until a patient develops dual-resistant virus, the combination of AZT and 3TC generally does continue to have anti-HIV activity.

Guidelines for the use of antiretroviral agents in HIV-infected adults and adolescents are available on the web site of the HIV/AIDS Treatment Information Service (ATIS) and can be reached at http://www.hivatis.org.

antiretroviral therapy   See ANTIRETROVIRAL.

antisense   A synthetic segment of DNA or RNA that will bind to a specific DNA or RNA sequence, interfering with the functioning of that particular gene. Antisense drugs are designed to block viral genetic instructions, marking them for destruction by cellular enzymes, in order to prevent the building of a new virus or the infection of new cells. Antisense therapy, a type of GENE THERAPY, and the first to enter clinical studies, attacks the RNA of the HIV virus.

An understanding of the antisense mechanism requires an understanding of VIRAL INFECTIONS. All viral infections, including AIDS, can be described as acquired GENETIC diseases. Viruses are packages of genetic material that insert themselves into DNA, the double-stranded chain of genes inside the nucleus of every cell, and transform the cell into a factory for producing new copies of the virus. Each sequence on the DNA provides the blueprint for the production of a specific protein. In order to produce proteins, the DNA must transmit its information to a messenger RNA (mRNA) molecule, also known as the sense strand. The mRNA uses this information to organize the building and assembly of proteins into the finished product, usually essential cellular components but, in the case of infected cells, new copies of HIV. An antisense drug carries the opposite message to a specific sense strand. Antisense drugs attach to mRNA, and thereby block the production of particular proteins at the genetic level.

Traditional drugs that attack proteins in anti-HIV treatments include reverse transcriptase, protease, and other familiar drugs. However, proteins are large, complex structures that are produced in massive quantities by infected cells. In order to be successful, traditional drugs must disable every copy of the protein. Traditional drugs often attack healthy, normal proteins as well, in a process known as toxicity. Antisense technology, by attacking a single mRNA strand that is responsible for producing large quantities of single protein, may be a more efficient way of eliminating large quantities of unwanted proteins at once, and, since an antisense drug binds only with its exact opposite, it is extremely specific and should produce minimal toxicities.

While proteins are large and complex, RNA is composed of various combinations of just four well-known amino acids—adenosine, cytosine, thymidine, and guanosine. Since the genes of HIV have been extensively studied by molecular biologists, researchers can design antisense compounds aimed at specific mRNA molecules that produce proteins essential to HIV's survival. Antisense has not yet become clinical reality, due partly to technological and partly to fiscal challenges. Few clinical trials have actually begun, and clinical efficacy is far from certain. Nonetheless, the pharmaceutical industry has devoted significant resources to antisense. Its proponents believe it will radically transform medicine and open new possibilities for the treatment of AIDS and other viral diseases.

antisense therapy   See ANTISENSE.

antiviral   Tending to destroy a virus or inhibit its replication; a drug that has such activity. Among the antiviral agents studied or in use against the HIV virus are AL-721, AMPLIGEN, Ansamycin, ACYLOVIR, DESCICLOVIR, GONCICLOVIR, AZIDOTHYMIDINE (AZT), RETROVIR, Compound S, BWA S900, ZIDOVUDINE (ZDV), ddC, 8-bromoguanasine, FOSCARNET, HPA-23, ALPHA-INTERFERON (IFN-A), RIBARIN, RIBABUTINE, silicotungstate, PEPTIDE T, susamin, and tilorone.

antiviral resistance   The developed resistance of a virus to a specific ANTIVIRAL agent.

antiviral therapy   See ANTIVIRAL.

anus   Terminal opening of the alimentary tube for the elimination of feces. Slang terms include asshole, butt hole and bung hole.

anxiety   Anxiety is a normal reaction to any serious illness. In the case of AIDS, anxiety is compounded by a number of factors including the current state of the epidemic, the cost of medical care, limited therapy options, the number and severity of potential HIV-associated infections and conditions, the corresponding complication of otherwise common complaints, and the difficulty of obtaining accurate and up-to-date information about health maintenance and prevention.

anxiolytic   Active against anxiety; or agent that has affect. See ANTI-ANXIETY DRUGS.

APC   See ANTIGEN PRESENTING CELL.

aphtha (pl. aphthae)   Single or multiple recurrent, well-circumscribed ulcers that develops on nonkeratinized oral mucous membraness. Aphthae are usually white. They are painful and may last for two weeks. Ulcers that persist longer should be biopsied in order to rule out cancer. In addition to the mouth, they occasionally appear in the ESOPHAGUS.

aphthous   Pertaining to, or characterized by, APHTHAe.

apoplexy   See CEREBROVASCULAR ACCIDENT; STROKE.

apoptosis   A metabolic process driven by cellular enzymes, in which a cell's chromosomes and then the cell itself breaks down into fragments—a part of cellular suicide. In the immune system, apoptosis is a process that eliminates unneeded cells. Some researchers believe that accidental apoptosis may be the way that CD4 cells become depleted in HIV disease, rather than through direct killing by HIV.

appeals council   The Social Security Administration's in-house "supreme court" for further appeals of decisions made by ADMINISTRATIVE LAW JUDGEs after hearings. Appeals almost always consist of file reviews rather than new in-person hearings.

appellate court   Any court above the trial court level in either a state or the federal court system; it hears cases on appeal from the trial court.

APTD   See AID TO THE PERMANENTLY AND TOTALLY DISABLED.

ARA-A   See VIDARABINE.

ARA-C   See CYTARABINE.

ARC   See AIDS-RELATED COMPLEX.

ARDS   See ADULT RESPIRATORY DISTRESS SYNDROME.

arenavirus   Any of a group of RNA viruses consisting of multishaped virions that have four large and one to three small segments of single-stranded RNA. The presence of ribosomes gives the virions a sandy appearance. The principal virus in this group is the lymphocytic choriomeningitis (LCM) virus. Also included are the American hemorrhagic fever viruses and the Lassa fever virus. The LCM virus rarely infects humans, but when it does, the disease is usually a mild form of meningitis. The Lassa virus causes a highly contagious, severe febrile illness and may be fatal. Rodents typically serve as hosts for these viruses.

arm   One of two or more treatment alternatives in a drug trial.

aromatherapy   ALTERNATIVE TREATMENTs using essential oils (the volatile oils distilled from plants) to treat emotional disorders such as stress and anxiety as well as a range of other ailments. Applied by a massage method, the essence is directly inhaled and is said to circulate over the pathways of the nerve centers of the spine. The oils are also absorbed into the body through the skin. This method is thought to work better than ingesting the oils in pill form. Although this process is of unproven medical value, many of the herbs and other plants are known to have medicinal properties have long been used in traditional medicine, and their derivatives in modern drugs. Aromatherapy is often used in conjunction with massage therapy, acupuncture, reflexology, herbology, chiropractic, and other holistic treatments.

artemisia An herb (*Artemisia annua*, also known as qing hao), that has been used as an antimalaria treatment in China since before A.D. 340. More recently, an extract of the herb, artemisinin, or qinghaosu (QHS), has shown efficacy against malaria. Studies have suggested that artemisinin and its derivatives may also have a place as antitoxoplasmic agents.

arthralgia Pain in a joint.

arthritis A clinical condition characterized by inflammation of the joints. It is associated with a large number of different disease processes.

artificial insemination The introduction by instrumental means of semen containing viable spermatozoa into the vagina or uterus to induce pregnancy. To be safe, sperm banks are requested to test sperm donors for HIV at the time of donation, freeze and quarantine the sperm, and test the donor again six months later. If both HIV tests are negative, the sperm can then be thawed and used. It is generally recommended that all women who want to use artificial insemination to become pregnant should be certain that the donor—whether known to them or not—has been screened for HIV antibodies. Individuals considering artificial insemination should talk to their doctors or call their sperm banks to discuss the procedures they use to protect their clients from HIV infection. Women inseminated with HIV-positive semen are at risk of getting the infection and passing it on to their babies.

ARV See AIDS-ASSOCIATED RETROVIRUS.

ascending disease Certain sexually transmitted diseases (STDs) that start in the CERVIX and move up to the pelvic organs.

asceticism See ABSTINENCE.

ascomycetes The largest class of Eumycetes, the true fungi. They are characterized by a sac that encloses the spores. Included in this group are yeasts, mildews, blue molds and truffles.

aseptic meningistis See MENINGITIS, ACUTE ASEPTIC.

ASO See AIDS SERVICE ORGANIZATION.

aspartate aminotransaminase (AST) A LIVER ENZYME that plays a role in PROTEIN metabolism. Elevated SERUM levels of AST are a sign of liver damage from disease or drugs.

AST also is known as serum glutamic oxaloacetic transaminase (SGOT).

aspergillomycosis See ASPERGILLOSIS.

aspergillosis An infection caused by the fungus *Aspergillus*, characterized by granulomatous lesions in the tissues or on any mucousal surface. Symptoms include fever, chills, difficulty breathing and coughing up blood. The infection can spread through the blood to other organs and cause lesions of the skin, ear, nasal sinuses, or lungs, as well as occasionally the bones, meninges, heart, kidneys, or spleen. If the infection reaches the brain, it may cause dementia. Also called *aspergillomycosis*.

Aspergillus A genus of fungi in the family Moniliaceae. After sexual development, it is classed with the asomycetes. This genus includes several species of molds, some of which are opportunistic pathogens. See ASPERGILLOSIS.

aspirin An anti-inflammatory drug (acetylsalicylic acid, a derivative of salicylic acid). It occurs as white crystals or powder. It is one of the most widely used ANALGESICS and antipyretics. Because it is so widely available, it is often misused. Prolonged use will cause gastrointestinal irritation and bleeding in some individuals.

assay The chemical analysis of a substance or mixture to determine its constituents and the relative proportion of each. In biology, the estimation of the strength of a drug or substance by comparing its effects in test animals to a reference standard.

asset level The standard used in needs-based programs to determine eligibility for benefits. Only those with assets below the set amount are eligible.

assets The total value of money and personal and real property owned by a benefits applicant.

AST See ASPARTATE AMINOTRANSAMINASE.

asthma A condition characterized by recurring sudden attacks of paroxysmal shortness of breath, accompanied by coughing and wheezing. The wheezing is caused by spasmodic contractions of the bronchi (bronchial tubes) or by swelling of the bronchial mucous membrane. Asthma may be an allergic reaction or be caused by other factors, such as physical, mental, or emotional stress; fatigue; and pollutant irritants. Severe attacks may be life-threatening.

astragalus An herb (*Astragalus memranaceious*) used in China, reportedly for the purpose of "boosting" the immune system and preventing chemotherapy-related bone marrow suppression and nausea. In the former Soviet Union and in Japan it is used to treat heart attacks and strokes. The active substances are taken from the root of the plant. Studies have reported that an extract of astragalus, Fraction 3 (F3), has stimulated immune responses in the test tube and in animal studies. Clinical trials of astragalus in people will determine whether such effects can be duplicated in the body. Astragalus is believed to be nontoxic, but there are reports that it can trigger low blood pressure and increase the amount of urine produced, resulting in dizziness and fatigue. Overdosing of astragalus may cause immunosuppression, and plants from different sources may vary in quality and produce different results.

asymptomatic   The absence of symptoms of a disease or infection. An asymptomatic person feels healthy, and may be healthy. It is possible, however, to be ill and be asymptomatic; this condition is generally associated with the early stages of an infection. See ASYMPTOMATIC INFECTION.

asymptomatic infection   An early stage of an infection in which the patient has no physical symptoms. Long-term asymptomatic HIV infection has been associated with high levels of antibodies to HIV core proteins and the absence of HEPATITIS B markers. No association with unsafe sex has been found. Additionally, no association between psychological coping skills and slower disease progression has been found.

ATEU   See AIDS TREATMENT EVALUATION UNITS.

athlete's foot   A fungal infection of the foot caused by various dermatophytes.

atopic dermatitis   A chronic inflammation of the skin of unknown cause and characterized by severe itching leading to scratching or rubbing, which in turn produces lesions. Individuals affected generally have a hereditary predisposition to irritable skin. Also called ALLERGIC DERMATITIS and ALLERGIC ECZEMA.

atopic diathesis   An allergic condition that makes the body tissues more susceptible to certain diseases.

atopic eczema   See ATOPIC DERMATITIS.

atopy   A genetically determined state of hypersensitivity to common environmental allergens, mediated by IgE antibodies.

atovaquone   Trade name Mepron. A recently licensed oral drug for treatment of mild-to-moderate cases of PCP as well as for salvage treatment of TOXOPLASMOSIS. Its absorption is highly dependent on ingestion with food, especially fatty food, which increases its absorption four or fivefold. Atovaquone is known to have many drug interactions, some of which result in synergistic or additive effects against the toxoplasma parasite. It is known to be synergistic with AZITHROMYCIN, CLARITHROMYCIN, PYRIMETHAMINE, and RIFABUTIN against this parasite. Atovaquone should be used with caution along with FLUCONAZOLE and RIFAMPIN, since they can lower atovaquone blood levels. Atovaquone itself can lower AZT blood levels, though to date the clinical significance of this reduction remains unknown.

atrophy   A wasting away; a decrease in the size of a cell, tissue or organ; to undergo or cause atrophy. Atrophy may result from death and resorption of cells, diminished cellular proliferation, pressure, ischemia, malnutrition, decreased activity or hormonal changes.

attenuation   Thinning or weakening of strength or virulence of pathogenic microorganism. An attenuated virus is a weakened virus whose ability to infect or produce disease is potentially reduced.

atypical squamous cells of undertermined significance (ASCUS)   Abnormalities in the cells on the surface of the CERVIX, an aberration that turns up on PAP TESTS. Three approaches to managing this mild abnormality include COLPOSCOPY (a procedure in which the clinician examines the cervix through a lighted, binocular-like magnifying instrument and biopsies abnormal areas), "watchful waiting" (repeating the Pap test every six months), and testing the cells in the smear for the strains of HUMAN PAPILLOMA VIRUS (HPV) that are associated with progression to cancer.

In 1997, the National Cancer Institute launched a nationwide study to evaluate these three approaches. Its two principal purposes are to determine whether watchful waiting is a reasonable alternative to colposcopy (if so, many women would be spared the inconvenience and discomfort of the procedure) and to discern whether HPV testing can predict which types of cells will revert to normal and which will progress to high-grade SQUAMOUS INTRAEPITHELIAL LESION.

autoantibody   An antibody produced by B CELLS in response to an altered self antigen on one type of the body's own cells, that attacks and destroys these cells; an antibody to self-antigens (autoantigens). Autoantibodies are the basis for autoimmune diseases.

autocatalysis   A phenomenon in which the rate of a chemical reaction is increased through the catalytic action of the products of the reaction itself. Autocatalysis is the process by which PROTEASE is able to cut itself loose from the other components of the larger, inactive viral protein.

autocrine system   The process by which a cell produces a hormone that then influences the cell's own growth.

autoimmune disease   An ailment caused by an IMMUNE RESPONSE against an individual's own tissues or cells. Among many such diseases are rheumatoid arthritis, diabetes mellitus, multiple sclerosis, and lupus.

autoimmune mechanism   The response that produces AUTOIMMUNITY, in which the body recognizes itself as foreign and forms antibodies against its own tissues. See ANTIBODY.

autoimmunity   Immunity to self-ANTIGENS (autoantigens); the loss of normal tolerance by the immune system of self-antigens on the surface of the body's own cells. B CELLS are activated to produce autoantibodies against these autoantigens, causing the destruction of normal tissue. Exactly why LEUKOCYTES do not normally react with self-antigens is not known.

autologous transfusion   See TRANSFUSION.

autopsy   An examination of the body after death, including organs and tissues, in order to determine the cause of death or pathological changes. Also called NECROPSY or POSTMORTEM EXAMINATION.

autovaccination   Vaccination with autogenous vaccine, or autovaccine, made from organisms taken from a patient's own tissues; vaccination resulting from the transfer of a virus or bacteria from a sore of a previous vaccination to a break in the skin elsewhere.

availability   In regard to health care, the degree to which services, including facilities and personnel, are in place and readily accessible to all consumers.

Avlosulfon   See DAPSONE.

award letter   Letter or form from a government agency informing an applicant of approval for benefits and, if applicable, how much those benefits will be. SOCIAL SECURITY DISABILITY INSURANCE (SSDI), SUPPLEMENTARY SECURITY INCOME (SSI) and DEPARTMENT OF VETERANS AFFAIRS (VA) notifications almost always state that disability is a basis for eligibility. AID TO FAMILIES WITH DEPENDENT CHILDREN (AFDC), GENERAL ASSISTANCE (GA), MEDICAID and FOOD STAMP PROGRAM award letters may not explicitly state that incapacity or disability is a basis of eligibility.

Ayurveda   An Indian spiritual tradition more than 5,000 years old. Ayurvedic tradition holds that illness is a state of imbalance among the body's systems that can be detected through such diagnostic procedures as reading the pulse and observing the tongue. Nutrition counseling, massage, therapy, natural medications and other modalities are used to address a broad spectrum of ailments, from allergies to AIDS.

azathioprine   An immunosuppressive agent (trade name Imuran) created from a cytotoxic chemical substance and used for the prevention of transplant rejection in organ transplantation. It is also under investigation for use in the treatment of autoimmune diseases.

azidothymidine (AZT) [zidovudine (ZDV)]   The first and best-known anti-HIV drug, and still the primary ANTIVIRAL agent used against HIV. Though the nomenclature has changed—the correct name for this drug is now zidovudine (ZDV)—it is still almost universally referred to as AZT, a practice followed in this dictionary. See AZT.

azithromycin   An ANTIBIOTIC drug that prevents the growth and multiplication of susceptible organisms by interfering with their formation of essential proteins. It is used in the treatment of certain upper respiratory tract infections (streptococcal pharyngitis and tonsilitis), certain lower respiratory tract infections (acute bronchitis and PNEUMONIA), certain skin infections, and non-gonococcal URETHRITIS and CERVICITIS due to CHLAMYDIA *trachomatis*. It may also have

activity against MAC, TOXOPLASMOSIS, and CRYPTOSPORIDIOSIS. Possible side effects include nausea, diarrhea, dizziness, sensitivity to sunlight, and vaginal CANDIDIASIS. It is marketed under the trade name Zithromax.

AZT (azidothymidine) [zidovudine (ZDV)]   A NUCLEOSIDE ANALOG used to slow replication of HIV. AZT was the first and is still the primary ANTIVIRAL drug used to combat the human immunodeficiency virus. AZT is a synthetic THYMIDINE (one of the basic components of DNA), and inhibits the virus's growth and development.

AZT is approved for the initial treatment of HIV infection in adults with CD4 counts of less than 500 and for children over three months old. It is also approved for preventing maternal-fetal HIV TRANSMISSION. Multiple investigations have shown that ASYMPTOMATIC patients with absolute CD4 counts of less than 500 benefit from taking AZT, slowing the decline in their CD4 counts and delaying the development of opportunistic infection, but it has not been demonstrated to prolong long-term survival. AZT is indicated for symptomatic HIV disease and is superior to DIDEOXYINOSINE (ddI) and DIDEOXYCYTIDINE (ddC), as first-line therapy. While there is still some controversy regarding the optimal time to initiate therapy, offering asymptomatic patients the option of initiating AZT when their CD4 counts are under 500 is recommended. Patients with CD4 counts of more than 500 may also benefit from AZT.

It is known that AZT and other nucleosides lose effectiveness over time, especially in advanced HIV disease. The reasons for this are not fully understood, but appear to relate to incomplete suppression of viral replication and consequent development of DRUG RESISTANCE, decreased drug PHOSPHORYLATION, and the development of syncytium-inducting (SI) viral phenotypes.

AZT is especially vulnerable to the emergence of genetic mutations that produce resistance because it belongs to a class of drugs known as REVERSE TRANSCRIPTASE INHIBITORS. These drugs block HIV's reverse transcriptase enzyme, which the virus uses to help insert its genes into the genetic material of healthy, uninfected cells. Reverse transcriptase inhibitors thus impede the spread of HIV into new cells, but they do nothing to stop the production of new virus in cells that already harbor their viral agents. Moreover, it is now clear that there are large numbers of HIV-containing cells at nearly every stage of infection, especially in the LYMPH NODES, and therefore a steady production of new HIV particles, some of which inevitably contain mutations conferring resistance to AZT.

At first it seemed a good idea to administer as much AZT as possible as early as possible in HIV infection, but this intuitive notion has run up against the complex realities of an interaction among a limited and toxic therapy, a rapidly mutating virus, and a declining immune system. Real-world experience indicates that AZT has an impact on health and survival that lasts for a year or so and then fades, no matter at what stage of immune deficiency the treatment is started. Another intuitive notion that has proven not to be true is that patients with HIV could benefit from AZT for a year or so and change to another drug, with equal results. Experience has shown, however, that such patients do poorly on their second drugs. The reason these replacement drugs perform comparatively poorly is not clear. The continued toll of HIV and opportunistic infections plus AZT's accumulating side effects may leave the immune system less functional than before AZT therapy, regardless of actual CD4 count. Also, AZT-resistant HIV may be more mutable than AZT-sensitive strains of the virus, making resistance to new drugs emerge more quickly.

The primary toxicity of AZT is hematologic. When AZT treatment is first started, patients seem to get a boost to their immune system, but then, inevitably, there's a rapid decline. This is called a rebound effect. AZT is a toxic chemical, and when a TOXIN is introduced into the blood, the supply of red blood cells is killed off. To compensate for that loss, the bone marrow,where the blood cells are made, produces at a higher level. The loss increases, however, as long as treatment with AZT is continued, until the supply is below the level it was at before treatment. So for the short term, if the bone marrow is in reasonably good shape, it can compensate for the initial loss. But as cells are continually killed off, the damage exceeds the ability of the remaining intact cells to produce more. Patients develop ANEMIA, with fewer white and fewer red cells than before AZT treatment. The time it takes for this decline to occur varies among individuals.

Patients tolerant of AZT generally develop a mild macro-CYTOSIS with or without anemia in two months. This is not a reason to discontinue treatment with AZT. Normocytic anemia may develop and is of greater concern because it may precede severe anemia. In cases of severe anemia, AZT is reduced or discontinued, and TRANSFUSIONS given as needed. Severe persistent anemia may respond to ERYTHRO-POIETIN. There may also be other causes of anemia, particularly infections. Patients with persistent or severe recurrent anemia are candidates for alternate ANTIRETROVIRAL therapy such as ddI or ddC.

In pregnant women, AZT may reduce transmission to babies by lowering HIV levels, though it is not clear when in pregnancy or labor it should be administered. Most mother-to-child transmission seems to take place at the time of birth, but a significant amount of IN UTERO transmission is also thought to occur. AZT may function as a primary prophylaxis in fetuses and newborn babies, preventing infection of any of their cells. This would argue for administering AZT prior to birth as well as afterward. The long-term dangers AZT poses for birth defects and other health problems for children is unknown.

Major side effects, such as NEUTROPENIA, limit therapy. Recent studies indicate that AZT may be continued safely until the absolute neutrophil count declines to below 750. GROWTH stimulating FACTORs may be considered at this point, but alternative therapy with ddI or ddc may be preferable.

Common side effects of AZT include headache, insomnia, and gastrointestinal symptoms and are often seen soon after beginning therapy. They generally resolve in a few weeks with symptomatic treatment, but will occasionally require discontinuation of AZT (see AZT INELIGIBILITY). Some clinicians initiate therapy at a low dose and increase it gradually until the target dose is reached, a practice that appears to mitigate some of the headaches and gastrointestinal distress.

Taking AZT with meals may also minimize such complaints, and these can be affected by other drugs taken simultaneously. Drugs that decrease AZT concentrations may decrease antiretroviral activity. Insufficient viral inhibition and lack of a CD4 response may be a sign of this problem. Drugs that lower AZT levels include RIFABUTIN and CLARITHROMYCIN, the two most common agents used for MAC prevention.

Drugs that increase AZT concentrations in the blood reinforce AZT's suppression of bone marrow, resulting in increased hematologic toxicity, producing anemia and neutropenia. Drugs that increase AZT levels include Bactrim, FLUCONAZOLE, and probenecid.

Drugs with hematologic toxicity similar to AZT's have to be used with caution, since if given simultaneously, the combination may lead to enhanced anemia or neutropenia. Such drugs include Bactrim, DAPSONE, FLUCYTOSINE, GANCICLOVIR, INTERFERON, PENTAMIDINE, PYRIMETHAMINE, and SULFADIAZINE and CHEMOTHERAPIES such as DOXORUBICIN.

AZT/ddI treatment   COMBINATION THERAPY with AZT and ddI. Both drugs appear to prevent the AIDS virus from replicating, and ddI is in fact a chemical relative of AZT. Their relationship may also be synergistic, meaning that the combination may work better than would be indicated merely by adding their separate efficacies. There does not appear to be cross resistance—strains of the virus which have become resistant to AZT are not automatically resistant to ddI, so ddI may be effective in patients for whom AZT no longer works well.

AZT-experienced   Having taken AZT or other ANTIVIRAL drugs. See also AZT-NAIVE.

AZT failure   The status of a patient who has taken at least 500 mg per day of AZT for more than six months and whose condition is worsening.

AZT ineligibility   The status of an HIV-infected patient who may not be administered AZT owing to a condition such as low WHITE BLOOD CELL count or severe ANEMIA, or the simultaneous administration of an incompatible drug.

AZT ineligible   Prohibited from taking AZT for medical reasons. See AZT INELIGIBILITY.

AZT intolerance   Abnormal SENSITIVITY or ALLERGY to AZT; inability to endure treatment with the drug. AZT intolerant patients may experience the same common side effects of AZT (headaches, nausea, hypertension, and a general sense of feeling ill) as AZT tolerant patients, but these do not disappear after a few weeks of therapy as they generally do in the AZT tolerant. The AZT intolerant may also experience more serious side effects (ANEMIA, GRANULOCYTOPENIA, MYOPATHY). AZT intolerance may occur in people with a known allergy to the drug and in those with kidney or liver disease.

AZT intolerant   Abnormally sensitive to, and unable to endure treatment with, AZT; patients who have such sensitivity. See AZT INTOLERANCE.

AZT monotherapy The administration of zidovudine (AZT) to an HIV-infected person, unaccompanied by other drugs. The effectiveness of monotherapy is known to decline over time, since the HIV virus gradually becomes resistant to the drug. There is now research evidence that combination drug therapies will so reduce HIV replication that strains resistant to multiple medications may not evolve. See also MONOTHERAPY, SEQUENTIAL MONOTHERAPY, and COMBINATION THERAPY.

AZT-naive Never having taken AZT or any other ANTI-RETROVIRAL drug; those who have never taken such drugs. See AZT-EXPERIENCED.

AZT resistance The ability of the body to resist the effects of AZT. Resistance to AZT may predict more rapid disease progression. Studies have shown that the presence of AZT-resistant HIV in the body translates into poorer physical health in general, even in individuals who have switched to another drug. The reasons for this continue to elude researchers. It may be that AZT resistance is a sign that the virus has gained greater mutability, helping it to respond quickly to challenges posed by new drug therapy or immune defenses.

One way to get around the problems posed by resistance to AZT and related drugs, researchers speculate, is to find a therapy that attacks the virus at a different, more vulnerable point in its life cycle. Protease inhibitors block the assembly of HIV particles as they bud out from an infected cell and hold promise as such a therapy. Simultaneous resistance to different protease inhibitors may be more difficult for HIV to achieve. Studies of protease inhibitor compounds have reported that viral resistance may develop at a slower pace than with NUCLEOSIDE ANALOGS such as AZT, ddI, and ddC.

AZT resistant Having developed resistance to the antiviral activity of AZT; those HIV-positive patients in whom the virus has developed such resistance and for whom the drug is no longer working well.

It is believed that the AIDS virus may develop resistance after a year or more, though this point is still under investigation. It is not feasible to do viral cultures for every potential subject to prove that viral resistance to AZT has in fact developed. There may be other reasons that explain the declining effectiveness of AZT in any given case. See AZT RESISTANCE.

AZT tolerance The ability to tolerate treatment with AZT without serious side effects (anemia, granulocytopenia, and myopathy). They may experience the drug's more common side effects (or symptoms due to anxiety about taking it), including headaches, nausea, hypertension and a general sense of feeling ill, but these generally disappear after a few weeks. Side effects occur more frequently in people taking high doses of AZT or in people with more advanced disease at the time therapy is started. See AZT INTOLERANCE.

AZT tolerant Able to endure treatment with AZT; patients who have this tolerance. See AZT TOLERANCE; AZT INTOLERANCE.

AZT worrisome An informal term for those who are on AZT and not intolerant, but who show signs, short of a major opportunistic infection, that the drug is beginning to fail; those apprehensive about AZT generally and the implications of taking it.

Patients on AZT therapy may continue to experience HIV-related symptoms, OPPORTUNISTIC INFECTIONS, and declining IMMUNE-SYSTEM function, in addition to the side effects of the drug itself. Controversies exist about when to begin AZT therapy, continue it and add or change to other therapies. All these factors—added to the trauma of being infected with HIV in the first place—create understandable unease, anxiety, and apprehension. The AZT worrisome may also include friends and family of patients who are using this drug.

B

b₂-microglobulin   A protein associated with the outer membrane of many cells, including lymphocytes, that functions as a structural part of the class I HISTOCOMPATIBILITY ANTIGENS on cells.

B & D   Also written as B/D and BD. Short for bondage and discipline, a sexual practice that involves sadomasochistic (S & M) activities such as whipping or flogging. Even though partners usually signal when an activity exceeds pleasurable limits, such practices expose participants to considerable risk. Emotional and physical safety and disease prevention are increasingly common subjects of discussion in S & M literature and such practices are increasingly common during those who participate in such activities.

Bleeding, abrasion, infection, and bruises can result from whipping or flogging. Any time the skin is broken, there is the risk of disease transmission and infection. This can be minimized by cleaning the area and the hands, by using sterile instruments, and by using a whip only on well-cushioned body parts such as the buttocks, thighs, and upper back. Breasts and soles of feet can be lightly flogged; abdomen or kidneys never. Whippings that break the skin will require a cleaning of the abrasions or cuts with a disinfectant afterward. The whip should also be cleaned and then oiled.

B cell   See B LYMPHOCYTE.

B lymphocyte   A type of white blood cell (also called a B cell) responsible for producing antibodies to attack certain diseases. B lymphocytes are distinct from T lymphocytes (including CD4 cells, also called T4 cells), which are also part of the immune system, but work against a different group of microbes using different mechanisms. B lymphocytes are formed from pluripotent stem cells in the BONE MARROW that migrate to the spleen, lymph nodes, and other peripheral tissue where they come into contact with foreign antigens and become mature functioning cells. Mature B cells independently identify foreign antigens and differentiate into antibody-producing plasma cells or memory cells. Plasma cells are the only source of immunoglobulins (antibodies).

baboon bone marrow   See BONE MARROW TRANSPLANTATION.

bacille Calmette-Guérin (BCG) vaccine   A vaccine containing a bovine-derived live attenuated strain of mycobacterium that has been used in countries other than the United States as immunization against human tuberculous.

baclofen   A drug used to control muscle spasms. The most common side effect is drowsiness and, in large doses, severe sedation, lack of coordination and lowered functioning of the heart and lungs. Sold under the trade name Lioresal.

bacteria   A class of single-celled MICROORGANISMS characterized by a lack of distinct cellular components. They may be aerobic or anaerobic, motile or nonmotile, and may exist independently, in decaying matter or as parasites. Those that can cause disease in humans are called pathogenic bacteria.

bacterial culture   See CULTURE.

bacterial infection   The state or condition in which the body or part of it is invaded by bacteria that have multiplied and caused injurious effects.

bacterial pneumonia   An inflammation of the lungs caused by bacteria. Although PNEUMOCYSTIS CARINNI PNEUMONIA (PCP) is more widely associated with AIDS, bacterial pneumonia also occurs frequently among HIV-infected persons. Community-acquired bacterial infections of all sorts often affect persons with HIV, both women and men. Bacterial pneumonia is also common in pregnancy and may be more common in HIV-positive pregnant women. Symptoms of bacterial pneumonia include fever, wet cough, and chest pain. Some infections are easily treated with standard oral or intravenous antibiotics, while some lead to life-threatening complications. Pneumococcal vaccination (along with annual influenza vaccination) has been recommended for people with HIV disease with more than 200 T4 cells, although its effectiveness in HIV disease is unknown. Other strategies for dealing with persons at risk include cessation of smoking, the use of trimethoprim-sulfamethoxazole, immunoglobulin therapy, and antimicrobial prophylaxis. See PNEUMONIA.

bacterial vaginosis Inflammation of the vagina due to *Gardnerella vaginalis*. Prior to identification of this organism, this form of vaginitis was classed as nonspecific.

bacteriophage A virus that infects bacteria. Bacteriophages are found throughout nature and have been isolated in excrement, polluted water, and sewage. They are regarded as "bacterial viruses." The phage particle consists of a head composed of either RNA or DNA and a tail by which it attaches to a host cell.

bacterium See BACTERIA.

Bactrim See TRIMETHOPRIM-SULFAMETHOXAZOLE (TMP-SMX).

bad debt In the medical industry, unpaid hospital bills, which may include in-house charity care, Hill-Burton cases, and balances in which a hospital charges more than MEDICARE, MEDICAID, or insurance contracts allow.

bad sex Cultural analysis fueled by the AIDS epidemic often pits "good sex" against "bad sex." These terms refer not to the subjective quality of a sexual experience but, in this context, to "safe" and unsafe practice.

People do not "catch" AIDS. They may be infected with HIV, which over a period of time may or may not cause AIDS, but they will do so only through very intimate physical contact, when bodily fluids are passed from one body to another. People do not "catch" HIV through causal social contact. With the proper precautions, nobody has to "catch" HIV. Current AIDS prevention activities, rather than emphasizing the negative aspects of bad or unsafe sex, emphasizes the positive aspects of good or safe sex. The positive approach stresses that even if sexual behavior patterns have to be changed to prevent infection, they can still lead to satisfaction and complete erotic fulfillment, and may even lead to greater intimacy and mutual understanding between partners. While bad or unsafe sex can also lead to satisfaction and erotic fulfillment, it increases the risk of contracting HIV (as well as other sexually transmitted diseases) during sexual contact. Bad sex includes such behaviors as impromptu, unprotected sexual encounters or engaging in frequent, nonrelational unprotected sex. In this context, bad sex is also approaching sex with fear and anxiety, avoiding the facts, and making negative choices about how one lives one's life.

BAL See BRONCHOALVEOLAR LAVAGE.

barbiturates Drugs derived from barbituric acid and commonly used to treat insomnia, anxiety, and seizures. All barbiturates affect the central nervous system. Low doses cause mild sedation, and high doses can lead to deep coma. When barbiturates are used for sedation, they remain effective for only about two weeks. As a result, alternative drugs are generally preferred to treat insomnia. Barbiturates' most impor-

tant role may be controlling anxiety. The major side effects are symptoms of central nervous system depression, including drowsiness, depression, lethargy, and hangovers, as well as stomach pain, allergic reactions, and fever. Prolonged use of high doses of the drug can cause physical dependence, psychological dependence, and tolerance. Discontinuing use of barbiturates can cause withdrawal symptoms similar to those experienced by an alcoholic who has abruptly stopped drinking. Examples of barbiturates include amobarbital (trade name Amytal), penibarbital (trade name Nembutal), phenobarbital, and secobarbital.

bareback sex UNPROTECTED SEX among HIV-positive gay men, many of whom appear to believe that we are in the twilight of the AIDS epidemic and that they will not be infected with HIV—or if they are, that they won't die.

"Bareback sex" is very much a phenomenon of the late 1990s (and has become a popular topic of discussion on the Internet). The late 1990s have witnessed better HIV treatment—and alarming rates of new HIV infection among gay men. There is generally believed to be a connection, even if it is impossible to say that it is one of direct cause and effect. Regardless of the precise role of new combination therapies and the new class of drugs known as PROTEASE INHIBITORS, there is little doubt that attitudes towards AIDs have been changing, and that some gay men are engaging in unsafe sex at higher rates than before. Unprotected sex can have serious consequences. Even if infected, one partner may not have developed opportunistic infections, and he may contract one. Another major concern is that someone with a strain of HIV that responds well to drugs could have the virus change to a drug-resistant one introduced by a sexual partner. AIDS educators fear that unsafe behavior may have an effect on HIV-negative men as well, by eroding their negative views about being HIV-positive. For men longing to return to condomless intimacy, this trend only accentuates that attitude. Some argue, however, that some unsafe sex has been occurring all along and that the availability of protease inhibitors and combination therapies may simply be focusing attention on it.

Baridol See BARIUM SULFATE.

barium A soft metallic element of the alkaline earth group. Barium sulfate is used as a contrast medium in X-ray examinations of the gastrointestinal tract. The barium outlines the anatomical forms, allowing irregularities to be spotted.

barium sulfate A radiopaque barium compound used in roentgenography of the gastrointestinal tract.

barrier See CONTRACEPTIVE; SAFE SEX.

Bartholin's duct A duct that drains one of the two BARTHOLIN'S GLANDs, located at either side of the vaginal opening; also called the *ductus sublingualis major*. CYSTS may form in Bartholin's duct as a result of an acute infection such as GONORRHEA or CHLAMYDIA, or as a recurrent or chronic

ABSCESS, secondary to obstruction in the duct. The cystic mass may be small or large, sterile or infected, asymptomatic or very tender. Treatment is with local heat or sitzbaths, along with a broad-spectrum antibiotic where purulence is noted.

Bartholin's gland   One of a pair of glands located at either side of the vaginal opening; drained by BARTHOLIN'S DUCT. Also called the *glandula vestibularis major*.

basal cell   A type of cell found in the innermost layers of the skin.

basal-cell carcinoma   The most common, and least lethal, form of skin cancer. It usually develops on areas of the skin exposed to sunlight. It commonly appears as a small nodular bump that is raised from the surrounding skin and has a pearly quality. It can also appear as a firm scarlike patch. Basal-cell skin cancer is very slow-growing and seldom fatal. Diagnosis requires the removal of some tissue for a biopsy (a microscopic examination for cancer cells). Frequently, if the cancer is small, the biopsy also removes the cancer. However, if the area is sizable, more tissue may have to be removed until there are "clean margins." Treatment depends on the size of the tumor, the type of tumor and the general health of the patient. Treatment is generally surgery to remove the cancer. The main cause of basal-cell carcinoma of the skin is ultraviolet radiation from the sun.

baseline   The beginning point of a CLINICAL TRIAL, just before a volunteer starts to receive the experimental treatment undergoing testing; the point at which BASELINE VALUEs are determined.

baseline CD4 count   The BASELINE VALUE of CD4 at the start of a clinical trial or the beginning of a course of treatment. The CD4 COUNT was once believed to be a complete SURROGATE MARKER, but current diagnostic and prognostic technology suggest otherwise.

baseline value   The initial measurement of a crucial SURROGATE MARKER or indicator, made at the start of a clinical trial or a course of treatment as a reference point for later measurements, allowing for assessment of results.

basic research   Basic or pure research in the sciences; not product oriented.

basket   Slang term for the protuberance of the male sex organs.

basophil   A blood cell that has high-affinity RECEPTORS for IgE and generates inflammatory mediators in ALLERGY; a granular leukocyte characterized by the possession of coarse, bluish black granules of varying size that stain intensely with basic dyes. Also, an endocrine found in the anterior lobe of the pituitary gland, which produces the substance that stimulates the adrenal cortex to secrete adrenal cortical hormone.

bathhouse   The gay liberation movement of the 1970s spawned a sex industry, with bathhouses and sex clubs, back-room bars, bookstores, porno theaters, and other businesses, all of which advertised in local gay papers. Of these, bathhouses and sex clubs remained major centers of gay sexual activity through the mid-1980s and were vital to the social cohesiveness and economic viability of gay communities in large cities like Los Angeles, New York, Paris, and San Francisco.

Bathhouses were sex emporiums, sprawling sex palaces characterized by a complete focus on the physical aspect of sex. Labyrinthine hallways, private rooms with doors, private cubicles, dark back rooms, dim lights that encouraged orgies, and dormitories where group sex was conducted were commonplace. Sex was oriented toward eroticism and the exchange of semen. Frequent, nonrelational, anonymous sexual behavior was de rigueur. Bathhouses were also havens for anal intercourse. The only limit to promiscuity was stamina.

Bathhouses were designed to make many partners available to all—ensuring that everyone had a high chance of being infected. By the early 1980s, virtually every study on sexually transmitted diseases had shown for years that gay men who went to bathhouses were far more likely than others to be infected with whatever venereal disease was going around. While AIDS would have crept through the United States without bathhouses, bathhouses guaranteed the rapid spread of AIDS among gay men. By the early to mid-1980s, common sense dictated that they be closed down. The inevitable impassioned bathhouse controversy is one of the gay political landmarks of the early to mid-1980s. The controversy pitted bathhouse owners against public health officials, businesspersons against politicians, spokespeople of the gay rights movement against "concerned individuals," community leaders against physicians, government against media. The challenge of balancing public health and private rights was at the heart of the controversy. The issue ultimately became one, however, not of civil liberties, but of money. In his book *And the Band Plays On*, Randy Shilts writes, "The bathhouses weren't open because the owners didn't understand they were spreading death. They understood that. The bathhouses were open because they were still making money."

In the early 1980s many bathhouse owners agreed to put out brochures and post notices about AIDS. Others rallied against steps to impede bathhouse sex. In the face of increasing pressures (to support AIDS education, to impose regulations to ban high-risk sexual activity, to shut down), many owners joined forces and formed organizations such as the Northern California Bathhouse Owners Association, protesting that gay businesses should not be singled out for harassment during the AIDS crisis. Inspections of bathhouses increased, as did publicity, and attempts to close them down. By the mid-1980s, support for the facilities had steadily dropped within the gay community. Gay America's changing response to the AIDS epidemic, and the subsequent business decline, ultimately proved lethal for many bathhouses and private sex clubs.

BCG   See BACILLUS CALMETTE-GUÉRIN.

bedsore   A sore most often due to pressure from confinement in bed or from a cast or splint. There are six stages of manifestation. First is skin redness; second, redness, edema and induration; third, necrosis extending through the skin to subcutaneous fat; fourth, necrosis extending through skin and fat to muscle. Extensive fat and muscle necrosis characterize the fifth stage, and in the sixth bone destruction begins, progressing ultimately to osteomyelitis, or inflammation of the bone.

Emaciated or weak HIV/AIDS patients and those who must remain immobile because of orthopedic or similar problems are especially likely to develop bedsores. These are generally located in areas over bony prominences only thinly covered with flesh, such as the end of the spine, hips, heels, elbows, and shoulder blades. Persons with HIV/AIDS are likely to develop bedsores if they have any of the predisposing causes: injury or illness that weakens circulation of the blood and interferes with mobility; prolonged fever; paralysis; cardiac diseases; nephritis; diabetes; or anemia. Poor nutrition, poorly made beds, beds containing irritating bits of debris, lack of cleanliness, and infrequent changes of position also contribute substantially to the development of bedsores.

Treatment includes keeping the bed dry and clean, relieving pressure as soon as the first signs of redness appear, and use of prescribed medication strictly as directed. Maintenance of proper nutrition, chemical or surgical debridement of ulcers, use of sheepskin or a substitute under vulnerable area, and use of a special air bed are also generally recommended.

behavior, risky   See RISK BEHAVIORs.

beneficiary   The person(s), institution(s), trustee(s), or estates named to receive death benefits, if any, from insurance or annuity contracts.

benefit   SOCIAL SECURITY, welfare, MEDICAID, MEDICARE, food stamps, housing, and drugs are among the financial, health care, nutrition, and other public welfare benefits that are available to persons with HIV/AIDS. These benefits are also available to the indigent, disabled, or elderly who are eligible for them. Unlike the traditional poor, disabled, and elderly who have long had institutional support to help them access benefits, persons with HIV/AIDS and their advocates often have virtually no personal knowledge of public benefit programs or their eligibility rules. Today, most persons with HIV/AIDS and their advocates are aware that the programs available to them are often complicated and obscure and vary widely from jurisdiction to jurisdiction. Working within the current American social benefits system is often difficult, frustrating, and enormously intimidating.

Major federal benefits programs include AID TO FAMILIES WITH DEPENDENT CHILDREN (AFDC); AZT DRUG ASSISTANCE; EMERGENCY ASSISTANCE (EA); the FOOD STAMP (FS) PROGRAM; GENERAL ASSISTANCE (GA); GENERAL MEDICAL ASSISTANCE; the HILL-BURTON PROGRAM; LOW INCOME HOME ENERGY ASSISTANCE (LIHEA); MEDICAID; MEDICARE; the SOCIAL SERVICES BLOCK GRANT program; SOCIAL SECURITY DISABILITY INSURANCE (SSDI); SUPPLEMENTAL SECURITY INCOME (SSI); STATE SUPPLEMENTARY PAYMENTS (SSPs); and the TEMPORARY EMERGENCY FOOD ASSISTANCE (TEFA) PRO-

GRAM. Benefits may also be obtained from the DEPARTMENT OF VETERANS AFFAIRS (VA).

benign   In medicine, noncancerous (of a growth).

benwa balls   A sex aid consisting of small metal or plastic balls that are placed in the vagina.

benzodiazepine   Any of a class of drugs commonly used to treat anxiety, insomnia, seizures and painful muscles. In general, all benzodiazepines act in similar ways and seem to be equally effective. Most physicians prefer benzodiazepines to BARBITURATES and MEPROBAMATE for treating anxiety and tension. When given at effective doses, they are less addictive and produce less sedation. Major side effects are drowsiness, loss of coordination, confusion, dizziness and fainting. People taking benzodiazepines should be aware that the drug may impair their ability to perform activities that require mental alertness and physical coordination. Benzodiazepines can also cause physical dependence and symptoms of severe withdrawal if stopped suddenly after regular use over a substantial time. These drugs include alprazolam (trade name Xanax), diazepam, flurazepam hydrochloride (trade name Dalmane), lorazepam (trade name Centrax), temazepam (trade name Restoril) and triazolam (trade name Halcion).

benzoyl peroxide   A class of skin cleaners that are used in the treatment of skin infection and acne due to their ANTIBACTERIAL and ANTIFUNGAL properties.

bequest   Personal property left to another by will.

bestiality   Sexual interest in/or contact with animals. Also called *zoophilia.*

beta-2 microglobulin (B2M)   A LYMPHOCYTE membrane protein that is tightly bound to the surface of all cells with a nucleus. B2M is released into the blood when a cell dies. Elevated B2M levels occur in a variety of diseases and cancers. Although B2M is nonspecific for HIV infection, there is a correlation between elevated B2M levels and progression of HIV disease.

beta-2 microglobulin test   A test that doctors use to monitor the immune status of someone who has the HIV virus.

beta carotene   A hydrocarbon that is converted to VITAMIN A in the body. Beta-carotene is a red-orange substance found in leafy dark green vegetables like spinach, beet greens, and kale and yellow or deep orange vegetables and fruits like butternut squash and cantaloupe. Carotene is the primary pigment of these deeply colored vegetables (the green comes from chlorophyll), and unlike nutrients from animal sources, it must undergo conversion within the body before it can be absorbed. There are 500 carotenoids. (ANTIOXIDANTS that work to destroy FREE-RADICAL–causing disease agents), of which 50 are known to go through the conversion process. The best-known is the carrot, which gives the group its name.

While small increases in dietary vitamin A may stabilize blood cells so their immune abilities may be enhanced, an excess of vitamin A may harm immune response. For this reason, vitamin A should be replaced with beta-carotene, which as an antioxidant, has its own potential to fight disease. The body excretes any excess amounts not absorbed, eliminating the risk of toxicity experienced with vitamin A. In laboratory tests, beta-carotene can stimulate immune cells so that they are better able to fight off such infections as CANDIDA ALBICANS, the sort that multiply in AIDS patients. Adding beta-carotene to suspensions of immune cells called NEUTROPHILS more than doubled the kill rate of *Candida.*

beta cell   One of the cells making up the islets of Langerhans, in the PANCREAS. Beta cells secrete the HORMONE insulin. BASOPHILIC cells in the anterior lobe of the pituitary are also called beta cells.

BHT   See BUTYLATED HYDROXYTUOLENE.

bi   See BISEXUAL.

bicyclam   A class of compounds that inhibit fusion of HIV cells with healthy cells. How bicyclams work is the subject of research; their properties have obvious value for use against HIV and other viruses. Bicyclams are thought not to work on the CHEMOKINE RECEPTOR.

bidirectional transmission   See TRANSMISSION.

bilirubin   The orange-colored or yellowish pigment in bile. It is carried to the liver by the blood. It is produced from hemoglobin of red blood cells by RETICULOENDOTHELIAL CELLS in bone marrow. It is changed chemically in the liver and excreted in the bile via the duodenum. As it passes through the intestines, it is converted into urobilinogen by bacterial enzymes, most of it being excreted through the feces. If urobilinogen passes into the circulation, it is excreted through the urine or reexcreted in the bile. The accumulation of bilirubin leads to jaundice in many cases. An elevated level in blood serum is an indication of liver disease or drug-induced liver impairment.

bioavailability   The extent to which an oral medication is absorbed in the digestive tract and reaches the intended target via the bloodstream.

bioenergetics   A kind of psychoytherapy based on the idea that repressed emotions and desires create chronic muscular tension, diminish vitality and energy, and thereby wound the psyche. Through physical exercises, breathing techniques or other forms of emotional-release work, combined with "talk therapy," therapists attempt to loosen "character armor" and restore natural well-being.

biofeedback   A technique of monitoring minute, normally imperceptible metabolic changes in one's own body, such as temperature changes, heart rate and muscle tension, with the aid of sensitive machines, for the purposes of exerting control over them consciously. By visualizing, relaxing, or imagining, while observing light, sound, or metered feedback, one is said to be able to learn to make subtle adjustments to achieve a more balanced internal state. For some people this can be an effective way of controlling pain. The technique is also used for stress-related conditions, such as asthma, migraines, insomnia and high blood pressure.

biological cofactor   Any physico-chemical variable, such as the effect of a toxin or vitamin deficiency on the rate of HIV progression, that influences the pace, and perhaps the direction, of HIV's course.

biological response modifier (BRM)   Any agent that boosts the body's immune system by stimulating it, modifying it, or restoring it. There are many types of BRMs, some produced naturally in the body, others made synthetically. The major biological response modifiers are antibodies, MONOCLONAL ANTIBODIES, VACCINES, COLONY-STIMULATING FACTORS, and CYTOKINEs, which include the INTERFERONs and INTERLEUKINs.

biological warfare   An alternative theory of the origin of AIDS holds that AIDS is the result of the deliberate manipulation of human genes to defeat the body's immune response, as part of a program of biological warfare. The culprits are said to be the Pentagon or the now defunct Soviet Union. Today, the theory that AIDS is biowarfare, a descendant of any of a number of germ warfare programs, has been banished beyond the periphery of respectability by the accumulated weight of medical research, reported by the medical establishment and the press, including many "alternative" publications that cover AIDS extensively.

biomaterial dumping   The sale in bulk and at a price below the domestic market price of a natural or synthetic substance that is compatible with living tissue and is suitable for surgical implantation, especially in a foreign market.

biomedical discourse   See BIOMEDICINE; CULTURAL ANALYSIS AND AIDS.

biomedicine   The practice of medicine based on the application of the natural sciences, especially biology and physiology.

biopsy   A procedure in which a small sample of some tissue or organ is removed for laboratory examination under a microscope. The microscopic changes in tissue often indicate a diagnosis, and stains and CULTURES for MICROBES will often reveal the infecting organism. Many biopsies are performed with long needles with special tips that are pushed into an area or organ. A biopsy may be performed on an outpatient basis when the area to be biopsied is near the surface or in the lungs or gastrointestinal tract and can be reached with an ENDOSCOPE, an instrument passed through the mouth or anus. The biopsy of organs deep within the body may require a surgical procedure. Means of obtaining tissue for biopsy include aspiration (by use of a needle attached to a syringe); needle (by use of a needle with a hollow point);

punch (by use of a hollow punch); brush (by use of a brush); and endoscopic.

birth control pill A drug taken by women to achieve contraception. It works by preventing ovulation.

birth defect A congenital anomaly.

birth rate The number of live births in one year for each 1,000 persons in the population.

bisexual Although most people are exclusively heterosexual or homosexual in orientation during their entire adult lives, there is also a vast number of people who are both—those whose sexual desires are aroused, often or occasionally, in fantasy or in fact, by both men and women. People in this group are known as bisexuals. Slang terms include bi, versatile, and AC/DC.

biting In October 1995, the *New York Times* reported that a 91-year-old man in Florida, had become infected with HIV after a prostitute bit his hand. Prior to that incident, there was apparently only one previous case on record of HIV being transmitted through a bite. Health officials do not believe that the 1995 case will significantly change the way scientists think the disease is spread. Apparently, both cases involved the spreading of blood between the persons involved. The CENTERS FOR DISEASE CONTROL AND PREVENTION claims that no cases of HIV TRANSMISSION are clearly attributable only to saliva, and states that there has been a number of reports of bites from people infected with HIV that did not spread the infection. Officials at the CDC do not keep statistics on such bites, as they do on cases in which people are stuck by needles that have been used by someone infected or presumed to be infected with HIV. If bites and saliva were important in the transmission of HIV, however, many more cases attributable to such facilities would have been identified among the cases reported to date.

Bites by children rarely draw blood or break the skin. Federal health recommendations say the type of educational and health care setting in which children with HIV are placed should be determined by their behavior, neurological development and physical condition, and by the way they could be expected to interact with other children in a given setting. The recommendations call for the decision to be made on a case-by-case basis by a team including the child's doctor, parents or guardians, public health workers, and school officials.

bitter melon "Bitter melon" (*Momordica charantia*) is the fruit of a vine-type climbing plant and is a relative of Chinese cucumber (*Tricosanthes kirilowii*), the source of the drug COMPOUND Q. Extracts of bitter melon fruit, seeds, and vine have been used in Asia to induce abortion and to treat diabetes, gastrointestinal complaints, and some cancers and viral infections. Scientists have extracted several active proteins from bitter melon, including MAP-30, alpha-momorcharin, and beta-momorcharin.

In the test tube, MAP-30 has been shown to inhibit the ability of HIV to infect cells and to replicate, as assessed by

expression of the HIV core protein P24 and by levels of REVERSE TRANSCRIPTASE in certain cell cultures. It also inhibited syncytia formation. No toxic effects on human cells were seen in these studies. A crude extract from bitter melon fruit has shown anti-tumor activity in mice, and a seed extract inhibited herpes virus-1 and poliovirus in human cells.

blackout A sudden loss of consciousness; condition characterized by a temporary loss of consciousness and failure of vision due to reduced blood circulation to the brain; a period of total memory loss induced by prolonged ingestion of alcohol and drugs.

bladder A membranous sac or receptacle for a secretion, as the GALLBLADDER. Used alone, the term commonly refers to the urinary bladder.

blanc fixe See BARIUM SULFATE.

bleach Ordinary chlorine bleach is highly effective in killing HIV within minutes. It is recommended for killing any virus or other microbe that may be present in such body fluids as blood, saliva, and stool. Mixed in water at a strength of 1:10 (one part bleach in ten parts of water), it can be applied to surfaces or on clothes.

bleomycin A chemotherapeutic drug used in the experimental treatment of AIDS-associated KAPOSI'S SARCOMA (KS). Specifically, any of a group of antibiotics produced by a strain of *Streptomyces verticillus*. Commonly used in conjunction with other chemotherapies for treatment of HODGKIN'S DISEASE and NON-HODGKIN'S LYMPHOMAS, squamous cell carcinomas of the head and neck, testicular carcinoma, and uterine cervix carcinoma. Fever, nausea, and vomiting are common side effects. Other side effects include occasionally fatal dose-related pneumonia, pulmonary fibrosis, and severe skin reactions.

blind test A trial of a drug or form of therapy in which one group of patients will receive the drug or therapy being tested and another group will be given a placebo or ineffective therapy; neither group knows which is which. In a "double blind" test those conducting the test are also "blinded." Blind tests are designed to prevent patients' or testers' judgment from being influenced by their expectations.

blinding See BLIND TEST.

blindness The leading causes in the United States are cataract, glaucoma, and age-related macular degeneration, but it also occurs in the late stages of AIDS.

blood The fluid that circulates through the heart, arteries, veins, and capillaries, carrying nourishment, ELECTROLYTES, HORMONES, vitamins, ANTIBODIES, heat, and oxygen to the tissues, and taking away waste matter and carbon dioxide. Human blood is composed of fluid (plasma) in which are suspended red blood cells (erythrocytes), which carry oxygen; white blood cells (leukocytes), which help make up the immune system; platelets (thrombocytes), required for coagulation; fat globules; and a great variety of chemical substances, including carbohydrates, proteins, hormones and gases such as oxygen, carbon dioxide, and nitrogen. Blood consists of approximately 22 percent solids and 78 percent water. See also BLOOD PLASMA.

blood bank   A facility for the collection, processing and storage of whole blood and certain derived components for transfusion.

Blood is mixed with adenine-supplemented citrate phosphate dextrose and is stored at 4°C (39°F). Heparin may be used as a preservative. Banked blood should be used as soon as possible because the longer it is stored, the fewer red blood cells survive in usable form. Ninety percent of the red cells survive up to 14 days of storage, but only 70 percent remain after 24 days.

blood-brain barrier   The barrier between circulating blood and brain tissue, formed by astrocytes (fibrous cells) and brain capillaries, which prevents harmful substances in the blood from damaging brain neurons. The phrase also refers to the relative resistance to diffusion of molecules across the unfenestrated capillaries of the brain, whose cells have tight junctions, and the fatty astroglial cell sheath surrounding the capillaries. The latter obstructs polar solutes more than it does such lipid solutes as psychoactive drugs. This presents a problem in treating HIV infection in the brain because treatments must cross it to be effective. Research is being done to find ways to disrupt the barrier temporarily so that drugs and other treatments can penetrate it.

blood cell differential   Changes in the amount of each type of white blood cell (LEUKOCYTE) and changes in the size and shape of red blood cells (ERYTHROCYTES) can be of greater importance than changes in the total white and red blood cell counts. Ascertaining changes in the proportions of the different kinds of white blood cells helps to diagnose different disease processes.

blood clot   A coagulated mass of blood. See COAGULATION.

blood count   The number of red and white blood cells and platelets in a unit of blood. It is determined by a relatively simple, inexpensive standard test, in which the red blood cells are stained as well as counted, to reveal their size, shape and hemoglobin content. Blood for testing is usually taken from a vein, but a drop from the heel, fingertip, or earlobe may also be drawn. The blood is examined through a microscope and counted manually or electronically. Normal red cell counts may vary from 4 to 6 million per unit (one cubic millimeter [cu mm], for men; for women, slightly lower; and for newborn babies, higher. A low red cell count is called ANEMIA; a low white cell count is called LEUKOPENIA; a low platelet count is called THROMBOCYTOPENIA. People infected with HIV commonly have low red counts, low white counts, and low platelet counts. A normal white cell count is 5,000 to 10,000 per unit for adults; children may have higher values.

Although blood counting is believed to be 90 percent accurate, there is recent evidence that electronic counting may yield false undercounts.

blood donation   Giving blood to be used for transfusion. Today, the Centers for Disease Control and Prevention, the Food and Drug Administration, and blood-banking organizations advise those in the following groups to refrain from the donation of blood and plasma: persons with clinical or laboratory evidence of HIV infection; men who have had sex with another man at least once since 1977; persons who have been prostitutes since 1977; users of intravenous drugs for nonmedical purposes; hemophiliacs who have received clotting factor concentrates; residents of sub-Saharan Africa or the islands off the coast of Africa (unless known to be HIV-1 and HIV-2 negative); those with sexual contact with any member of the above groups. The following additional groups are asked to refrain from blood donation because there is a small, but real, risk that they may be infected with HIV: recipients of a blood transfusion or a blood component; those with tattoos, ear piercing, or acupuncture performed with a nonsterile needle; persons stuck with a needle in a health care setting; persons who have had sexual contact with a prostitute.

A frequently asked question in the first decade of the AIDS epidemic was "Can I get AIDS from donating blood?" There is a big difference between donating blood and receiving a blood transfusion. Donating blood involves having blood taken out of one's own body. The needle used is sterile and is never reused. The only blood a donor comes into contact with is his or her own. It is not possible to catch anything that one doesn't already have, including HIV/AIDS, from donating blood.

blood plasma   The liquid part of the blood, containing minerals and proteins. See BLOOD SUPPLY; PLASMA.

blood pressure   The pressure exerted by the flow of blood on the wall of the arteries. The flow is determined by a number of factors: the force of each heartbeat, the elasticity or resilience of the walls of the arteries, the amount of blood flowing through the arteries at any time, the viscosity (thickness) of the blood, the amount of various substances in the blood (such as protein, sodium, and certain hormones and enzymes, including adrenalin and renin), and the functioning of the autonomic or sympathetic nervous system in response to changes in posture, emotional stress, and other stimuli, as well as age and general state of health.

The blood pressure is altered during every heartbeat, reaching its highest point when the heart muscle is most contracted and its lowest point when the heart muscle relaxes after each heartbeat. In medicine, the heart muscle contraction is called *systole*, and the highest point of one's blood pressure is known as *systolic*. The momentary resting phase of the heart is called *diastole*, and the low point of one's blood pressure is called *diastolic*. The difference between these two pressures is called the blood pressure.

blood product   Any natural or artificial substance taken or derived from the blood, to be used in medical procedures. There are two major types of blood products. The first type is obtained from whole blood itself and includes both blood cells (red cells, platelets, and buffy coat elements) and plasma. The second type is derived from separating the plasma (a process called *fractionation*) into components such as albumin, immune serum globulin, and factor VIII (anti-hemophilia factor).

Today, decreasing the transmission of HIV through blood and blood products remains an issue of prevention. Four key methods have been identified: donor selection, laboratory testing, appropriate usage, and viral inactivation. When relying on the general population for blood donations, no screening method will ever be totally fail-safe. However, appropriate education, counseling, and well-designed questionnaires are all emphasized. In additional, voluntary blood donation has proved to be much safer than paid or otherwise remunerated donations.

All donors should be tested for HIV. In practice, however, this is thwarted by lack of structures, services, funding, and coordination. When HIV prevalence is especially low in the general donor population, other approaches—such as pooling samples of blood for testing—may be considered.

Guidelines should be strictly followed to ensure that blood and blood products are not used unless absolutely necessary. In many countries, for example, transfusions are prescribed in situations where blood substitutes such as volume expanders could have been used instead, but these alternatives are not always available or affordable.

As a final measures, heat processing can ensure viral inactivation of certain blood products, including plasma.

Each of the foregoing models—donor selection, laboratory testing, appropriate usage, and viral inactivation—are interdependent; one cannot be ignored without reducing the efficacy of the others, thus the need for comprehensive, coordinated blood transfustion services. See BLOOD, BLOOD BANK, BLOOD DONATION, BLOOD SUPPLY.

blood splash   An accidental scattering of blood that comes into contact with an individual.

blood screening   Each year 12 million units of blood are donated in the United States. Every single unit is tested to make certain that it is not infected with HIV and other diseases. If infected blood is found, it is destroyed.

blood sugar   Glucose dissolved in the blood. Normal level is from 60 to 100 mg per 100 ml; it may rise after a meal to as much as 150 mg/100 ml.

blood supply   The amount of blood stored in blood banks and hospitals and available for use. Blood and blood products are exchanged and sold through an international network. The major commercial interest is in PLASMA, and the industry is well developed, particularly in the United States. The American plasma industry has been strongly criticized in the past, particularly for its practice of obtaining plasma in developing countries.

The practice of obtaining plasma from donors in poor countries for the benefit of those in rich countries is considered morally abhorrent by many and has been less free, and in some places eliminated altogether, in recent years. The lack of a universal labeling or an enforced marketing code for blood also works to increase potential for abuses.

blood supply safety   The advent of HIV has raised new concerns about the safety of the BLOOD SUPPLY in the United States. Although safety has been a concern since the practice of TRANSFUSION began, AIDS places a serious stress on the supply system. Early in the epidemic, suspicions arose that AIDS could be transmitted by transfusion. In the spring of 1983, cases of AIDS diagnosed among HEMOPHILIACS were thought to be related to CLOTTING FACTOR concentrates made from contaminated blood. Although the etiologic or causative agent of AIDS had not been identified in the early 1980s and no specific diagnostic tests were available, these cases prompted BLOOD BANKs and collection organizations to institute a variety of precautions. These included efforts to exclude donors who were members of groups at high risk for AIDS, tests that measured factors considered to be surrogate markers for AIDS (such as ANTIBODY to HEPATITIS B core ANTIGEN and T-LYMPHOCYTE ratios), increased use of AUTOLOGOUS transfusion, and the reduction of unnecessary transfusions. After HIV, the etiologic agent of AIDS, was identified and blood tests became available in 1985, HIV ANTIBODY TESTs became standard as well.

Despite the high sensitivity of these tests, they do not detect all infected blood. A variable length of time elapses between infection with HIV and development of a detectable antibody response. Generally, this is no more than a few months, but studies have found that it may be as long as three years. Blood collected from an infected donor during this so-called "window" period may test negative and thus go undetected. For this reason, although HIV antibody tests have vastly improved the safety of the blood supply, they cannot eliminate all possibility of transfusion-associated HIV infection.

Additional methods to detect infected blood continue to be explored to increase the sensitivity of serologic testing. These include methods based on recombinant-DNA technology, synthetic peptides, and gene-amplification techniques. Other safeguards involving improved donor screening and recruitment are also being evaluated and implemented.

The major organizations active in efforts to improve global blood supply are the Red Cross, the World Health Organization, and the International Society of Blood Transfusion.

blood test   A diagnostic laboratory analysis of a sample of blood taken from a vein, usually in the arm, to determine the chemical, physical, or serological characteristics of the blood or some portion of it. Blood tests can help in the diagnosis and treatment of a host of conditions and to monitor a patient's progress once in treatment.

Specific blood tests are performed to ascertain blood cell differential, blood pressure, clotting factors, blood grouping, blood type, and blood matching, volume, and as a measure of electrolytes, fats, gases, blood urea nitrogen, and viscosity.

blood transfusion   The process of replacing blood in the body with whole blood or blood products, taken from others. See TRANSFUSION.

blotting   Any of several techniques for analyzing a tiny portion of the primary structure of genomic material (DNA or RNA). Northern blot techniques are used to analyze small portions of RNA. Southern blot analysis techniques are used in molecular genetics to analyze small portions of DNA. The WESTERN BLOT TEST is for analyzing PROTEIN ANTIGENS and is often used to confirm a diagnosis of AIDS. See GENE; GENETIC RESEARCH; AIDS-DEFINING DIAGNOSIS.

blue balls   A painful condition of the testicles resulting from prolonged sexual stimulation without ejaculation.

blue-green algae   A generic name for the algae (*Cyanobacteria*) found in most wet places. Spirulina is an edible variety commonly available as a food supplement at health food stores. Scientists have reported that extracts from *L. lagerheimmi* and *P. tenue*, two specific types of blue-green algae found only off the islands of Hawaii and Palau, contain sulfolipids that have a cytotoxic (cell-killing) effect on HIV and have reduced HIV replication in the test tube. It is unknown whether spirulina contains such sulfolipids. It has not been shown to possess any direct benefit against HIV, though it is rich in amino acids and minerals.

BLV   See BOVINE LEUKEMIA VIRUS.

board-and-care home   A publicly or privately operated residence that provides personal assistance, lodging and meals to two or more adults unrelated to the operator. Also called custodial, domiciliary, personal-care, adult foster-care, congregate, old age, community and rest homes. Rents are paid from residents' private incomes, and—for the needy—with SSI and SSPs.

body fluids   The total amount of water in the human body varies from 50 percent of body weight in obese individuals to 70 percent in the non-obese. The principal compartments for body fluids are intracellular and extracellular. A much smaller segment, the transcellular, includes fluid in the tracheobronchilial tree, the gastrointestinal tract, the bladder, cerebrospinal fluid and the aqueous humor of the eye. Of the various liquids found in the human body, such as blood, breast milk, cervical secretions, saliva, semen, sputum, sweat, tears, urine and vaginal secretions, only blood, breast milk, semen, and vaginal secretions have been found to contain concentrations of HIV high enough to infect another person. Saliva, sweat, tears and urine have not been shown to transmit HIV.

boil   A furuncle, or acute circumscribed inflammation of the subcutaneous layers of the skin, glands or hair follicles. The deeper tissue inflammation is so severe that blood clots in the vessels and forms a "core." This is the cause of the acuteness of the pain. The core is ultimately expelled or reabsorbed. Boils are most commonly due to localized infections with staphylococci.

bone marrow   The inner, spongy substance in the center of the bones that produces all of the red blood cells (ERYTHROCYTES), most of the white blood cells (LEUKOCYTES) and all of the platelets (THROMBOCYTES). It is now believed that all blood cells derive from primitive stem cells in the bone marrow. Damage to the bone marrow makes an individual far more susceptible to infections. Bone marrow is located throughout the skeletal system.

Bone marrow plays a significant role in the development, diagnosis, and treatment of cancer. Bone marrow can be withdrawn (by placing a needle in the hip bone) and analyzed to detect abnormalities in the production of red blood cells, white blood cells, or platelets.

bone marrow depression   See BONE MARROW SUPPRESSION.

bone marrow suppression   Bone marrow suppression (or depression) is a condition characterized by the decreased ability or inability of the bone marrow to make white blood cells, red blood cells, and platelets. Such reductions result in anemia, bacterial infections, and spontaneous or excess bleeding. Bone marrow suppression is a side effect of many anticancer and antiviral drugs, including AZT and a major factor in determining the frequency of treatment and the amount of such drugs given to patients. Bone marrow suppression is usually reversible.

Because persons with below-normal blood levels are at greater risk for infections, anemia, and serious bleeding they are generally advised to take the following preventive measures: wash hands frequently, always before eating and after using the bathroom; avoid crowds and people who have infectious diseases; do not tear or cut nail cuticles; avoid using a hard toothbrush or dental floss; use an electric shaver rather than a razor, to prevent cuts; do not squeeze or scratch pimples; take a warm shower daily and pat your body dry rather than rubbing it briskly; clean any cuts or scrapes immediately with warm water and soap; after bowel movements clean the rectal area gently but thoroughly.

bone marrow transplantation   A supportive treatment in which healthy bone marrow is removed from a donor and transfused into a recipient. Bone marrow transplantation is an effective treatment for some cancers, among them LEUKEMIA and LYMPHOMA. The main purpose of the treatment is to enable the patient to be given very large, and potentially more effective, doses of chemotherapy or radiation. Such doses cause severe damage to the bone marrow; by replacing the damaged marrow, the patient regains the ability to fight off infections. There are three types of bone marrow transplant: autologous (the patient's own marrow is harvested prior to chemotherapy, cryopreserved and reinfused); allogeneic (the marrow comes from a sibling, parent or compatible unrelated donor); and syngeneic (the marrow comes from an identical twin). Side effects, usually shortterm, of the high doses of anticancer drugs and/or radiation therapy can include nausea, vomiting, irritation of the lining of the mouth and gastrointestinal tract, lowered blood count, damage to vital organs, hair loss and loss of appetite. Longterm side effects, which are usually results of anticancer drug and radiation treatment, can include infertility, early menopause, cataracts and secondary cancers. A patient may experience any of several complications as a result of this treatment, including infections and bleeding, most often from the nose or mouth, under the skin or in the intestinal tract. Liver disease may also develop in the weeks and months following the treatment.

According to Dr. Suzanne Ilstad, baboons are immune to HIV and cannot get AIDS; if an infected patient's body does not reject the transplants, cells from the bone marrow of a baboon might help battle HIV and restore the immune system by replenishing its depleted army of white blood cells. (By contrast, the drugs currently used to treat AIDS merely slow the rate of immune-system destruction.) Human bone marrow doesn't work very well against AIDS; human white blood cells are the very cells the HIV virus attacks, so giving a patient more does not help in the long run.

Many scientists, however, have doubts about the effectiveness of cross-species transplants. One potential problem is that the immune system might recognize the transplanted cells as "invaders" and attack them, a problem common with all transplants. There is also a chance that the donated non-human cells will identify the human body tissues as "foreign" and try to destroy them. And there have been more dire predictions. Such an experiment could start an epidemic, or outbreak of another disease; the patient might pick up a nonhuman disease from the donated bone marrow and spread it to other humans. In the end, Dr. Ilstad and others managed to convince the FOOD AND DRUG ADMINISTRATION that no dire consequences would result, and to approve an experiment. In December 1995, Jeff Getty, an Oakland, California AIDS activist and former policy analyst at the University of California at Berkeley, who had already survived AIDS for fifteen years and by all medical evidence was living on borrowed time, received a bone marrow transplant from a baboon.

The transplant was successful; whether the treatment has been, however, is not so clear. Prior to the transplant Getty received radiation treatments and chemotherapy to suppress his immune system, in order to reduce the possibility of his body's rejecting the transplant. But in this weakened state, Getty would also be less able to fight off any baboon diseases, or baboon immune cells attempting to destroy his body.

Eight weeks after the transplant, Getty was alive and feeling better than he had in years. His white blood cells had increased in number. His chronic asthma had cleared up. And doctors found no evidence that he had picked up a baboon disease. But they didn't find any baboon immune cells either; Getty may not have benefited as a result of the transplant. Researchers speculated that Getty's immune system destroyed the baboon cells. Or that the baboon cells were there, but in numbers too low for tests to detect. Dr. Ilstad has been unable to draw any sure conclusion; it is possible that some other part of the experiment improved Getty's health.

Jeff Getty, meanwhile, continues to thrive. He credits this mainly to the radiation phase of the treatment and to his use of PROTEASE INHIBITORS, drugs that have revolutionized HIV treatment.

booting The procedure practiced by intravenous drug users in which blood is withdrawn into the drug-filled syringe prior to injecting the entire contents. The process is supposed to enhance the drug-induced high. Booting increases the risk for transmission of the HUMAN IMMUNODEFICIENCY VIRUS by providing increased contact between the blood and the syringe.

bootleg drugs Drugs which are produced, carried or sold illegally.

bottom In SEXUAL INTERCOURSE, a slang term for the partner whose body is penetrated by the other.

In regard to sexually transmitted diseases, *bottom mentality* means wanting not to have to deal with negotiation over safety; it's the job of the top to be responsible for that. See also TOP.

bottom mentality See BOTTOM.

bovine leukemia virus (BLV) A virus found in cattle that is similar in structure to the human T-CELL LEUKEMIA virus.

brachioproctic intercourse Penetration of the rectum with the hand and forearm to induce sexual stimulation. Also called FISTING or FIST-FUCKING.

brain cancer Any primary cancerous tumor in the brain. Brain cancer is relatively rare. There are many different types of brain tumors, only some of which are cancerous. A malignant tumor can spread to other parts of the brain; while a benign brain tumor does not spread, it can be just as devastating because the skull cannot expand to accommodate the mass growing inside. Some benign tumors become malignant.

The symptoms of a brain tumor can vary depending on what part of the brain is affected. The most frequent signs of a brain tumor are subtle changes in personality, memory, and intellectual performance that may go unnoticed. A common symptom is a headache, not necessarily persistent or severe. Nausea and vomiting unrelated to food consumption occur in about a quarter of people with a brain tumor. Some of the procedures used in the diagnosis of brain cancer are X RAYS, CT SCAN, EEG, MRI, cerebral angiography, pneumoencephalography, and SPINAL TAP.

Brain cancers are classified according to the types of cell in the tumors and their histologic grade (how different the tumor cells are from the cells that are near it). Childhood brain tumors are generally classified by location within the brain rather than by stage. Treatment depends on cell type, location of the tumor, the general state of health of the patient, and other factors. The three types of treatment currently being used are surgery, radiation therapy, and chemotherapy; biological therapy is being studied in clinical trials. Traditionally, the treatment for childhood brain tumors has been surgery and radiation therapy, with chemotherapy only on a limited basis.

brain imaging The use of X-RAY or nuclear techniques to produce an image representative of the brain.

brain lesion Any abnormality in the brain tissue.

brain scan A form of brain imaging using radioactive isotopes injected into the circulation to detect abnormalities in structure and function of the brain.

brain tumor A growth of tissue in the brain. See BRAIN CANCER.

branched DNA assay (bDNA)   A test for the presence of HIV. It measures HIV RNA using branched DNA signal amplification technology. The assay yields reproducible results and is relatively simple to perform. It uses a light-detecting system to find HIV RNA in virus particles in a blood sample. The bDNA test does not count actual HIV RNA particles directly, but assesses the amount of HIV genetic material present; the intensity of light generated by the captured particles is proportional to the amount of HIV RNA. Results are recorded as the number of viral "copies" or "equivalents" per unit measure.

This test caused some excitement at the first conference on human retroviruses and related infections, held on December 12–16, 1993, in Washington, DC. Early studies reported that this test is precise and amenable to routine laboratory use. Another early study suggested that the branched DNA assay may be useful in predicting progression to AIDS. If these results are confirmed by other studies, the branched DNA test is likely to be a considerably simpler and less expensive means of measuring HIV viral load than the POLYMERASE CHAIN REACTION (PCR) test. In addition, researchers reported that branched DNA technology can be used to detect TB bacteria in sputum samples within 24 hours. Moreover, the assay does not cross-react with other MYCOBACTERIA, such as MAI.

breast   Area of the chest surrounding the nipple. In women this area may be enlarged and is the source of milk production.

breast cancer   Malignant growth (neoplasm) of the breast. In the United States, breast cancer is the leading cause of death in women between the ages of 30 and 50 and is second only to heart disease as a cause of death in women over 50. Approximately one woman in 10 will develop breast cancer in her lifetime. About 1,000 men develop breast cancer each year. See BREAST TUMOR.

breast-feeding   Since the first reports of possible HIV TRANSMISSION through breast milk, concerns have been raised about the continued safety of breast-feeding, particularly in the "developing" world. Because breast-feeding is the only practical way to feed a baby adequately in much of the world, the stakes are high. If breast-feeding were to decline precipitously in favor of expensive or inappropriate commercial infant formulas, especially where the water supply is not always safe, child mortality could double or triple in many places. If the risk of HIV transmission through breast-feeding is substantial, hundreds of thousands more infants could potentially be infected.

In 1987, the U.N. World Health Organization (WHO) recommended that HIV-infected women should continue to breast-feed where "safe enough" feeding alternatives were unavailable. Although this recommendation clearly supported continued breast-feeding in developing countries, its implications for the industrialized countries were less clear. Several major health institutions in these countries, including the United States Centers for Disease Control and Prevention (CDC), have recommended against breast-feeding for HIV-infected women.

Initial concern about postnatal transmission (transmission from HIV-infected mother to infant after childbirth) was raised when HIV was found in COLOSTRUM and BREAST MILK. However, finding the virus in breast milk did not mean that breast-feeding would become a significant transmission route. Several reasons for this have been proposed, including the inability of HIV to survive in the inhospitable environment of the digestive tract, the presence of anti-HIV antibodies in breast milk and the fact that not all viruses may be transmitted in this way. For example, while both CYTOMEGALOVIRUS and HTLV-I are commonly transmitted via breast milk, breast-feeding does not appear to be a common mode of transmission for either rubella or hepatitis B.

Debate over the extent of HIV transmission via breast-feeding grew heated as transmission was documented in case reports on four continents. Although these reports provided evidence that HIV can and has been transmitted via breast milk, the extent, rates, and precise circumstances of transmission remain unknown. Most of these reports focused primarily on infants, but we now know that the mother's general health, well-being and outlook for survival are also factors that must be considered. Past studies have questioned whether pregnancy accelerates the progression of HIV disease; studies are needed to examine the impact of breast-feeding on an HIV-infected mother's immune status, nutritional condition and disease progression.

Why not simply recommend, as did the WHO, that HIV-infected women should breast-feed where bottle feeding is not "safe enough?" The trouble is in defining "safe enough." The trend today is to formulate recommendations that take account of conditions at a local level, given the great variations in the risk of bottle feeding within individual countries and between different regions and local populations. Specific strategies must be developed for the smallest areas for which data on child mortality rate (CMR) and HIV infection rates are available. In any case, more research is needed because the precise role of breast-feeding in transmitting HIV is unclear. Several studies have found a 14 percent increased risk of HIV transmission from mother to baby in women who breast-feed.

breast mass   See BREAST TUMOR; BREAST CANCER.

breast milk   See BREAST-FEEDING.

breast tumor   A growth of tissue, or neoplasm, in the breast. Most such breast masses are found either by a woman on self-examination or inadvertently by her sexual partner. Routine breast exams will also uncover breast tumors. The majority are benign. It is currently unknown if breast cancer rates, which have been increasing, are altered by HIV infection.

Axillary lymphadenopathy may be associated with breast pathology. Many HIV-positive women have PERSISTENT GENERALIZED LYMPH ADENOPATHY (PGL), a condition common in cases of HIV, in which multiple lymph glands are swollen for a long period. Bilateral axillary nodes may be a part of PGL. However, a new node, singular node, or change in the size of a previously noted node may be significant and require node biopsy. It may represent pathology or infection in the breast, elsewhere in the chest, or systemically. The stage of HIV infection must be considered to generate an appropriate differential for evaluation of any singular lymph nodes. Breast exams are the key to management. At the time a breast exam is to be performed, inquiry should be made regarding breast pain, nipple discharge, axillary nodes, lumps, and changes in the skin of the breasts. A mammogram may be a useful adjunct to the diagnosis of a mass. Ultrasound is often used in differentiating a tumor from a cystic mass.

HIV-positive women should be offered routine mammography on the same schedule as other women. The most widely accepted schedule is baseline mammogram at age 35–40; annual or biannual mammograms for women in their 40s and annual mammogram for all women over 50. See MAMMOGRAPHY.

breathwork "Breathwork" is a general term for a variety of quasi-therapeutic techniques that use patterned breathing to promote physical, mental, and/or spiritual well-being. Some techniques use the breath in a calm, peaceful way to induce relaxation or manage pain, whereas others use stronger breathing to stimulate emotions and emotional release.

breeder Pejorative gay slang term for a HETEROSEXUAL.

brick Military slang for a pure crystallike block of packed virus particles that grows inside a cell. Also known as an *inclusion body*.

broad-spectrum In pharmacology, effective against a variety of MICROORGANISMS.

broad-spectrum antibiotic A substance that kills or inhibits the growth of a range of different organisms and can be used to combat diseases and infection. See ANTIBIOTIC.

bronchi See BRONCHUS.

bronchoalveolar lavage (BAL) The introduction, by use of a fiberoptic bronchoscope, of a sterile saline fluid into the lung in order to remove secretions, cells, and protein from the lower respiratory tract. BAL is used to treat cystic fibrosis, pulmonary alveolar proteinosis, and severe asthma with bronchial obstruction due to mucous plugging. It may also be used to obtain materials for diagnostic purposes.

bronchoscopy Examination of the bronchi through a bronchoscope, an endoscope designed to pass through the trachea to allow visual inspection of the tracheobronchial tree. Bronchoscopy is often used to detect PCP. The flexible fiberoptic tube is also designed to permit the passage of an instrument that can be used to obtain tissue for biopsy or to remove a foreign body from the tracheobronchial tree.

bronchus (pl. bronchi) One of the two main branches leading from the trachea to the lungs, providing the passageway for air movement.

brush biopsy Removal of tissue from the body by use of a brush. See BIOPSY.

BuCAST A recently developed antiviral drug, BuCAST is a butanoyl derivative of castanospermine, a naturally occurring plant alkaloid that has been shown to have inhibitory activity against HIV in laboratory experiments. BuCAST's mechanism of action seems to be inhibition of a viral enzyme called alpha-glycosidase. This enzyme is involved in the addition of sugar molecules to the HIV coat protein GP160. This "glycosylated" gp160 is the precursor to two other proteins, GP120 and GP41, which are essential components of the virus's envelope. gp120 serves as the binding site for the CD4 receptor and thus allows the virus to attach to T cells. Many other viral activities are also dependent on the integrity of the sugar molecules on the HIV membrane, such as virus absorption, syncytia formation, and cell-to-cell spread of HIV.

BuCAST and its major metabolite, castanospermine, make HIV less infectious and pathogenic by changing the sugar molecules of gp160. BuCAST has been shown in laboratory test-tube experiments to have activity against both laboratory and clinical isolates of HIV and to be synergistic with AZT, ddC, and ddI. Its potency in vitro seems to be similar to that seen with nucleoside analogs. BuCAST is rapidly converted to castanospermine when it is administered either orally or intravenously.

In humans, BuCAST has been tested in several dose and multiple dose studies to determine its safety, toxicity, and maximum tolerated dose. These studies, which involved HIV-positive asymptomatic volunteers, showed that the maximum tolerated dose was 400 mg per day. Above that dose, severe toxicities were observed. Follow-up pharmacokinetic experiments in humans noted that castanospermine appears in the blood as early as five minutes after BuCAST is administered orally, indicating that BuCAST is rapidly absorbed and metabolized to castanospermine. The drug is eliminated from the body in approximately 72 hours and does not seem to accumulate. Further studies are in progress to evaluate the safety and efficacy of BuCAST in HIV-infected patients.

budding A method of asexual reproduction common in lower animals and plants, including many of the fungi that invade the human body, in which a budlike appendage grows from the side or end of the parent and develops into a new organism. The bud may remain attached, or it may separate and live independently of the parent.

buddy Generally, a volunteer caregiver who works with a person with HIV or AIDS, providing or arranging for an array of services, such as home care, daily living needs (personal hygiene, clothing, bed linens, etc.), transportation, and personal or social support. A buddy provides comfort and assistance and helps a person afflicted with HIV/AIDS maintain as much personal dignity as is possible with this disease. Many AIDS service organizations support some form of buddy system. Buddies often begin working with persons with HIV or AIDS that they do not know. Often, more than one buddy will be assigned to a patient. A patient's needs, capabilities, and limitations from one day to the next generally determine the care and support that are provided. Buddy training and ongoing buddy education are often required of all persons who volunteer as caregivers. Most AIDS service organizations offer buddy support meetings to help buddies deal with stress and burnout, as well as their own grief.

buffered   Coated or encased in a special substance that allows easier absorption of a medication by neutralizing the acidic environment of the stomach.

bulletin board   See BULLETIN BOARD SYSTEM.

bulletin board system (BBS)   An online "space" where computer users can exchange information. Once connected to a BBS, users can post messages, read messages left by others and reply to them, and find and copy files. Other BBS services may include online games, chatting, and database searching. There are thousands of bulletin boards around the world, each with its own area of interest. Many offer access free of charge; for others there is a nominal fee. Online bulletin boards have been a major factor in the maintenance of an international AIDS community.

The growth of a network of AIDS-related computer bulletin boards in the early 1990s both constituted and fostered the emergence of a new kind of activism. They allow specialists to share information with other clinicians, patients, and the "lay learned"—individuals who, dissatisfied with the lack of progress in AIDS research, have taken it upon themselves to learn the basic science and engage credibly in the ongoing dialogue on AIDS therapies. The online bulletin boards also allow discussion between scientists and activists, as well as individuals attempting to develop alternative treatment options. The evolution of this dialogue has had a strong impact on the AIDS treatment development agenda. This global exchange disseminates instantaneously the latest research in immunology and other disciplines relevant to the design of AIDS treatments.

Many online bulletin board systems make available the texts of primary AIDS publications, abstracts of medical journal references on AIDS, government reports, and the daily summaries of the Centers for Disease Control and Prevention. Rather than having to wait for the lengthy process of medical journal publication, professionals and others in this way have available instantaneous peer review of their theories and proposed treatment regimens by tens of thousands of researchers and practitioners, as well as by knowledgeable PWAS. Many bulletin board systems also sponsor online AIDS-related conferences.

Burkitt's lymphoma   A small noncleaved (undivided) cell LYMPHOMA, also referred to as Burkitt's or Burkitt's-like lymphoma. It normally occurs in children and is rapidly progressive. In the United States, Burkitt's lymphoma makes up a significant portion of undifferentiated B-cell lymphomas in children. The most common sites of occurrence in Americans are the neck and the digestive system. It is often associated with the Epstein-Barr virus (a herpes-like virus) and chromosomal abnormality. Burkitt's is also seen as a form of aggressive lymphoma in AIDS patients. See also NON-HODGKIN'S LYMPHOMA.

burnout   A condition resulting from chronic stress, characterized by physical and emotional exhaustion and sometimes physical illness. As the number of people affected by AIDS continues to grow, the emotional, psychological, and physical toll on professional and volunteer AIDS caregivers also increases. Many are confronting burnout. Depression, anger, and despair are some of the emotional effects of AIDS-related burnout.

AIDS caregivers, both professionals and others, face unique demands and stresses. All must cope daily with the risk of accidental exposure, continuing social stigmata associated with the disease, inadequate resources, and the lack of effective treatments or cure, as well as complex ethical and legal issues and the devastating impact of watching young patients die. It is not surprising that emotional responses to these stresses—sometimes referred to as "bereavement overload" or "chronic mourning"—should affect them. Some may also be dealing with AIDS in their own lives, through the illness and death of friends, colleagues, and partners, or because they themselves are infected or ill.

The effects of burnout are both personal and institutional. Burned out caregivers may experience difficulty functioning, psychological distress, and poor health. Where the rate of staff burnout is high, institutions suffer low morale, communication breakdown, internal conflict, decreased productivity, absenteeism, and high turnover. Furthermore, when staff attempt to distance themselves emotionally, become cynical, or limit contact, AIDS patients and their families also suffer.

Strategies to address burnout include creating formal and informal support groups, developing coping and stress management skills, and providing professional development opportunities. All help individuals bolster or renew their inner resources. Institutional responses can also support both patients and staff, without requiring the costly overhaul of established systems. Such institutional responses include restructuring workloads, benefits and time schedules, improving communication at all levels, and acknowledging the difficulties facing staff.

Busse-Buschke disease   See CRYPTOCOCCOSIS.

butch   Slang term, formerly gay but now in common use, to describe someone or something as stereotypically masculine.

butyl nitrite inhalant   A liquid compound that dilates blood vessels and reduces blood pressure when inhaled. It is used recreationally to produce a brief high. Unlike AMYL NITRITE, butyl nitrite does not require a prescription. Also called RUSH and POPPERS. See ISOBUTYL NITRITE INHALERS.

butylated hydroxytuolene (BHT)   A food preservative widely used to prevent rancidity in fat-containing foods. It is believed to strip LIPID-coated viruses of their protective envelope, leaving them susceptible to recognition and destruction by the immune system. It is also thought to remove the binding proteins that viruses use to penetrate cell membranes. Medical researchers have found that BHT greatly reduces the progression of NECROSIS in doxorubicin-induced skin ulcers.

buy-in   The procedure, effectively mandatory since 1969, whereby state MEDICAID programs pay Part B MEDICARE premiums for those eligible for both programs; by extension, sometimes used to denote the pre-1989 practice whereby states paid Medicare deductibles and coinsurance, as well as premiums, for those on both programs. See QUALITY MEDICARE BUY-IN for the newly expanded mandatory buy-in provision.

buyers' club   A nonprofit group that makes available "underground" drugs (drugs not approved by the Food and Drug Administration and thus not available in the United States). Many of these drugs are used abroad for purposes not related to AIDS or HIV infection and their effectiveness as treatment for these conditions is only speculative. Many underground groups, some of which are approved in other countries and some not, carry nutritional supplements and vitamins, as well as minerals, enzymes, and herbal or Chinese therapies. Persons considering joining a buyers' group should ask questions and explore thoroughly the standards and procedures of any group offering unapproved therapies before buying a drug from them. Buyers' clubs offer those infected with HIV the opportunity to take drugs that might not otherwise become available for years, but the drugs are untested and could be useless or toxic.

The Food and Drug Administration has had long-standing concerns about buyers' clubs' activities. The lack of physician involvement in the medical care of their clients; the sale of injectable products of unknown purity, sterility and strength; the sale of products with unknown sources of manufacture; and the promotion, distribution, and commercialization of unproved and potentially dangerous products are among the agency's interests.

In 1993, it wrote to a number of AIDS buyers' clubs expressing official concern about "certain" activities. This was the first time the agency made a stab at formally defining its relationship with the clubs. The agency noted that it had, in the past, articulated a policy regarding importation of drugs for personal use, under which it may exercise what it refers to as "enforcement discretion." It noted further that many buyers' clubs have taken the position that their activities fall under the policy. And it announced several courses of action designed to "explore the feasibility of allowing continuation of the beneficial aspects of the personal use importation policy while at the same time, preventing serious abuses of this policy . . . " The agency claimed it would intensify communications with interested parties in an effort to catalog those products, not yet legally available in the United States, that may have the greatest potential for benefit to people with HIV. It also promised to explore alternatives.

Buyers' clubs were designed as guerrilla activity, intended to spark systemic reform. Issues of access and regulation of bootleg drugs acquired through the underground and increased access to genuine drugs through an expanded testing program have dominated this arena since the AIDS crisis began. Many argue that insofar as it is the government's responsibility to protect people with HIV (and others too) from being harmed or taken advantage of, regulation in this arena is appropriate and even welcome.

buyers' group   See BUYERS' CLUB.

bystander lysis   COMPLEMENT- or CYTOKINE-mediated LYSIS of cells in the immediate vicinity of an immune response, which are not themselves responsible for the activation. Also known as *bystander effect*.

cachectin   A factor present in serum; causes wasting and is identical to TUMOR NECROSIS FACTOR alpha.

cachexia   A state of ill health, malnutrition, and wasting that may occur in many chronic diseases, certain malignancies and advanced pulmonary tuberculosis.

cesarean section   A surgical procedure by which a fetus is removed directly from the mother's uterus.

CAF   See CELL ACTIVATED FACTOR.

calcitonin   A hormone from the thyroid gland important in bone and calcium metabolism.

calcium antacid   A compound used to neutralize stomach acid and relieve heartburn, acid indigestion, esophageal reflux disease, and other conditions related to stomach upset. Aluminum hydroxide is the ingredient most commonly used in antacids. Because it may cause constipation, aluminum hydroxide is often combined with magnesium, which has a balancing laxative effect. Calcium-containing antacids have become more popular recently, in part because their manufacturers have marketed them as calcium supplements to prevent osteoporosis in women. Some antacids also contain a chemical called simethicone, which is used to reduce the gas that may be caused by the reaction of the aluminum or magnesium salts with the stomach acid. In HIV disease, antacids should be used carefully because they reduce the absorption of a number of drugs that combat HIV or opportunistic infections and require acidity in the stomach.

calcium channel antagonist   See CALCIUM ENTRY BLOCKER.

calcium channel blocker   See CALCIUM ENTRY BLOCKER.

calcium entry blocker   Any of group of drugs that act by slowing the influx of calcium ions into muscle cells, resulting in decreased arterial resistance and myocardial oxygen demand. These drugs are used in treating angina hypertension and supraventricular tachycardia, but may cause hypotension. They have been shown to provide protection against coronary artery disease. Included in this group are nicardipine, nifedipine, verapamil and diltiazem.

call girl   See PROSTITUTE.

cancer   The uncontrolled, or malignant, growth of the cells of the tissues of any organ in the body. Cancers can destroy the tissues surrounding them by depriving normal cells of nourishment and space. Cancer cells can form a mass, or tumor, that can invade and destroy normal tissues, and can spread to different parts of the body through the bloodstream or lymphatic system. Cancers that arise in EPITHELIAL tissues are called CARCINOMAS. Cancers that arise from mesenchymal tissues are classed as SARCOMAS. Leukemias are also classed as malignant growths. Depending on the site, diagnosis is made by various means, including BIOPSY; roentgenography, including COMPUTERIZED AXIAL TOMOGRAPHY (CT scanning); MAMMOGRAPHY; ultrasound; cytology, such as the Papanicolaou test; and palpation for lumps. Some of these techniques and devices can detect an increase in the size or change in the shape of an organ, but cannot tell if such alteration is due to benign or malignant growth. There are various systems of classifying and staging cancers according to the extent and prognosis of tumors. There is no cure for cancer, but there are some effective methods of treatment, including surgery, chemotherapy, radium, and radiotherapy.

Candida   A group of yeastlike fungi that develop pseudomycelia (rootlike structures) and reproduce by budding. Part of the normal flora of the mouth, skin, intestinal tract and vagina, *Candida* can become clinically infectious in immunocompromised people. HIV-infected women have vaginal CANDIDIASIS more often than non-HIV-infected women; HIV infection should be considered a possibility in recurrent or severe cases.

Candida albicans   The most commonly found species of CANDIDA, and the most frequent cause of CANDIDIASIS.

candidemia   The presence of cells from a CANDIDA fungus in the blood, a result of a *Candida* infection, or CANDIDIASIS, in the MUCOUS MEMBRANE of the mouth, throat, intestines or vagina.

candidiasis   A condition produced by infection with a fungus of the genus CANDIDA, most often *Candida albicans,* that can affect the skin (dermatocandidiasis) and nails, MUCOUS MEMBRANES of the mouth (thrush or oral candidiasis), respiratory tract and lungs (bronchocandidiasis), esophagus (esophagitis or esophageal candidiasis), gastrointestinal tract and vagina (vaginitis or vaginal candidiasis), and other tissues. It is most often found in the mouth and esophagus and is usually nonlife-threatening and treatable. Candidiasis is commonly seen in people with suppressed immune systems, whether or not they are HIV-infected. Candidiasis of the esophagus, trachea, bronchi, or lungs is frequently the first opportunistic infection associated with AIDS. In people who do have HIV infection, candidiasis is especially common, sometimes severe, and likely to recur. In such cases patients may experience only temporary symptomatic improvement with the use of antifungal agents and require almost constant therapy for at least one year after presentation. Many women with HIV infection experience severe, recurrent vaginal *Candida* infections before any other signs of IMMUNE DYSFUNCTION. Among women with HIV infection, unexplained oral and vaginal candidiasis appear to indicate advanced disease and a severely compromised immune system. ULCERATIONS from these disorders may increase the risk of TRANSMISSION in the woman who is HIV negative.

The location of *Candida* infection indicates the state of the immune system. Vaginal candidiasis may precede oral candidiasis (thrush) and may be the first sign of immune dysfunction. As immune suppression becomes worse, the primary site of the *Candida* infection may change from the vagina to the mouth and pharynx and later to the esophagus and gastrointestinal tract in severely immunocompromised women. Vaginal candidiasis may be accompanied by generalized lymphadenopathy, localized HERPES SIMPLEX, depletion of T-HELPER CELLS, and ANERGY.

Despite the presence of oral LESIONS, patients are often asymptomatic during early stages of a candidal infection. Some complain of oral discomfort, a burning sensation when eating or an altered sense of taste. Oral candidiasis is commonly seen as whitish furry or cheesy exudates on the buccal mucosa, gingiva, tongue or palate. There may be an erythematous (reddish) base noted after scraping the lesion. Occasionally, the typical white exudate is absent and the only finding is inflamed or atrophic oral mucosa. Diagnosis is made by scraping the lesion and examining the collected material under a microscope. Mycelia will be evident. Several therapies are available for oral candidiasis: CLOTRIMAZOLE and NYSTATIN are commonly recommended topical therapies. Systemic therapy with KETOCONAZOLE, FLUCONAZOLE or ITRACONAZOLE is also available. Many clinicians are quick to institute therapy with fluconazole hoping that there may be some additional prophylactic effect against other fungal infections.

Esophageal candidiasis typically presents as ODYNOPHA-GIA or DYSPHAGIA. Many patients complain of anterior chest pain exacerbated by swallowing. Oral thrush may or may not be present. Esophageal candidiasis may occur in patients taking topical therapy for oral candidiasis. A presumptive diagnosis may be made in patients with odynophagia that responds to empiric treatment. Barium swallow may reveal esophageal ulcerations suggestive of candida, but it is not diagnostic. Definitive diagnosis is made by ENDOSCOPY with BIOPSY and pathologic or cytologic evidence of *Candida.* For most patients with odynophagia or dysphagia, fluconazole or ketoconazole are the treatments of choice. Patients who have had esophageal candida may relapse after treatment and may require continuous systemic low-dose prophylaxis.

When infection is extensive or involves deeper organs, it is sometimes necessary to treat it with intravenous AMPHO-TERICIN B. For vaginal candidiasis, exams every six months are warranted. Studies indicate that the ACIDOPHILUS bacteria found in yogurt may reduce candida infection in the vagina.

Candida species resistant to ketoconazole and fluconaxole have been reported. Amphotericin is required for treatment of resistant strains.

capitation   A method used by managed care plans to reimburse providers. Unlike the traditional fee-for-service system, which pays providers per service, the capitation system pays a fixed amount per capita, regardless of the type and amount of services provided. This means that doctors get the same amount of money for a person they never see as for someone to whom they provide many services. Capitation provides an incentive to avoid expensive procedures, in theory through early detection and preventive care. Managed care plans often lack adequate outreach and culturally appropriate health education and HIV prevention services.

carbohydrate   An organic molecule made up solely of carbon, hydrogen and oxygen. Carbohydrates may be made up of only one or two components (mono- or disaccharides, also called "sugars") or complex chains of repeating units (polysaccharides or "starches," also the "cellulose" in plant cell walls).

carcinoma   A NEOPLASM or malignant TUMOR that arises in the epithelial tissues. Carcinomas tend to infiltrate tissue and METASTASIZE. These abnormal growths may affect almost any organ or part of the body and spread by direct extension, through lymphatics or through the bloodstream. Generally differentiated by location of occurrence in the body, etiology, appearance, or composition, there are many different types of carcinomas. See also CANCER.

cardiac abnormalities   Abnormalities of the heart.

cardiomyopathy   Any disease of the MYOCARDIUM, the cardiac muscle that forms the walls of the chambers of the heart.

cardiopulmonary resuscitation (CPR)   The restoration of breathing and heartbeat in a person in which these have stopped. CPR is a form of first aid whose goal is to provide oxygen quickly to the brain, heart and other vital organs until appropriate, definitive medical treatment can restore normal heart and pulmonary function.

There is a prescribed sequence of steps for CPR. To be certain CPR is required, a patient's state of consciousness and cardiac and pulmonary function must be assessed. A patient may be questioned to test responsiveness. Once it is determined that CPR is necessary (and medical help is called for) the patient is positioned for access to face and anterior chest. Rescue breathing is begun using mouth-to-mouth techniques. In order to prevent transmission of disease from the patient to one administering CPR, a bag, valve, mask, or other device should be used rather than direct mouth-to-mouth contact. The Heimlich maneuver is often used to clear the airway of a foreign body. External chest compression is done if there is no pulse and there is cardiac arrest.

care   The provision of accommodation, comfort, medical treatment, protection and custodial concern, as needed. In medicine, the five basic types of care are ambulatory, emergency, primary, secondary, and tertiary.

care plan   A formal written plan for nursing, auxiliary services, and other services and activities for a patient to be conducted by hospital, home health agency, residential treatment center, or other health facility. It is used as a guide for treatment and rehabilitation and to evaluate the patient's needs and progress.

caregiver   Professional health care providers (physicians, nurses, social workers, therapists) or personal care providers (family, friends, spouses, significant others, volunteers) who work with persons who are ill or incapacitated.

Compassion, courage, and caring are attributes associated with those who care for people with AIDS. Training for volunteer caregivers often covers the medical aspects of HIV/AIDS coping (including stress and burnout), counseling, and practical matters, such as home care, paperwork, or dealing with institutions. Care of caregivers themselves is also a concern of nurses, social workers, and others who manage chronic patients. Generally, caregivers are in need of emotional support and comfort because of the extreme stress of their lives.

carrier   1. A person who shows no signs or symptoms of disease but who is infected with a contagious disease. This person is capable of spreading the infectious organism to others. 2. Anything that passively carries infectious organisms. 3. A substance that, when combined with another (transport) substance is capable of passing through cell membranes.

Infectious organisms may be carried by people, by animals, air, food, insects, soil and water. Carriers may be active, convalescent, genetic, healthy, incubatory, intermittent, or passive.

Carrisyn   See ACEMANNAN.

case   An instance of disease. A shorthand, somewhat depersonalized way to refer to a patient or client and the medical, psychological, or social problem he or she presents to a health care provider.

case advocacy   Argument on behalf of or attempts to find a solution for a person or persons with a unique set of problems or service needs. It is distinguished from class advocacy, which is arguing on behalf of or attempting to find a solution to the problems or service needs of an entire population.

case definition (of AIDS)   See AIDS CASE DEFINITION.

case control   In epidemiclogy, a study in which "index" cases are matched to comparison cases in an attempt to discover risk factors for exposure.

case history   The complete medical, family, social, and psychiatric history of a patient up to the beginning of treatment for his or her present illness. Case histories are used in the practice of medicine, psychiatry and psychology to help rule out and pursue probable cause of illness and disease.

case management   A system under which a patient's health care and social services are coordinated by one or more individuals familiar with both the patient's needs and community resources. Components of the system include patient or client assessment, treatment planning, referral, and follow-up. The goals of case management are the provision of comprehensive and continuous service and the coordination of payment and reimbursement for care in a manner designed to reduce inpatient costs by providing access to outpatient services and consideration by the insurer or other third-party payer of benefit reimbursement for services and supplies not typically covered. See also CASE MANAGER.

case manager   One who directs or coordinates CASE MANAGEMENT. Insurers or other third-party payers may have counterparts, also called case managers, who review treatment plans and authorize exceptional benefits in high-cost cases.

case summary   A summary of the essentials of a patient's illness, treatment, and prognosis. The interpretations of the health professional preparing the summary may be included.

casual contact   Contact with other people in the course of normal, nonintimate everyday activities and behaviors such as going to school, talking, working, eating, playing, studying, hugging, or shaking or holding hands. Casual contact is distinct from intimate, specifically sexual contact, which involves exposure to or sharing of body fluids.

Casual contact implies contact closer than chance passing on a street or sharing a seat on a bus. Being or dwelling in the same physical environment as an HIV-infected person, wearing that person's clothing, using that person's furniture, or touching or hugging or otherwise exposing the surface of the skin to that person's are all instances of casual contact. Casual contact can also include sitting on a toilet seat, touching a doorknob, or using a public telephone after someone who is HIV-positive or has AIDS. Casual contact is considered without risk of infection with HIV.

casual sex   Sexual intercourse with a person whose sexual history is not known and with whom one has not established a permanent, closed sexual relationship.

CAT   See COMPUTERIED AXIAL TOMOGRAPHY.

CAT scan   See COMPUTERIZED AXIAL TOMOGRAPHY.

categorically needy   In MEDICAID parlance, those who receive Medicaid because they receive, are eligible for, or are deemed eligible for AFDC, SSI, or SSPS.

cathartic   An active purgative, producing bowel movements.

catheter   A tube made of a flexible material, such as silicon rubber, which is used when it is medically necessary to introduce fluids to or drain fluids from the body. Many people with HIV illness need a catheter for intravenous infusions of medication or nutrition. A catheter is inserted directly into a sac, cavity or vein and can be used to administer drugs (it is this function that concerns us here). A peripherally inserted central catheter (PICC) line is usually inserted into a vein in an arm and is used for periods of up to three months. This type of catheter does not need to be surgically implanted and can be inserted at home by a trained nurse. For longer periods, catheters are surgically implanted directly into a central vein in the chest. These are called central venous catheters and can be used for months or years.

When infusions are begun, the first few administrations are usually given through a regular INTRAVENOUS (IV) line, not a catheter. An intravenous line is a small tube that extends about one inch into a vein and about half an inch outside the skin. It ends in a heplock, a small chamber that contains heparin, a substance that keeps blood from clotting, allowing the catheter to remain open. The heplock can be reused for two to three days. After that, a midline, long-line or peripherally-inserted central catheter is likely to be inserted. A midline catheter is inserted into a vein in the arm like an IV line, but the tubing extends about 6 inches. Midline catheters can be used for up to six weeks and cannot be used for long-term total parental nutrition, chemotherapy, or to draw blood. A long-line catheter consists of a tube inserted into the arm and then threaded up the arm into a big vein near the heart. Long-line catheters can be used for up to three months.

The most common complication of midlines and PICC lines is phlebitis (inflammation of the vein), in which the skin overlaying the vein becomes warm, red, and painful. The catheter will then usually be removed and replaced in another vein. The irritation may be caused by the catheter itself or by the medication. Over time, people may run out of good peripheral veins, and an indwelling central line (also known as a right atrial catheter or venous access device) becomes necessary. Another complication of both midlines and PICCs is that they can "migrate out," that is, the end of the catheter within the big vein near the heart can be dislocated to a smaller vein. When this occurs, the line usually has to be replaced.

The major complications of central venous catheters are bacterial infections. The catheter exit site and impurities in infusion liquids are potential ports of entry for bacteria. Local infections at the exit site, without tenderness along the tunnel, usually can be treated locally. Tunnel infections may require catheter removal and replacement on the other side of the chest.

The Hickman catheter is the most common of the indwelling central venous catheters. The Hickman catheter is a modification of an earlier catheter developed by a Dr. Broviac in 1973 for the purpose of infusing total parenteral nutrition. The Hickman has a wider tube and thicker tube wall than the Broviac catheter and is more widely used today. The Hickman consists of a long internal tube that extends from a vein above the heart through a "tunnel" in the chest to what is called an exit site. About one inch before the exit site there is a small Dacron cuff that serves as an anchor and barrier to infection.

Catheters may have one or more separate external tubes or "lumens" branching from the catheter outside the body. Each lumen is four or five inches long and ends in a rubber cap. When the catheter is used a needle is inserted in this cap. The lumens are looped and taped to the chest when not in use. Many catheters used today by people with HIV illness have two lumens so that two procedures can be done simultaneously. The Groshong catheter is a newer version of the Hickman, in which the internal catheter tip is closed. Instead of an open tube, there is a valve or slip on the side of the tube. The valve remains closed when not in use. During an infusion, the pressure of the incoming fluid opens the valve, letting the fluid enter the bloodstream. When suction is applied, this negative pressure causes the valve to open inward, letting blood flow through the catheter into the syringe. A Groshong catheter does not need heparin flushes, slightly simplifying routine maintenance procedures. The valve is intended to minimize blood backflow problems. The Groshong's tube is not as wide as the Hickman's. As a result, more time is needed for procedures such as infusions.

The internal tubing of the port is the same as that extending outside the body; a "port" made of metal or a synthetic material is placed mid-chest under the skin. The skin is punctured with special needles every time the port is used. There are no external components to the port. Initially, the skin over the port may be bruised and sore from the operation, but often becomes numb after a couple of weeks. Ports are most suitable for medication administered once or twice a month, but are now being used for daily procedures by people with HIV illness.

Ports are attached to four of five inches of silicone tubing with a clamp and rubber cap at one end and a needle at the other. The needle is inserted through the skin into the port, creating a temporary lumen. Medication is inserted by a needle into the tube's rubber cap, not the port itself. Ports are available with either one or two chambers, however the double size is somewhat large. When two "channels" are considered appropriate, surgeons often prefer to use an indwelling catheter instead of a port. A recent development is a port that can be placed in the forearm under the skin, instead of in the chest.

Institutional contracts with suppliers may determine whether Hickmans or Groshongs are used. Some hospitals do not consider PICC lines cost-effective, and patients go directly from intravenous lines to indwelling central venous catheters. Not all systems are available at every hospital.

There are some clear-cut advantages to one system or the other (catheters vs. ports), and also some relative advantages depending on medical indications. A significant disadvantage of the port is that it must be surgically removed. Also, an infected Hickman catheter can be removed on the spot in an emergency room, while a port requires transfer to an operating room for surgical removal. This can cause a delay in removing the source of the infection.

Some people don't like to stick themselves with needles, and so prefer catheters where the needle goes into the lumen through a rubber cap, not their skin. When made of stainless steel or titanium, ports interfere with diagnostic imaging (MRI and CT scans) and radiation. People with significant visual impairment cannot handle ports. When two lumens are indicated rather than one, surgeons often prefer Hickmans or Groshongs to ports, although double ports are available. At advanced stages of illness, people might not be able to insert the special needles used with ports and will need assistance. In addition, when people lose a lot of weight, the port becomes quite prominent, particularly if it has two reservoirs.

There are no absolute disadvantages to Hickman-type catheters. However, there are relative disadvantages. The lumens are visible to the patient and to others. More equipment is entailed. This involves keeping track of supplies (dressings, swabs, injection caps) and their delivery. These are also needed with ports, but in smaller amounts. Swimming with a Hickman is not possible. Nursing visits may be needed more often to check on procedures and the condition of the exit site. These are primarily practical and aesthetic disadvantages, and while far from trivial, they are not in the same league as potential port-related major medical problems. All of these disadvantages also apply to ports if the needle and attached tubing are left in place for several days at a time.

CD   See CLUSTER OF DIFFERENTIATION.

CD2 cell   See ACCESSORY MOLECULES.

CD4   A protein whose presence on the surface of a human cell allows HIV to attach to and enter, and thus infect, a cell. CD4 RECEPTORS are present on CD4 CELLS (HELPER T CELLS), MACROPHAGES, and DENDRITIC CELLS, among others. Normally, CD4 acts as an ACCESSORY MOLECULE, forming part of a larger structure through which T CELLS and other cells signal each other.

It has been hypothesized that CD4 alone is not able to allow HIV or HIV-infected cells to fuse with target cells and infect them. Several lines of evidence have suggested that one or more cofactors, presumably also molecules on the surface of target cells, are necessary for HIV fusion and entry. Recent data indicate that a second molecule, fusin, also is required for fusion and entry of certain strains of HIV into cells.

See also ANTIGEN; RECEPTOR.

CD4, synthetic   Soluble genetically-engineered CD4 designed to be injected into the blood to inactivate the HIV virus by covering all its "plugs" before they can find real "sockets." CD4 molecule is very expensive to make, and breaks down so fast that it has to be taken—by injection, every four hours.

The efforts to develop synthetic CD4 are the first attempts to develop a potential AIDS therapy by employing recombinant DNA technology (gene-splicing) to focus on a part of HIV's life cycle. Scientists have taken the CD4 protein's gene-encoding program and inserted it into cells that then manufacture more. The idea is that flooding the body with synthetic CD4 might decoy the virus, sparing healthy T-CELLS from infection and destruction. So far, at least, CD4 doesn't seem to be producing auto-antibodies (nor has it been found to be toxic).

CD4 cell   A white blood cell (LYMPHOCYTE) with CD4 molecules on its surface; a CD4-positive (CD4+) cell.

Each type of white blood cell plays a specific role in the immune system. The CD4 cell modulates the immune response to an infection through a complex series of interactions with ANTIGEN presenting cells (MACROPHAGES, DENDRITIC CELLS, and B CELLS) and other types of lymphocytes (B cells and CD8 CELLS). The CD4 cell is also known as the T-helper cell or HELPER T CELL.

CD4 cell count   The number of CD4 CELLS per cubic millimeter of blood. This measurement is the most commonly used SURROGATE MARKER for assessing the state of an HIV-infected patient's immune system. The CD4 cell count frequently indicates the stage of HIV infection. As the count declines, the risk of developing OPPORTUNISTIC INFECTIONS increases. The trend of several consecutive CD4 cell counts is more important than any one measurement.

Recent findings indicate that the immune system's army of CD4+ T cells not only declines in overall size during the course of HIV disease but also becomes progressively less diverse as specific CD4+ T cells programmed to fight different invaders are lost. Furthermore, these depleted cell types may not be immediately restored by therapies such as anti-retroviral drugs or interleukin-2 (IL-2) that can increase an HIV-infected person's overall CD4+ T cell count. Rather, such therapy, at least in the short term, appears to boost only the cells that were present when therapy began. These findings argue for treatment early in the disease, before elements of the immune system are significantly depleted. The data also suggest that drugs to prevent opportunistic infections may remain important even for patients with CD4+ T cell counts that are rapidly increasing in response to therapy, because these individuals may be missing part of their CD4+ T cell repertoires.

The normal range for CD4 cell counts is 500 to 1500 and patients should be tested every six to twelve months if counts are higher than 500. If the counts are lower, testing every three months is advised. The CD4 count is a relatively expensive test, but it is an important way of monitoring the state of the immune system. Counts vary considerably, however; the same laboratory performing multiple tests on the same specimen can find counts that vary by as much as 20 percent. The count is also influenced by a variety of other medical conditions apart from HIV infection. As a result, although the

CD4+ count is frequently used to assess progressive disease, changes in the count are sometimes difficult to interpret.

A few years ago, there seemed to be a sound scientific rationale for using CD4 cell counts to predict treatment response. They provided most of the evidence justifying the approval of ddI, D4T and ddC in combination therapy. Little, however, can be said definitively about the clinical benefit of these drugs, and it has become increasingly apparent that CD4 is a poor "surrogate" for predicting results. A 1994 study retrospectively analyzing the outcomes of a number of randomized trials found that CD4 cell counts actually obscured the clinical results, highlighting the importance of empirical validation in assessing the information derived from such tests.

CD4 lymphocyte A white blood cell with CD4 molecules present on its surface. See CD4 CELL.

CD4-positive (CD4+) A designation indicating the presence of CD4.

CD4-positive (CD4+) cell A cell on whose surface molecules of CD4 are present; a CD4 CELL.

CD4-positive (CD4+) cell count See CD4 CELL COUNT.

CD4-positive (CD4+) lymphocyte See CD4 CELL.

CD4-positive (CD4+) percentage The proportion of CD4+ CELLs in relation to the total number of LYMPHOCYTES in a quantity of blood (standard specimen unit is one cubic millimeter). As HIV infection progresses, the percentage decreases. A significant drop in the CD4 CELL COUNT reflects significant damage to the immune system.

CD4-to-CD8 ratio The ratio of CD4 to CD8 cells. A common measure of immune system status that is found in healthy individuals.

CD8 A protein present on the surface of some white blood cells, or LYMPHOCYTES. CD8 seems to be necessary to the CYTOTOXIC function of these cells, which are crucial to the working of the IMMUNE SYSTEM. See CD8 CELL; T-LYMPHO-CYTES.

CD8 cell A white blood cell (LYMPHOCYTE) with CD8 molecules on its surface; a CD8-positive (CD8+) T CELL. Most CD8 cells are thought to consist of SUPPRESSOR/CYTOTOXIC lymphocytes, which play a crucial role in determining IMMUNE RESPONSE. Some recognize and kill cancerous cells and those infected by intracellular pathogens (some bacteria, viruses, and mycoplasma).

In addition to killing HIV-infected cells directly by a process called CYTOLYSIS, these cells also secrete soluble factors that suppress HIV replication in blood and lymph nodes taken from HIV-infected people. It is hypothesized that part of the CD8 suppressor phenomenon is due to the secretion by CD8+ T cells of signaling molecules called beta-CHEMOKINEs, which normally recruit inflammatory cells to the site of an infection. Three of these molecules, known as

RANTES, MIP-1a and MIP-1B, apparently block HIV replication by occupying receptors necessary for the entry of MACROPHAGE-tropic strains of HIV into their target cells.

Halting of AIDS progression is thought to be associated with stable CD8 CELL COUNTS over time, despite declines, in some cases to zero, in CD4 CELL COUNTs. It is speculated that stable CD8 cell counts may be a common denominator in cases of long-term survival. As a result, therapies have been developed based on techniques of increasing CD8 cell counts in symptomatic individuals. Approaches have included a KAPOSI'S SARCOMA treatment called CD8 cell expansion, in which CD8 cells are removed from the blood and cultivated in culture by adding the protein INTERLEUKIN-2. The cultivated cells are then reinjected into the patients' bloodstream. Another method is modification of the body's biological response. DINITROCHLOROBENZENE (DNCB) is a powerful stimulator of an immune response called DELAYED-TYPE HYPERSENSITIVITY, which is known to control intracellular infections; topical application of it has been shown to raise the levels of CD8 cells and natural killer cells consistently and nontoxically among compliant patients.

CD8 cell count The number of CD8 CELLS per cubic millimeter of blood; an important measurement of IMMUNE SYSTEM status.

CD8 cell expansion A treatment that involves growing an HIV-infected patient's CD8 CELLs outside the body, in order to increase his CD8 CELL COUNT.

CD8 lymphocyte A white blood cell with CD8 molecules on its surface. See CD8 CELL.

CD8-positive (CD8+) A designation indicating the presence of CD8.

CD8-positive (CD8+) cell A cell on whose surface molecules of CD8 are present; a CD8 CELL.

CD8-positive (CD8+) cell count See CD8 CELL COUNT.

CD8-positive (CD8+) cell expansion See CD8 CELL EXPANSION; CD8 CELL.

CD8-positive (CD8+) lymphocyte See CD8 CELL.

CDC definition See AIDS CASE DEFINITION.

ceftriaxone A broad-spectrum antibiotic. Ceftriaxone is used for bacterial infections of the lower respiratory tract, skin, urinary tract, bones and joints, abdomen, and blood. It is also used for PELVIC INFLAMMATORY DISEASE and MENINGI-TIS. It is generally not the first-choice therapy for most bacterial infections because it cannot be taken orally. It is particularly useful against infection in the brain or other part of the central nervous system, when the bacteria is resistant to penicillin or the oral cephalosporins. Ceftriaxone weakens the cell walls of newly formed bacteria. Common side effects include pain, tenderness, or hardness at the injection site. Rash, itching, fever or chills, blood-clotting disorders, and deficiencies in red or white blood cells occur less frequently. (Trade name Rocephin.)

cefuroxime   An antibiotic used to treat bacterial infections of the ear, respiratory tract, skin, sinuses, bones and joints, and urinary tract. Cefuroxime belongs to the cephalosporin class of antibiotics. The most common side effects include diarrhea, nausea, vomiting, and abdominal pain; these occur more frequently at higher doses. This drug works by preventing susceptible bacteria from building strong cell walls.

Cefuroxime is available in tablet, oral suspension, and injectable solution form. These are taken up differently by the body and require different doses. The oral suspension is intended primarily for children. Tablets are used for mild-to-moderate infections and injection for more serious infections. (Trade names Ceftin, Kefurox, and Zinacef.)

celibacy   Abstention from sexual intercourse. Also, in a somewhat old-fashioned usage, the state of being unmarried.

cell   A microscopic unit of protoplasm containing a nucleus and bounded by a membrane. The cell is the smallest independent unit of life that is capable of performing all living functions, and the smallest unit making up larger living organisms.

cell-activated factor (CAF)   A so-far unidentified substance that cells produce to keep HIV in check. Not long after HIV was identified, researchers noticed that it was very difficult to culture it from the blood of many infected people, particularly those free of symptoms. Investigating this phenomenon, Dr. Jay Levy of the University of California, San Francisco, determined that activated CD8 CELLS in these cultures were responsible. Dr. Levy found that activated CD8 LYMPHOCYTEs from HIV-negative donors and from SIV (simian immunodeficiency virus)-infected primates, also halted the growth of HIV in cell cultures. This effect was not due to CD8 cells directly killing HIV-infected cells; rather, something that these cells produced, which Dr. Levy referred to as the "cell antiviral factor," was keeping the virus in check.

Since proportionately more CD8 cells are required to block the virus in cultures derived from patients with advanced HIV disease, Dr. Levy concluded that these CD8 cells were not producing as much CAF. He reported that CAF could be what is responsible for the long period of clinical latency that most HIV-infected people experience and for the continued health of many long-term survivors. He also believes that production of CAF ebbs before CD4 CELLs become depleted and symptoms develop. CAF's chemical identity has proved to be extremely elusive. No one substance secreted by CD8 cells had been isolated that could effect this dramatic suppression until late 1995, when two groups of researchers separately claimed to have done so (see *Nature*, December 7, 1995, p. 563 and *Science*, December 15, 1995, pp. 1811–15). Their claims, however, have not been verified.

cell cycle   The phases that a cell goes through in dividing, and specifically the period during which events involved in nucleation and reproduction are completed. In proliferative cells this includes all the events taking place between the completion of one round of mitosis and CYTOKINESIS and the next. Cells that have begun to differentiate have generally left the cell cycle for good.

The molecular details of the cell cycle have been the subject of intense research in recent decades, not least because of their implications for our understanding of the origins of many cancers. In both normal and cancer cells a cell growth cycle can be divided into discrete phases. The two key phases of the cell cycle are the S phase, during which DNA is synthesized, and the M phase, the period of actual division, or mitosis. Both of these points can be measured or marked on an individual cell. Active cells are dynamic, and cancer may be thought of as a disorder of cells that are constantly dividing. Chemotherapy is thought to be effective only when cells are dividing, and certain drugs target this phase of the cell cycle in a specific way. On a basic cellular level, this is how anticancer drugs work.

cell line   A collection of cells that divide continuously in culture. They may be either monoclonal or polyclonal and may have been transformed naturally or be an artificial hybridization.

cell-mediated immunity (CMI)   See CELLULAR IMMUNITY.

cellular immunity   The mechanism of immunity that does not involve antibody production, but rather the destruction of foreign antigens by the activities of T CELLS and MACROPHAGES. The human immune system, which protects the body from infections and tumors, consists of two "arms," HUMORAL IMMUNITY (effected by soluble antibodies secreted by B CELLS into the body fluids) and cellular, or cell-mediated immunity (effected by cells, especially T cells, and their secretions). The primary effector cells are activated macrophages, NATURAL KILLER CELLS, and CYTOTOXIC T CELL lymphocytes. It is the natural function of these cells to destroy all infected and abnormal cells, including HIV-infected CD4 cells. These effector cells are activated by DELAYED-TYPE HYPERSENSITIVITY (DTH). Cellular, or cell-mediated, immunity is critical in controlling and clearing the agents that cause OPPORTUNISTIC INFECTION AND DISEASE in AIDS; these and the neoplasms seen in AIDS, as well as HIV itself, are cellular infections and can be controlled only by cellular immunity.

Defective cellular immunity was the first recognized hallmark of AIDS in 1981 and is a prerequisite to disease progression. Researchers have concluded that the opportunistic infections and neoplasms seen in AIDS, including HIV, flourish when cellular immunity is suppressed and humoral immunity is dominant. They also believe that an imbalance between the two, with humoral immunity dominant, may actually predispose individuals to HIV infection. Successful treatments for AIDS must therefore be able to stimulate cellular immunity and suppress humoral immunity. Stimulation of cellular immunity will probably be the only means by which HIV infection may be made a chronic, rather than fatal, disease. Most of the current approved treatments and prophylaxis for HIV and opportunistic infections are IMMUNOSUPPRESSIVE—they impair cellular immunity.

central nervous system (CNS)   The part of the nervous system that controls intelligence and emotion. In human beings and other vertebrates it consists of the brain and the spinal cord and the protective membranes (meninges) surrounding them. See PERIPHERAL NERVOUS SYSTEM.

central nervous system lymphoma   See PRIMARY CENTRAL NERVOUS SYSTEM LYMPHOMA.

cerebrospinal fluid (CSF)   The fluid found within the cavities of the brain and surrounding both the brain and the spinal cord. A sample of this fluid is often removed from the body for diagnosis purposes by a lumbar puncture (SPINAL TAP). The fluid is analyzed for cancer cells or evidence of other disorders.

cerebrovascular accident (CVA)   A STROKE. A general term most commonly applied to cerebrovascular conditions that accompany either ischemic or hemorrhagic lesions. These conditions are usually secondary to atherosclerotic disease, hypertension, or a combination of both. Also called APOPLEXY or simply a "shock."

Centers for Disease Control and Prevention (CDC)   The federal public health agency serving as the center for preventing, tracking, controlling, and investigating the epidemiology of AIDS and other diseases. The agency performs epidemiological study and surveillance of disease, mortality and morbidity, and develops and conducts programs for disease prevention. The CDC AIDS CASE DEFINITION of AIDS can be understood as the legal definition of AIDS; it is the standard for reporting AIDS cases in the United States and for determination of eligibility for welfare and health benefits.

Center for Infectious Diseases (CID)   A constituent part of the CENTERS FOR DISEASE CONTROL AND PREVENTION (CDC).

cervical atypia   Abnormalities or irregularities in cervical cells.

cervical cancer   Malignant neoplasm (growth) in the CERVIX, or neck of the uterus. Cervical cancer may occur at any age from puberty on. The mortality rate increases with age. Risk factors include early age at first intercourse, multiple sexual partners, more than five pregnancies, and a history of SYPHILIS or GONORRHEA. Women whose mothers took DES while pregnant are also at risk. It is suspected that an oncogenic factor, most probably a virus, is transmitted sexually, and the HUMAN PAPILLOMA VIRUS is thought to be an important factor. COLPOSCOPY and regular PAP (Papanicolaou) tests after a woman becomes sexually active are two means of diagnosis.

Cervical cancer may be present for up to ten years before symptoms appear. The most common symptom, when the cancer is at a more advanced, invasive stage, is abnormal bleeding (which can be a symptom of other diseases as well).

Cervical cancer develops progressively in several stages through which it spreads throughout the cervix, the pelvic areas and other parts of the body. Treatment depends on the stage of the cancer, general state of health of the patient, and other factors. As with other cancers, radiation, surgery, and cytotoxic agents are used.

The best way to screen HIV-positive women for cervical cancer has long been a matter of debate. Medical reports through the years have documented that women with HIV have a greater risk of cervical cancer than noninfected women, and that it progresses more rapidly and tends to recur after treatment. The accuracy of the Pap smear, the standard method for detecting abnormalities that might develop into cervical cancer, has recently been called into question, particularly in the case of women with HIV. These women frequently have lower genital tract infections that may obscure test results. In colposcopy, a low-power microscope (colposcope) is used to examine the cervix, and if suspect tissue is observed, a biopsy is performed for further evaluation. Colposcopy has traditionally served only as a corroborative test in women with abnormal Pap smears, but in recent years some medical authorities have urged that cervical colposcopy be part of the routine management of HIV-positive women regardless of the findings of previous Pap smears.

Cervical cancer is now regarded as a totally preventable disease. AIDS activists and many health care providers believe that cervical cancer represents not an individual or a medical failure, but a system failure. They believe that all women should receive gynecological care as part of their routine primary care.

cervical cap   A contraceptive device for women that works like a small diaphragm over the CERVIX. It is held in place by suction.

cervical disease   Any disease of the cervix, particularly HUMAN PAPILLOMA VIRUS (HPV), a sexually transmitted virus certain strains of which are known to cause precancerous growths in the cervix (CERVICAL INTRAEPITHELIAL NEOPLASIA, or CIN). See also CERVICAL CANCER.

cervical dysplasia   An abnormality in the size, shape, or organization of the cells lining the cervix, which can be detected through a PAP SMEAR. If undetected, cervical dysplasia may progress to a more severe lesion; thus any abnormal finding should prompt further examination. See also CERVICAL INTRAEPITHELIAL NEOPLASIA and CERVICAL CANCER.

cervical intraepithelial lesion   Localized damage or abnormality, resulting from disease or trauma, in the tissue of the CERVIX. Such LESIONS can be benign (noncancerous) or malignant (cancerous).

cervical intraepithelial neoplasia (CIN)   DYSPLASIA of the basal layers of the squamous EPITHELIUM of the uterine CERVIX. It may progress to involve deeper layers of the epithelium. It is classified to severity; grades 1, 2 and 3 represent progressive stages of pathology. Grade 3 (CIN 3) represents CARCINOMA in situ, i.e. stage 0 of cancer of the cervix (see CERVICAL CANCER). CIN is generally revealed by PAP SMEAR or COLPOSCOPY.

Although there are few well-controlled studies, evidence suggests that HIV-infected women are at high risk of cervical dysplasia, particularly in advanced stages of disease (with low CD4 CELL COUNTS) or when there is coexistent infection with HUMAN PAPILLOMA VIRUS (HPV). At least one study suggests that Pap smears in HIV-infected women may not be as sensitive as those in HIV-negative women. Colposcopy is advised if a Pap smear shows any cellular atypia (including persistent inflammation). Invasive cervical carcinoma is now considered an AIDS-DEFINING DISEASE in the presence of HIV infection. There is evidence that HIV-infected women have a higher incidence of cervical neoplasia, and present at a more advanced stage of disease.

cervical secretion   HIV was first detected in the cervical secretions of HIV-infected women in 1986. Scientists reported that the virus might be cultured from secretions throughout the menstrual cycle, an indication that the presence of virus was not solely the result of contamination with menstrual blood. The probable source of HIV in cervical secretions is infected cervical tissue. The cells most often infected were MONOCYTE/MACROPHAGES and ENDOTHELIAL cells. In male-to-female TRANSMISSION of HIV, contact with infected semen could lead to local infection of susceptible cervical cells. Replication of the virus in those cells might precede systemic infection with HIV. Female-to-male transmission probably results from the sloughing of infected cervical cells into cervical and vaginal fluids. HIV infection of the uterine CERVIX might also explain some cases of viral transmission from mother to newborn.

cervical squamous cell abnormalities   See SQUAMOUS CELL CARCINOMA.

cervicitis   Inflammation of the CERVIX. Cervicitis may be asymptomatic and is generally diagnosed by inspection. Symptoms, when present, include vaginal discharge that increases just after menstruation, intermenstrual bleeding, postcoital bleeding, a burning sensation during urination, and low back pain. The cervix appears red and friable on examination. It often bleeds when touched with a cotton applicator or cervical spatula. A purulent exudate is often observed. CERVICAL CANCER can also give this appearance. Most infectious cervicitis is due to sexually transmitted infection, often CHLAMYDIA, GONORRHEA, or TRICHOMONAS. In HIV-positive women, viral infections may be isolated from cervical secretions and may cause local infections including CYTOMEGALOVIRUS, HERPES SIMPLEX virus, and even HIV itself. All vaginal infections should be treated and followed up.

cervix   The lower end of the uterus which protrudes into the vagina. Various contraceptive devices, such as the cervical cap and the diaphragm, do their job by blocking off this cervical opening and thus preventing the egg-hunting sperm from entering the uterus. Also called *cervix uteri*.

cesarean section   The removal of a fetus by means of an incision into the uterus, usually by way of the abdominal wall. It may be performed by an extraperitoneal or intraperitoneal abdominal route. Indications for cesarean section include an abnormally large fetus (too large to be delivered through the pelvic outlet), an abnormally small pelvis, or a combination of these factors. A breech presentation of the fetus may also be an indication that a cesarean section is needed.

chancre   A primary sore or lesion at the site of entry of the bacteria that causes SYPHILIS.

chancroid   An ulcerative lesion caused by *Haemophilus ducreyi*. Chancroids usually begin with a sensitive and inflamed pustule or ulcer with multiple, abrupt edges, a rough floor, and yellow exudate, purulent secretion. The incubation period is approximately three to five days. Chancroids may affect the penis, urethra, vulva, or anus. Multiple lesions may develop by autoinoculation. Types include transient, phagedenic, giant, and serpiginous. Chancroids usually present as painful ulcers accompanied by tenderness and inguinal lymphadenopathy. Women with cervical chancroid tend to have multiple ulcers, with an average of four. Diagnosis based only on history and physical exam is often inaccurate. Culture for *H. ducreyi* is warranted for both diagnosis and reporting purposes. SYPHILIS, HERPES SIMPLEX, and HIV coinfection should also be considered in the differential diagnosis.

Chancroid lesions have been identified as a major risk factor for heterosexual spread of HIV through ulceration. Genital ulcers are thought to act as portals of entry for the virus from male genital secretions. Women may be unaware of the presence of ulcers.

ERYTHROMYCIN or CEFTRIAXONE usually satisfactorily treat chancroid. Treatment failure is more common in HIV-infected patients, especially single-dose treatment. As the susceptibility of *H. ducreyi* varies by geography, response should be monitored clinically and by susceptibility patterns.

charbon   Infection with *Bacillus anthracis*. See ANTHRAX

charity care coordinator   A financial counselor.

chastity   The state or quality of being chaste, or abstention from sexual intercourse or sexual relations. In a more general sense, chastity also refers to moral purity.

chemokine   One of a class of proteins found in the blood that is known to direct LYMPHOCYTES to the cite of an infection or inflammation.

In late 1995, a group of researchers led by Drs. Paulo Lusso and Robert Gallo (one of two that separately claimed to have identified CAF [cell antiviral factor]), argued that CAF was not one but three substances acting in concert to keep the virus in check. Dr. Gallo's team took a CD8 CELL LINE that was particularly effective at suppressing HIV, removed the actual cells, and separated the remaining substances in the culture. They found three proteins that had potent anti-HIV activity at nontoxic levels in cell culture. These proteins belonged to the chemokine family. The researchers then added antibodies that deactivate the individual chemokines to see which chemokine was primarily responsible for the CAF activity. The antibody of only one seemed to reverse the suppressive effect, and only partially. Yet when antibodies to all three chemokines were added, all of the anti-HIV activity was eliminated. The same result was observed when the antibodies were added to cell cultures taken from HIV-infected people; the researchers concluded that all three of the chemokines are required to keep the virus under control. Further research is being done to determine which aspect of the viral life cycle is disturbed by the chemokines and whether there may be some way to trigger the local secretion of chemokines. The hope is to develop altered forms of chemokines that suppress HIV but do not have the potential side effects of the natural forms.

The systemic administration of chemokines, however, poses certain problems. Since the known function of chemokines is to direct white blood cells to the site of infection, systemic administration might cause immune cells to wander aimlessly, confused by conflicting signals and not certain to respond when secondary infections occur.

chemotaxis The movement of additional white blood cells to an area of inflammation in response to the release of chemical mediators by NEUTROPHILs, MONOCYTEs, and injured tissue. For instance, the movement of LEUKOCYTEs toward the chemicals produced by an immune reaction.

chemotherapy The use of chemical agents in the treatment or control of disease, generally malignancies. Used colloquially most often to refer to the treatment of cancer with anticancer drugs, highly toxic medications that destroy cancer cells by interfering with their growth or preventing their reproduction. Generally, the smaller the tumor the more effective the chemotherapy is. The larger the tumor, the greater the number of cancer cells and the greater the possibility that some of the cells will become resistant. Chemotherapy may also be used to prolong life when a cure is improbable and to provide palliation (relieve symptoms).

There are a number of types of chemotherapy drugs, including alkylating agents, antimetabolites, anticancer antibiotics, plant alkaloids, hormones, and others. To be as effective as possible, different types of chemotherapy drugs are frequently used together (COMBINATION CHEMOTHERAPY). In that way, as many cell phases as possible will be vulnerable at the same time. In addition, chemotherapy can be used alone or along with other treatments such as radiation therapy, surgery, and/or biological therapy. When chemotherapy is used along with other treatments, it may be given before surgery to reduce the size of the tumor so that the surgery can be more effective. Chemotherapy may also be given after the primary treatment, as adjuvant therapy, to destroy any remaining cancer cells. The type of chemotherapy given a patient, and the dose, is determined by a number of factors, including the kind of cancer, the stage it has reached, the objective of the treatment, and the medical condition of the patient. Chemotherapy has many side effects, ranging from unpleasant to life-threatening, depending upon, among other things, the degree of toxicity of the particular drug. Nausea, vomiting, diarrhea, and constipation are common.

Chemotherapy can treat cancer throughout the body, systemically. Administration may be oral, by IV, by injection (into a vein, the membrane lining the abdomen, a muscle, an artery, a body cavity, or the spinal fluid), or by topical application. Chemotherapy may be given on any schedule that has proved to be effective.

child and family services Social services provided to children and their parents, such as counseling, home chore aid, child rearing, housekeeping training, and abuse treatment. Child and family services may be provided to welfare recipients and may also be provided to other modest-income families, by government agencies or private charitable or social service organizations.

childbearing age The period of a woman's life between puberty and menopause during which she is capable of bearing a child.

children and HIV/AIDS HIV is predicted to become a major cause of death among children by the end of the century, yet the pandemic is still perceived as largely an adult issue. When the initial impact of HIV becomes apparent in a particular region, the effects on children may not be immediately obvious. Sick adults are noticed first, and infected adults may be identified through testing and screening programs. In contrast, infants infected with HIV die early, usually without being diagnosed. When parents have AIDS the effect on their children is cumulative and not easy to see at first. These children may receive less nutrition and have to leave school, assume adult responsibilities, face the trauma of the death of their parent (s), and carry the stigma of being labeled AIDS ORPHANs. Children who lose their parents and grow up outside a family environment are more likely to become sexually active early, to get sexually transmitted infections, and to become infected with HIV.

chimpanzee Because of their genetic similarity to humans, chimpanzees have often been used in HIV and other medical research (chimps are the only other primates that can be infected with HIV-1, although it does not make them ill). However, because of habitat destruction in their native Africa, theirs is an endangered species. Decreased numbers and high cost have limited their use in recent years.

Chinese herbs Herbs used routinely in therapy, including treatment of HIV, by practitioners of traditional CHINESE MEDICINE. Some commonly used natural herbal products—ASTRAGALUS *mongholicus, Acanthopanax senticosus* and *Eleutheroccocus senticosus, Panax notoginseng,* aconitum, *Artemisiae annua, Tripterigium wilfordii,* and *Echinacea purpurea*—are clearly active immunologically, and can modulate, potentiate or suppress immune response. It is important to note that the immunological effects may not be due to the purified versions or extracts of the herbs, but to their entire compositions, possibly including unknown and unrecognized substances. Many researchers and clinicians observe that Chinese medicine can hope to function in full partnership with Western medicine only if it heeds the most recent discoveries in immunology. To date, critical analyses of the use of Chinese herbs for HIV are lacking, and the jury is still out on the use of Chinese therapeutics for HIV.

Chinese medicine The practice of the Chinese system of medicine dates back more than two thousand years, making it the oldest medical tradition in the world. Chinese medicine combines empirical experience with a philosophical theory.

Unlike Western medicine, which is derived solely from scientific methods of observation and investigation of physical disease, Chinese practice is founded on a holistic view of the mind-body's innate ability to maintain health and to heal itself should illness occur. This view sees the universe as a living organism, and the human body as a microcosm of that larger organism. In contrast, Western medicine tends to view the human body mechanistically and has evolved its practice based on the assumption that the body is a machine with essentially separate but linked components. Rather than dealing only with discrete components of the human organism, the Chinese approach is one of "aligning" the functions of the organs and internal systems as a whole, promoting the dynamic balance of energy polarities crucial to good health and well-being. Much Western research on certain aspects of Chinese medicine, particularly on the properties of traditional herbs, has been conducted in recent years, but so far it has not led to the development of any useful therapies for HIV/AIDS.

chiropractic   The chiropractic system of physical therapy is based on the premise that the spine, literally the backbone of the body, is also the "backbone" of health: subluxation (misalignment) of the vertebrae caused by poor posture or trauma or pressure on the spinal nerve roots, which may lead to diminished function and illness. The chiropractor seeks to analyze and correct these misalignments through spinal manipulation or adjustment.

Though chiropractic has its roots in nineteenth-century pseudoscientific theories, it has proved of same use for those with ailments specifically related to muscle tension, pinched nerves, and so forth.

chlamydia   A sexually transmitted bacterial infection that is now the most common STD among heterosexuals in the United States. It causes infection in the cervix and often spreads to the pelvic organs. Often asymptomatic in women, it can cause great damage to pelvic structures, resulting in PELVIC INFLAMMATORY DISEASE, tubo-ovarian abscesses, and tubal infertility. It can be transmitted perinatally and is a frequent cause of conjunctivitis and pneumonia in newborns.

chlamydial infection   See CHLAMYDIA.

chloral hydrate   Chloral hydrate is a sedative used to treat insomnia. It is usually taken fifteen to thirty minutes before bedtime. Using chloral hydrate regularly for more than two weeks often reduces its effectiveness. Major side effects include stomach irritation, residual sedation, and hangover. Chloral hydrate should be used with great caution by people who are depressed, who are suicidal, or who have a history of drug abuse.

chloramphenicol   A broad-spectrum antibiotic used to treat a number of bacterial infections, including salmonella, meningitis caused by *Haemophilus* influenza, rickets, and cholera. Chloramphenicol prevents multiplication of susceptible bacteria by preventing them from making strong cell walls and essential proteins. There are significant toxicities with chloramphenicol, so it should only be used when necessary, for serious infections caused by organisms that are resistant to other antibiotics or when other antibiotics are not tolerated.

In HIV-infected people, chloramphenicol is most frequently used to treat salmonella infections that cause severe diarrhea. Salmonella is more common in people with AIDS than in the general population. In people with healthy immune systems the infection is rarely treated, but symptoms tend to be much more severe in immunocompromised people and require intervention. Chloramphenicol is available in tablet, ointment and injectable form. Although rare, the most serious side effect of chloramphenicol is BONE MARROW SUPPRESSION. (Trade names Chloromyecitin and Elase-Chloromycetin.)

Chloromycetin   See CHLORAMPHENICOL.

chlorpheniramine   An antihistamine used to treat allergic reactions such as hay fever, hives and inflammation of the eye, among others. It is also taken to prevent or treat allergic reactions to blood transfusions or compounds taken to enhance X-ray images. Occasionally it is used as a supplementary therapy to EPINEPHRINE for the treatment of ANAPHYLACTIC SHOCK. In people with HIV, the drug is used to reduce certain drug-induced allergic side effects, including skin rashes, redness, swelling, hives, and breathing difficulties. The drug is available in a wide variety of formulations, including capsules, tablets, syrup, and oral suspension. Drowsiness is the most common side effect. (Trade names Alermine, Aller-Chlor, Chlor-Trimeton, Comtrex, Histex, and Teldrin.)

cholera   A severe contagious infection of the small intestine characterized by profuse watery diarrhea and dehydration, caused by *Vibrio cholerae* bacteria, and commonly transmitted through contaminated drinking water.

chronic   A term denoting symptoms and diseases that last for an extended period of time without noticeable change. Distinguished from acute.

chronic fatigue syndrome   A viral disease of the immune system, usually characterized by debilitating fatigue and flu-like symptoms.

chronically infected cells   HIV cells that carry the blueprints of the virus in them and therefore continually make new HIV.

CID   See CENTER FOR INFECTIOUS DISEASES.

cidofovir   A NUCLEOSIDE ANALOG that has recently been approved as a treatment for CYTOMEGALOVIRUS (CMV) infection. Studies have indicated that cidofovir is effective in the treatment of CMV retinitis and that its toxicities may be alleviated. Cidofovir's primary advantage over the other approved medications (GANCICLOVIR and FOSCARNET) is that it need be infused into patients only on a weekly or biweekly basis, compared to once or twice daily for the others. This dosing schedule also removes the need for an indwelling catheter. Cidofovir is now on a par with the two older drugs and may be administered either as initial treatment or as a salvage therapy.

Like those drugs, cidofovir is toxic. Like foscarnet, it can cause irreparable, life-threatening kidney damage. Usage guidelines now clearly state that cidofovir should not be used together with other drugs that are toxic to the kidneys or in patients with impaired kidney function. Laboratory tests for kidney malfunction must be undertaken both before and 48 hours after starting cidofovir. In addition, users of other kidney-toxic drugs, such as foscarnet, must terminate them at least a week before starting cidofovir. Also, the guidelines mandate strict adherence to the schedule for administering probenecid and intravenous hydration on the day of the cidofovir infusion.

Activists feel that the clarity of the new guidelines is perhaps overdue. Studies have shown that the drug can be safely and effectively used, but the close monitoring that participants in drug trials receive is rare in general medical practice. When cidofovir was being considered for approval by the Food and Drug Administration, many activists were concerned that in the real world, patients would not be followed rigorously enough, resulting in adverse event rates not seen in the cidofovir trials.

A few years ago, cidofovir appeared too dangerous to be useful as a systemic therapy, but researchers learned that the toxicity could be attenuated with hydration therapy and four grams of probenecid on the day of the infusion. Even with probenecid and hydration, the drug at standard dose should not be administered to patients with proteinuria or elevated serum CREATININE levels, both ·ndications of kidney impairment. Additionally, probenecid produces its own side effects, including transient fevers, nausea, and rashes. To date, studies are lacking that directly compare cidofovir to ganciclovir or foscarnet. Unless intravenous cidofovir is shown to be superior to other CMV therapies, or until there is more clinical experience with the drug, most clinicians will use it only as a second or third choice, when other approaches fail.

cimetidine   A drug that blocks the action of HISTAMINE (H-2), a substance secreted by MAST CELLS, and thus inhibits the ability of the stomach to make acid. Once acid production is decreased, the body is able to heal itself. Benefits include control of hypersecretory stomach disorders and effective treatment of peptic ulcer disease, reflux esophagatis, and heartburn. The drug has been shown to have some stimulating effects on the immune system and has been proposed as a treatment for the immune suppression associated with HIV. Trade name is Tagamet.

cipro   See CIPROFLOXACIN.

ciprofloxacin (Cipro)   An oral antibiotic approved for the treatment of many common bacterial infections. It is sometimes administered to treat MAC in combination with other drugs. Possible side effects include gastrointestinal upset, seizures, and rash. Concomitant administration of antacids like Mylanta or Amphogel that contain aluminum or magnesium hydroxide can lead to the formation of insoluble chelates (heterocyclic chemical compounds) that prevent the drug's absorption, reducing its level in the blood. Sucralfate, a stomach ulcer remedy, has a similar effect and should not be taken with ciprofloxacin. Ciprofloxacin, in contrast, can increase the absorption and blood levels of theophylline, an asthma remedy.

circulating immune complexes   Circulating immune complexes are formed in the blood when antigens are present in excess amounts. The host produces antibodies against these, forming antigen-antibody complexes. These can mask the surface of a tumor cell and, for example, prevent LYMPHOCYTES from reacting. Immune complexes can cause diseases, such as nephritis and kidney failure.

circumcision   The surgical removal of the end of the prepuce, or foreskin, of the penis. Circumcision is a social or religious custom, usually performed on newborn babies at the request of the parents. It has been suggested that there is a relationship between absence of circumcision and HIV.

Studies seem to support such an association but must be interpreted cautiously because evidence may be unavoidably confounded with other factors.

Since the late 1800s, it has repeatedly been found that men with SEXUALLY TRANSMITTED DISEASES (STDS) are more likely to be uncircumcised than are men without STDs. Modern investigators have reported that uncircumcised men were more likely than circumcised men to be infected with gonorrhea or syphilis, less likely to have genital warts and equally likely to have herpes virus infection. Recently several investigators have reported that uncircumcised men may be more susceptible to HIV infection than are circumcised men. Some researchers believe the evidence may be strong enough to warrant considering circumcision for HIV prevention. Published articles and abstracts are few, however, and conclusions are not certain.

civil liberties   Fundamental rights of citizens, such as freedom of speech, often guaranteed by law. Also the freedom of individuals to exercise such rights without state interference.

Some of the responses to the AIDS epidemic have included proposals for drastic legal curtailments of individual rights and liberties, purportedly to stop the spread of the disease. Even without such legal action, people with AIDS or HIV have been discriminated against in employment, housing, public accommodations, government services, and other areas. Despite these deplorable actions, which have largely been based on ignorance and fear, there are serious questions about appropriate public response to AIDS, with implications for civil liberties. Why shouldn't employers be allowed to fire people who have AIDS or who test positive for the AIDS virus? If people who carry the virus can infect others through sexual contact, why shouldn't the government require citizens to be tested? Why shouldn't the government have the name of everyone who carries the AIDS virus? Blood tests to detect sexually transmitted diseases have been required as a prerequisite for a marriage license; why is testing for AIDS different? What should be done about a person known to be infected who refuses to refrain from activities that could transmit the virus? Isn't education about AIDS offensive and, for many, obscene?

Civil Rights Act of 1964   The most comprehensive civil rights legislation in the history of the United States. The Civil Rights Act of 1964 mandates equality for all persons in access to public accommodations and facilities, education, and employment, as well as federally assisted public programs of all kinds. Title VII of the act is regarded as the most all-inclusive source of employment rights. All employers who have at least fifteen employees, including state and local governments and labor unions, are subject to its provisions, but it does not apply to the federal government, Indian tribes, certain agencies in the District of Columbia, private clubs, and religious organizations. Its principles have been extended to federal employment, however, by executive order.

Civil Rights Act of 1968   This act proscribes discrimination in the sale, rental and financing arrangements of most housing. It applies to agents and brokers as well as to owners of properties.

Civil Rights Act of 1991   This law amends the CIVIL RIGHTS ACT OF 1964 to provide greater protection against employment discrimination. The act repudiates recent U.S. Supreme Court decisions limiting civil rights; grants women and disabled persons the right to recover money damages under Title VII of the Civil Rights Act of 1964; and grants congressional employees the protection of Title VII. The 1991 act was a direct outgrowth of the failed Civil Rights bill of 1990, which President Bush had vetoed. The section of the act that raised the greatest concern dealt with money damages for victims of intentional discrimination or harassment based on sex, religion, national origin, or disability. Unlike claims of racial discrimination, claims of these types of Title VII discrimination could result in awards of back pay and reinstatement on a job.

clap   See GONORRHEA.

clarithromycin   An anti-infective macrolide used in the treatment of certain upper respiratory tract infections, some lower respiratory tract infections, certain skin and skin structure infections and MYCOBACTERIUM AVIUM COMPLEX (MAC) infections, and in the prevention of disseminated *Mycobacterium avium* complex in advanced HIV. Other generally accepted uses include combination antibiotic treatment of duodenal ulcer disease caused by *H. pylori*. Clarithromycin can also have a role in combination therapy of some TOXOPLASMOSIS infections. It works by preventing the growth and multiplication of susceptible organisms by interfering with their formation of essential proteins. Possible risks include mild gastrointestinal symptoms, drug-induced colitis (rare), and superinfections (rare). Brand name is Biaxin.

client   An individual who has retained or consented to treatment or receipt of services from a professional. In general, the term "*client*" is used by those educated in social services, where *patient* is used by professionals educated in the medical sciences.

client advocacy   See CASE ADVOCACY.

client-centered therapy   A method of psychotherapy or counseling pioneered by the American psychologist Carl Rogers in which the therapist refrains from advising, suggesting, or persuading but tries instead to establish empathy with the client by clarifying and reflecting back the client's expressed feelings; the therapist tries to convey an attitude of "unconditional positive regard" in the context of a permissive, nonthreatening relationship; hence this method of psychotherapy is also called NONDIRECTIVE COUNSELING or therapy.

client oriented   Directed toward the client's or patient's needs and interests; used of medical and social services.

climax   See ORGASM.

clindamycin   An antibiotic effective against anaerobic pathogens, microbes that can grow without the presence of free oxygen. In HIV therapy, clindamycin is used primarily in combination with the antimalarial drug primaquine to treat mild-to-moderate PCP in people who have failed with or cannot tolerate TRIMETHOPRIM-SULFAMETHOXAZOLE (TMP-SMX). People with mild cases of PCP often take the oral from of clindamycin immediately. People with moderate cases of the disease sometimes initially receive clindamycin intravenously and then switch to the oral drug. Clindamycin has also proved effective in treating ENCEPHALITIS caused by the protozoal pathogen *Toxoplasma gondii*. Clindamycin has also been used effectively in combination with SULFADIAZINE and PYRIMETHAMINE to treat TOXOPLASMOSIS. For PELVIC INFLAMMATORY DISEASE, intravenous clindamycin can be combined with intravenous or intramuscular injections of gentamicin to treat acute infection, followed by GENTAMICIN as maintenance therapy to prevent recurrence.

The most common side effect of clindamycin is diarrhea, caused by the growth of a bacterium called CLOSTRIDIUM DIFFICILE. *Clostridium* infection can lead to a condition called pseudomembranous colitis, characterized by abdominal pain, blood diarrhea, fever and dehydration. *Clostridium* requires direct treatment with oral vancomycin or Flagyl. Use of any agent that just slows intestinal motility may prolong or worsen pseudomembranous colitis by delaying elimination of the toxin made by the bacteria. Furthermore, use of antidiarrheal agents that contain kaolin or attapulgite (Kaopectate) may decrease the absorption of clindamycin, leading to subtherapeutic effects. ERYTHROMYCIN also interacts with clindamycin, by interfering with its mechanism of action against bacteria.

The most significant side effect associated with the use of clindamycin is severe COLITIS, which is a potentially fatal superinfection caused by *Clostridia*. Severe and persistent diarrhea (occasionally bloody) and severe abdominal cramps are the first signs of colitis.

clinic   A facility or part of a facility used for the diagnosis and treatment of medical outpatients. Depending on context, "clinic" may include physicians' offices, facilities that serve poor or public patients, or facilities in which graduate or undergraduate medical education is provided. More broadly, clinics may also include complete inpatient and outpatient facilities and resources. Here, the term describes a group practice of specialty and general health care practitioners who have banded together to share resources and increase the marketability of their services.

clinical   Directly observable; diagnosable by observation.

clinical endpoint   The measure of clinical improvement in a DRUG TRIAL.

This subject has been at the center of an ongoing debate about testing and approving new drugs for deadly diseases, particularly AIDS. At issue are the speed with which drugs are evaluated and approved for use, and the criteria for drug efficacy and effectiveness. Traditionally, the Food and Drug Administration (FDA) has evaluated experimental drugs, not by improvements in the patients who receive them, but by the occurrence of OPPORTUNISTIC INFECTIONS (OIs) or death in those who do not. Because the FDA will not approve a drug based solely on SURROGATE MARKERS, such as reduction in P24 antigen or a rise in T-cell count, because it wants statistical proof that a drug is helping people, and because the FDA has traditionally insisted on the slowest measure of clinical improvement—clinical endpoints—trials often take a long time. Activists and researchers as well as scientists have long questioned whether the best way to prove a drug is to wait for deaths and OIs in those who do not receive it. They do not see why a potentially useful drug should be withheld for months or years pending conclusive proof of benefit, after it is already clear that it does show substantial clinical benefit. And many fear that a return to survival as the sole endpoint in studies would also require a return to the routine use of placebo controls, a guarantee of death for the untreated.

clinical trial   A carefully planned scientific study done to test an experimental medicine in human beings to see if it is safe and effective. Some trials seek to evaluate safety (phase 1), others test effectiveness and short-term safety (phase 2), and others test safety, effectiveness, and dosage level (phase 3). Phase 1, 2, and 3 clinical trials differ in terms of number of patients, length, and method.

At hospitals across the country, the National Institute of Allergy and Infectious Diseases (NIAID), the research arm of the United States PUBLIC HEALTH SERVICE, has set up a group of research centers called AIDS CLINICAL TRIALS UNITS (ACTUs), where these tests take place. These ACTUs together make up the AIDS CLINICAL TRIALS GROUP (ACTG). In addition, doctors who are part of NIAID's COMMUNITY PROGRAMS FOR CLINICAL RESEARCH ON AIDS conduct studies of AIDS drugs at hospitals and clinics in the communities where the impact of the AIDS epidemic is severe. Clinical trials are also sponsored by drug companies, other government agencies, and private research organizations.

clitoris   A small, complex organ located where the inside lips of the vagina meet. It becomes erect, or blood-filled, during sexual excitement. Slang terms include clit, little man in the boat, and jewel in the lotus.

clofazimine   An antileprosy agent sometimes administered in combination with other drugs to treat MAC. It can

decrease the rate of RIFAMPIN absorption and thus reduce its effects. In addition, it lowers dilantin levels, which has led to breakthrough seizures. Possible side effects include gastrointestinal upset, skin discoloration, and rashes. (Trade name Lamprene.)

clonal anergy   The downregulation of the immune response by lack of proliferation of effector and memory LYMPHOCYTES.

clonal deletion   Physical deletion of immune cells such as LYMPHOCYTES from the peripheral repertoire. Also known as *programmed cell death* or APOPTOSIS.

clonal selection   The fundamental basis of LYMPHOCYTE activation, in which an antigen selectively stimulates only those cells to divide and differentiate which express receptors for it.

clonazepam   An antiseizure drug that is used alone or in combination therapy to prevent and treat epileptic seizures. Clonazepam belongs to a class of psychoactive drugs known as benzodiazepines. In general, these drugs are used to treat anxiety and insomnia, but clonazepam is used almost exclusively as an anticonvulsant in people who have not responded to standard therapy. Many develop a tolerance for clonazepam, and the drug often loses it effectiveness after a few months of therapy. To counter the effect, the drug's dosage may be increased or therapy switched to a different anticonvulsant. Seizures may be caused by any of the CENTRAL NERVOUS SYSTEM disorders or infections associated with HIV infection. Toxoplasmosis is the most common cause of seizures in people with AIDS. Clonazepam treats the symptoms of the neurological disorders, not the underlying causes. When seizures are being caused by an opportunistic infection of the central nervous system, therapy should also include appropriate antibiotic, antifungal, or antiparasitic treatment. Clonazepam is available in tablet form for oral administration. The most common side effects are drowsiness, dizziness, unsteadiness, increased salivation, and altered behavior.

clone   A cell, cell product, or organism that is genetically identical to the unit or individual from which it was asexually derived. Colloquially, by extension, a person or thing that duplicates, imitates, or closely resembles another in appearance.

cloning   The process of producing a clone.

Clostridium difficile   A microbe that is a relatively common, and particularly severe, cause of diarrhea in people who take antibiotics. Almost any antibiotic can cause this complication, but the ones that do so most frequently are AMPICILLIN, AMOXICILLIN, CLINDAMYCIN, and a group of drugs called cephalosporins that includes cefixime, cefuroxime, cephalexin and cefaclor. People who develop diarrhea while taking these or any other antibiotics should stop taking them and call their physicians. A test of stool will determine if Clostridium difficile is the cause. If it is, it can be treated with METRONIDAZOLE or vancomycin hydrochloride.

clot   See BLOOD CLOT; COAGULATION.

clotrimazole   An antifungal drug used primarily during HIV infection as a topical agent for oral and vaginal CANDIDI-ASIS. (Trade names Gyne-Lotrimin Letrimin and Mycelex.)

clotting   See BLOOD CLOT; COAGULATION.

clotting factor   A substance in the blood consisting of proteins essential to COAGULATION. Absence of these proteins may lead to prolonged, uncontrollable bleeding, as in HEMO-PHILIA.

clotting factor products   See COAGULATION FACTORS.

cluster of differentiation (CD)   One or more cell surface molecules, detectable by MONOCLONAL antibodies, that define a particular cell line or state of cellular differentiation.

CMI   See CELLULAR IMMUNITY.

CMV   See CYTOMEGALOVIRUS.

CMV colitis   See CYTOMEGALOVIRUS COLITIS.

CMV esophagitis   See CYTOMEGALOVIRUS ESOPHAGITIS.

CMV gastritis   See CYTOMEGALOVIRUS GASTRITIS.

CMV nureolotical disease   See CYTOMEGALOVIRUS NEUR-OLOGICAL DISEASE.

CMV pneumonia   See CYTOMEGALOVIRUS PNEUMONIA.

CMV polyradiculopathy   See CYTOMEGALOVIRUS POLYRADICULOPATHY.

CMV retinis   See CYTOMEGALOVIRUS RETINIS.

CNS   See CENTRAL NERVOUS SYSTEM.

CNS lymphoma   See PRIMARY CENTRAL NERVOUS SYSTEM LYMPHOMA.

coagulation   The process by which a liquid becomes a viscous or solid mass; clotting. Normal blood contains chemical compounds, called COAGULATION FACTORs, whose sequential interactions comprise the process of blood clotting. Those with HEMOPHILIA lack these factors. The blood's ability to clot may be impaired by infection.

coagulation factor   Any of the chemical compounds in the blood which interact to create the coagulation process, or blood clotting. Factors are designated by Roman numerals and names. They include Factor I, fibrinogen; Factor II, prothrombin; Factor III, tissue factor; Factor IV, calcium ions; Factor V, proaccelerin, an unstable protein substance; Factor VII, proconvertin or serum prothrombin conversion accelerator; Factor VIII, antihemophilic factor; Factor IX, Christmas factor; Factor X, Stuart-Prower factor; Factor XI, plasma thromboplastin antecedent; Factor XII, Hageman or glass factor; Factor XIII, fibrin stabilizing factor. Other factors include prekallikrein, also called Fletcher factor; high molecular weight kininogen, also called Fitzgerald, Falujenc, or William factor, or contact activation cofactor.

When HEMORRHAGE occurs in patients with HEMOPHILIA A, coagulation factor IX is given. Factor VIII is given when hemorrhage occurs in patients with hemophilia B. These factors are available from various sources and special care has been taken to be as sure as possible that they are free of HIV and hepatitis viruses. Many hemophiliacs learn to self-administer these factors to control bleeding episodes.

coalition building   See ACTIVISM.

coalition politics   See ACTIVISM.

cocaine   A bitter white crystalline alkaloid obtained from coca leaves, used medically as a local anesthetic. It is also widely used illicitly for its stimulant and euphoric properties.

coccidioidomycosis   A respiratory infection, often accompanied by a skin rash, caused by inhaling spores of coccidioides fungi, common in semiarid regions. Also called *desert fever*.

coccidiosis   An intestinal infection mainly of birds and domestic animals, caused by *Isospora belli,* a parasite protozoan of the order Coccidia. Occasionally this parasite causes infection in the small intestine and colon in humans. It is generally asymptomatic. When symptoms appear, they may manifest in severe, watery mucous diarrhea.

cock ring   A device placed around the base of the PENIS and TESTICLES that aids men in getting and maintaining an ERECTION, thus prolonging sex.

code   In a hospital or medical setting, a coded message used to transmit information, usually about a medical emergency, especially when broadcast over a public address system. "Code blue," for instance, alerts an emergency care team to a particular type of emergency, generally cardiac arrest.

coenzyme Q10   First isolated in cow heart cells, coenzyme Q10 (Co-Q10) is a substance that assists in the oxidation of nutrients within cells to create energy. It is also highly efficient at protecting internal and external cell membranes against oxidation and is sometimes proposed as a complementary therapy to combat AIDS-related conditions. Co-Q10 is found in mammalian tissue, with the highest concentrations in the heart, liver, kidney, and muscle. Co-Q10 levels are abnormally low in people with congestive heart failure and in populations with HIV, muscular dystrophy, periodontal disease, immune dysfunction, and immunosuppression caused by the cancer chemotherapy DOXORUBICIN. To date, no toxicities have been reported from Co-Q10 use.

cofactor   A factor other than the basic causative agent of a disease that activates or furthers the action of a disease-causing agent, thereby increasing the likelihood of developing that disease. Cofactors may also increase the progression of a particular disease. Cofactors may include the presence of other microbes, proteins, hormones, genes, genetic predispositions, psychosocial factors such as stress, or environmental issues. With HIV infection, cofactors are only suspected but may include other viruses (like CYTOMEGALOVIRUS), age, genetic resistance or predisposition and certain hormone-like substances called CYTOKINES, released by LYMPHOCYTES.

cognitive function See AIDS DEMENTIA COMPLEX; ENCEPHALITIS.

cohort In medical research, a group of individuals sharing a demographic or clinical characteristic that is the subject of a study of the EPIDEMIOLOGY or natural course of a disease.

cohort studies Studies that follow groups of similar individuals over time, noting who develops a disease and who does not, and comparing the groups at the end of the study to determine COFACTORS and other elements that may influence outcome. Cohort studies of gay men in San Francisco have determined that behavior modification can influence incidence of HIV infection and reduce the number of new cases.

coil An INTRAUTERINE DEVICE (IUD), a type of contraceptive device considered an effective form of birth control.

coinfection The condition of an organism or individual cell infected by two pathological microorganisms simultaneously. It has not yet been determined whether an additional "super infection" (or "reinfection") with a second strain of HIV occurs at a period of time after initial infection.

coinsurance Under MEDICARE and most health insurance plans, the percentage of allowable charges for a given class of medical care that the patient must pay.

coitus SEXUAL INTERCOURSE. The term is often used with a modifier to distinguish type (e.g., anal coitus, interfemoral [between the thighs] coitus). Slang terms include ball, FUCK, or hump.

coke See COCAINE.

colitis Inflammation of the COLON, the lower part of the large intestine. It is a chronic condition that causes abdominal pain, diarrhea, and other symptoms.
Colitis caused by CYTOMEGALOVIRUS is a common development in HIV-infected patients. Cytomegalovirus infects the colon in slightly more patients than it does the esophagus. While there is no typical pattern of CMV-caused gastrointestinal disease, it is often associated with intermittent or persistent diarrhea with cramping, lower abdominal pain, involuntary rectal spasms, and weight loss. The stool may be watery, semi-formed or formed, and may be accompanied by bleeding. In some patients, diarrhea can be quite severe, with up to twenty bowel movements each day, resulting in severe loss of fluid and electrolytes from the body; other patients may have no discernible diarrhea at all. Fevers are common in patients with CMV colitis.
The diagnostic procedure of choice for colitis is COLONOSCOPY, in which an ENDOSCOPE is inserted into the colon through the rectum for a visual examination. A

colonoscopy is performed only after the stool has been examined several times for evidence of other pathogens that may be responsible for the symptoms. The colons of patients with colitis appear diffusely inflamed and bleed easily on contact with the endoscope. A BIOPSY is necessary to rule out possible causes.

colon The part of the large intestine between the cecum and the rectum. The colon and the small intestine are commonly the sites of infections that cause diarrhea. To diagnose problems in the colon, common procedures are COLONOSCOPY and SIGMOIDOSCOPY. These procedures permit observation and BIOPSY of the colon by passing a tube through the rectum.

colonization The presence of a microorganism in or on a host without associated disease.

colony-stimulating factor (CSF-1) A protein present in human serum that promotes MONOCYTE differentiation. G-CSF and GM-CSF have similar efficacy, but G-CSF is significantly better tolerated, according to a study that compared the two colony-stimulating factors as acute salvage therapy in advanced HIV-infected individuals with NEUTROPENIA.

coloproctitis Inflammation of the COLON and RECTUM.

colostrum Breast fluid that may be secreted from the second trimester of pregnancy onward, but is most evident in the first two or three days after birth and before the onset of true lactation. This thin yellowish fluid is rich in proteins, calories, antibodies and lymphocytes, and is low in fat and sugar.

colposcope A magnifying instrument in the form of a flexible fiberoptic tube, used in COLPOSCOPY.

colposcopy Examination of the VULVA, VAGINA and CERVIX by means of a COLPOSCOPE.
A more accurate alternative to the PAP TEST, colposcopy is a procedure in which the surface of the uterine cervix is examined for cancerous growths through a colposcope, a flexible fiberoptic tube. Colposcopy requires specialized training, as practitioners must be able to recognize diseased tissue visually through the colposcope lens. There have never been enough expert colposcopists to examine regularly every woman with HIV.
When the CENTERS FOR DISEASE CONTROL AND PREVENTION (CDC) began drafting gynecological guidelines for HIV-positive women in 1993, the CDC's advisory group had to choose between a schedule of regular Pap smears and/or colposcopy. The agency settled on recommending repeat Pap smears as a way of countering false-negative individual Paps. AIDS activists feared that HIV-positive women who had to wait six months or more for testing of abnormal Paps would risk contracting cervical cancer and insisted on colposcopy examinations for all HIV-positive women. Health care providers and activists generally agree, however, that, as a practical matter, it may be a more effective use of resources to create the best conditions for successful use of the low-tech Pap test than to put them into the more sophisticated colposcopy technique.

combination therapy   The use of two or more therapies administered alternately or simultaneously, in order to achieve maximum results. Different drugs have different ways of working and different side effects; by combining drugs, it is often possible to come up with a more effective treatment with reduced side effects and less risk of developing drug-resistance. Combination therapy is distinguished from MONOTHERAPY (one drug used alone) and SEQUENTIAL MONOTHERAPY (two or more drugs used sequentially, one at a time, with the change either after a fixed amount of time or after a drug has become ineffective). Research has shown that existing therapies such as the NUCLEOSIDE ANALOGS AZT, ddI, ddC and D4T progressively lose their effectiveness when used alone. There is evidence that combining therapies reduces HIV replication, preventing the evolution of strains resistant to multiple medications. See also CONVERGENT COMBINATION THERAPY.

According to comprehensive *Guidelines for the Use of Antiretroviral Agents in HIV-Infected Adults and Adolescents*, made available by the Department of Health and Human Services in 1997, all people with CDC-defined AIDS should receive combination ANTIRETROVIRAL therapy, preferably with three drugs, including a PROTEASE INHIBITOR. The *Guidelines* recommend starting treatment with three drugs and changing at least two when there are indications that treatment is failing. Treatment with only two drugs is, in general, considered less than optimal. Treatment with only one drug is not recommended. However, zidovudine (AZT) monotherapy is recommended as prophylaxis to prevent HIV TRANSMISSION to newborn babies. It should not be given during pregnancy to healthy HIV-infected women who do not require antiretroviral drugs for their own treatment.

Two drugs have also been shown to be better than one for treating children with symptomatic HIV. Initial therapy using zidovudine (AZT) combined with either LAMIVUDINE (3TC) or DIDANOSINE (ddI) has been shown to be far more effective at staving off disease progression or death in children with symptomatic HIV disease than treatment with ddI alone.

combination antiretroviral therapy   See COMBINATION THERAPY.

communicable   Capable of transmission from person to person (said of a disease or disease-causing organism).

Community Acquired Immune Deficiency Syndrome (CAIDS)   One of the names proposed in 1981–82 for AIDS.

community-based organization   Community-based organizations are those organized at a local level, within a community, as close as possible to the individuals they serve. Those concerned with AIDS issues are also called AIDS ADVOCACY ORGANIZATIONs and AIDS SERVICE ORGANIZATIONs (ASOs). They provide services to people with HIV infection, as well as education and prevention programs for the whole community. The leaders of community-based organizations are lay people, not doctors or government officials, although many have physicians as advisers and have a

paid professional staff as well as volunteers. Funding usually comes from state governments, private donations, and local fund-raising events.

community norms   As a disease associated with activities regarded by many as violations of public morality, AIDS is a controversial subject. Discussion of AIDS is often disturbing, and rational discussion difficult, for this reason. It challenges, or seems to challenge, the boundaries of community norms of behavior and discourse. Any attempt at AIDS prevention through programs of public education has to deal with this problem.

Broadly speaking, there are two positions on disseminating information about AIDS and AIDS prevention. The first may be called the public health viewpoint and advocates providing complete information as widely as possible. The second, more moralistic view is that since the activities that lead to getting AIDS are morally unacceptable, information about them should not be widely publicized. Among people holding this view, advocating abstinence or saying no to drug use are strongly, even exclusively, favored as AIDS prevention techniques. For those holding the first view, vocabulary is important because it may determine the success of any attempt to overcome public discomfort or hostility to honest and open discussion. The language of AIDS has therefore been evolving toward a more neutral or medical-sounding usage. Examples include: prostitutes (now referred to as commercial sex workers); AIDS patients/victims (PEOPLE WITH AIDS); drug addicts (INJECTION DRUG USERs); promiscuity (multiple sex partners).

Community Programs for Clinical Research on AIDS (CPCRA)   The Community Programs for Clinical Research on AIDS is sponsored by the National Institute of Allergy and Infectious Diseases of the National Institutes of Health. It was established in 1989 to involve community physicians and their patients in studies of treatments for HIV and comprises 17 research units, consisting of consortiums of primary care physicians and nurses located in 13 American cities. These research units represent a significant geographic, racial, and RISK-GROUP diversity. Through this diversity, the CPCRA extends greater opportunity for participation in clinical research to those persons underrepresented in traditional, university-based HIV studies.

community residence home care   The term for BOARD-AND-CARE HOME services used by the US DEPARTMENT OF VETERANS AFFAIRS.

comparison trial   A trial in which experimental drugs are tested against each other or against an approved drug.

compassionate use   A FOOD AND DRUG ADMINISTRATION classification that allows use of an experimental drug by very sick patients who have no treatment options, even though there is insufficient data about the drug's effectiveness to allow licensing. Drugs are provided free under this program, which is also called Open Study Protocol. Often, specific approval of individual cases must be obtained from the FDA for compassionate use of a drug.

compensation   In biology, the improvement of any defect by the excessive development or action of another part of the same structure.

competence   In psychological evaluation, having the ability to manage one's affairs and to perform in a manner adequate to the demands of a situation; to interact effectively with the environment.

In cell biology, the capacity of embryonic cells to differentiate into a variety of cell types. Also, a cell able to take up DNA and be transformed is described as "competent."

complacency   Despite increasingly grim projections concerning the AIDS pandemic and its demographic, economic, and social impact, many people involved in the international AIDS effort believe that the sense of urgency that marked the late 1980s has abated noticeably, at least in industrialized countries. This apparent complacency has been identified by the Global Commission on AIDS as one of the critical issues for the 1990s.

There appears to be a number of factors contributing to this phenomenon: unrealistic expectations that the problem will soon be solved by vaccines and drugs; a public view that the epidemic has leveled off or peaked and is declining in industrialized countries; the belief that spread of AIDS among heterosexuals is not a serious problem in industrialized countries; and fatigue about AIDS on the part of the media, politicians, and the public.

In some seriously affected countries, this apparent complacency may actually be a form of denial, as the true dimensions of the disaster become apparent. In other countries, complacency may be the result of the mistaken belief that certain societies are virtually immune to HIV/AIDS because of cultural factors, including religious beliefs and practices. Whatever its roots, complacency is extremely dangerous. It leads to the failure not only of individuals to protect themselves, but also of governments to sustain a high level of commitment and action, especially in regard to public education and other preventive efforts, such as condom distribution. There is particular danger that public complacency in wealthy countries, combined with economic recession, will result in failure to increase the bilateral transfer of funds to poor countries or to sustain or increase contributions to international efforts against AIDS, at the very time when needs are increasing dramatically, especially for the care of the sick and orphaned. In less affluent countries, complacency may lead officials to ignore the need to shift priorities in national spending, perhaps from military and police to health and social services.

Because the mass media clearly have been the major source of public information about AIDS, they obviously have a critical role in combating complacency. Yet the media's primary role is to report information not to persuade the public. Governments and nongovernmental organizations need to persevere in developing and promoting both general and targeted AIDS information to increase public knowledge and maintain public concern.

Finally, organized advocacy must continue to be one of the cornerstones of the AIDS effort if the danger of complacency is to be overcome and AIDS is to remain high on the national and international agendas.

complement   See COMPLEMENT SYSTEM.

complement fixation test   A diagnostic test that distinguishes between forms of serum antibody proteins (called complement) in the blood to identify specific diseases.

Antibodies are formed when the body is exposed to infections. If the antigens (specific causes) of a disease are mixed with a patient's serum, along with specially prepared sheep red blood cells, the antibodies and antigens will combine, and the blood cells will remain whole. If the patient's serum does not contain complement antibodies to a disease, the sheep red blood cells will dissolve (a process called HEMOLYSIS).

complement system   Collectively, the 20 plasma proteins involved in specific and nonspecific IMMUNE RESPONSES. The three main functions of the complement system are CHEMOTAXIS (release of chemicals that attract phagocytic cells to an invasion site), opsonization (the coating of an invading cell for easy recognition by phagocytic cells) and the formation of membrane adherence complex (making the invading cell vulnerable to LYSIS).

Complement activation occurs when antibodies bind to an antigen, causing an amplifying cascade of reactions as each complement protein is activated sequentially.

complete blood count (CBC)   A measurement of the most important cellular components of the blood. A CBC includes total white blood count, counts of specific types of white blood cells, red blood cell count, hemoglobin level, and platelet count.

compound Q   A substance (also called GLQ223) whose active ingredient is a protein called tricosanthin, extracted from the root tuber of a Chinese cucumber, *Trichosanthes kirilowii*. It is used in China to induce abortions and to treat ectopic pregnancy, hydatidiform moles, and a type of cancer, choriocarcinoma. In China there are three different grades of trichosanthin prepared for injection: crude extract, purified extract, and crystallized, the highest purity. Only the crystallized form can be used safely; the others cause severe side effects.

In late 1988 and early 1989 compound Q generated enormous public and scientific interest, and was touted as an important treatment to watch. In April 1989 there was widespread publicity about a severe adverse reaction to an injected bogus "compound Q," apparently homemade from roots obtained from a health food store. It was also reported that some health food stores were exploiting the situation by promoting a dried root or extract that, they suggested, contained compound Q. The public was warned that the root also contains lectins, which are poisonous when injected (they cause blood cells to clump together, potentially causing heart attacks or strokes). Moreover, compound Q is almost certainly destroyed by drying, so the dried root available in health food stores does not contain the active ingredient anyway.

A potential benefit of compound Q is that trichosanthin, unlike other treatments, kills HIV-infected cells; thus it has the potential to reduce the total amount of infection and not just slow its spread. Physicians and researchers continue to be concerned about toxicity, however. Two kinds have been found. One appears to be dose-related and the other seems to depend on the condition of the patient. Clearly not enough is known to determine the most beneficial use of this substance, or to predict its value as a treatment.

Comprehensive AIDS Resource Emergency Act of 1990
See RYAN WHITE COMPREHENSIVE AIDS RESOURCES EMERGENCY (CARE) ACT OF 1990.

comprehensive care   Care that includes the full spectrum of health, educational, social, and related services.

compromised   Weakened, as in compromised immunity, a decreased ability to resist infection.

computer bulletin board   See BULLETIN BOARD SYSTEM.

computerized axial tomography (CT)   A noninvasive method of examining the brain or other organ by means of scanning it with an X-RAY beam repeatedly from different angles, enabling a computer to build up a visual image. This procedure is known as a CT (formerly CAT) scan. CT scans are more detailed than conventional X-ray images, which provide only a two-dimensional view. CT scans can be done of the entire body or of parts of it.

A person undergoing a CT scan first receives an injection of a "CONTRAST AGENT" material that shows up well in X-ray images. (Some people have allergic reactions to contrast agents.) He or she is next put into a cylindrical chamber around which a scanner moves, producing three-dimensional images in parallel sections of an inch or less. CT scans, first developed in the 1970s, are an excellent method for detecting tumors, infections, or other changes in the anatomy of the brain, chest or abdomen.

Concorde   The Concorde study was a landmark clinical trial that examined the long-term effect of AZT on the survival of HIV-infected but asymptomatic patients. Concorde began in October 1988 and was organized by the British Medical Research Council and the French National AIDS Research Agency, and was conducted in Britain, France, and Ireland. The trial was the largest randomized, double-blind placebo-controlled AZT study ever conducted. Neither the clinicians nor the participants knew who was given AZT and who was given placebo. Preliminary results were released in a letter to the *Lancet*, the leading British medical journal, on April 3, 1993.

Concorde addresses a fundamental question: does early AZT therapy truly prolong the lives of asymptomatic people?

The study followed nearly 1,800 subjects for an average of three years. At the start, all were HIV-positive and asymptomatic, with a broad range of CD4 counts. Eight hundred and seventy-seven individuals were randomized to receive 1,000 mg per day of AZT from the start, regardless of their CD4 levels ("immediate treatment") and eight hundred and seventy-two were given placebo ("deferred treatment") until they developed symptomatic disease (AIDS or ARC). The two groups were similar in age, sex (15 percent were women),

and immunological markers. The trial was designed to show whether it is beneficial to begin AZT treatment of HIV-positive people before symptoms appear. The trial was not designed to provide information on the usefulness of taking AZT for symptomatic HIV disease.

In 1989, an American study was halted after one year when it found that AZT seemed to delay progression of disease in people with a CD4 count of below 500. (This study was too small and too short to examine the effect of AZT on ultimate survival.) The Concorde study was then modified on ethical grounds to allow all participants with a lower-than-500 CD4 count to begin taking AZT. Those who chose to begin AZT once their CD4 count fell below 500, along with those who began AZT because they developed symptomatic disease, were included in the preliminary analysis.

After an average of three years, survival rates did not differ significantly, nor was there a significant difference in disease progression. However, there was a statistically significant difference in CD4 levels between the two arms of the study, which was sustained up to three years. No new or unexpected toxicities were seen.

The authors of the study concluded that "Concorde has not shown any significant benefit from the immediate use of zidovudine (AZT) compared with deferred therapy in symptom-free individuals in terms of survival or disease progression, irrespective of their initial CD4 counts."

Criticisms of Concorde were numerous. Some noted, for example, that the protocol change in 1989, which allowed open label use of AZT for those with less than 500 CD4 cells, may have skewed the results by causing a significant number of those in the deferred treatment arm to receive the same therapy as those in the immediate treatment arm. It was therefore not surprising that there was no significant difference between the two arms. Others noted that since Concorde did not use what is believed to be the optimum dose of AZT, the results did not provide an accurate indication of the potential benefits of AZT. It was also noted that Concorde was a study of AZT MONOTHERAPY, rather than COMBINATION THERAPY, which is widely believed to provide the most beneficial results in anti-retroviral therapy.

Concorde results challenged the belief that the NUCLEOSIDE ANALOGS (the class of compounds that includes AZT, ddI, and ddC) would transform AIDS into a so-called chronic manageable condition. Some of the basic assumptions underlying AIDS drug development evidently needed to be reexamined. Consensus on the central questions in AIDS research was lost.

Concorde also raised questions about the applicability of the current expedited drug approval criteria to treatments for asymptomatics as well those with AIDS disease symptoms. The question was becoming urgent as more and more companies were taking advantage of regulations to develop new therapeutic vaccines, new antiretrovirals, and immunomodulators for asymptomatics as well as those with AIDS disease symptoms. On a broader level, Concorde raised disturbing questions regarding the American AIDS research effort as a whole. Had the point of diminishing returns been reached with the nucleosides? Would it be wiser to use limited AIDS research dollars to develop and test new, more promising classes of compounds? Was there an overall strategy and program for developing anti-HIV therapies? Was the federal government ensuring that the country's AIDS research effort was as effective as it could be? Some activists felt there was evidence of a conspiracy by the manufacturer of AZT to manipulate scientific evidence.

conditional eligibility The status of those applicants granted temporary SSI benefits even though they have slightly too much in assets, while they attempt to sell some assets. They are required to repay program benefits out of the proceeds. By extension, this term is sometimes applied to situations in which an applicant is granted eligibility, in the SSI or MEDICAID program, despite excess assets, if the assets are essentially unsalable (for instance rural property for which there is no market).

condom A flexible shield made of latex or lambskin that is placed over the penis or sex toy during penetration to prevent conception and sexually transmitted diseases. The HIV virus will not go through latex; if a condom does not leak, break, or fall off, it will block the virus. Correct use of a latex condom during every act of intercourse greatly reduces, but does not eliminate, the risk of infection with HIV. Lambskin or "natural" condoms do not offer protection because they are too porous. Also called bag, boot, french letter, jimmy hat, latex sheath, prophylactic, rubber, and raincoat.

Latex condoms have been proved to be the most effective contraceptive as well as the best protection against sexually transmitted diseases, including HIV. Some are lubricated with a spermicide, NONOXYNOL-9, which decreases the risk of pregnancy if some semen spills outside the condom. However, the extent of decreased risk has not been established. The condom should not be used alone, but always in combination with a vaginal spermicide. Condoms seldom break when used correctly, but pulling out before ejaculating will add further protection. (Condoms can fail: No condom or contraceptive works 100 percent of the time. The only absolutely sure way to prevent pregnancy and sexually transmitted diseases is not to have sex.) Condoms should be used for vaginal, anal, or oral sex, and a new condom should be used for each sex act. Both men and women should learn how to use a condom properly. All latex condoms sold in the United States must meet minimum standards for strength and quality.

Here are the basic instructions for using a condom: Open the package carefully so that the condom is not torn or a hole made with a fingernail. Testing the elasticity will only make it weak. Do not unroll the rubber until putting it on. A drop of water-based lubricant inside the tip of the rubber will make the penis feel better during sex. The shaft of the penis should be free of lubricant, to keep the condom from falling off. Hold the tip of the condom to squeeze out the air; excess air can cause the condom to break. This leaves room for the semen after ejaculation. When the penis is hard (before sexual contact), place the condom on the tip and roll down all the way. If uncircumcised, the foreskin should be pulled back first.

In vaginal or anal intercourse, use plenty of water-based lubricant like ForPlay, Kimono Aqua Lube, K-Y Jelly, or Wet. Baby oil, cocoa butter, cold cream, Crisco, hand creams or lotions, massage oil, mineral oil, or petroleum-based prod-

ucts like Vaseline can break down the latex within minutes. This will increase the risk of breaking the condom or injuring internal and external body tissue, which could leave an opening for infection. Lubricants with alcohol in them can also damage latex. Read the label to make sure there is no oil or alcohol in the jelly or lubricant. A lot of lubricant should be used on the outside of the rubber. This will make it slide easier so it won't break. Jelly or lubricant can also be put on the vagina or anus. Water-based lubricants may become dry during sex. If this happens, put a little water on the rubber and it will be slippery again. More jelly or lubricant can also be used. If during intercourse you or your partner sense burning or itching, discontinue use of the condom and try another type.

After ejaculation but before losing the erection, pull the penis out gently. Hold the condom at the base of the penis while pulling out so that it doesn't leak or fall off. Take it off carefully so the semen doesn't spill. Roll it off starting at the base of the penis. Throw the condom away. Never wear the same condom twice. Finally, because no one knows for sure how long a virus lives outside the body, it is good to wash after having sex. Avoid further sexual contact with your partner until both of you wash your sex organs and any other areas that come in contact with body fluids.

If a condom is sticky or brittle or looks damaged, do not use it. Store condoms in a cool, dry place. Do not keep condoms in a wallet, pocketbook, or glove compartment of a car for a long time. Keep condoms out of direct sunlight; heat can make them weak. Condom packages have a date on the outside, the inner wrapping or on the condom itself. This is the date of manufacture, not an expiration date. If condoms are kept in a cool, dry place, they will last about four years, but unless you know exactly how and where a condom has been stored, don't use it more than two years after the date stamped on it.

condyloma acuminatum A projecting warty growth on the external genitals or the ANUS caused by infection with the HUMAN PAPILLOMAVIRUS (HPV). It is usually benign or noncancerous. Condyloma acuminatum is also referred to as GENITAL WART or verruca acuminata.

condyloma lata The genital lesion that occurs during the secondary stage of SYPHILIS.

confidential information Confidential HIV-related information is information that a person has been the subject of an HIV-related test, or has HIV, HIV-related illness or AIDS, or any information which identifies or reasonably could identify an individual as having one or more of these conditions, including information pertaining to the individual's contacts. In general, confidentiality laws require written authorization for information to be released. This requirement serves to extend the law's coverage beyond the realm of health and social services, because anyone who obtains information pursuant to a written release is fully bound by the law. See CONFIDENTIAL TESTING; PRIVACY.

confidential testing In regard to HIV testing, confidential testing means that the results of a test are formally restricted to the person being tested and the person or facility performing the test. Confidential test results however, are permanently recorded in a patient's medical charts, and there is always the risk that they may be disclosed without his or her permission. ANONYMOUS TESTING precludes that risk.

confidentiality   See PRIVACY.

congenital syphilis   A syphilis infection that is present at birth.

congregate living   Any one of a number of housing, shelter, or confinement arrangements in which a number of individuals live together.

conjugate   A combination of two molecules, such as hapten and a protein, that can initiate an immune response.

conjugated protein   A protein to which a non protein portion is attached.

conjugation   A union of bacterial cells in which two individual bacteria or filaments fuse together to exchange or donate genetic material.

conjunctivitis   An inflammation of the conjunctiva, the thin protective membrane on the inner surface of the eyelids and the outer surface of the eye. There are many different types of conjunctivitis, and treatment varies depending on the specific type of infection.

conservator   See SURROGATE.

conservatorship   See SURROGACY.

constitutional symptoms   Symptoms caused by the impact of an illness on the entire body or constitution are frequently referred to as constitutional symptoms. These include loss of weight, fatigue, fever, diarrhea, night sweats, and malaise over a period of months. Constitutional symptoms are present in many types of infectious diseases, tumors, and other medical conditions, ranging from the serious to the trivial. For people with HIV infection, constitutional symptoms may be a result of HIV infection itself or the result of such opportunistic illnesses as PNEUMOCYSTIS pneumonia, TUBERCULOSIS, or widespread CMV infection.

consumer   An individual who uses a product or service. In the health care setting, a more general term for *client* or *patient*.

contact infection   An infection resulting from direct or indirect contact with a person who is infected. A contact infection may be transmitted through physical contact with those afflicted with COMMUNICABLE diseases or with utensils handled by them.

contact sensitivity   A type of delayed hypersensitivity reaction in which sensitivity to simple chemical compounds is manifested by skin reactivity.

contact tracing   A technique used in the treatment of AIDS and other sexually transmitted diseases, involving finding and notifying an HIV-positive person's recent and current sexual contacts, either with or without identifying the infected individual.

contagion, fear of   Fear of contracting a disease, by either direct or indirect contact with infected individuals, carriers, or objects they may have touched or passed near. During the early years of the AIDS epidemic, the fear experienced by the uninfected was compounded by the seriousness of the disease, the degree to which it was associated with unpopular or marginal social groups, and misinformation coupled with inadequate efforts to educate the public about the disease and methods of prevention.

contagious   The term is used of diseases, referring to the capacity of being spread from one person to another through casual contact. All contagious diseases are also infectious; but some diseases, like TOXIC SHOCK SYNDROME, are infectious but not contagious. HIV is both infectious and contagious, but it is contagious only with specific types of contact.

contain   In medicine, to prevent or limit the advance, spread, or influence of a disease.

contamination   In medicine, the introduction of disease germs or infectious material into sterile environments or onto sterile objects.

continuity of care   Uninterrupted health care provided from initial contact with a physician or clinic through all phases of a patient's medical care needs. The term is frequently applied more narrowly to mean the provision of care from initial contact through recovery from a given illness.

continuous care   In health care services, care that is maintained without interruption despite changes in site, caregiver, or method of payment.

continuous infusion   Uninterrupted introduction of fluid other than blood into a vein.

contraceptive   Against conception; a drug (ORAL CONTRACEPTIVE, INTRAMUSCULAR PROGESTERONE), BARRIER (creams, gels, suppositories, foams, sponges), physical alteration (surgical sterilization), or device (INTRAUTERINE DEVICE, DIAPHRAGM, CONDOM) that tends or serves to prevent conception or impregnation. For HIV-positive women, there are pros and cons of the various choices that need to be taken into consideration. Oral contraceptives have known and unknown interactions with other medications and possibly reduce immune function in immune-compromised women. Diaphragms with spermicide or cervical cap do not prevent, although they may limit, transmission of STDs. Other barriers, such as creams, gels, suppositories, foams, and sponges may be inadequate for contraception or STD prevention unless used with condoms. Intrauterine devices are not a good choice for immune-compromised women because the risk of PID is high. Decisions for permanent sterilization should not be made in the early months, and perhaps the first year, after diagnosis with HIV infection, and in any case bilateral tubal ligation does not prevent the transmission of STDs. Progesterone implants have uncertain hormonal interaction in HIV illness, a slight risk of infection at the site of insertion which may be increased in conditions of compromised immunity, and uncertain interaction with medications commonly used in treatment of HIV infection and they do not prevent the transmission of STDs.

contraindicated   In medicine, inadvisable; used of drug therapies or other treatments and procedures.

contrast agent   A contrast agent blocks X rays and thereby silhouettes the body parts of interest, allowing their visual imaging. Different contrast agents are used for different procedures; the methodologies for administering contrast agents also vary. Some contrast agents may be administered by way of an INTRAVENOUS (IV) drip; others can be taken orally. In general, contrast agents and not the X rays cause the complications arising from gastrointestinal exams. Allergic reaction is a major consideration when using any contrast agent.

control arm   The group of participants in a clinical trial who receive standard treatment or a PLACEBO, against which those receiving the experimental treatment are compared.

control group   In experimental design, a comparison group of subjects who, when the independent variable is manipulated, are not exposed to the treatment that subjects in the experimental group are exposed to, but who in other respects are treated identically. This group provides a baseline against which to evaluate the effects of treatment.

controlled study   A study in which doctors give a new drug being tested to one group of people, the treatment group, and give another drug or no drug to a second group of people with the same type of illness, the CONTROL GROUP. Then they compare the results of the two groups. Simply put, if people taking the new drug get better and people taking the other drug or no drug do not, the new drug works. If the treatment group does not improve more than the control group, the new drug does not work, or not better than the treatment the control group was taking. If many people in the treatment group get sicker and people in the control group do not, the new drug is not safe.

controlled trial   See CONTROLLED STUDY.

convergent combination therapy   An experimental form of COMBINATION THERAPY based on the 1992–93 research of Yang-kung Chow, a medical student in Boston. Chow's research suggested that a combination of three drugs—AZT, ddI and either NEVIRAPINE or the pyridinone L679,661— could stop HIV replication completely. The significance of the finding was limited, however, since successful test tube experiments with new drugs often fail in the nonideal condition of the human body. Nevertheless it was a promising line of investigation.

The idea behind convergent combination therapy is to turn one of the virus's greatest strengths—its ability to mutate quickly and become resistant to anti-HIV drugs— against itself. By 1993, it was well documented that HIV can become resistant to single-drug therapy with AZT or ddI, perhaps even simultaneously. However, Chow's research suggested that there may be a limit to HIV's ability to mutate. The combination of three drugs forces the virus either to mutate to resist all three drugs, resulting in a genetically defective virus, or to remain susceptible to at least one of the drugs' antiretroviral action. In either case, HIV replication will be inhibited.

Chow's findings were later contradicted when the virus proved capable of producing viable strains resistant to all three drugs at once. Ambiguous results from a federally funded clinical trial also demonstrated that the virus can sidestep convergent therapy. However, convergent therapy attracted attention back to a class of compounds known as NONNUCLEOSIDE REVERSE TRANSCRIPTASE INHIBITORS (NNRTI), which include a number of different types of drug, including the pyridinones, the BHAP drugs, and the thiobenzimidazolone (TIBO) derivatives. In 1991 these drugs were found to induce resistance rapidly in HIV, leading to serious doubts about their usefulness. Convergent combination therapy raised hopes that the NNRTIs may ultimately prove beneficial in combination.

cookers   Equipment used in the preparation of some injectable illicit drugs. See WORKS; DRUG ADDICTION; DRUG PARAPHERNALIA LAWS; NEEDLE SHARING; TRANSMISSION.

Cooley's anemia   ANEMIA resulting from inheritance of a recessive trait responsible for interference with the rate of hemoglobulin synthesis.

Coomb's test   A test for antiglobulins in the red cells used in diagnosing various hemolytic anemias.

copayment   The amount an insured patient pays for a health service, beyond the amount paid by the insurance or health plan. By extension, a synonym for COINSURANCE.

coping   Dealing effectively with the stress of daily life and the unusual challenges posed by chronic disease, disability, and pain.

copper-7   One of several CONTRACEPTIVE devices known as INTRAUTERINE DEVICES (IUDs).

copralalia   Talking dirty, usually in an attempt to be sexually arousing.

coprophilia   A sexual interest in feces.

corticosteroid   A steroid synthesized in the adrenal cortex from cholesterol. Some are potent hormones. Corticosteroids are immunosuppressive; synthetic corticosteroids are used as short-term treatments for a host of AIDS-related conditions, such as NEUROPATHY, esophageal ulcers, skin rashes, and THROMBOCYTOPENIA. They are combined with other drugs to treat AIDS-related KAPOSI'S SARCOMA (KS), acute PNEUMO-CYSTIC CARINII PNEUMONIA, and tuberculosis and to reduce intracranial pressure caused by TOXOPLASMOSIS or CNS LYMPHOMA. Corticosteroids include prednisone, corticosterone, cortisone, and aldosterone and are available in preparations for use intravenously, orally, or by direct application to the skin. The effects of corticosteroids on primary HIV infection have been given little formal study.

Long-term use of corticosteroids has been associated with reactivation of herpes viruses, *Pneumocystis carinii*, tuberculosis and various fungal infections. Corticosteroid use has also been associated with the development of AIDS-KS, although rarely with the development of KS in other diseases, and it remains unclear if their use increases the risk of developing KS for people with HIV.

Using high doses of corticosteroids for a long time can be dangerous. They reduce the immune system's defenses against certain infections and are sometimes considered especially dangerous for people whose immune defenses are already weakened. Nevertheless, many of the complications of HIV infection appear to result from an abundant but misdirected immune response; these complications respond well to corticosteroids. In any case it is considered best that these drugs be taken at the lowest possible dose for the shortest possible period.

cortisol   A glucocorticoid hormone secreted by the adrenal gland to moderate stress. Among other things, glucocorticoids promote the breakdown of protein stores in the body to produce sugar (glucose) and can decrease immune system activity. Cortisol levels are high in people with HIV infections, and the hormone has been implicated in WASTING SYNDROME. Recent studies have found that blocking cells' glucocorticoid receptors reduces the proliferation of KAPOSI'S SARCOMA tissue, and that blocking these receptors also might inhibit HIV itself.

cortisone   A CORTICOSTEROID often used to reduce inflammation in the body caused by various illnesses.

Corynebacterium   A genus of the family Corynebacteriaceae. The bacteria are rod shaped, gram-positive and nonmotile. Though many species of this genus are pathogens in domestic animals, birds, reptiles and plants, the most important is the species *C. diptheriae*, the causative agent of diphtheria in humans.

Cotrimoxale   See TRIMETHOPRIM-SULFAMETHOXAZOLE.

cotton-wool spots   Fluffy-looking white patches on the retina; small areas that have lost their blood supply due to blockage of local vessels. Also called *cotton-wool patches*.

counseling   The providing of advice and guidance to a patient by a health professional.

countable income   The amount of a potential enrollee's income needs-based programs use to determine eligibility, after exemption of specified amounts or percentages of gross income.

crab louse   A species of louse (*Phthiru pubis*) that infests the pubic area of the human body. Often called simply *crab*.

crack   A crystallized derivative form of cocaine that is ingested by being smoked. Crack is cheap and extremely addictive. Its use become epidemic in the late 1980s and early 1990s and is said to be receding in the late 1990s.

crack house   A indoor place where individuals gather to smoke crack.

Cranston-Gonzalez National Affordable Housing Act of 1990   A federal housing law that includes a block grant program designed to encourage state and local governments to provide housing for people with HIV. This provision was intended as a measure against discrimination in housing against people with HIV.

cream, spermicidal   Like spermicidal jelly, foams, and vaginal suppositories, spermicidal creams are a form of birth control that are really designed for use with a BARRIER such as a diaphragm, cervical cap, or INTRAUTERINE DEVICE (IUD). Like jellies and vaginal suppositories, creams can be used for extra protection with a condom. Creams come in a tube with a plastic applicator. While jellies are clear, creams are white. Like condoms and jellies, creams are available without prescription at most drugstores. Deposited just outside the entrance to the cervix at the top of the vagina, cream keeps sperm from entering the cervix and kills them as well. Like jellies, creams increase protection against gonorrhea and chlamydia.

creatinine   A substance produced by the breakdown of creatine, an important molecule involved in energy transfer within muscle cells. The level of creatinine in the blood and urine provides a measure of kidney function.

Creutzfeldt-Jakob disease   A central nervous system disease that causes presenile DEMENTIA, myoclonus, and distinctive EEG changes. Etiology is unknown but is assumed to be a slow virus. The infectious agent has been isolated but not identified. To date, there is no treatment, and the course of the disease is fatal. The causative agent of this disease is extremely resistant to most sterilization procedures; thus the same precautions as used for AIDS should be exercised when handling body fluids and tissues from patients with this disease.

crisis intervention   Problem-solving activity intended to correct or prevent the continuation of a crisis. Often this is provided by telephone by professional or paraprofessional medical or social workers.

cross-reaction   A reaction between an antibody and an antigen other than the one that precipitated its development. The antigen in such cases is closely related to the original antigen.

cross-resistance   A phenomenon in which a microbe that acquires resistance to one drug through direct exposure also becomes resistant to one or more other drugs to which it has not been exposed. Cross-resistance occurs because the mechanism of resistance to each drug is the same and arises through identical genetic mutations.

cryoprecipitate   A substance obtained from blood, rich in the clotting factors absent in a common form of HEMOPHILIA.

cryosurgery   A method involving freezing for removing GENITAL WARTS and treating cervical problems. See CRYOTHERAPY.

cryotherapy   The use of liquid nitrogen to freeze and destroy a lesion or growth, sometimes used to induce scar formation and healing to prevent further spread of a condition.

cryptococcal infection   A fungal infection in the central nervous system.

Acute cryptococcal infection can be treated with intravenous AMPHOTERICIN B followed by oral FLUCONAZOLE. Lifelong maintenance therapy, usually with fluconazole, is necessary to inhibit resurgence of the *Cryptococcus* fungus. Oral FLUCYTOSINE (100 to 150 mg per kilogram of body weight per day) may be used in conjunction with amphotericin, but both drugs have side effects that can limit their use. Liposomal amphotericin has been tried as a safer alternative. Fluconazole and ITRACONAZOLE are other possible options.

cryptococcal meningitis   The most common fungal infection attacking the central nervous system in HIV-infected persons. Symptoms include severe headache, confusion, sensitivity to light, blurred vision, fever, and speech difficulties. Left untreated, the disease can lead to coma and death. Diagnosis is established by cerebral spinal fluid tests or blood tests. A major problem is elevated intracranial pressure, which can be relieved by various drainage techniques. Treatment with acetazolamide also has been effective. In addition, CORTICOSTEROIDS are being tested for this purpose. See also CRYPTOCOCCAL INFECTION.

cryptococcosis   Cryptococcosis is an infection caused by the fungus CRYPTOCOCCUS NEOFORMANS. In people with HIV it is especially severe, frequently causing MENINGITIS. Common symptoms include headache, fevers, vision problems, and seizures. The diagnosis is usually made by analyzing CEREBROSPINAL FLUID obtained with a SPINAL TAP. The disease is treated with INTRAVENOUS AMPHOTERICIN B or oral FLUCONAZOLE. When treatment is stopped, the disease tends to recur so that long-term treatment is generally necessary.

Cryptococcus   A usually harmless fungus that causes MENINGITIS in persons with AIDS. Cryptococcal infections are difficult to cure because they keep recurring and the drug treatment is very toxic.

Cryptococcus neoformans   A ubiquitous fungus that is found in soil. When inhaled by those in normal health, the fungus is contained in the lungs. In immunosuppressed peo-

ple, it can cause disseminated infection. *Cryptococcus* can cause pulmonary, central nervous system, or disseminated infection. In people with AIDS, the most common presentation is MENINGITIS. Cryptococcal infections may be fatal if untreated.

Onset is insidious with fever, nonspecific fatigue, nausea, and vomiting. Headache may be diffuse, frontal, or temporal. ENCEPHALITIS may occur with altered mental status, subtle behavioral changes, memory loss, and confusion. Photophobia, cranial nerve palsies, PNEUMONIA, and painless skin LESIONS may occur. Prostatic abscesses may serve as a reservoir for recurrent infections. Diagnosis is by serum cryptococcal antigen or lumbar puncture. Treatment is generally with AMPHOTERICIN B followed with FLUCONAZOLE. It is believed that there are some patients who, once disease is diagnosed, may be treated initially with oral fluconazole rather than intravenous amphotericin. These patients generally have earlier disease and milder symptoms. Patients with increased intracranial pressure tend to have poorer outcomes. Elevated pressure readings may be managed with frequent lumbar punctures, mannitol, or CORTICOSTEROIDS. Both liposomal amphotericin and itraconazole for treatment of cryptococcosis are currently in clinical trials.

cryptosporidiosis   A highly contagious infection caused by an opportunistic protozoan, the CRYPTOSPORIDIUM, which is found in human and animal feces and which may contaminate public water supplies by way of untreated sewage. Cryptosporidiosis is must commonly seen in cattle and cattle handlers. It usually causes a diarrhea whose severity varies; in persons with normal immune systems the diarrhea is self-limiting, lasting a week or two, but in persons with AIDS, it is severe and results in enterocolitis that can lead to dehydration and malnutrition. Other symptoms of cryptosporidial infection in AIDS can include weight loss, nausea, vomiting, cramping, abdominal pain, and fever. Infection by the parasite usually occurs in the small intestine, but infection of the colon and other areas of the gastrointestinal tract have been observed. In cryptosporidial infection of the bile duct, nausea and vomiting may be more severe. Cases of respiratory cryptosporidiosis have been documented in immunocompromised individuals. In the lungs, cryptosporidiosis resembles PCP.

A diagnosis of cryptosporidiosis is usually established by simply examining the stool under a microscope to detect the parasite. Since it was first identified in people with AIDS in 1982, more than 70 therapeutic agents have been tested, without success. Cryptosporidiosis was originally classified as a veterinary pathogen, or an organism that affects and causes diseases in animals only. Relatively recently recognized as a common cause of diarrhea in humans, *Cryptosporidiosis parvum* is poorly understood. Without a clear understanding of the biology of the parasite, attempts to design rational therapy for the disease have been nearly impossible. Using animals as models for human cryptosporidiosis has, to date, largely been unsuccessful. *Cryptosporidium* does not grow well in the test tube, making it difficult to determine a drug's potential for animal and human testing. The presence of multiple disease-causing organisms in the gastrointestinal tracts of PWAS also confounds efforts to assess the efficacy of anticryptosporidiosis drugs. Severe immune dysfunction may also contribute to the stubborn nature of cryptosporidiosis infections to people with AIDS.

There are no standard treatments, but proposed drug therapies include PAROMOMYCIN SULFATE (Humatin), AZITHROMYCIN (zithromax), letrazuril, and various forms of concentrated cow and chicken antibodies. Controlling and minimizing diarrhea while maintaining fluid and electrolyte balance and nutritional status are key components of treatment. Intravenous nutrition is commonly required to provide sufficient calories and hydration. Prophylaxis is debatable, since there is no clear indication of effectiveness. However, some have recommended prophylaxis of 250 mg of Humatin twice a day for people with AIDS and fewer than 50 T4 CELLS, especially those who have diarrhea, weight loss, or previously diagnosed cryptosporidiosis.

Cryptosporidiosis is highly contagious and can be spread from person to person, as well as through contaminated water and food. Transmission can occur through any contact with fecal matter, so good hygiene is crucial. A latex barrier should be used for all forms of anal sex.

Cryptosporidium   A protozoan parasite (plural *Cryptosporidia*) that causes severe, protracted diarrhea. In persons with normal immune systems, the diarrhea is self-limiting and lasts one to two weeks. In AIDS patients, the diarrhea often becomes chronic and may lead to severe malnutrition. Commonly used medications for *Cryptosporidium* include paromomycin or antidiarrheal medications such as loperamide.

crystallography   The study of crystal structure. Used in the study of crystallized viruses.

CSF   See CEREBROSPINAL FLUID.

CT   See COMPUTERIZED AXIAL TOMOGRAPHY.

CT scan   See COMPUTERIZED AXIAL TOMOGRAPHY.

cultural activism   See ACTIVISM.

cultural analysis and AIDS   AIDS is not just an illness. Like every other social or cultural phenomenon, it is represented and understood in language, images, and ways of thinking that are characteristic of a particular culture, or way of life, and within that culture, ways of considering different aspects life (social, sexual, moral) or defining and approaching formal disciplines of study (medical, literary), each with its own set of terms, theoretical concepts and basic viewpoints. (These are sometimes called discourses.) It might be said that AIDS is not only an epidemic of a transmissible lethal disease, but simultaneously an "epidemic" of cultural signification. Cultural analysis seeks to engage AIDS and its meanings in a broad cultural context, beyond the unreflective "news and public affairs" level of discussion, beyond what has been called the tyranny of images circulating endlessly in every medium, to understand what the epidemic and our responses to it tell us about ourselves and our deepest beliefs. Highly visible public information about

AIDS (AIDS education in schools, public service announcements on TV, posters in buses or subways, etc.) is a frequent subject of cultural analysis, as is the representation of the epidemic and people with AIDS, in the movies and on TV and in other mass media. Cultural analysis examines the "meaning" of AIDS in the variety of formal and informal discourses in which it has its cultural (as distinct from physical) existence. The discourses of medicine, science and sexual morality are often explored as sites where meaning is constructed. Key words and phrases often under scrutiny include virus, carrier, condone, family, community, general population, gay/homosexual, heterosexual, lesbian, prostitute, PWA (person with AIDS), risk group, risk practice, spread, and victim. On a practical level, such analysis can help us to challenge automatic assumptions, and may help us to modify social responses and avoid the kinds of difficulties that have so far confronted all practical attempts to control the epidemic.

culture   In medical terms, a medium in which MICROBES can grow. HIV is grown in cultures containing LYMPHOCYTES. If a sample of a person's blood is put into such a culture, and HIV grows, the person is infected with HIV.

cunnilinctus   See CUNNILINGUS.

cunnilingus   The use of the tongue or mouth to stimulate the VULVA.

curcumin   The main active ingredient in tumeric, a major ingredient of curry. Curcumin was touted as a "new kind of HIV ANTIVIRAL" and an important treatment possibility in the mid-1990s, when it was one of a class of newly discovered anti-HIV compounds that appear to inhibit the LONG TERMINAL REPEAT (LTR) sequence of HIV. Three substances were thought to have potential: curcumin, topotecan, and beta-lapachone. The most powerful may be topotecan, shown in studies to be active against HIV in very small concentrations, and reasonably well tolerated in cancer patients. Early laboratory studies found that curcumin was less active, but it may be more important because it is a readily available food additive (its medical use would be an economic benefit as well for those countries where tumeric is grown). Curcumin has also been studied as an anti-inflammatory, as a possible cancer inhibitor, and for other potential medical uses. It has also been used for various purposes in traditional Indian, Chinese, and Western herbal medicine.

cure   A means of healing or restoring to health; remedy. Although the gloom that has pervaded AIDS research for more than a decade has begun to lift a bit, and progress is occurring on several fronts, no one talks of an imminent cure. Scientists in the lab and doctors treating the disease believe they may be drawing closer to a secondary goal, making the disease manageable.

curette   A spoon-shaped scraping instrument for removing foreign matter from a cavity in the body (curetting).

curse   See MENSTRUATION.

cyclophosphamide (CY)   An IMMUNOSUPPRESSIVE DRUG that at high doses has been used in cancer chemotherapy regimens. In low doses, the drug has well-documented immunomodulatory properties and has been used to treat several immune disorders, including lupus and Wegener's granulomatosis. In people with HIV, cyclosphosphamide is most commonly used in combination therapy for AIDS-related lymphoma. CY has a greater suppressive effect on B CELLS than on T CELLS, and CD8 CELLS are more sensitive to the drug than other T cell subsets.

CY is an alkylating agent, which means that it works by attaching to biologically important molecules such as DNA and RNA, interfering with cell growth and division. Alkylating agents are toxic to rapidly dividing cells, like those in a tumor or in the bone marrow (where blood cells are continually being replaced). CY is one of the most widely used chemotherapy drugs, in part because its toxicity is more specific to malignant cells and less likely to cause severe bone-marrow toxicity than many other alkylating agents. Although CY can be used alone in chemotherapy, it is used more frequently in combination with other drugs. For the treatment of AIDS-related lymphoma CY is routinely used in a combination of drugs called CHOP (CY, doxorubicin, vincristine, and prednisone). It is also used in a combination called m-BACOD (methotrexate, bleomycin, doxorubicin, CY, vincristine, dexamethasone, and leucovorin). People with less progressive disease, no prior AIDS-defining illness, and no bone marrow or central nervous system involvement are more likely to respond. The CD4+ count at the time the lymphoma is diagnosed is the most important predictor of success: people with CD4+ counts above 200 have the best chance of a positive reaction. CY is available in the form of tablets for oral administration and solution for injection.

Side effects are numerous, ranging from sterility, possibly irreversible (in both sexes), to toxicity to the lungs or kidneys. Menstrual irregularity commonly occurs in women who use the drug; this usually reverses after treatment stops. Damage to the bladder is also a common side effect of CY and appears to be related to the size of dose and duration of therapy. Heart damage has been reported, primarily in those receiving high doses—120 to 270 mg per kg of body weight, administered over a few days. In a few instances, severe and fatal congestive heart failure has occurred. Nausea, vomiting, and temporary hair loss occur frequently. Bone-marrow toxicity that causes reductions in white blood cell count are common. Reductions in the number of platelets and red blood cells develop occasionally but are reversible after therapy stops. Finally, severe toxicity to the lungs or kidneys also occurs occasionally. Rarely, allergic reactions, and death have been reported.

cycloserine   A broad-spectrum antibiotic that has been used in combination with other drugs in treating tuberculosis. It is contraindicated in patients with epilepsy and in those with depression or anxiety. Trade name is Seromycin.

cyclosporine   An IMMUNOSUPPRESSIVE DRUG used to prevent graft rejection in organ transplants. The drug acts specifically against T CELLS in the early stages of activation.

Reports on the use of this drug in people with HIV are contradictory. Also called cyclosporine A, CsA for short.

cyst   A closed sac or pouch, with a definite wall, that contains fluid, semifluid, or solid material. It is usually an abnormal structure resulting from developmental abnormalities, obstruction of ducts, or from a parasitic infection. See also BARTHOLIN'S DUCT.

cysteine   An amino acid, one of three components of GLUTATHIONE (GSH). See N-ACETYLCYSTEINE.

cystitis   An infection of the urinary bladder, usually occurring secondary to ascending urinary tract infections. Associated organs (kidney, prostate, urethra) may be involved. May be acute (with frequent and painful urination) or chronic (secondary to another lesion) possibly with pyuria as the only symptom. Antibiotics are useful in treating the infection, but more definitive therapy will be required if the basic cause is a renal calculus (kidney stone) or other obstruction in the urinary tract.

cytarabine   A drug compound (cytosine arabinoside) originally developed as an antileukemic agent and now being used in treating HERPES virus hominis infections that cause either keratitis or ENCEPHALITIS. The first well-controlled clinical trial found that treatment offers no benefit to patients with progressive multifocal leukoencephalopathy (PML). These results came as no surprise, since there were reports that patients treated with cytarabine die faster than those who received no treatment. There has been at least one published case of cytarabine *causing* PML in a person with cancer by suppressing the immune system. Also called ARA-C.

cytokine   A generic classification for a soluble molecule that mediates interactions between cells, some of which boost HIV replication and some of which suppress it. Cytokines normally involved in inflammatory responses include TUMOR NECROSIS FACTOR-alpha, INTERLEUKIN-1 beta and interleukin-6. These cytokines can upregulate the virus.

HIV actively replicates in cultures of immune cells taken from HIV-infected people. The addition of antibodies that block these inductive cytokines, which are produced by the cells in culture, shuts down HIV replication. Recent research has shown that naturally occurring suppressive cytokines, such as interleukin-4, interleukin-10 and transforming growth factor-B can block the inductive cytokines in cell culture, thereby stopping HIV replication.

Some inflammatory cytokines, such as tumor necrosis factor (TNF) and interleukin-1, have been associated with metabolic dysregulation and wasting. Their chronic release during HIV infection seems to play a major role in HIV-related wasting.

cytolin   Cytolin is the trade name for an experimental drug under development by CytoDyn, a biotechnology firm. It reportedly consists of a specific mice-derived antibody that is infused over twenty minutes, with repeat administration every four weeks. The mouse antibodies that make up

Cytolin do not recognize or bind to HIV at all. They recognize and bind to a specific protein only, known as S6F1, found on the surface of a subgroup of CD8 cells that help control viral infections. In theory, Cytolin should not interfere with the critical functions provided by other immune cells that lack the S6F1 surface proteins.

As would be expected with the introduction into the body of a nonhuman protein-based substance, Cytolin causes serum and protein sickness. Some patients experience mild flu-like serum sickness reactions, such as low-grade fever, swollen lymph nodes, and body aches, within hours of Cytolin injection. Temporary mood changes, such as depression, irritability, and anxiety lasting for several days have also been reported, as well as much more serious allergic or anaphylactic reactions. Critics have also warned that Cytolin can neutralize the critical role that CD8 cells possessing S6F1 play in killing cancerous or virus-infected cells. Cytolin may promote the spread of LYMPHOMAS or EPSTEIN-BARR VIRUS, for example.

Proponents of Cytolin have claimed that both increases in CD4 counts and improvements of immune responses, as measured by delayed-type hypersensitivity skin tests, have occurred in treated patients with early HIV disease. Apparent resolutions of MOLLUSCUM CONTAGIOSUM, a skin condition associated with HIV infection, were seen in some Cytolin recipients.

Distribution of cytolin is currently taking place outside FOOD AND DRUG ADMINISTRATION–sanctioned channels. It is noted that products arising in such an unregulated environment are frequently rushed into human use without the proper lab and animal studies to gather preliminary safety and efficacy information. To date, reliable data on Cytolin is lacking. The medical experience of individuals on Cytolin has not been recorded in a precise or uniform manner.

cytological screening   Testing for cell pathology for diagnostic purposes. Cytological tests can detect and identify both normal and abnormal cells, especially cancer cells, in areas that cannot be easily and directly examined. Specimens to be examined may be obtained from body excretions, secretions, and tissue scrapings. Tests make possible a very early diagnosis and treatment of cancer. They can also indicate hormone activity in the body as well as specific infections and the effect of radiation.

cytology   The study of cells. See CYTOLOGICAL SCREENING.

cytomegalovirus (CMV)   A virus belonging to the herpes family, and a major PATHOGEN in people with AIDS. Before the appearance of AIDS, it was most commonly associated with severe congenital infection in infants and with life-threatening infections in patients who had undergone bone marrow transplants and other procedures requiring suppression of the immune system. CMV's most common target is the retina— the light-sensitive-tissue at the back of the eyes. If left untreated, CMV RETINITIS causes blindness in the affected eye 90 percent of the time. CMV also infects the gastrointestinal tract, and may involve the entire tract, from mouth to anus, including the liver and pancreas. Most cases of CMV gastrointestinal disease involve the esophagus or colon. CMV can also cause PNEUMONIA or CERVICITIS in women. There have also

been reports of CNS and adrenal disease, although the frequency and significance of these conditions are unclear. As a result of these infections, CMV produces considerable illness and greatly affects the survival of patients with AIDS.

Approximately half of the American population over 50 has evidence of past CMV infection, but prevalence appears to be even higher among homosexual men. Most patients who have CMV disease are infected with it long before they become HIV-infected. CMV is typically contracted in infancy and childhood, but patients may also become infected through sexual contact or after receiving infected blood products. In individuals with intact immune systems, infection either goes unnoticed or may provoke a self-limited one-time illness. After infecting a patient, the virus becomes "latent," hiding in the host's cells. Under conditions of immunosuppression, such as with AIDS, the virus may "reactivate" and cause symptomatic disease. This does not usually occur until a patient's CD4 cell count falls below 100, and more typically below 50. CMV infection of the gastrointestinal tract commonly results in inflammation, erosions, and ulceration of the mucosal linings. This may be quite destructive, and occasionally leads to damage throughout the entire wall of the gut; it may cause perforation of the gastrointestinal tract.

Symptoms and physical findings of cytomegalovirus vary from disease to disease. Symptoms of chorioRETINITIS include unilateral visual field loss, blurring of vision, or scotomata. Examination generally reveals whitish areas with perivascular exudates and hemorrhages. A careful search of the entire fundus (base) of the eye is required. Generally, in gastrointestinal disease, COLITIS is associated with abdominal pain and diarrhea. Fever may also be present. ESOPHAGITIS and GASTRITIS most commonly present with pain from the involved structures. Endoscopy reveals ERYTHEMA, submucosal hemorrhage, and diffuse mucosal ulceration. While CMV may be isolated from pulmonary secretions, it is generally believed that it rarely has a true pathologic role in HIV-infected patients. Diagnosis must be confirmed by lung BIOPSY demonstrating histologic evidence consistent with invasive disease. Finally, ENCEPHALITIS, cranial nerve dysfunction and neuropathies may occur. CMV polyradiculopathy is rare, but characterized by lower extremity weakness, numbness and bladder dysfunction.

Rapid diagnosis of CMV disease may lead to improved survival. A variety of diagnostic methods have been attempted, but the most useful is microscopic examination of biopsy samples. CMV infection of human cells results in characteristic changes found in these biopsies. CMV-infected cells become enlarged with a so-called owl's-eye appearance; they are typically found in areas with considerable inflammation. Special tests, which involve such staining techniques as IMMUNOFLUORESCENCE and DNA in situ hybridization may be used by experienced pathologists to confirm the presence of CMV cells. Newer procedures, such as POLYMERASE CHAIN REACTION (PCR), which identifies minute quantities of CMV DNA in body fluids and tissue samples, may be helpful. Culture of CMV from bodily fluids probably adds little diagnostic information. Use of radiographic techniques such as barium exams and CT SCANS may reveal defects in the esophagus, stomach, or intestines, but without biopsy of those lesions, diagnosis is uncertain, and treatment premature.

In the absence of therapy, CMV disease is progressive and is associated with a high mortality rate. Early treatment is essential and may alter the course of the disease, including its spread to other locations in the body. Treatment may also prevent severe consequences of CMV disease such as perforation and hemorrhage, which may result in death. The two most commonly used drug treatments for CMV infection are GANCICLOVIR and FOSCARNET. Both are approved by the United States FOOD AND DRUG ADMINISTRATION. Both result in the suppression of CMV, but not elimination. Ganciclovir has been shown to be effective in the treatment of both CMV esophagitis and colitis in patients infected with HIV, resulting in increased time until relapse and increased survival. Ganciclovir causes adverse side effects that lead to discontinuation of therapy in about one third of patients. The most common adverse effects are on the bone marrow, resulting in a decrease in the number of NEUTROPHILS. Ganciclovir may also cause lowering of the platelet count, which can increase the risk of bleeding because of decreased clotting ability of the blood. The risk of toxicity is worsened when ganciclovir is given with AZT. Adverse reactions are decreased when either DDI or DDC are used instead of AZT. Other side effects include headaches, confusion, nausea, vomiting, diarrhea, and possibly testicular damage.

Foscarnet has also been found to be effective in treating CMV disease and appears to inhibit HIV as well. It is as effective as ganciclovir in the treatment of CMV gastrointestinal disease and can be used both in newly infected patients and in patients who have relapsed after therapy with ganciclovir. Foscarnet has a different side effect profile than ganciclovir. While foscarnet does not affect the bone marrow tissues, and therefore can be used concurrently with AZT, it does have a toxic effect on the kidneys that results in passage of excess electrolytes into the urine. Other adverse effects associated with foscarnet include nausea, vomiting, diarrhea, oral and penile ulceration, and seizures.

Standard treatment of CMV disease usually begins with several weeks of ganciclovir. If there is no elimination of the virus from biopsies taken during repeat ENDOSCOPY, or the patient continues to experience severe symptoms, he or she is switched to foscarnet. If there is only a partial response to ganciclovir, the patient can be reinduced with ganciclovir for several more weeks. It may also become necessary to switch between medications when serious toxicity begins.

Maintenance therapy appears to be necessary for the long-term control of symptoms as well as prevention of CMV dissemination to other sites. Maintenance therapy is controversial for CMV gastrointestinal disease, though, in contrast to CMV retinitis. Progression during maintenance therapy requires reinduction. If both medications fail to result in improvement of gastrointestinal CMV disease, then combined treatment is often recommended.

Treatment of CMV disease with oral agents is being considered. This will permit home therapy and decrease the dangers of infection due to permanent indwelling catheters. The benefit of oral therapy on quality of life could be enormous. Both agents appear to have problems with absorption via the oral route. Newer agents, such as a precursor of the anti-herpes drug ACYCLOVIR, called valacyclovir, are also being studied for treatment and prophylaxis. Valacyclovir is better absorbed than ganciclovir and is completely metabolized to acyclovir, resulting in serum concentrations similar to that achieved by intravenous administration of acyclovir. Another drug called HPMPC is also being studied but appears to be too toxic for routine use. It is associated with severe damage to the kidney, although concurrent use of probenicid may help prevent this.

cytomegalovirus (CMV) disease Disease caused by infection with CYTOMEGALOVIRUS. See also: COLITIS; ESOPHAGITIS; GASTRITIS; NEUROLOGICAL DISEASE; PNEUMONIA; POLYRADICULOPATHY; RETINITIS.

cytomegalovirus gastritis GASTRITIS caused by CYTOMEGALOVIRUS (CMV).

cytomegalovirus esophagitis ESOPHAGITIS caused by CYTOMEGALOVIRUS (CMV).

cytomegalovirus colitis COLITIS caused by CYTOMEGALOVIRUS (CMV).

cytomegalovirus neurological disease NEUROLOGICAL DISEASE caused by CYTOMEGALOVIRUS (CMV).

cytomegalovirus pneumonia PNEUMONIA caused by CYTOMEGALOVIRUS (CMV).

cytomegalovirus polyradiculopathy CYTOMEGALOVIRUS infection of the peripheral nerves and the spinal roots, leading to generalized weakness and paralysis.

cytomegalovirus retinitis RETINITIS caused by CYTOMEGALOVIRUS (CMV).

cytopenia A reduction in the number of cells found in a clinical specimen.

cytophilic Having a propensity to bind to cells.

cytopreservation A technique for preserving cells by freezing (especially CD8 cells) taken from the blood of an AIDS patient for the use by the same patient at a later stage of the disease, when the cells in the patient will have been destroyed or damaged.

cytosine arabinoside See CYTARABINE.

cytostatic Having the ability to stop cell growth.

cytotoxic Having the ability to kill cells; poisonous to cells.

cytotoxic T lymphocyte A type of CD8 or, less often, CD4 LYMPHOCYTE that kills diseased cells infected by a specific virus or other intracellular microbe. CTLs interact with MAJOR HISTOCOMPATIBILITY COMPLEX (MHC) class I receptors on infected cells and have the prime role in CELL-MEDIATED IMMUNITY.

cytotoxin An antibody or toxin that attacks the cells of particular organs.

D4T (stavudine) A NUCLEOSIDE ANALOG similar in structure to AZT, approved for use in patients intolerant to, or unsuccessful on, AZT. These drugs work by inhibiting REVERSE TRANSCRIPTASE and stopping DNA production that is essential in spreading HIV. Nucleoside analogs have never had more than a mediocre record, and D4T, despite early promise, appears to be no exception. Possible side effects include mental confusion and peripheral neuropathy. (Trade name Zerit.)

dantrolene Dantrolene is a muscle relaxant. Its most common side effect is muscle weakness that usually disappears after taking the drug for several days. Other side effects include diarrhea, gastric intolerance, depression, insomnia, and frequent urination. Also sold as Dantrium.

dapsone An antibacterial sulfone administered orally that inhibits or retards bacterial growth in a variety of GRAM-NEGATIVE and GRAM-POSITIVE organisms. It is used in the treatment of dermatitis herpetiformis and leprosy and in the prophylaxis of falciparum malaria. Dapsone is also commonly used for the treatment and prevention of PNEUMOCYSTIS CARINII PNEUMONIA (PCP) in sulfa-intolerant persons, and occasionally for the treatment of mycobacterial or other protozoal infections in people living with HIV. Possible side effects include skin rash, fever, and gastrointestinal upset. In persons who have the hereditary condition GLUCOSE-6-PHOSPHATE DEHYDROGENASE (G6PD) DEFICIENCY, dapsone can cause destruction of red blood cells (hemolysis), resulting in severe anemia. Deaths have been associated with this use. Dapsone also causes reduced absorption of ddI.

Because it stops certain bacteria from multiplying, but does not kill them, dapsone is usually considered backup therapy for the treatment of mild-to-moderate PCP in those who cannot tolerate the preferred drugs such as TRIMETHO-PRIM-SULFAMETHOXAZOLE (TMP-SMX) or INTRAVENOUS PENTAMIDINE. Similarly, dapsone is considered second-line therapy for the prevention of PCP. All HIV-infected people are at risk for PCP and should consider some form of preventive therapy. This includes anyone who has already had PCP or any other AIDS-related condition and asymptomatic HIV-infected people with consistent CD4+ counts below 200 or whose percentage of CD4+ cells is 15 percent or below. In addition, many physicians recommend PCP prophylaxis for HIV-infected individuals with CD4+ counts greater than 200 who also have symptoms of oral thrush or HIV-related constitutional symptoms. There is no clear consensus on the best dose of dapsone to use to prevent PCP.

Dapsone is known to interact with various drugs, including probenecid, RIFAMPIN, and TRIMETHOPRIM. Dapsone used with AZT or ganciclovir may increase the risk of bone-marrow toxicity. Dapsone may decrease the effectiveness of CLOFAZIMINE and increase the risk of PERIPHERAL NEUROPATHY when used with ddC, ddI, or D4T. The most serious side effect of dapsone is anemia, accompanied by shortened red blood cell life span and a rise in abnormal hemoglobin. These side effects are dose-related and occur to some extent in almost all people taking the drug, but it is uncommon for them to be severe enough to stop therapy. Peripheral neuropathy is an unusual side effect of dapsone. Other side effects include muscle weakness, nausea, vomiting, abdominal pain, inflammation of the pancreas, vertigo and blurred vision.

dapsone/trimethoprim A drug therapy combining dapsone and trimethoprim. This combination is common outpatient regimen for the treatment of PNEUMOCYSTIS CARINII PNEUMONIA.

Daraprim See PYRIMETHAMINE.

databases The federal government provides unlimited free access to its AIDS-related electronic databases. These are maintained by the National Library of Medicine (NLM), a unit of the National Institutes of Health in Bethesda, Maryland, and the largest health sciences library in the world. The library's four AIDS-related databases are Aidsline, which lists references to journal articles, books, audiovisuals, and conference abstracts; Aidstrials, which contains up-to-date information about clinical trials of drugs and vaccines that have been or are being tested; Aidsdrugs, a dictionary of licensed anti-HIV. drugs and experimental chemical and biological agents that are being evaluated in clinical trials; and Dirline, which lists organizations and services that provide information to the public about HIV and AIDS. Free access to this information is the result of recommendations made at the

National Institutes of Health HIV/AIDS Information Services Conference in June 1993, to increase AIDS outreach, and to reduce barriers to AIDS information. Increases in the National Library of Medicine's AIDS funding enabled the Library to offer this service. Additionally, the National Library of Medicine plans to create a new electronic database to cover publications on research concerning health services.

date of onset   The date on which an SSDI, SSI, or MEDICAID applicant first becomes disabled within the meaning of the SOCIAL SECURITY ACT; almost always before the application, first treatment, or even work-cessation date.

daunorubicin hydrochloride   An antineoplastic drug used in treating acute leukemia. Daunorubicin is a modified form of an antibiotic isolated from a species of fungus-like bacteria called *Streptomyces coeruleorubidus*. A potent bone marrow suppressant, the drug inhibits the synthesis of nucleic acids, preventing cancer cells from dividing. An increased risk of opportunistic infection or bleeding generally occurs. When used in people taking AZT or ganciclovir, colony-stimulating factors are often used as well to limit bone-marrow suppression. With standard INTRAVENOUS administration, fatal congestive heart failure may occur either during therapy or months to years after the drug was used. The risk increases proportionately to the total cumulative dose. Severe MYELO-SUPPRESSION occurs when daunorubicin is used in either its standard intravenous form or when encapsulated by liposomes. Reversible hair loss occurs in most people treated with standard daunorubicin. Acute nausea and vomiting occur but are usually mild. Diarrhea has occasionally been reported. Rarely, allergic reactions occur, including fever, chills, and skin rash. Daunorubicin may temporarily make the urine red. (Trade name Cerubidine.)

DaunoXome   Liposomal DAUNORUBICIN, DaunoXome, is currently being tested in clinical trials for KS. In a mechanism that is not completely understood, encapsulating daunorubicin in liposomes increases the concentration of the drug at the tumor site significantly without increasing the concentration of the drug in the blood or other healthy tissues. In theory, it should target more drug against the cancer while limiting the drug's side effects. As yet, large clinical trials have not produced conclusive evidence of the effectiveness of this formulation. DaunoXome's main side effect is NEUTROPENIA, which can be managed with G-CSF (Neupogen).

ddC   See DIDEOXYCYTIDINE.

ddI   See DIDEOXYINOSINE.

DDS   See DAPSONE.

DD214   The military discharge certificate (Department of Defense form 214) that all veterans must present when applying for VA services.

death   Permanent cessation of all vital functions; total irreversible cessation of cerebral function, spontaneous function of the respiratory system, and spontaneous function of the circulatory system; final and irreversible cessation of perceptible heartbeat and respiration. Indicators of death include the cessation of the heart's action; absence of reflexes; cessation of electrical activity in the brain as determined by EEG; manifestation of rigor mortis.

death benefit   The amount payable to a beneficiary at the annuitant's, or insured's death. Also called the survivor benefit.

death rate   The number of deaths per 1,000 of the population occurring in a given area within a specified time.

death with dignity   A natural death allowed to occur humanely with no attempt made to prolong life by artificial means. The concept arose in reaction to the ability of modern medical technology to maintain vital functions in, without improving the condition of, persons who are at the point of death.

decubitus ulcer   An ulceration of the skin due to prolonged pressure on the affected area in a patient allowed to lie too long in the same position in bed; a bedsore. The tissues in the area die from lack of blood supply. Areas with prominent bones are at greatest risk. If not treated properly, such an ulcer can progress to the deeper layers of the skin and may eventually affect the underlying muscle and bone.

deductible   The medical costs a patient must incur before MEDICARE or health insurance coverage begins, usually on an annual basis.

"deeming" income and assets   The procedure of lumping together the income of separate nuclear family members who live together in common households (even if they claim not to be sharing income), in determining the eligibility of one of them for a needs-based program. For example, the incomes of spouses, or parent and child, living together are mandatory combined and measured against a two-person eligibility level, rather than to two separate one-person levels.

defendant   The person or entity against whom or which a lawsuit or criminal indicment, is brought.

defense mechanism   A term originating in psychoanalysis, widely used in psychology and psychiatry, for a pattern of feeling, thought, or behavior that arises in response to perceptions of psychic danger, thus enabling a person to avoid conscious awareness of conflicts or anxiety-arousing stressors. Among the most common defense mechanisms are denial, displacement, intellectualization, projection, rationalization, reaction formation, regression, and repression.

definitive diagnosis   A diagnosis established with certainty, without question, as distinct from a presumptive diagnosis, one based on reasonable grounds established by previous experience.

dehydroepiandrosterone (DHEA)/dehydroisoandrosterone
Produced by the adrenal glands, DHEA is the most dominant

steroid hormone in the body. The body converts this mother hormone to whatever particular hormone is needed at any specific time. It has recently been found that the long-term survival of some with HIV may be due to high levels of DHEA in their blood. In HIV patients, AIDS did not develop until the DHEA blood levels dropped. Blood levels of DHEA decrease in the body after the age of 20, and by the age of 80, levels of this substance are 5 percent of that of a 20-year-old. The decline of DHEA in the body appears to allow age-related diseases to appear. DHEA appears to be especially beneficial in treating problems related to memory loss, recall, long-term memory, and Alzheimer's. The hormone increases both estrogen levels in women and testosterone levels in men to those found in younger people, reduces body fat, and reduces risk of breast cancer and cardiovascular disease. It also decreases incidences of strokes, chronic fatigue, multiple sclerosis, and Parkinson's disease, and in general protects against early death. All these conditions affect the elderly population. DHEA is nontoxic and is available in synthetic form by prescription. An all-natural form that is absorbable by the intestine is called Proteusterone. Phytochemicals and meditation increase DHEA levels and are highly recommended.

delavirdine   A nonnucleoside reverse transcriptase inhibitor that, like other NNRTIs, chemically combines with HIV's reverse transcriptase enzyme to block the virus' infection of new cells. Despite its potency when coadministered with indinavir and the fact that adding delavirdine to indinavir makes the latter potent as well, there are several reasons why delavirdine is not a very attractive drug. In the first place, resistant HIV emerges within a few weeks of taking the drug due to a single mutation. That mutation most often occurs at reverse transcriptase's amino acid 103. This same mutation also reduces HIV's sensitivity to Du Pont Merck's experimental and much more active NNRTI DMP 266. Researchers comment that it would be a shame to lose some of the advantages of DMP 226 through previous use of delavirdine. Largely because of its resistance problem, delavirdine provided no statistically significant benefit in two of the three clinical trials that led to its approval.

Then there is the problem that delavirdine therapy requires taking four 100 mg pills three times a day. This comparatively large burden, of course, comes in addition to the other antiviral drugs with which delavirdine must be taken—delavirdine monotherapy is strongly advised against. With the recommended regimen, delavirdine blood levels vary considerably from person to person, and on average women achieve 31 percent higher levels than men.

Thirdly, delavirdine is metabolized by the liver and inhibits the same CYP3A hepatic enzyme that the protease inhibitor ritonavir does, although not to the same extent. Like ritonavir, delavirdine comes with a long list of warnings concerning drugs whose blood levels delavirdine raises due to this suppression of liver metabolism. Delavirdine also causes skin rashes that are usually, but not always, temporary in about 20 percent of patients. Finally, it causes birth defects in rats.

delayed-type hypersensitivity (DTH)   A CELL-MEDIATED immune response producing a cellular infiltrate and edema

that are maximal between 24 and 48 hours after antigen challenge. This term includes the delayed skin reactions associated with type IV hypersensitivity. DTH, which is the process involved in the reaction to poison ivy and poison oak, is often used in tests of immune system function.

delirium   A state of mental confusion and disorder characterized by the inability to focus attention, disorientation, incoherent speech, sensory misperceptions, disturbance in motor skills, and memory impairment. Forms of delirium vary with the cause (infection, fever, drug overdose or side effect, shock, trauma, or metabolic disturbance).

delta-9-tetrahydrocannabinol (THC)   The psychoactive ingredient in MARIJUANA. A synthetic version is sold as a drug under the name DRONABINOL as an appetite stimulant for HIV/AIDS patients and to relieve the side effects of cancer chemotherapy.

deltacortisone   See PREDNISONE.

dementia   An organic mental disorder characterized by a loss of intellectual abilities interfering with social or occupational function. AIDS DEMENTIA COMPLEX (ADC) is a complicated syndrome made up of different nervous system and mental symptoms found somewhat commonly in people with HIV disease. The frequency of ADC increases with advancing disease. It is thought to be fairly uncommon in persons with early HIV disease but is found more frequently in AIDS patients with system-wide symptoms.

AIDS dementia affects not only the survival times of people with AIDS, but their quality of life as well. The course of AIDS dementia is variable, and currently there is no way to predict the pace of its progression. It may progress rapidly to severe deterioration and death, or there may be prolonged periods of stability. Intercurrent illnesses and infections may precipitate delirium and induce forgetfulness, mental slowing, loss of concentration, social withdrawal, and loss of physical coordination. In the late stages of the disease there is significant global deterioration of cognitive and motor functions and severe psychomotor retardation. These symptoms are likely to be present at the same time as systemic AIDS-related opportunistic infections, further complicating treatment.

ADC consists of many progressive conditions that can be mistaken for symptoms of other problems, such as depression, drug-induced side effects, or opportunistic infections that affect the brain, like TOXOPLASMOSIS or LYMPHOMA. Symptoms of ADC may include poor concentration, forgetfulness, loss of short- or long-term memory, social withdrawal, slowed thinking, short attention span, irritability, apathy, weakness, poor coordination, impaired judgment, and personality change, to name a few. Because there are many different manifestations of ADC, the syndrome is poorly understood and has been reported and described in a variety of conflicting ways.

Since 1985, when the term was coined, AIDS dementia complex has been added to the list of AIDS-defining illnesses and the concept further refined for by the CENTERS FOR DISEASE CONTROL AND PREVENTION. Even so, diagnosing the illness is still dependent on the keen judgment of doctors. The main way to detect and evaluate ADC is a test called the mental status examination, which is designed to reveal problems such as short- or long-term memory loss, disorientation, lack of concentration, and mood swings. In addition, certain laboratory tests can be useful, including examination of CEREBROSPINAL FLUID (CSF) obtained by a SPINAL TAP. Most patients with ADC have mild elevations of certain proteins and of white blood cells, which are detected by CSF\ examination.

CAT scans, MRI scans, and SPECT scans are also helpful in the detection of ADC. CAT scans usually show signs of atrophy of brain tissue. MRI (magnetic resonance imaging) is a sensitive but very expensive brain scan used when CAT findings are inconclusive. MRIs usually detect white matter disease in the brain. SPECT scans (single photon emission computed tomograms) use a radioactive material to measure blood flow in the brain and may be useful to detect early HIV dementia. SPECT scans can also follow the response of senses to antiviral therapy by determining whether the therapy has improved the blood flow in the brain. These tests can also help differentiate ADC from other brain disorders such as CRYPTOCOCCAL MENINGITIS, toxoplasmosis, lymphoma, or PML.

The cause of AIDS dementia remains unknown, and the direct role of the HIV virus in it is unclear. In general, such central nervous system and mental disorders are caused by the death of nerve cells, and it has been demonstrated that HIV does not directly infect nerve cells. It is thought that it is somehow able to kill them indirectly. Because of this lack of understanding, and the absence of reliable data on the incidence of ADC, treatments have been extremely slow in coming, even compared to treatments for other AIDS-related conditions. Agents that have been identified as useful in treating ADC include the anti-HIV drug AZT, which has been shown to reduce the risk of productive HIV infection of the brain (it is also known that early discontinuance of AZT leaves patients vulnerable to HIV ENCEPHALITIS). ddI and ddC also need to be thoroughly evaluated for their usefulness in treating ADC. To treat the symptoms of persons with ADC, the full range of psychoactive drugs is used, including antipsychotics, antidepressants, anxiolytics, psychostimulants, antimanics, and anticonvulsants. These drugs, however, do not affect the underlying condition or stop its progression.

demography   The statistical and quantitative science dealing with the age, density, distribution, growth, size, and vital statistics of human populations. Demographic study has shown that rates of disease progression and survival among HIV-infected individuals are determined by access to good medical care, rather than by factors such as race, gender, drug use, income, level of education, or insurance status.

demyelinate   To remove or destroy the myelin sheath surrounding a nerve or nerves, interrupting the transmission of nerve impulses.

dendrite   One of many cytoplasmic processes branching from the cell body of a nerve cell and synapsing with other neurons. Several hundred boutons may form synaptic connections with a single cell and its dendrites.

dendritic cells   A set of antigen-presenting cells present in EPITHELIAL structures and LYMPH NODES, SPLEEN, and (at low levels) BLOOD. Dendritic cells are particularly active in presenting antigen and stimulating T CELLS. Four types of dendritic cells are recognized: follicular dendritic cells in the lymph nodes, lymphoid dendritic cells, interdigitating cells, and Langerhans cells of the skin.

denial   The conscious refusal to admit something; an unconscious defense mechanism in which the existence of anxiety-producing realities are kept out of conscious awareness.

Elisabeth Kübler-Ross, the prominent student of death and dying, believes there are five stages people go through after they learn they are dying. These are denial and isolation; anger; bargaining; depression; and acceptance. Kübler-Ross notes that denial, at least partial denial, occurs in almost all patients, not only during the early stages of illness or immediately following an explicit diagnosis but also later on from time to time. She notes that denial functions as a buffer after unexpected shocking news, allows the patient to collect him- or herself, and, with time, mobilize other less radical defenses. Denial is temporary and is replaced by partial acceptance. Kübler-Ross adds that denial maintained until the end does not necessarily bring increased distress, but that most patients do not maintain it too long.

dental dam   A 150 mm (6-inch)-square piece of thin latex, available in dental and medical supply stores made for use in oral surgery. Dental dams are widely used as a barrier for oral, vaginal or anal sex, by men and women. After being rinsed to remove any talc or other substance, and then dried, the dam is stretched across the entire VULVA (including the CLITORIS, VAGINA, and LABIA) for CUNNILINGUS or the ANUS for ANILINGUS and held in place with the fingers. A water-based lubricant smeared on the side of the shield against the vulva increases sensation and helps to keep the dam in place. Oil-based lubricants weaken latex and can cause dams or condoms to break. Generous lubrication of the vagina or anus also helps to increase pleasure. Dental dams prevent blood, vaginal secretions, or fecal matter from being transferred between partners. Turning the dam inside out during sex will totally defeat the purpose. Similarly, moving the barrier back and forth between the vagina and anus can transfer infections.

Safer sex guidelines targeted toward women who know that their HIV status is positive and who have sex with men stress the use of dental dams and more private barrier methods, such as a sponge, diaphragm, or spermicidal creams or foams, to help decrease infection. Safer sex guidelines for women who know that their HIV status is positive and who have sex with women advise the use of dental dams to cover the vagina or anus for oral sex. Plastic wrap is often recommended as a substitute for a dental dam, if the latter cannot be found. Women who are sensitive or allergic to latex will need to use alternatives.

Some guidelines suggest a dental dam should be used only once, then discarded. Most sources, however, describe ways of cleaning it safely for reuse. Washing it in a 10 percent bleach solution is often recommended, but can cause skin irritation, so washing in a warm solution of mild detergent followed by a cold rinse may be preferred. Dry flat on a clean towel or tissue. Check for holes by holding up against the light. Color codes for each partner can help identify which one is whose. Marking one side avoids confusion over which side should be in contact with the mouth.

deoxynojirimycin   A plant alkaloid that, in the laboratory, inhibits cell-to-cell spread and formation of nucleated protoplasmic mass induced by the HUMAN IMMUNODEFICIENCY VIRUS.

deoxyribonucleic acid (DNA)   A self-replicating molecule, the major constituent of chromosomes, containing the hereditary information transmitted from parents to offspring in all living organisms apart from some viruses (including the AIDS virus). DNA consists of two strands coiled into a double helix linked by hydrogen bonds between the complementary chemical bases that encode the genetic information—between adenine and thymine and between cytosine and guanine. Recombinant DNA is a hybrid DNA formed by joining pieces of DNA from different organisms.

Department of Health and Human Services (HHS)   The cabinet-level federal agency responsible for almost all health and welfare programs; includes the Health Care Financing Administration, PUBLIC HEALTH SERVICE, and SOCIAL SECURITY ADMINISTRATION.

Department of Housing and Urban Development (HUD)
The cabinet-level federal agency that operates the public housing, rent supplement, low-income housing assistance, and FEDERAL HOUSING ACT and HUD mortgage insurance programs.

Department of Veterans Affairs (VA)   A cabinet-level federal agency that operates a variety of income and medical care programs for certain disabled veterans, some other veterans, and in some cases, their dependents.

dependent variable   See VARIABLE.

Depo-Provera   MEDROXYPROGESTERONE acetate.

depression   A decrease or lowering of a functional activity or vital function; a mental state denoted by an altered mood and characterized by feelings of despair, discouragement, guilt, hopelessness, helplessness, the inability to cope, low self-esteem, and sadness. Depression often results in withdrawal from activities usually found to be pleasurable. It may also cause sleep disturbances and changes in eating patterns and energy levels; it may range in intensity from a general feeling of "the blues" to major clinical depression.

The term *depression* is used to describe various conditions, including transient moods, mild but persistent sadness, and clinical illness. Clinical depression is defined as a cluster of symptoms that occur together daily for a certain period of time. The main forms of depressive disorder are major depression, which is often episodic, and dysthymia, which is a milder chronic condition.

The diagnosis of major depression, as defined in current psychiatric standards, requires the presence of at least five of nine specific symptoms during one two-week period. These must include either the first or second of the following: depressed mood; markedly diminished interest/pleasure in almost all activities; significant unintentional weight gain or loss; insomnia or oversleeping; fidgeteness or slowed movement or speech; fatigue or loss of energy; feelings of worthlessness or excessive or inappropriate guilt; diminished ability to think or concentrate; and recurrent suicidal thoughts. The task of diagnosis in an HIV-positive person is complicated, since several of these symptoms could be caused by the HIV virus, HIV-related conditions, or even HIV medications. Furthermore, the diagnosis cannot be made if the disturbance is a "normal reaction" to the death of a loved one. However, if focused queries are made by a clinician with experience in depression and HIV illness, it is possible to obtain a reliable diagnosis in the context of HIV.

It has been suggested but not demonstrated that HIV itself causes mood changes and that AIDS-related DEMENTIA induces depression. Another important question is whether HIV drugs such as AZT induce mood changes. In practice, it is extremely difficult to distinguish between the symbolic effects of starting antiviral treatment with its direct chemical effects. In later stages of HIV illness it becomes even more difficult to identify effects of any one medication on mood, since as a rule many are taken simultaneously. Patients may experience mood changes in association with medication, but no specific impact on mood has been documented.

Clinical depression is the most commonly observed psychiatric disorder among people with HIV illness. The available research literature indicates that HIV-positive depressed patients can tolerate standard doses of antidepressant medications such as Prozac. Psychostimulants, such as methylphenidate (Ritalin) or dexedrine, have also been prescribed. Therapy and group therapy can also be of benefit to patients with depression.

dermatitis   Inflammation of the skin.

dermatitis medicamentosa   See DRUG ERUPTION.

desensitization   The process of reducing a patient's allergic responsiveness to an antigen through a protocol of repeated injections of that allergen, or modified allergen. Desensitization procedures have become common when administering BACTRIM for the first time. Also known as *hyposensitization*.

desmopressin acetate   A VASOPRESSIN analog with antidiuretic (water retention) properties used in the treatment of DIABETES INSIPIDUS. Also used before surgery to increase FACTOR VIII (the factor contributing to the intrinsic value of blood coagulation) in hemophiliacs or patients with Von Willebrand's disease. Desmopressin acetate has greater antidiuretic activity than vasopressin but less pressor activity. Trade names are DDAVP and Stimate Injection.

detoxification   Reduction of the toxic properties of a poisonous substance; the process of reducing the physiological effects of a drug or other toxic substance in an addicted individual.

detumescence   The process of losing an erection; deflation of the penis.

developmentally oriented care   Care based on an individual's functional level and chronological age. Functional level includes physical, cognitive, psychosocial, and communicative development.

dexamethasone   A synthetic steroid hormone, similar to those produced by the adrenal glands. Like other CORTICO-STEROIDS, dexamethasone has a wide range of biological actions. It is used most frequently for its anti-inflammatory effects, but it is also a potent inhibitor of certain immune responses. Dexamethasone is used to treat a variety of conditions, including arthritis and other rheumatic diseases, connective-tissue disease, respiratory disease, skin disorders, allergic reactions, inflammation of the eyes, certain blood disorders, inflammation of the brain, and, as a palliative, in certain cancers. In people with HIV it is commonly used alone to counteract allergic drug reactions and as part of a combination chemotherapy for the treatment of AIDS-related lymphoma. Dexamethasone is available in a number of formulations, including tablets or liquid, topical creams or lotions, ointments for administration to the eyes, inhalants, and as a solution for injection. Stomach upset, indigestion, and weight gain are common side effects of dexamethasone. More serious side effects usually occur only with high doses taken for prolonged periods. Trade names are Decadron and SK-Dexamethasone.

dextran sulfate   A complex sugar compound used in Japan to treat atherosclerosis, and which showed promise in the test tube as a potential synergizer of the effects of AZT. Such an effect would allow for the use of lower, presumably less toxic doses of that drug. In a trial, however, the drug demonstrated no antiviral or clinical immunological efficacy. In addition, physicians in clinical practice have observed severe side effects such as gastrointestinal bleeding, since dextran sulfate breaks down in the body into sulfuric acid.

dextroamphetamine sulfate   Dextroamphetamine sulfate is an amphetamine, which, as with METHYLPHENIDATE hydrochloride (RITALIN hydrochloride), stimulates the brain. It is usually given to people with AIDS dementia complex to counter the symptoms of apathy and social withdrawal. The most common side effects are nervousness and insomnia. Both can usually be controlled by decreasing the dose and by not taking the drug late in the day.

DHEA   See DEHYDROPIANDROSTERONE (DHEA)/DEHYDRO-ISOANDROSTERONE.

DHPG   See GANCICLOVIR.

DHT   See DELAYED-TYPE HYPERSENSITIVITY (DTH).

diabetes   A general term for diseases characterized by excessive urination. The term usually refers to diabetes mellitus, a chronic disorder of carbohydrate metabolism, characterized by hyperglycemia and glycosuria and resulting from inadequate production or utilization of insulin.

diabetes insipidus   A metabolic disorder caused by damage to the neurohypophyseal system (the main portion of the posterior lobe of the pituitary gland). This results in deficient production or release of antidiuretic hormone (vasopressin). As a result, the individual experiences uncontrollable excessive thirst and urination. In almost half of all cases, the cause is unknown. Trauma to the head that causes pituitary damage and tumors in the pituitary region account for the remainder of cases.

diacetylmorphine   The chemical designation for HEROIN.

diagnosis   The determination of the nature of a medical condition; the recognition of the presence of a specific disease or infection, usually accomplished by evaluating clinical symptoms and laboratory tests. For AIDS, the presence of antibodies to HIV in the blood is a sign of HIV INFECTION. These antibodies do not destroy the virus, they simply serve as markers of infection. AIDS is diagnosed when opportunistic infections in sites other than the skin and mucous membranes are present.

In 1993, the original classification for HIV infection was revised and the surveillance case definition for AIDS among adolescents and adults was expanded. These changes are important to people who do, indeed, have AIDS but under the original criteria were denied certain medical and economic assistance. The revised criteria include persons who have 200 or fewer CD4 cells or T CELLS per cubic mm of blood. The normal level is about 1,000 per cubic mm. See also AIDS-DEFINING ILLNESS.

There are issues specific to HIV-infected women—gynecologic concerns, gynecologic infections, menstrual disorders, cervical dysplasia and neoplasia, etc., as well as issues specific to pregnant HIV-infected women—prenatal care, intrapartum considerations, postpartum considerations, etc. However, the revised classification for HIV infection and expanded surveillance case definition for AIDS among adolescents and adults does not include a different definition for women. There are in the revised classification, conditions that women present and men do not, such as, for example, cervical cancer.

diagnostic   A means by which to measure or evaluate a patient's medical condition.

dialysis   The process of separating out materials in solution by forcing the solution through a semipermeable membrane. Separation is accomplished because different substances have different rates of diffusion. See also HEMODIALYSIS and PERITONEAL DIALYSIS.

diaminodiphenylsulfone   See DAPSONE.

diapedesis   Passage of blood cells, especially leukocytes, by ameboid movements through the unruptured wall of a capillary vessel.

diaphragm   A contraceptive device in the form of a round or dome-shaped latex object resembling a cap or a cup, which is inserted in the vagina to cover the cervix. It is most effective when used with spermicide. It can also be used as part of an STD risk-reduction strategy. For example, safer sex guidelines for HIV-positive women who have sex with men often suggest that if a man won't use condoms that a diaphragm or other barrier method be used, with spermicidal creams or foams, to prevent pregnancy and to help decrease the risk of infection.

diarrhea   A disturbance in bowel movements characterized by abnormally frequent, loose, or watery stools. Diarrhea is often related to a disturbance in the gastrointestinal system.

diarrhea-wasting syndrome   A term sometimes used to refer to the severe diarrhea characteristically associated with HIV INFECTION. The syndrome (diarrhea persisting for at least a month, accompanied by otherwise unexplained weight loss of 10 percent) in conjunction with HIV infection composes an AIDS-defining illness.

dideoxycytidine (ddC)   A NUCLEOSIDE ANALOG similar to ZIDOVUDINE, but exhibiting less toxicity, that inhibits infection of new cells by HIV. ddC is approved for advanced (CD4 CELL count less than or equal to 300 cells per cubic millimeter) HIV infection in adults who do not tolerate ziduvudine or have progression of their disease while receiving AZT. The drug is not approved for use in patients with CD4 counts less than 150 cells per cubic millimeter. This drug is not a cure for AIDS, and it does not reduce the risk of transmission of HIV infection to others through sexual contact or contamination of blood. Other (unlabeled) generally accepted uses: combination treatment with saquinavir (Invirase) decreases death from AIDS by 70 percent versus single agent treatment with either medicine alone, and ddC may have a role in pediatric AIDS. An orally administered antiviral, ddC works by interfering with essential HIV enzyme systems, and is thought to prevent the growth and replication of HIV particles within infected cells, thus limiting the severity and extent of HIV infection; it is also used in combination with AZT for the treatment of advanced HIV disease. It is thus similar in effect to other nucleoside analogues such as AZT, ddI, d4T, and 3TC. While ddC works by a mechanism similar to AZT, it is not as effective as AZT in delaying disease progression. However, ddC has different side effects and may be useful for people who cannot tolerate AZT. PERIPHERAL NEUROPATHY, which is nerve damage that typically includes numbness, tingling, or sharp burning pain in the feet, legs, or hands, is the most serious side effect of ddC. ddC may also cause severe disease of the pancreas (pancreatitis), which has been fatal in some cases. Other significant, but rare, side effects of ddC include ulcers in the mouth or esophagus, cardiomyopathy/congestive heart failure, and arthritis. Trade name is Hivid. Also called Zalcitabine.

dideoxyinosine (ddI)   A NUCLEOSIDE ANALOG that inhibits infection of new cells by HIV. Clinical studies have determined that ddI is not as effective as AZT in adults who have not previously used antiviral drugs, but it offers an option to individuals intolerant of or failing on AZT or who have taken AZT for sixteen weeks or more. It is also approved for children over six months of age with advanced HIV infec-

tion who cannot tolerate AZT or who have experienced disease progression while on AZT. Side effects can include nerve damage in the hands and feet (peripheral neuropathy), damage to the pancreas (pancreatitis), and diarrhea.

Many physicians don't wait until AZT fails to switch patients to ddI or to add it to their regimen. It is becoming more common for physicians to prescribe a combination of AZT and ddI. This approach is based on studies that show that some forms of resistant virus are less likely to develop on the combination than when either drug is used alone. Results from a number of clinical trials have suggested that switching from AZT to ddI after a number of months of AZT therapy is more effective at slowing disease progression than continuing with AZT, although there is no known "right" time to switch therapies.

ddI can be taken orally as chewable tablets or as a powder dissolved in water. The drug mimics a naturally occurring building block of DNA and works by interfering with HIV replication, thus reducing the production of new virus and slowing the progression of infection. ddI is similar to AZT, but has different side effects. Also called didanosine. Trade name is Videx.

didox   A relatively new drug, which, like TRIMIDOX, is a much more potent inhibitor of ribonucleotide reductase (RR) than hydroxyurea. As of September 1995, trimidox was not yet in clinical trials, but didox had been well tolerated in clinical trials for breast and other cancers. Also as of this date, the drug had not been given to people on a daily chronic basis, but chronic use is well tolerated in baboons with sickle-cell anemia.

diet supplements   There are many different causes for nutrient deficiencies in people living with HIV: the high demand for antioxidants, the increased metabolism that begins in the earliest disease stages, malabsorption because of damage to the intestines, decreased intake of food because of mouth or throat problems, loss of appetite, loss of taste, fever, nausea, and vomiting. The resulting deficiencies are often of important nutrients critical for supporting immune function. The use of antibiotics and other medications that destroy the body's "friendly" gastrointestinal bacteria also cause nutrient deficiencies. Gastrointestinal bacteria are necessary for the breakdown and absorption of certain food substances. Without them, foods cannot be digested properly and become useless to the body as a source of nutrients. Moreover, maldigested food may cause other problems, including diarrhea. Gastrointestinal bacteria also produce several different vitamins, including thiamin, riboflavin, niacin, pantothenic acid, vitamin B_6, VITAMIN B_{12}, folic acid, choline, biotin, and vitamin K.

People with HIV are usually advised to take a multiple vitamin–mineral supplement that supplies the basic level of nutrients most important to body function. Many nutritionists believe that additional supplements are necessary. Symptoms that may be related to nutrient deficiencies and may be reversible with appropriate supplementation include serious fatigue, memory loss or other cognitive dysfunction, skin problems, NEUROPATHY, weight loss, loss of the senses of smell or taste, appetite loss, muscle pain or cramps, digestive problems, night blindness, canker sores, constipation, DEPRESSION, anxiety, menstrual cramps, and menopausal problems. Many other symptoms in people living with HIV may be related to nutrient deficiencies.

diethylcarbamazine citrate   A drug used in treating filarial infections.

differential diagnosis   Diagnosis based on comparison of symptoms of two or more similar diseases to determine the cause of illness.

digital-anal sex   Erotic stimulation of the anus with a finger or fingers.

dihydroxpropoxymethyl (DHPG)   See GANCYCLOVIR.

diiodohydroxyquin   See IODIOQUINOL.

dildo   An artificial erect penis used as a sexual aid.

Dinacrin   See ISONIAZID.

dinitrochlorobenzene (DNCB)   A potent topical contact sensitizer, DNCB has been used as an alternative treatment for HIV since 1986. Studies have shown that, when used regularly, DNCB will boost the immune response resulting in increased numbers of CYTOTOXIC T LYMPHOCYTEs (CTL) and NATURAL KILLER CELLs. DNCB is one of the very few therapeutic agents that have been observed to have a direct impact on the generation and activation of cytotoxic T cells, a goal of cellular immunology. DENDRITIC CELLS in the tissue were identified in the early '90s as the primary antigen-presenting cells of the body and are now known to carry a significantly large portion of the body's viral burden of HIV and other disease-causing agents. Impairment of these cells' activity by the loss of delayed-type hypersensitivity is one of the earliest and most consistent symptoms of HIV infection after SEROCONVERSION.

Topical application of DNCB modulates the activity of epidermal Langerhans and dendritic cells, initiating a systemic delayed-type sensitivity reaction throughout the body. The Langerhans cells in the skin at the application site pick up the DNCB antigen, migrate from the skin, change into veiled dendritic cells, continue their migration to the nearest lymph node, and change into interdigitating dendritic cells. Once in the lymph nodes, they present the DNCB antigen to CD4 helper cells, initiating what is called alternately a Th1 response, cell-mediated immune response, or Type IV delayed-type hypersensitivity response.

The CD4 helper cells proliferate forming more CD4 helper cells, which then circulate and activate effector cells (primary macrophages) to rid the system of the DNCB antigen. At the same time, CD4 memory cells are produced, adding to the CD4 memory pool for the DNCB antigen. Each time DNCB is applied, these memory cells are activated thus initiating a systemic Th1 response to DNCB. The longer DNCB is used, the faster, more potent, and more effective the response becomes, as there are more circulating DNCB CD4 memory cells to initiate the immune response.

The result of this specific systemic TH1 RESPONSE to DNCB is the nonspecific activation of macrophages. Many of these macrophages are infected with HIV and other intracellular pathogens that cause AIDS but are unable to present these pathogens antigens due to infection. The microbial pathogens of AIDS are of the facultative or obligate intracellular type. The activation of these macrophages results in proteolysis of the pathogens, which are then presented by macrophages to CD4 and CD8 memory cells specific for the presented pathogen. The activated helper and cytotoxic T lymphocytes initiate specific systemic responses to destroy the presented pathogens. This results in more activated macrophages, more pathogens presented, more T-memory cells activated, more infected cells destroyed, ad infinitum.

Antibiotics, nucleoside analogs, and other drug treatments can interfere with the cell-mediated immune response and negate the systemic action initiated by DNCB. Drugs required for the treatment of infections must be continued until the infections are cleared or controlled. Prophylactic drugs can impair the immune response and might interfere with the immune boosting properties of DNCB. Individuals with AIDS must use PCP prophylaxis. The need, amount, and dosing schedule for other prophylactic drugs and treatments that suppress absolute CD8 counts should be given serious consideration.

Further investigation into its apparent ability to slow or eliminate decline in AIDS is warranted. Its negligible cost, easy accessibility, and lack of toxicity make DNCB a treatment worth serious consideration by anyone living with HIV. Research in the early '90s showed that there is no latency period in HIV infection, as was previously thought. Since the virus is continually replicating in the lymph nodes, initiation of treatment with DNCB is recommended by researchers as early as possible after sero-conversion.

Diodoquin   See IODOQUINOL.

dipstick test   A test to determine the presence of protein, glucose, or other substances in urine by dipping a chemically impregnated strip of paper into a urine sample.

dipyridamole   A blood-thinning drug long used in heart disease, which has also been shown to potentiate the activity of NUCLEOSIDE ANALOG by reducing the entry of competing natural nucleosides into the cell. Further studies are needed to establish the long-term safety and effectiveness of dipyridamole in combination with AZT, although researchers have been unable to secure financial support from the manufacturer, possibly because the drug's patent has expired.

direct fluorescent antibody staining   A specific test (performed on a biopsy sample) for TREPONEMA PALLIDUM, the organism that causes SYPHILIS. The presence of *T. pallidum* organisms in lesions of early acquired or congenital syphilis is the definitive means of making a diagnosis of syphilis.

directly observed therapy (DOT)   A process by which a patient takes a medication while under direct observation by another individual. Usually used in antituberculosis treatment.

disability   Qualification for disability benefits under Social Security is based on an individual's medical condition. An individual is considered disabled if, because of such condition, he or she is unable to earn a "substantial" income in work for which he or she is suited. Usually, monthly earnings of $500 or more are considered substantial. Inability to work must be expected to last at least a year, or the condition must be so severe that the victim is not expected to live. The Social Security Administration also decides how a condition affects children's ability to function—to do the things and behave in the ways that other children of the same age normally would.

Social Security works with an agency in each state, usually called a Disability Determination Service (DDS), to evaluate disability claims. At the DDS, a disability evaluation specialist and a doctor follow a step-by-step process that applies to all disability claims, thus assuring a consistent national approach. First, the DDS specialists decide whether an individual's impairment is severe. This simply means the evidence must show that the disability interferes with the individual's ability to work. The next step is deciding whether the impairment is included in an approved list. This list describes, for each of the major body systems, impairments that are considered severe enough to prevent an adult from doing any substantial work, or in the case of children under the age of 18, impairments that are severe enough to prevent a child from functioning in a manner similar to other children of the same age.

Because HIV research is a dynamic process and medical knowledge concerning the disease and its symptoms is constantly growing, Social Security continually updates its evaluation criteria for HIV infection. If an individual has symptoms of HIV infection that are not specifically included in (or equivalent to) Social Security's current guidelines, then DDS disability specialists will evaluate all medical evidence to determine ability to work. They will be looking for documentation of signs, symptoms, and laboratory findings that can result from HIV infection. They will also look for evidence of restrictions in daily activities caused by HIV infection. If a disability decision cannot be made on medical factors alone, the DDS specialists evaluate a variety of physical and/or mental limitations that may prevent an individual from working.

Recent developments in Social Security's evaluation process include guidelines that recognize that HIV can show up differently in women than in men, and differently in children than in adults, and differently in younger than in older children (13 or above). When assessing the degree to which the disease affects a woman's ability to function, DDS disability evaluators consider gynecological problems such as vulvovaginal candidiasis, GENITAL HERPES, PELVIC INFLAMMATORY DISEASE and CERVICAL CANCER.

disability discrimination law   In the early 1980s, there was no existing body of legal precedent regarding discrimination based on a contagious medical condition. As the epidemic progressed and such discrimination increased against people with HIV/AIDS, the courts and legislatures responded by adapting disability discrimination law to this new problem. The process culminated in 1990 with the enactment of the federal AMERICANS WITH DISABILITIES ACT

(ADA), which has become the basic law governing HIV-related discrimination in employment, public services, and public accommodations as its various provisions have gone into effect during the 1990s. The act applies broadly to businesses and individuals providing goods and services to the public, employers of fifteen or more employees, and most federal and state agencies.

Under the REHABILITATION ACT OF 1973, an "individual with handicaps" is "any person who (i) has a physical or mental impairment which substantially limits one or more of such person's major life activities, (ii) has a record of such an impairment, or (iii) is regarded as having such an impairment." The ADA defines a "disability" as "(A) A physical or mental impairment that substantially limits one or more . . . major life activities. . .; (B) a record of such an impairment; or (C) being regarded as having such an impairment." HIV infection and AIDS have come to be considered handicaps or disabilities by most administrative agencies and courts considering discrimination claims.

disability-related inquiries   What prescription drugs are you currently taking? Have you ever been treated for mental health problems? How many days were you sick last year? Do you have a disability that may affect your performance on the job? Do you have AIDS?

Historically, many employers have felt free to request such information concerning a job applicant's physical or mental condition. However, with the passage of the Americans with Disabilities Act, these questions may not legally be asked at an initial interview. Employers may not ask about the existence, nature or severity of a disability, or require a medical examination, until after a conditional offer of employment has been made. At the preoffer stage, the employer is entitled to ask only about an applicant's ability to perform the essential functions of the job. Congress intended the ADA's restriction against preemployment inquiries to prevent discrimination against individuals with "hidden" disabilities, like cancer, epilepsy, and HIV/AIDS. The ADA's prohibition against preemployment questioning and examinations ensures that the applicant's hidden disability is not considered prior to the assessment of the applicant's nonmedical qualifications. After a conditional offer is made, employers may require medical examinations and may make disability-related inquiries, if they do so for all entering employees in that job category.

disability insurance   Insurance that replaces income for individuals unable to work because of accident or sickness.

discharge   To release from care by a physician, other medical care worker, or a medical care facility.

The secretion or excretion from the body of pus, feces, urine, etc.; the material thus ejected.

disclosure   The revelation of a diagnosis of HIV or AIDS. Disclosure of such a diagnosis to someone other than a person with the illness involves issues of public health, social convention, and civil liberties. See PRIVACY.

disclosure counseling   The news that one has been infected with HIV isn't easy to receive. Individuals who have tested positive will have many questions about their condition and its impact on their lives. Post-disclosure counseling is intended to help them come to terms with their diagnosis and to prepare them to deal with their illness in a practical way.

Typical questions include: Why me? Am I contagious to others? Is my partner positive? Is he or she immune? What do symptomatic and asymptomatic mean? Whom should I tell? What should I tell my sexual or needle-sharing partners? What should I tell my doctor and dentist, my family, my employer, my insurer? Will information in my medical records be confidential? Advice is offered concerning medical follow-up, staying healthy, and stopping the spread of the disease. The complexities of disclosure may also be addressed. See PRIVACY.

discourse   See CULTURAL ANALYSIS AND AIDS.

discrimination   Disadvantageous treatment, either overt or insidious, of individuals or groups that results in the unequal treatment of or the denial of opportunities to these people. The stigma associated with AIDS has prompted, and continues to prompt, a wide range of individual and social reactions to persons with AIDS and HIV infection. HIV-infected people have the same civil and social rights as the noninfected. Examples of these rights include access to justice; public benefits (programs such as Social Security Disability Income and Supplemental Security Income); confidentiality (as regards testing, donor disclosure, and access to donor medical records, etc.); education (the rights of both HIV-infected students to be able to attend public schools and of HIV-infected teachers to be able to remain the heads of their classes, etc.); employment (the rights of persons with HIV/AIDS to work as long as they are able, etc.); free speech (the right to publish and disseminate AIDS education materials, etc.); housing; immigration; insurance (the right to coverage for health care costs, the right to life insurance coverage, etc.); public accommodations; and professional regulation.

Laws related to AIDS, such as statutes enacted and cases reported, are the most visible evidence of how U.S. society is dealing with AIDS- and HIV-related discrimination. Discrimination laws provide a legal foundation for the rights of people with HIV infection and AIDS. Whether or not this foundation is really adequate to ensure that people with HIV infection and AIDS receive the humane treatment to which everyone is entitled as a basic human right is another issue entirely. The statutes provide limited remedies, and their administration frequently takes more time than people with HIV infection or AIDS can afford to wait. Examples of federal protections include the Americans with Disabilities Act, which passed the United States Senate on September 7, 1989, and the Fair Housing Rehabilitation Act of 1973, Public Law 93–12, Section 504. In addition to federal protections, there are a myriad of state and local protections; for example, all 50 states and the District of Columbia have statutes that parallel the federal Rehabilitation Act prohibiting discrimination against handicapped persons.

disease   A pathological condition of the body that presents a group of clinical signs and symptoms and laboratory findings peculiar to it and that sets the condition apart as an abnormal entity differing from other normal or pathological body states. Disease is usually tangible and may even be measured. Illness is highly individual and personal.

disease classification   Disease classification is one of many public health measures that are considered technical, yet have direct consequences for human rights. Classification of a disease as contagious, communicable, transmissible, infectious, or sexually transmitted is only the beginning of a process entailing the application of previously existing laws that may mandate compulsory medical examination or hospitalization, restrictions on travel or immigration, or isolation. Classification can also lead to social stigma, as evidenced by the frequent so-called analogies between AIDS and leprosy.

Even though the scientific literature has pleaded for consistency and precision in disease classification, there is still no uniformity regarding AIDS and HIV infection. Some countries classify HIV/AIDS as a communicable disease, others as infectious disease, still others as a viral disease. Many countries have classified AIDS as a sexually transmitted disease. The World Health Organization (WHO) seems to have passively endorsed this latter approach, arguing that most HIV infections are acquired and transmitted sexually. From the human rights viewpoint, this classification gives public health authorities wide-ranging powers under already existing STD legislation. Coercive and compulsory measures are envisaged in STD; laws are broad, and the stigma associated with sexually transmitted disease means that these laws are rarely challenged.

The main feature of legislation on STDs is their effort to prevent the spread of infection by denying rights to infected individuals. The traditional measures for controlling STDs include compulsory examination, contact tracing, restrictive measures against carriers to prevent further transmission, compulsory treatment and/or hospitalization, and extensive case finding through premarital and prenatal screening. Additionally, immigration regulations enacted for STDs have been applied to AIDS in order to exclude persons who are HIV infected, thus reviving "certificates of freedom from venereal disease."

disease progression   The process of growth, spread and development of symptoms and affects. The median time from HIV infection to development of AIDS in adults is 10 years. Individuals of similar age have highly variable rates of disease progression, a phenomenon that has remained unexplained. A recent study, reported in *Nature* in April 1996, has found multiple genes or gene combinations in human DNA that appear to influence how long a person with HIV infection remains disease free. The genes encode HUMAN LEUKOCYTE ANTIGEN (HLA), molecules that help regulate the immune response to HIV-1. The study focused on products of the MAJOR HISTOCOMPATIBILITY COMPLEX (MHC), a cluster of genes that includes the HLA region. The MHC is important for immune recognition and for immune responsiveness to foreign antigens such as might derive from HIV-1. HLA (or MHC) class 1 markers, found on the surfaces of all nucleated cells and blood platelets, determine the immunologic acceptability of transplanted tissue. HLA (or MHC) class II markers, expressed on B CELLS, MACROPHAGE, and other immune system cells, are required to initiate an immune response to foreign antigens such as HIV-1. Pieces of these foreign antigens are transported across the cell's interior by products of TAP genes (also in the MHC). This study provides further support to the belief that the immune response to HIV is an important factor in determining the rate of HIV-mediated disease progression.

disinfection   The act of freeing from PATHOGENIC organisms, or rendering such organisms inactive, by physical or chemical means. The term is generally used of inanimate objects. Methods of disinfection include moist heat, radiation, filtration, physical cleaning, and the application of chemical substances, including quaternary ammonia compounds (both tincture and aqueous), mercurials, formaldehyde, glutaraldehyde, germicidal soaps, and formaldehyde gas. Three levels of disinfection are covered in the Centers for Disease Control's *Guidelines for Prevention of Transmission of Human Immunodeficiency Virus (HIV) and Hepatitis B Virus (HBV) to Health-Care and Public Safety Workers.* High-level disinfection destroys all forms of microbial life except high numbers of bacterial spores; intermediate-level disinfection kills MYCOBACTERIUM TUBERCULOSIS, vegetative bacteria, most viruses, and most fungi, but not bacterial spores; and low-level disinfection kills most bacteria, some viruses, and some fungi but not mycobacterium tuberculosis or bacterial spores. The *Guidelines* also spells out methods for cleaning, disinfecting, and sterilizing equipment and surfaces at each level.

disorientation   The loss of normal relationship to one's surroundings; confusion about time, place, and identity.

disregards (of assets or income)   Amounts, values, or percentages of an applicant's assets or income that needs-based programs do not count in determining eligibility for benefits.

disseminated tuberculosis   MYCOBACTERIUM TUBERCULOSIS that has spread from the primary focus of infection through the blood or LYMPHATIC SYSTEM.

distal   Remote, away from the point of origin.

distal symmetric polyneuropathy (DSPN)   A disease of the nerves that manifests as subacute onset of numbness or tingling in the fingers or toes. Early clinical signs are bilaterally depressed ankle reflex and impaired sensation in the toes.

disulfiram   In orally administered drug used in the treatment of alcoholism. Ingestion of alcohol after taking this drug causes severe reactions, including nausea and vomiting, and may endanger the life of the patient. Disulfiram is widely known under its proprietary name, Antabuse.

diuretic   A drug or other agent that promotes excretion of urine, resulting in the loss of water from the body.

DNA   See DEOXYRIBONUCLEIC ACID.

DNA polymerase alpha   An enzyme essential to the life of a cell for its synthetic and repair functions.

DNA polymerase beta   An enzyme with repair functions in the life of a cell.

DNA polymerase gamma   An ENZYME consisting of cells that contain small granules or rod-shaped structures found in differential staining of the cytoplasm.

DNAR   See DO NOT ATTEMPT RESUSCITATION.

DNCB   See DINITROCHLOROBENZENE.

DNR   See DO NOT RESUSCITATE.

dogfish shark   Any of several small sharks that are destructive to food fishes. A compound isolated from dogfish shark has been found to dramatically inhibit HIV replication in the test tube without disrupting CD4+ T cell proliferation and other normal cellular activities. The compound works by blocking a process central to cellular activation—the exchange of ions across the cell membrane. The compound is known as MSI-1436.

do not attempt resuscitation (DNAR)   An order somewhat more precise than DO NOT RESUSCITATE (DNR). DNAR indicates resuscitation efforts should not be attempted regardless of expected outcomes of those efforts.

do not resuscitate (DNR)   An instruction given by a patient or family member not to administer cardiopulmonary resuscitation to the patient on the apparent cessation of life. Such an order can be made effective both within and outside a hospital setting. DNR implies that if a resuscitation attempt is made, the patient could be revived.

donor insemination   See ARTIFICIAL INSEMINATION.

dormancy   The period when an infectious organism is in the body but not yet producing ill effects. See LATENCY.

Dornan Amendment   Attached to the 1996 defense authorization bill, a regulation put forth by Rep. Robert K. Dornan (R-Calif.) that would have discharged military service members with HIV and denied them medical benefits. President Clinton reluctantly signed the defense bill into law, but said the Dornan measure was unconstitutional and ordered governmental lawyers not to oppose legal challenges to it. In April 1996, the leadership of both the Senate and House turned against the measure and killed it after it became clear that the U.S.'s military's entire command structure opposed it. Service members with HIV have been banned from combat and overseas duty since the mid-1980s.

dosage   The size, frequency, and number of doses of a drug.

dose   The amount of a drug that is given at one time.

dose escalation   A preliminary clinical trial technique in which the amount of a drug is either periodically increased or increased with each new trial arm that is added. The test is done to determine how a drug is tolerated.

dose ranging   A drug trial technique in which two or more different doses of a drug are tested against each other to determine which works best and is the least harmful.

double blind   See DOUBLE-BLIND STUDY.

double-blind study   A kind of clinical study in which neither the experimenter nor the subjects know until after the data have been collected what treatment has been applied to which subjects. This type of study employing an experimental drug and a placebo, is used in drug trials to avoid contamination of the results from the biases and preconceptions of experimenters or subjects. Double-blind studies are believed to promote faster and more objective results, since they control for the possibility of bias.

double standard   See SEXUAL DOUBLE STANDARD.

douche   A liquid that is put into a woman's vagina and then expelled in order to flush out any loose material that may be inside. A douche may be used to rinse out a person's rectum, in which case it is called an ENEMA.

douching   Application of a DOUCHE.

Doxil   See DOX-SL.

doxorubicin   A wide-spectrum antineoplastic antibiotic agent. A long-lasting version of doxorubicin, DOX-SL, may prove beneficial to people whose KAPOSI'S SARCOMA does not respond to other approved treatments. Encapsulated in protective LIPOSOMES (fat globules), this drug tends to concentrate in KS lesions, where it is gradually released.

DOX-SL (Doxil)   An antibiotic agent used in chemotherapy for KAPOSI'S SARCOMA, consisting of a preparation of doxorubicin encapsulated in LIPOSOMES which deliver significantly greater quantities of doxorubicin to the KS lesions than the standard treatment while reducing the drug's side effects. DOX-SL incorporates so-called stealth liposomes, whose polyethylene glycol (PEG) coating gives them greater stability in the bloodstream. Side effects include nausea, vomiting, stomatitis, diarrhea, and hair loss. DOX-SL causes a significant amount of neutropenia, which can be managed with G-CSF (Neupogen).

doxycycline   A broad-spectrum antibiotic of the TETRACYCLINE group. Trade name Vibramycin.

DPT vaccine   A vaccine used for diphtheria, pertussis, and tetanus.

drip   See GONORRHEA.

dronabinol   An appetite stimulant composed of synthetic THC (DELTA-9-TETRAHYDROCANNABINOL), the psychoactive component of MARIJUANA. It is used to treat weight loss caused by loss of appetite in people with AIDS. It is also used to treat nausea and vomiting caused by cancer chemotherapy in people who have not responded to other treatment.

Dronabinol affects the central nervous system, altering appetite, mood, thinking, memory, and perception. The effects of dronabinol are the same as those of natural THC. They are dose related, and the response varies from person to person. Consequently, the dose must be adjusted for each person. The drug is a central nervous system depressant and may impair a person's ability to drive an automobile or operate dangerous machinery. It should not be used with alcohol or other depressants such as BENZODIAZEPINEs or BARBITURATEs. It should be used cautiously in people with a history of cardiac disease, since it may cause low blood pressure, rapid heartbeat, or fainting. Because dronabinol affects the nervous system, it may worsen mania, depression, or schizophrenia. Mood shifts, and less frequently, hallucinations, may occur. These effects are reversible and disappear when the drug is stopped. The most common side effects of dronabinol are of the central nervous system, including elation, easy laughing, dizziness, confusion, and drowsiness. Again, these are generally dose related and reversible when the drug is stopped. Trade names: Marinol and Deltanyne.

drug abuse   The (generally self-administered) use or overuse of a drug in a manner other than that for which it is intended or prescribed. A drug of abuse may be legal or illicit, addictive or not. (In common usage, the terms *drug abuse* and *drug use* are synonymous. Drug use is rarely used to refer to legitimate medical use of drugs.) Serious drug abusers are those in bad relationships with drugs, those who have great difficulty with them. A large proportion of drug abusers are compulsive, addicted, or chaotic drug users. There are six key relationships between drug use and HIV/AIDS. The first, and most obvious, is that HIV is efficiently transmitted by sharing drug injection paraphernalia.

The second relationship between drug use and HIV/AIDS involves the sex-drug link. The use of COCAINE, for example, in any form, has effects on the libido. In early cocaine use, the libido is stimulated, resulting in more sexual activity; with frequent high-dose use of cocaine, the neurochemical dopamine becomes depleted, resulting in a loss of sexual desire. Additionally, many high-dose users of cocaine, for example crack-cocaine users, begin to sell sex for crack or for money to buy crack. They are often young teenagers of both genders and various sexual orientations who enter into unprotected sexual encounters resulting in SEXUALLY TRANSMITTED DISEASES, including HIV INFECTION. There is a strong link between sexually transmitted diseases, particularly those that involve genital lesions, and HIV because these infections and lesions seem to facilitate HIV transmission.

A third link between drug use and HIV is that the use of any mood-altering substance often results in unsafe sexual activity. The effects of drugs can reduce inhibition, cloud judgment, result in memory lapses (called "blackouts"), and lead to false feelings of safety and lack of concern about HIV. This is an important link even for those who are experimenters with or only occasional users of drugs of abuse.

A fourth link between drug use and HIV involves the IMMUNOSUPPRESSIVE qualities of some drugs. Alcohol, cocaine, amphetamines, and inhalant nitrates are believed to damage the immune system, leaving frequent users immune-suppressed and possibly more likely to have HIV exposure result in HIV infection. In addition, if drug users do become HIV-infected, HIV spectrum disease may progress faster than in those who do not have a history of immune-suppressive drug use.

The fifth link between drug use and HIV/AIDS is the pediatric connection. The vast majority of pediatric AIDS cases in the United States have resulted from prenatal transmission in which one or both parents is or was a needle drug user.

Lastly, the role of injection routes and adulterated drugs should not be ignored. The needle route of drug administration results in a hole in the skin. Since drug users often reuse disposable syringes and needles without the proper sterilization, microorganisms can enter the body where the immune system must deal with them, adding stress to this system. In addition, due to the criminalization of drug use, illicit drugs are generally not pure but adulterated or "cut" with other substances, which increase the dealer's profit but may be harmful to the immune system of the user.

drug addict   A person who is physically dependent on drugs and unable to control his or her craving. See DRUG ABUSE; DRUG ADDICTION.

drug addiction   A dependency on a habit-forming drug, acquired through excessive or continued use. Symptoms of drug addiction are behavioral and physical and include change in personality, loss of appetite, dulled appetite, disturbance in normal sleep rhythm, and weight loss.

Drug addiction is a psychic and physical state encompassing a compulsion to take a given drug on a continuous or periodic basis in order to experience its pleasurable effects or avoid the discomfort of its absence. Tolerance may or may not be present, and a person may be dependent on more than one drug. Drug addicts run a number of serious risks; aside from organ damage and other long-term destructive effects, users may have serious reactions to unknown substances present in illicit drugs, and hepatitis and AIDS can be transmitted through the use of dirty needles and syringes.

drug administration   A regimen, generally ordered by a physician, for taking drugs or other medications. Most medications are taken orally as tablets, capsules, or liquids; some are administered by injection, through intravenous devices, or via inhalant; some may be applied as liquid or ointment directly to an affected area of the body.

drug approval process   The United States system of new drug approvals is perhaps the most rigorous in the world. The steps in development and approval of new medicine are preclinical testing, investigational new drug (IND) application, clinical trials (phase I, phase II, phase III), new drug application (NDA), and approval. Drugs are researched and developed, for the most part, by privately owned pharmaceutical manufacturers. The entire process is regulated and overseen by the Food and Drug Administration (FDA), part of the United States Department of Health and Human Services.

In preclinical testing of a new compound, laboratory and animal studies are done to show biological activity against a targeted disease, and the compound is evaluated for safety. These tests take approximately three and a half years.

After completing the preclinical testing, the developer files an investigational new drug (IND) application. The IND shows results of previous experiments, along with information detailing how, where, and by whom the new studies will be conducted; the chemical structure of the compound; how it is thought to work in the body; any toxic effects found in the animal studies; and how the compound is manufactured. In addition, the IND must be reviewed and approved by the FDA's Institutional Review Board, where separate studies will be conducted. Upon approval of the IND, which is effective in 30 days unless the FDA has an objection, the manufacturer may begin to test the new drug on humans. Progress reports on clinical trials must be submitted at least annually to the FDA.

Phase I clinical trials take about a year and involve 20 to 80 normal, healthy volunteers. These tests study a drug's safety profile, including the safe dosage range. The studies also determine how a drug is absorbed, distributed, metabolized, and excreted, and the duration of its action.

In Phase II clinical trials, controlled studies of approximately 100 to 300 volunteer patients (people with the targeted disease) assess the drug's effectiveness. This phase takes about two years.

In Phase III clinical trials, 1,000 to 3,000 patients in clinics and hospitals are administered the new drug and closely monitored by physicians to determine efficacy and to identify adverse reactions. This phase lasts about three years. Under a plan implemented by the FDA in early 1989, phases II and III may be combined to shave two or three years from the process for medicines that show sufficient promise in early testing and are targeted against serious life-threatening diseases.

Following the completion of all three phases of clinical trials, if the results successfully demonstrate safety and effectiveness, the developer files a new drug application (NDA) with the FDA. The application must contain all the scientific information that has been gathered. NDAs typically run 100,000 or more pages. By law, the FDA is allowed six months to review a new drug application. In almost all cases, the period between the first submission of an NDA and the final approval exceeds that limit. The average NDA review time for new synthetic molecular entities reviewed in 1991 was 30.3 months.

Once the FDA approves a new drug, it is made available for physicians to prescribe. The drug's manufacturer must continue to submit periodic reports to the FDA, including any cases of adverse reactions and appropriate quality control records. For some medications, the FDA requires additional studies to evaluate long-term effects.

The developer of a drug is also granted a patent on it that lasts for seven years from the time the drug is approved. During that period the patent holder has the exclusive right to manufacture and sell the new drug or to license it for manufacture and sales.

drug dependence   See DRUG ADDICTION.

drug development   See DRUG APPROVAL PROCESS.

drug dosage   See DOSAGE; DOSE.

drug-drug interaction   See DRUG INTERACTION.

drug efficacy   See EFFICACY.

drug eruption   See ERUPTION.

drug-fast   See DRUG-RESISTANT.

drug fever   The elevation of body temperature that occurs as an unwanted manifestation of drug action. Drugs can induce fever by several mechanisms; these include allergic reactions, drug-induced tissue damage, acceleration of tissue metabolism, constriction of blood vessels in the skin with resulting decrease in loss of body heat, and direct action on the temperature-regulating center in the brain. The most common form of drug fever is associated with allergic reactions. It may be the only allergic manifestation apparent, or it may be part of a complex of allergic symptoms that can include skin rash, hives, joint swelling and pain, enlarged lymph glands, hemolytic anemia, or hepatitis. The fever usually appears about seven to ten days after starting the drug and may vary from low-grade to alarmingly high levels. It may be sustained or intermittent, but it usually persists for as long as the drug is taken. In previously sensitized individuals, drug fever may occur within one or two hours after taking the first dose of medication.

drug interaction   The mutual pharmacological influence of two or more drugs taken concurrently. The influence may be antagonistic or synergistic and may be lethal in some cases. The chances of developing an undesired drug interaction increases rapidly as the number of drugs taken increases. People with HIV commonly take several medications at the same time to fight HIV and its related conditions. These drugs can interact, leading to more toxic side effects and reduced effectiveness. (Not all drugs interact in this way. Since may be combined without ill effect.)

Some interactions affect the way drugs are absorbed by the gastrointestinal system. Degree of absorption is highly dependent on stomach acidity and the rate of absorption; drugs that are not absorbed well will not achieve sufficient levels in the blood to exert their effects. Malabsorption can be caused by diarrhea, which is a side effect of some drugs; it can also happen if a coincident therapy increases or decreases the excretion or metabolism of a drug. Drugs with similar toxic effects will usually result in combined toxicity, which may contraindicate taking both drugs together.

For HIV-infected persons, the most common drug interactions are among antiretroviral drugs and drugs for PCP and fungal infections. Interactions among TOXOPLASMOSIS, TB, MAC, and CMV medications are also common. There are thousands of potentially significant interactions for patients with HIV infections.

drug overdose   Literally, any excess dose of a drug, but in ordinary usage, the self-administration, accidental or not, of a potentially lethal amount of a drug of abuse.

drug paraphernalia laws   In effect in virtually every state in the nation, drug paraphernalia laws make it a crime to deliver or possess with intent to deliver, virtually any item that could be used in connection with illegal drug use, with the knowledge that it will be so used. There must be criminal intent to supply or use such items for unlawful purposes in order for there to be a crime. Selling or distributing hypodermic needles and syringes without knowledge that they will be used to inject illicit drugs are not offenses under these statutes.

Drug paraphernalia laws erect formidable obstacles for illicit IV drug users, especially those attempting to comply with public health advice to use sterile injection equipment. (The definition of drug paraphernalia in these laws is so broad that it could conceivably be read to include bleach distributed with the intent that it be used to clean hypodermic needles.) Even if a user can buy sterile equipment over the counter, she or he may be prosecuted under these statutes if it is found in her or his possession. In order to escape prosecution a user must demonstrate that he or she has a valid medical purpose for it. Drug paraphernalia laws not only significantly limit the supply of sterile equipment on the street but also provide a marked disincentive for users to have sterile equipment. Drug paraphernalia laws therefore constitute a significant barrier to effective public health practices.

See also NEEDLE PRESCRIPTION LAWS.

drug reaction   Adverse and undesired reaction to a substance taken for its pharmacological effects.

drug receptor   See RECEPTOR.

drug regulation reform   The Kefauver Amendments passed by Congress in 1962 first vested the FOOD AND DRUG ADMINISTRATION, already responsible for the safety of drugs, with the responsibility to ensure their efficacy as well. This mandate is the cornerstone of drug regulation today. Well publicized debates between AIDS activists and the agency concerning the approval of AIDS drugs have attracted media attention since the beginning of the epidemic. Legislative proposals to significantly reshape the mandate of the FDA began to receive serious attention in Washington in 1995. Although the FDA has always claimed a mandate to advance the public health, the responsibility to keep harmful products off the market has always taken precedence over ensuring that helpful products reach the market. Now the balance is starting to shift the other way. Many of the current suggestions for reforming the FDA would significantly alter its authority. Among the items under discussion are measures that would shift more efficacy studies to a "post-market" setting; utilize local INSTITUTIONAL REVIEW BOARDS to review proposals for early human testing (phase I clinical trials) of drugs; privatize certain drug safety reviews by relegating them to independent testing or accrediting institutions; permit the promotion of FDA-approved drugs for "off-label" (not prescribed) uses; impose statutory time limits on FDA reviews; harmonize American with international standards; and remove export barriers for non FDA-approved drugs. Although AIDS activists sparked much of the discussion in the first place, their intention has never been to debilitate the agency; like many more traditional consumer groups, they are now worried that many so-called reform proposals would do just that—and what is worse, might actually diminish the number of effective drugs developed in the future. AIDS activists will both continue to play a major role in the FDA reform debate and be key players in the evaluation of FDA reform proposals from the standpoint of people with life-threatening disease.

drug resistance   The ability of disease-causing microorganisms to evade the drugs designed to eradicate them. Microbial resistance has emerged as one of the major problems in treating infectious diseases. Along with other factors (the emergence of new disease agents, HIV infection, and the use of therapeutic drugs that depress the immune system), microbial resistance has helped to raise the rate of illness and death from infectious diseases in the last 15 years. As germs have developed defenses to penicillin and other widely used antibiotics, diseases like pneumonia and tuberculosis, which were once simply and easily vanquished, have become more difficult to eradicate.

It is commonly believed that it is genetic agility that enables bacteria to become resistant. As single-celled organisms, bacteria divide many times a day, and every division provides an opportunity for a DNA mutation. Some mutations create new genes that are harmful to the bacteria. Others result in changes that are beneficial. Bacteria also occasionally pick up a few new genes from their fellows. They can do so through conjugation—a primitive form of sexual activity in which two cells join together and, in the process, may exchange plasmids—gene-carrying structures outside the chromosomes. Genes can also be transferred by viruses that infect bacteria.

Occasionally, genes acquired through mutation, plasmids, or viral infection confer bacterial resistance. Some genes enable the bacteria to make proteins like penicillinase, which deactivate antibiotics. Other proteins serve as pumps to clear antibiotics out of the bacterium before the drugs have a chance to do any damage. Genetic changes may also alter structural proteins that once served as entry or attachment sites for antibiotics, effectively locking the cellular doorway to these drugs. The end result is the same: drugs are ineffective against the bacteria. With antibiotics, most of the bacteria are wiped out, but the fraction that remain, because they carry the resistance gene, survive to reproduce. This scenario repeats to some degree each time an antibiotic is used. If the resistant bacteria become numerous enough to make themselves known, the original antibiotic is likely to be prescribed again. This time, however, it won't work as well; many of the bacteria are impervious to its effects. In this way, many drugs that were once considered fail-safe have been rendered ineffective. In some cases, bacteria that are resistant to one drug can be eliminated with another one. Eventually, though, strains that are resistant to the second antibiotic will spring up.

The proliferation of resistant microbes is a consequence of the overuse of antibiotics. Much of the problem has industrial and commercial origins. These drugs are routinely added to cattle and poultry feed to produce bigger and healthier livestock. However, the practice also turns the animals into a breeding ground for resistant bacteria. We ultimately consume these pathogens as we eat the meat on our tables.

Antibiotics are also more loosely regulated in some parts of the world. They are available over the counter in many countries, and the resultant overuse has produced resistant strains that have been disseminated via international travel.

Microbial resistance can be corrected. When antibiotics are not used for a time, the slower-growing resistant strains lose their advantage and gradually are eliminated. While we as individuals have little influence over the agriculture industry or foreign drug sales, there are a few things we can do to stem the time of bacterial resistance: (1) don't demand antibiotics for colds (most colds are the result of viral infections, which are unfazed by antibiotics); (2) don't take antibiotics to prevent infection (i.e., to ward off traveler's diarrhea or to prevent urinary-tract infections); (3) consider vaccination (immunization with a vaccine called Pneumovax can prevent not only pneumonia and meningitis, but ear and blood infections as well); (4) use antibiotics only as directed; (5) follow a healthy lifestyle; and (6) keep your hands clean.

drug-resistant   Resistant to the action of a drug or drugs; drug fast. Said of infectious agents or diseases. Drug-resistant disease, such as multiple-drug resistant tuberculosis and AZT-resistant strains of HIV, are well understood by modern medicine. A resistant bacterial strain can transfer its resistance to other bacterial strains through resistance transfer factors and transposons (transposable genetic elements). It is a public health imperative to prevent endemic levels of drug-resistant diseases through prudent prescription of antibiotics. A basic tenet of medical ethics requires that antibiotics never be prescribed before performing a "culture and sensitivity" test, a set of diagnostic techniques to determine the most effective antibiotic to be used in a given case and the briefest duration of treatment needed to control or cure the illness. Today, the dangers of physicians' presumptive diagnoses and excessive use of antibiotics, antifungals, antiprotozoals, and antivirals are evident in the increasing drug resistances of formerly treatable diseases. Two types of resistance are recognized—immunity and inherent resistance. Immunity is resistance associated with the presence of antibodies having a specific action on infectious microorganisms. Inherent resistance is the ability to resist disease independently of antibodies.

Many of the antimicrobial drugs used indiscriminately today as prophylaxis for HIV/AIDS opportunistic infections were originally intended to be used only for brief periods, for the treatment of specific disorders proved susceptible to given drugs through culture and sensitivity testing. A closer look at these drugs, many of which are frequently used for lifetime duration in people with AIDS, may be needed. Concern has been expressed, for example, about the immunosuppression inherent in many of these drugs (especially antibiotics and antivirals) and the fact that they are commonly used in combinations of three or more in an already immune-compromised subject.

drug tolerance   A condition in which the body develops the ability to withstand or overcome the effects of a drug and therefore greater and greater amounts are needed to be effective. This can develop, for example, in patients being treated with painkillers or undergoing chemotherapy.

drug trial   Also known as a CLINICAL TRIAL; the clinical experiment through which researchers determine the effectiveness of different forms of treatment.

drug use   The issue of drug use, particularly in the face of HIV/AIDS. In ordinary usage, synonymous with DRUG ABUSE.

drug user   See DRUG ABUSE.

dry kiss   Also called a social kiss; a kiss with no exchange of saliva.

dry sex   Sex that doesn't involve mucous membrane or secretion contact.

DSPN   See DISTAL SYMMETRIC POLYNEUROPATHY.

DTC   See DIETHYLDITHIOCARBAMATE; IMUTHIOL.

DTH   See DELAYED-TYPE HYPERSENSITIVITY.

durable power of attorney   See POWER OF ATTORNEY.

duty to warn   Within the context of AIDS, there exists both the patient's duty to warn and the practitioner's duty to warn. The standard says that it is the responsibility of a person who is HIV positive or has AIDS to notify one's sexual partner, or partners, that she is infected with a sexually transmitted disease; this notification must occur before engaging in activities by which a disease might be transmitted. Similarly, this standard requires warnings prior to sharing needles. Some argue that this duty is increased if a pregnancy could result from the unprotected sexual encounter because of the risk of transmission of HIV to the fetus. An individual's duty to warn is probably paramount to the therapist's duty to protect, except in those cases where the patient is mentally incompetent to understand the duty to warn or is actually unable to warn his or her partner. It is generally advised that practitioners should educate clients about the duty to warn their prospective partners and to engage only in safe behavior. Practitioners should also encourage and monitor their clients progress in the fulfillment of these duties. If a patient appears uneasy about informing sexual or needle-sharing partners, then the therapist should offer his or her services to counsel the partners of the patient.

Today, there is probably no issue that causes as much consternation among mental health practitioners as does the "duty to warn" or *Tarasoff* duty. At issue in the *Tarasoff I* case is the basic balance between safeguarding the confidentiality of a patient and protecting others from a patient's violent tendencies. Justice Tobriner of the California Supreme Court said in the *Tarasoff I* case, "Protective privilege ends where public peril begins." The case of *Tarasoff v. Regents of the University of California (UC)* (1976) involved a voluntary psychiatric outpatient evaluated and treated at the UC Berkeley Student Health Service. The patient, Prosenjit Poddar, revealed during therapy with a staff psychologist that as a part of his obsession with a Berkeley student, Tatiana Tarasoff, he had fantasies about

harming and perhaps even killing her. In addition, a friend of Poddar's revealed to the psychologist that Poddar planned to purchase a gun. During this period, a staff psychiatrist who had originally evaluated Poddar appropriately prescribed a neuroleptic drug. Despite this intervention, both the psychologist and the psychiatrist became concerned about Poddar's violent tendencies. When Poddar discontinued therapy, the two professionals became particularly concerned and determined that Poddar should be evaluated for hospitalization. Upon their request, the campus police went to see Poddar and questioned him about his intentions toward Tarasoff. When Poddar denied any desire to harm her, the police left. Two months later, Poddar stabbed and killed Tarasoff. Tarasoff's parents sued the practitioners and the UC police for the wrongful death of their daughter, arguing that the university had the duty to protect their daughter from the harm threatened by Poddar during his therapy sessions, despite the privacy privilege Poddar could have asserted. The Supreme Court ruled that the Student Health Service could be found negligent in its duty to protect Tarasoff because it failed to take the necessary steps to insulate her from the harm fantasized by Poddar in therapy sessions. The Court established the basic standard that "When a therapist determines . . . that his patient presents a serious danger of violence to another, he incurs a serious obligation to use reasonable care to protect the intended victim from such danger."

The standard of *Tarasoff*, as later codified in a California statute, allows warning the third party of the patient's threatened violence only when there is a genuine psychotherapist-patient relationship, when the patient has communicated to the therapist a serious and imminent threat of physical violence against another, and when the threat is against a reasonable identifiable victim or victims. In the absence of these elements, the duty to warn or to protect the third party does not arise, and the therapist should be free from liability. If there is a duty to warn or protect under these limited circumstances, the duty shall be discharged through the therapist's reasonable efforts to communicate the threat to the intended victim or victims and to an appropriate law enforcement agency.

Rulings in other duty to warn cases also help to understand how the *Tarasoff* standard applies in the AIDS crisis. A discussion of duty to warn and a decision tree is available in "Assessing dangerousness and responding appropriately: Hedlund expands the clinician's liability established in Tarasoff" by B. H. Gross, M. J. Southard, H. R. Lamb, and L. E. Weinberger (*Journal of Clinical Psychiatry* 48: 1, 1987). Rulings on this question indicate that the *Tarasoff* duty to protect is a fairly limited one, subject to considerations of the clarity of the patient's threat, the actuality of danger to another, the identification of the potential victim(s), the imminence of danger, and the suitability of the patient to other psychosocial intervention to prevent the threatened harm.

Applying these standards to the issues raised by AIDS requires additional analysis. The risk of HIV infection—the "imminent danger"—is still medically unclear. As concerns "unsafe sex" and "unsafe intravenous needle use," what behavior threatens others with "imminent or impending danger"? In addition, although there are clinical reports of people who were infected after one exposure to the virus, there is still a debate about how many sexual or needle exposures are necessary to cause infection. In this context, it is extremely difficult to say what constitutes "imminent danger." Similarly, "imminent danger" cannot include past exposures to HIV. The standard only refers to those future dangers that the practitioner can prevent. A therapist cannot be held liable for failing to prevent infection in those cases in which a patient has exposed a partner to HIV prior to the therapist's knowledge of the possible danger to the partner. Even if a couple becomes aware of the situation, the therapist will probably not be held liable for the HIV infection of the partner, since the partner cannot prove that HIV transmission occurred after the therapist became aware of the couple's sexual practices. The window period after HIV transmission during which antibodies have not formed but HIV is present and may be transmitted complicates the definitive establishment of infection. If testing occurs during the window period, an infected person may test antibody negative.

The standard of "imminent danger" is also obscured by judicial decisions in other states. These courts have interpreted *Tarasoff* more broadly to require psychotherapists and physicians to warn others of the danger their patients may pose if the risk of disease transmission is merely foreseeable. It appears that, at least for now, before a therapist can be held liable for failing to warn the other party of the "imminent danger," he or she would have to know the following facts: the patient is HIV infected; the parties engage in unsafe behavior on a regular basis; such behavior is actually unsafe; the patient intends to continue such behavior even after being counseled to desist by the therapist; HIV transmission will likely occur in the future. Exposure to HIV in any other context would not be an "imminent danger" invoking the practitioner's duty to warn.

A final complicating factor involves the identification of parties. If a patient names only one or a few sexual or needle-sharing partners, a practitioner can easily identify those people who may be warned about a possible exposure to HIV. But when a patient engages in frequent anonymous contacts with large numbers of people, the practitioner probably cannot be held liable for failure to warn these unknown persons. Nonetheless, therapists do have a duty to treat obsessive or compulsive behavior that may endanger the world at large, and, if this therapy fails, they have a duty to take whatever steps toward legal intervention are available in their communities.

Other issues relevant to the duty to warn include liability for improper warning, the disclosure of HIV-related information by medical doctors, standards of knowledge for different types of practitioners, and partner notification or contact tracing.

dying   The condition in which death is imminent.

dying trajectory   A graphic representation of the dying process. Time is recorded along the horizontal axis and nearness to death along the vertical axis. The condition of a dying individual is plotted across time, with the resulting curve being the dying trajectory.

dyke   A sometimes pejorative term, depending on context, for LESBIAN.

dysfunction   In medicine, abnormal, disturbed, impaired, or inadequate function of an organ or system or failure to function. The term is often used to denote sexual problems and is also applied to social structures, such as the family.

dyspareunia   Occurrence of pain in the labial, vaginal, or pelvic areas during or after sexual intercourse. Dyspareunia is caused by infections in the reproductive tract; inadequate vaginal lubrication; uterine myomata; endometriosis; atrophy of vaginal mucosa; psychosomatic causes; and vaginal foreign bodies. Treatment includes specific therapy for the primary disease and counseling with respect to appropriate vaginal and vulval lubrication.

dyspepsia   Digestive upset, which may include flatulence, heartburn, nausea, or vomiting.

dysphagia   Difficulty in swallowing. The most common cause of dysphagia is an infection by CANDIDA ALBICANS, a fungus that can be easily treated. Less frequent causes are HERPES or CMV infections. In some cases dysphagia has no readily apparent cause. The usual method of finding the cause of dysphagia is ENDOSCOPY, a procedure in which a tube is placed in the esophagus to view and biopsy the lesions. X-ray examinations are also employed. In many cases, neither of these tests is considered necessary; a patient is presumed to have a candida infection if he or she has thrush and if swallowing is painful.

dysplasia   Abnormal growth in cells and tissues.

dyspnea   Difficult or labored breathing; shortness of breath. Dyspnea is sometimes accompanied by pain.

dysuria   A burning feeling during urination.

E

EA   See EMERGENCY ASSISTANCE.

ear piercing   Since the needle used to pierce ears does come into contact with blood, it is possible to become infected with HIV if the needle was previously used on an HIV-infected person and not properly cleaned and sterilized. Most places that pierce ears, however, clean their equipment with alcohol before each use, so the risk of contracting the virus this way is very small.

early access   Early access to drugs and therapies for the treatment of HIV infection. This also includes access to promising new drugs and therapies. See EARLY INTERVENTION.

early cases   See EARLY HIV INFECTION.

early HIV infection   The stage of HIV infection during which no major physical health symptoms are yet present, though emotional or psychological difficulties are likely to develop. Today, considerable attention is paid to early HIV infection for several reasons. First, it is widely recognized that the evaluation and management of early HIV infection is of critical importance. Second, recognition of early infection is becoming more common, due in large part to more widespread HIV testing and earlier diagnosis. Third, the prevalence of early HIV infection is increasing in proportion to later stages of infection. Fourth, early medical and psychosocial intervention is most effective in delaying the onset of life-threatening symptoms and diseases and in maintaining good health. Finally, early patient education often facilitates increased patient involvement in treatment and better access to services and helps prevent further spread of the disease.

Essential components of early HIV care include assessment of immune function; initiation of antiretroviral treatment and prophylaxis for *Pneumocystis carinii* pneumonia; evaluation and management of infection with mycobacterium tuberculosis and syphilis; oral, eye, and gynecologic assessment; and reproductive counseling. Evaluation usually begins with a medical, sexual, and substance-use history, followed by a physical examination with attention to HIV-related complications. Providers caring for adolescents or children need to consider a range of age-specific issues, including assessment of physical maturity, psychosocial aspects of adolescence, and impediments to assessing care. Providers caring for women, including pregnant women, need to be cognizant of a range of gender-specific issues. Finally, providers caring for infants need to be aware of the fact that HIV infection frequently progresses more rapidly in infants and children than in adults, and the disease characteristics are different. Early diagnosis and evaluation of the immune system are vital, and the disease must be managed aggressively.

early intervention   Action taken to protect the health of an HIV-infected person before his or her immune system becomes seriously weakened and opportunistic infections develop. Because early HIV infection presents itself differently in adults, adolescents, children, and infants, treatment recommendations vary from group to group. Guidelines for primary care providers as well as adults with early HIV infection generally pertain to monitoring CD4 lymphocytes, initiating antiretroviral therapy and PCP prophylaxis, testing and preventative therapy for tuberculosis, and testing, and treatment for syphilis. Special considerations for treating early HIV infection in women include Pap smears, pregnancy counseling, and access of women with HIV infection to clinical trials and investigational treatments. Because HIV-infected individuals experience a range of unique oral conditions in addition to dental problems common to all individuals, both specialized and routine oral care is required by individuals with HIV infection. Similarly, because of the wide range of ocular complications associated with HIV disease, specialized and routine eye examinations are required by individuals with HIV infection.

early treatment   See EARLY INTERVENTION.

eat   See ORAL SEX.

Ebola   See EBOLA VIRUS DISEASE.

Ebola virus   See EBOLA VIRUS DISEASE.

Ebola virus disease   A disease caused by a virus classed as a member of the family Filoviridae. It is an acute condition characterized by sudden onset of a high fever, prostration, vomiting, and diarrhea, followed by uremia, rash, hemorrhaging, and central nervous system damage. It is usually fatal. The disease can be transmitted by handling tissues and cells from African green monkeys, but in some cases the source of infection is unknown. Its first known victim come from a village near the Ebola River in Zaire (Congo) in 1976.

Clinically, this disease is almost identical to that caused by the MARBURG VIRUS, but the two viruses are not antigenically related. The virus has three subtypes: Ebola Reston, Ebola Sudan, and Ebola Zaire. There is no specific therapy to date.

EBV   See EPSTEIN-BARR VIRUS.

Echinacea   The leaves and root of the herb *Echinacea* (*Echinacea angustifolia* or *E. prupurea*) have been used by Native Americans for a broad range of pains and illnesses. Echinaecein is the substance that knits skin and prevents germs from penetrating tissues. Possibly the most important aspect of *Echinacea* is its immuno-stimulant capability for infectious diseases and other conditions like tonsilitis, bladder infections, colds, flu, and boils. The roots of this herb are used as a tonic and blood purifier, as well as for a variety of other conditions, and other pains and wounds. It is an effective antibiotic and anti-inflammatory for arthritis and rheumatism. Vaginal yeast infections are also helped. *Echinacea* also helps preserve white blood cells from radiation therapy and some anticancer activity is being looked into (leukemia and tumor). Advocates of the therapeutic value of *Echinacea* have cited test tube and animal studies to support these claims. Injections of purified *Echinacea* are believed to be relatively nontoxic even at high doses, although there have been reports of skin rashes and insomnia. Few clinical trials have been performed using either injected polysaccharides or oral over-the-counter *Echinacea* supplements, the most common form of this remedy, and its effects and ideal dosing are, to date, unknown.

Immune-stimulating herbs such as *Echinacea* have become controversial in HIV therapy. A stimulus to CD4+ cells might help the body or might lead to increased replication. Boosting some of the immune system's chemical messengers (cytokines) may help the body, while boosting others may lead to disease progression. Further research in people with HIV is needed.

echocardiography   A noninvasive diagnostic technique for examining the heart by directing beams of ultrasonic waves through the chest wall to produce a graphic record of internal cardiac structures. All cardiac valves can be visualized, and the dimensions of each ventricle and the left atrium can be measured. Also called ULTRASONIC CARDIOGRAPHY.

ecstasy   "Ecstasy" is the popular name for methylenedioxymethamphetamine (MDMA), an illicit recreational drug widely used by some urban populations, including an unknown number of gay men and HIV-infected people. MDMA is an AMPHETAMINE ("speed") with hallucinogenic properties. Most people who use MDMA believe the drug is safe. However, MDMA has caused serious toxicities, and in rare cases has been linked to death. Although there are no conclusive data on the long-term toxicities of the drug, some researchers believe that frequent, long-term MDMA use can cause brain damage or complicate underlying psychiatric disorders. Possible MDMA-related toxicities include tachycardia (rapid heartbeat), hypertension progressing to hypotension, hyperthermia (highly elevated body temperature), hypertonicity (increased pressure of body fluids), intravascular coagulation, kidney failure, hallucinations, and rhabdomyolysis (serious muscle degeneration). Possible residual effects of MDMA include flashbacks, anxiety attacks, persistent insomnia, psychotic reactions, and depression. Researchers do not agree whether MDMA is addictive. MDMA is manufactured illegally by underground chemists. Thus no regulations govern its manufacture; as a result, there is no certainty that street MDMA is actually MDMA.

MDMA was unsuccessfully developed as a weight-loss pill by a German drug company in 1912. The drug remained obscure and forgotten until its psychedelic properties were rediscovered in the 1960s. MDMA emerged fully into public view in the late 1970s and early 1980s when a group of psychotherapists openly advocated its use as an adjunct to therapy and underground chemists began producing it for recreational users. Its possession, distribution, and manufacture were criminalized in 1985 by the Drug Enforcement Agency (DEA), the federal government's lead agency in the "war against drugs."

The DEA classifies ecstasy as a Schedule I drug, which means that it has no medical use and a high potential for abuse. (Studies have shown that recreational drug use, of MDMA in particular, may be related to unsafe sexual practices and HIV infection among gay men. See DRUG ABUSE.)

ecthyma   An ulcerative inflammation of the skin caused by infection and marked by lesions with crusts or scabs. Variable scarring and pigmentation may result.

ectopic pregnancy   Ectopic pregnancy occurs when a fertilized egg attaches itself to tissue outside the uterus. There is usually a poorly developed decidual reaction in the uterus. Symptoms may include amenorrhea; tenderness, soreness, pain on affected side; pallor, weak pulse, signs of shock or hemorrhage; reflected shoulder pain; bluish discoloration of the umbilicus. Ectopic pregnancy may occur in the free abdominal cavity, in the interstitial portion of the tube, in the ovary, or in the fallopian tube (in the interstitial, ampullar, or isthmic portion). Ectopic pregnancy may be unruptured or ruptured. Irregular hemorrhage, vague pains in the abdomen (usually on one side), and amenorrhea may or may not be present in unruptured ectopic pregnancies. Diagnosis at this stage can be made by the usual biological tests for pregnancy. For ruptured ectopic pregnancies without a severe hemorrhage there is severe pain in the lower abdomen with repeated fainting spells. Diagnosis is made by a transvaginal needle puncture into the peritoneal cavity. This will reveal free blood. If bleeding is severe and surgical therapy is not instituted without delay, death may result.

ectropion   A condition in which the outer CERVIX is covered by cells that would normally be found in the inner cervix.

edema   A local or generalized swelling characterized by excessively large amounts of fluid in the body tissues. It may result from increased permeability of the capillary walls; increased capillary pressure due to venous obstruction or heart failure; lymphatic obstruction; disturbances in renal functioning; reduction of plasma proteins; inflammatory conditions; fluid and electrolyte disturbances; malnutrition; starvation; and chemical substances. It may also occur by diffusion.

Education for All Handicapped Children Act   Congress passed the Education for All Handicapped Children Act in 1975 to meet the special educational needs of children who are mentally retarded, hard of hearing, deaf, speech impaired, visually handicapped, seriously emotionally disturbed, or orthopedically impaired, or other health impaired children, including children with AIDS, or children with specific learning disabilities.

EEG   See ELECTROENCEPHALOGRAM.

efavirenz   DuPont Merck's new NON-NUCLEOSIDE REVERSE TRANSCRIPTASE inhibitor that is heading for FDA consideration in 1998. Efavirenz, like ABACAVIR, is marked by PROTEASE INHIBITOR–like potency. The older non-nucleoside reverse transcriptase inhibitors, NEVIRAPINE and DELAVIRDINE, suffer from the ease by which HIV develops resistance to them. Resistance to either requires only a single mutation, which can occur after a few weeks of monotherapy. Efavirenz is not as much an exception to this pattern as first appeared, and once again the rule holds that broad cross-resistance can arise for a given class of drugs.

effector cells   The active cells of the immune system responsible for destroying or controlling foreign antibodies. Also cell or organ by which an animal responds to internal or external stimuli, often via the nervous system.

effervescent tablet   A tablet that fizzes to dissolve when placed in water.

efficacy   Effectiveness; the power or ability to produce intended effects or results, for example the ability of a drug to control or cure an illness. Efficacy should be distinguished from activity, which refers to a drug's immediate effects on a microbe triggering a disease.

eflornithine   An antineoplastic and antiprotozoal drug. It has been used to treat African sleeping sickness. Trade name Ornidyl.

EIA   See ENZYME IMMUNOASSAY.

ejaculate   To release seminal fluid through the penis; the fluid emitted during ejaculation.

ejaculation   The release of semen from an erect penis, during orgasm.

electroencephalogram (EEG)   A record of the electrical activity of the brain obtained by placing electrodes at various locations on the scalp in order to measure the electrical potential. The recording device is called an *electroencephalograph*.

electroencephalography   Amplification, recording, and analysis of the electrical activity of the brain. This technique has proved useful as a diagnostic tool in studying convulsive disorders such as epilepsy and in locating cerebral lesions. The record obtained is called an ELECTROENCEPHALOGRAM (EEG).

electrolyte   A solution that is a conductor of electricity; a substance that yields ions in solution so that its solutions conduct an electric current. Also ionized salt in blood, tissue fluids, and cells, including chloride, sodium, and potassium.

electrolyte abnormality   A deviation from the normal condition in electrolytes.

electron microscope   A large and very powerful microscope that uses a beam of electrons to enlarge the image of a very small object, such as a virus, and replicate it on a screen.

elephant leg   See ELEPHANTIASIS.

elephantiasis   A disease characterized by enlargement of parts of the body, especially the legs and genitals, and by hardening and ulceration of the surrounding skin. Elephantiasis may be congenital (Milroy's disease) or the result of metastatic invasion of the lymph nodes by tumor cells. Inflammatory elephantiasis results from filariasis or local infection of the lymph nodes. Elephantiasis is caused by infection of the lymphatics by one of three filarial parasites of man: *Wuchereria bancrofti, Brugia malay,* or *Brugia timori.* There is no completely effective therapy, but diethylcarbamazine reduces the number of organisms in the peripheral blood. Surgery to treat hydrocele is indicated. Surgery is not effective in treating lymphedema of the legs.

eligibility criteria   The conditions that determine a person's suitability for a clinical trial or research study. Examples include age, symptoms exhibited (of HIV or other illness), results of certain lab tests, overall health, and past treatments undergone. To be right for a study, a person's health picture has to match all the study's needs. He or she must meet not only the research plan's inclusion criteria (conditions that must be present), but the exclusion criteria (conditions that must be absent). Both the "must have" and the "can't have" checklists help doctors get clear research results.

ELISA   See ENZYME-LINKED IMMUNOSORBENT ASSAY.

emaciation   State of being extremely lean. An emaciated person is excessively thin or lacking in normal amount of tissue.

embryopathy   Any pathological condition in an embryo.

Emergency Assistance (EA)   A federal-state welfare program that makes onetime crisis payments to or on behalf of low-income families with children and, in many states, the poor aged and disabled.

empiric therapy   Treatment based on a clinician's judgment of the patient's symptoms and signs, offered before a diagnosis has been confirmed.

employee benefits   Benefits, given to an employee, apart from salary, as part of his or her employment. Healthcare and financial benefits are the most common employee benefits. These are distinct from public benefits such as Social Security, Medicaid, Medicare, food stamps, and housing. Persons with HIV/AIDS should be aware what benefits are offered by their employers, who is eligible for them, where and how to apply for them, and how to appeal decisions to deny them.

employment discrimination   In the first decade of the epidemic, as AIDS and AIDS hysteria spread, reports of cases involving loss of jobs due to AIDS, or to perceived AIDS, were frequent. Hostility and fear were particularly marked in the workplace and in prisons, where transmission of the disease was particularly feared. Today, as the newest additions to the Lambda list of AIDS cases in court for trial demonstrates, employment discrimination, particularly as a way to sever the lifeline of health care benefits, is a primary problem for people living with AIDS. In decisions under the AMERICANS WITH DISABILITIES ACT emerging from the courts in greater numbers in recent years, there has been a perceptible trend toward a rigid, literal definition of the ADA's terms, shrinking the pool of those who can sue. Additionally, large employers have sought to limit the ability of ex-employees on COBRA or disability to sue over job-related discrimination, as have organizations representing employers' interests, such as the Equal Employment Advisory Council. Some argue that fired employees with asymptomatic HIV infection are not "disabled" enough to invoke the ADA. Others have flipped the argument, insisting that those with AIDS and presumptive eligibility for SSI benefits are too disabled to be "qualified employees" under the ADA.

empowerment   For persons who have concerns about staying well in the age of AIDS, empowerment means their taking control, or taking charge, of their own mental, spiritual, and physical health. Most programs of support and guidance for persons with HIV/AIDS, those at risk of infection or those who care for people with HIV or AIDS stress the importance of empowerment.

Taking control or taking charge can, of course, mean different things for different individuals. Research has shown that emotional and mental patterns affect outcome in chronic and life-threatening diseases. Current data strongly suggest that people who succeed in preventing illness or surviving illness longer have certain characteristics in common and employ similar approaches. Rejecting notions of victimhood, making a commitment to life and to wellness, accepting one's true circumstances, and releasing negative emotions are among the strategies most usefully employed by such people.

enabling   Any action by a person or an institution that intentionally or unintentionally has the effect of supporting or reinforcing an individual's self-destructive behavior.

encephalitis   An infection of the brain of viral or other microbial origin. Encephalitis commonly causes headaches, fever, seizures, and neurological problems. The diagnosis is frequently made on the basis of symptoms exhibited combined with the results of an examination of the brain by such methods as COMPUTERIZED TOMOGRAPHY SCAN (CT SCAN), MAGNETIC RESONANCE IMAGING (MRI) or ELECTROENCEPHALOGRAM (EEG). Diagnosis can also be made by analyzing the CEREBROSPINAL FLUID obtained by a spinal tap. Encephalitis may be due to a specific disease entity, be caused by an arthropod-borne virus, or occur as a sequela of influenza, measles, German measles, chicken pox, HERPES VIRUS infection, smallpox, vaccinia, or other diseases. In people with HIV infection, the usual causes of encephalitis are infection with HIV itself or such opportunistic illnesses as TOXOPLASMOSIS or lymphoma. Encephalitis is distinct from MENINGITIS, which is an infection of the meninges, the membrane surrounding the brain and spinal cord.

encephalopathy   Any progressive, degenerative disease of the brain.

encephalopathy, acute   Any degenerative disease of the brain, or reversible deterioration of mental status or cognitive function, with a short or relatively severe course.

endemic   Widespread or very common only in a particular place or population. The term may be used of an organism such as a plant, that is native to a region, as well as of disease. Of disease it is used in contrast to EPIDEMIC, which indicates widespread generally.

endocarditis   A bacterial infection that causes inflammation of the heart valves that, if left untreated, may lead to heart failure and death. The most common cause is a bacteria called *Staphylococcus aureus*. Endocarditis may also be due to an abnormal immunological reaction. Endocarditis has long been associated with INTRAVENOUS drug use and is a serious problem for HIV-positive men and women who are IV drug users. The most common symptom is fever; other symptoms include heart murmurs, irregular heartbeat, chills, headache, back and chest pain, stomachache, nausea, and vomiting. Endocarditis can lead to many complications in the circulatory system, central nervous system, lungs, kidneys, and brain. Treatment is with antibiotics. Prophylaxis is usually indicated only in persons who have had endocarditis in the past and who need to have a surgical or dental procedure during which bacteria may enter the blood.

endocervix   The lining of the canal of the CERVIX.

endocrine   A hormone; pertaining to an internal secretion, or to a gland that secretes directly into the bloodstream.

endocrine abnormality   Any deviation in hormonal secretions.

endocrine gland   Any ductless gland, such as the adrenal gland or the pituitary gland, that secretes hormones directly into the bloodstream. The endocrine system functions as an elaborate signaling system within the body, alongside the nervous system.

endocytosis The process whereby material external to a cell is internalized within a particular cell. The cell wall invaginates to form a space for the material and then closes to trap the material inside the cell.

endometrial biopsy A test in which a small sample of tissue is removed from the uterus, often to see if infection is present.

endometriosis The presence of ectopic endometrium, in various sites throughout the pelvis or in the abdominal wall. Pelvic pain, adnexal mass, and infertility are common symptoms.

endometrium The mucous membrane lining the inner surface of the uterus.

endorphins Proteins called polypeptides, produced in the brain, that act as opiates and produce analgesia by binding to opiate receptor sites involved in pain perception.

endoscope An instrument consisting of a tube and optical system for visually examining the inside of a hollow organ or cavity. See BIOPSY; ENDOSCOPY.

endoscopic Performed by means of an ENDOSCOPE; pertaining to ENDOSCOPY.

endoscopy A diagnostic procedure in which an instrument called an ENDOSCOPE, consisting of a flexible tube and optical system, is passed through the mouth, the rectum, or a small incision to examine an internal organ or to obtain a BIOPSY. In people with HIV infection, the most common types of endoscopy are done to examine the lungs (bronchoscopy) and the digestive system. Upper endoscopy of the digestive system involves passing an endoscope through the mouth to examine the esophagus, stomach, or upper small intestine. Lower endoscopy involves passing an endoscope through the rectum to examine the large intestine or colon. Endoscopy requires the expertise of a specialist and can be done on an outpatient basis. See BIOPSY.

endothelium A form of SQUAMOUS epithelium consisting of flat cells that line the blood and lymphatic vessels, the heart, and various other body cavities.

endotoxin A bacterial toxin confined within the body of a BACTERIUM, freed only when the bacterium is broken down.

endpoint A category of data used to compare the outcome of different arms of a clinical trial. Common endpoints are severe toxicity, disease progression, or such surrogate markers as CD4 count, but sometimes death is used as an endpoint. Usually when an endpoint reaches a certain set magnitude of change from BASELINE, a trial participant is removed from the trial and given an open-label therapy (either a standard treatment or the experimental one being tested).

enema The injection of a solution into the rectum or colon for the purpose of stimulating bowel activity, for therapeutic or nutritive purposes or to aid in roentgenography; also, a solution so introduced.

energy level The position of electrons within an atom. Specifically, one of a quantized series of states in which matter may exist, each having constant energy and separated from others in the series by finite quantities of energy. Energy levels in individuals who are HIV-positive or have AIDS vary depending on the stage of HIV infection, medical, psychological, and social interventions, the special conditions of each patient, and other variables.

enteric Pertaining to the intestines.

enteric coating A type of drug formulation in which tablets or capsules are coated with a special compound that will not dissolve until the pill is exposed to the fluids in the small intestine.

enteric disease Any pathological condition involving the small intestine.

enteric pathogen Any microorganism or substance capable of producing a disease in the small intestine.

enteritis An inflammation of the small intestine. In people with HIV infection, the microbes that usually cause enteritis are CRYPTOSPORIDIA, MICROSPORIDIA, MYCOBACTERIUM AVIUM-INTRACELLULARE, and CMV. These can be detected by examining stools under a microscope or performing a BIOPSY of the small intestine. The most common symptom is diarrhea.

enterotoxin A toxin produced by or originating in the intestinal contents; an exotoxin specific for the cells of the mucosa, produced by certain species of bacteria that cause various diseases, including food poisoning and TOXIC SHOCK SYNDROME.

envelope The outer covering of a virus, sometimes called the coat.

envelope gene The gene that encodes the major virion surface envelope glycoprotein (for the human immunodeficiency virus, this glycoprotein is GP160) and is then processed to form a transmembrane segment (GP41) and a glycosylated external segment (GP120).

envelope glycoprotein The glycosylated external segment (GP120) of the human immunodeficiency virus. The envelope glycoprotein is the major target for the HIV-neutralizing antibody.

enzyme A cellular protein whose shape allows it to hold together several molecules in close proximity to each other. In this way, enzymes are able to mediate and promote chemical reactions in other substances with little expenditure of energy and without themselves being altered or destroyed.

enzyme immunoassay (EIA)   Any of several rapid enzyme testing methods for detecting the presence of an antibody or an antigen in tissue by using an enzyme covalently linked to an antigen or antibody as a label. The resulting complex will retain both immunological and enzymatic activity. The pressure of the antigen or antibody indicates infection by a virus or germ. The two most common methods are ENZYME-LINKED IMMUNOSORBENT ASSAY (ELISA) and enzyme-multiplied immunoassay technique (EMIT).

Solid-phase immunoassay involves fixing antibody to the antigen on a polyvinylchloride sheet, putting on a drop of serum (or urine) and washing off after the antigen-antibody complex has had time to form, and then adding a second labeled or fluorescent antibody, this time specific to a different epitope of the antigen. The amount of the second antibody that binds is proportional to the amount of antigen present.

ELISA is similar, but an enzyme instead of the label is attached to a second antibody. This can convert a colorless substance to a colored product, or nonfluorescent to fluorescent, when added. Sensitivities of both methods can be extremely high.

These assays are quite sensitive and specific as compared with the radioimmune assay tests and have the advantage of not requiring radioisotopes and the expensive counting apparatus.

enzyme-linked immunosorbent assay (ELISA)   The most common blood test used to detect antibodies against HIV. When the body is exposed to a germ or a virus, the immune system mounts an attack against it and makes antibodies (the molecules that help fight it off) for the specific agent. The presence of these antibodies are indicative of ongoing infection. The ELISA test determines whether antibodies to the AIDS virus are present in the blood, which they usually are within several months of infection.

The ELISA is the first of two standard tests done together to detect antibodies to HIV. It is extremely sensitive but not very specific. Sensitivity means that the test specifically detects a particular infection and no other. With ELISA, people who have HIV infection will rarely test falsely negative, but people who do not have HIV infection will often test falsely positive. As a result, the ELISA is used as a screening test; blood samples that test positive are tested again with the western blot test. This combination is more than 99 percent accurate in both sensitivity and specificity.

These tests are generally offered free of charge by most health departments. Tests may be anonymous, meaning that the person being tested is not identified, or confidential, meaning that privacy is honored but a record is kept identifying by name the test result.

The ELISA is easily performed, but the western blot is more complicated and often done only by reference laboratories or on certain days of the week. For this reason, the combined results may not be available for several days or even weeks. Test results are usually either positive or negative, but occasionally western blot tests yield results that cannot be clearly interpreted and are considered indeterminate. The usual recommendation for people with indeterminate results is to have the test repeated in two or three months. People at low risk for HIV and with indeterminate results almost never turn out to have HIV infection. The cause of the indeterminate results is not known.

eosinophil   Bone marrow-derived GRANULOCYTES (nondividing granular cells) with a limited life span in the blood. They have both secretory and phagocytic functions and may play a specific role in defense against parasites. Eosinophils are readily stained with eosin, a synthetic red dye used to stain tissues for microscopic examination.

eosinophilic   Pertaining to eosinophils; readily stainable with eosin.

eosinophilic folliculitis   An inflammatory reaction around the hair follicles, characterized by very itchy papules that may grow together to form plaques. The cause of this condition in people with AIDS has yet to be established, although the condition obviously involves invasion of the follicles by eosinophils. Partially successful treatment has been reported with ULTRAVIOLET LIGHT, STEROIDS, ANTIHISTAMINES, and ITRACONAZOLE.

epidemic   Occurring in many more people than would be statistically expected during a given time. (Generally used of a disease the term may also be applied to injuries or other events that endanger public health.) Also, a disease that so occurs. We say there is an AIDS epidemic because the disease is spreading very quickly to many segments of the population. Distinct from ENDEMIC, which indicates restriction to a particular place or population. See also PANDEMIC.

epidemiology   A branch of medical science encompassing the study of the relationship of various factors in the incidence and distribution of a disease or of diseases in a human environment.

epididymitis   Inflammation of the epididymis, a tube that lies against the back wall of a testicle and serves as a storage facility for sperm.

epinephrine   A hormone secreted by the adrenal medulla in response to stimulation of the sympathetic nervous system. It causes some of the physiological expressions of fear and anxiety and has been found to be in excess in some anxiety disorders. Epinephrine, which has been synthesized, is also produced by tissues other than the adrenal. Used as a vasoconstrictor to treat cardiac dysrhythmias and to relax bronchioles. It is also used to check local hemorrhaging, to relieve asthmatic attacks, and to prolong the action of local anesthetics. Trade names are Adrenalin, Bronkaid Mist, Primatene Mist, and SusPhrine.

epistasis   In genetics, the suppression by a gene of the effect of another gene that is not its allele (one of two or more alternative forms of a gene occupying the same position on matching chromosomes; an individual usually has two alleles for each trait, one from either parent).

epistaxis   Hemorrhage in the nose.

epithelial cell   An irregularly-shaped cell that has a single nucleus. Frequently two or three are joined together.

epithelium   The layer of cells forming the epidermis of the skin and the surface layer or mucous and serous membranes. The cells rest on a basement membrane and lie closely approximated to each other with little intercellular material between them. The epithelium may be simple, consisting of a single layer, or stratified, consisting of several layers. Cells making up the epithelium may be flat (squamous), cube-shaped (cuboidal), or cylindrical (columnar). Epithelium serves the general purpose of protection, absorption, and secretion, and specialized functions such as movement of substances through ducts, production of germ cells, and reception of stimuli. Its ability to regenerate is excellent, and it may replace itself as frequently as every 24 hours.

epitope   The simplest form of an antigenic determinant present on a complex antigenic molecule, which combines with antibody or T-CELL RECEPTOR.

Epogen   See ERYTHROPOIETIN.

Epstein-Barr virus (EBV)   A herpeslike virus that lies dormant in the lymph glands and causes one of the two kinds of mononucleosis (the other is caused by CMV). EBV is also thought to be responsible for CHRONIC FATIGUE SYNDROME. It has been implicated as a causal factor in the development of BURKITT'S LYMPHOMA in Africa. It has also been linked with nasopharyngeal cancer, a common cancer in China. EBV is a common virus which can be a serious opportunistic infection when associated with AIDS. The virus manifests itself in LYMPHADENOPATHY, LYMPHOMA, KAPOSI'S SARCOMA, and other illnesses. EBV has been hypothesized as a CO-FACTOR for AIDS.

erection   The engorgement of the PENIS with blood and consequent enlargement and stiffening. Erection can be a sign of sexual excitement.

erogenous zone   Any area of the body that when stimulated increases sexual excitement.

erogeny   Sexuality and sensuality.

erotic   Sexually stimulating; relating to sexual activity or feeling.

erotophobia   The irrational hatred or fear of anything sexual, or guilt over erotic desire. The development of erotophobia has been the response of both the infected and the uninfected to the AIDS crisis.

eruption   An inflammation of the skin characterized by itching, redness, and skin lesions; may be caused by medication as well as by illness. A drug eruption is also called *dermatitis medicamentosa*.

Erythrocin   See ERYTHROMYCIN.

erythrocyte   A circulating red blood cell; a mature red blood cell or corpuscle shaped in the form of a nonnucleated, yellowish, biconcave disk. It consists of a respiratory pigment (hemoglobin) enclosed in a membrane of proteins and lipoid substances. By the nature of its composition, the erythrocyte is adapted to transport oxygen throughout the body.

erythrocyte sedimentation rate (ESR)   The rate at which ERYTHROCYTEs (the circulating red blood cells) settle in a well-mixed specimen of blood. The ESR is an indicator of inflammatory disease and other conditions in which the rate is usually elevated.

erythrocytophagy   The consumption or engulfment of ERYTHROCYTEs by other cells, for example histiocytes of the RETICULOENDOTHELIAL SYSTEM.

erythromycin   An antibiotic produced by streptomyces erythreus, which appears as a yellowish, crystalline powder. Administered orally, it is effective against many GRAM-POSITIVE and certain GRAM-NEGATIVE bacteria. It may also be applied topically in the treatment of certain infections. It is used to treat patients who are allergic to penicillin and in the treatment of penicillin-resistant infections. Trade name Erythrocin.

erythrophagocytosis   See ERYTHROCYTOPHAGY.

erythroplakia   A reddened velvety patch that may appear in the mouth. It is a precancerous condition. See ORAL CANCER.

erythropoietin (EPO)   A protein, made primarily by the kidney, that stimulates red blood cell production. A genetically engineered version has been approved as a treatment for HIV-related anemia and has had a significant impact on treatment of HIV. Anemia, which is frequently seen in people with HIV, can be caused by HIV infection itself or as a side effect of treatment. By reducing the need for transfusions, erythropoietin has allowed people to continue antiviral therapy even when the drugs they are taking cause anemia. Additionally, reducing the need for transfusions has reduced the risk of blood-borne disease.

The only alternative therapy routinely used for treatment of anemia in HIV-infected people is transfusion. Those with AZT-induced anemia may also stop AZT therapy or decrease the dosage until their red blood cells recover. The problem with this option is that dose reductions may decrease AZT concentration in the blood to levels that are ineffective in stopping HIV replication. Transfusions also involve risks, such as infections and allergic reactions.

EPO should not be used by people with uncontrolled high blood pressure, known allergy to mammalian-cell-derived products, or known allergy to human albumin. Because EPO causes an increase in blood pressure, blood pressure must be closely monitored and controlled in those treated. During hemodialysis, people treated with EPO may have an increased risk for blood clotting. EPO will not be effective if anemia is caused by iron deficiency, infection, cancer, blood loss, vitamin deficiency, aluminium poisoning, or inflammatory bone disease. It is not an appropriate therapy for severe anemia and cannot replace the need for blood transfusions. Early treatment of mild anemia with EPO may prevent the onset of severe anemia and the need for blood transfusions.

The recombinant version of EPO is available as a solution for IV injection under the trade names Epogen and Procrit.

Escherichia coli (E. coli)   Bacteria in the feces that causes most CYSTITIS.

esophageal candidiasis   Serious fungal infection in the conduit between the mouth and the stomach (the ESOPHAGUS). Esophageal candidiasis is caused by the same yeast infection that can also infect both the mouth and the vagina. It may start with an infection in the mouth (oral thrush) and spread to the esophagus, causing pain when swallowing, weight loss, and vomiting. Many professionals speculate that controlling and preventing yeast infections in the vagina may also prevent esophageal candidiasis.

esophagitis   Disease of the esophagus is very common in patients with AIDS and CYTOMEGALOVIRUS can be the responsible agent. Its most common physical symptoms are painful swallowing or the sense of food sticking in the throat. Patients sometimes complain of chest pain or hiccups. These symptoms may result in decreased food intake in patients with normal appetites, dehydration, weight loss, and malnourishment.

The diagnostic procedure of choice for CMV esophagitis is upper ENDOSCOPY, in which a lighted scope is passed through the mouth into the esophagus. The CMV-infected esophagus often appears inflamed and ulcerated, though CMV esophagus can occasionally take the form of a mass resembling a cancer. Since other esophageal infections in AIDS patients may manifest themselves in a similar manner, biopsies must be taken to confirm the diagnosis.

esophagoscope   A flexible or rigid instrument, equipped with an optical system, inserted into the esophagus for diagnostic and therapeutic purposes (obtaining or removing foreign substances).

esophagoscopy   An ENDOSCOPIC examination of the ESOPHAGUS using an ESOPHAGOSCOPE.

esophagus   A muscular canal extending from the pharynx to the stomach. The esophagus carries swallowed food and liquids from the mouth to the stomach.

esophotrast   See BARIUM SULFATE.

ESR   See ERYTHROCYTE SEDIMENTATION RATE.

estrogen   Any natural or artificial substance that induces estrogenic activity; more specifically, the estrogenic hormones estradiol and estrone, produced by the ovary; the female sex hormones.

ethambutol hydrochloride   A drug used in treating TUBERCULOSIS. It is used in combination with ISONIAZID. Trade name Myambutol.

ethics   A system or set of moral principles. Also, the rules of conduct recognized in respect to a particular class of human actions or governing a particular group, culture, or profession, such as medical ethics. AIDS research and policy development have from the very beginning involved serious ethical issues. Some of the earliest had to do with blood screening policies, the conduct of epidemiological research and surveillance, risk to health care providers, and the duty to warn people with HIV, patient confidentiality, and the conduct of drug trials. Many of these issues are still with us, although in different forms and some with lesser importance. For example, there are no longer debates about screening donated blood, but the questions around clinical trials have broadened, particularly concerning the inclusion of women and minorities. Additionally, because ethicists, at least in the United States, were involved very early on in policy discussions, the response of public health agencies reflected concerns about individual patient rights and standard infectious disease control measures.

Future ethical challenges include managed care, home care, and physician-assisted suicide. Issues raised by managed care, for example, include coverage for new therapies, coverage for alternative treatments, coverage for mental health treatment, and coverage for preexisting conditions. The challenge of optimizing the quality of life raises a range of ethical issues for health care professionals and AIDS service providers, in addition to family and friends of persons with HIV/AIDS. Attention to psychosocial issues and issues of death and dying are as important as both medical management of HIV infection and careful attention to financial matters. The practicalities of self-deliverance and assisted suicide for the dying aside, there are a number of ethical issues raised by physician-assisted suicide. Today, against a backdrop of a heated national debate on the issue of physician-assisted suicide, it is generally recognized that people with terminal illness have choices, choices on how—and when—to end their suffering. In his landmark book *Final Exit* (New York: Dell, 1991), Derek Humphry addresses the dilemmas facing the terminally ill, including shopping for the right doctor, the hospice option, the cyanide enigma, storing drugs, and insurance. He also raises questions such as Who shall know? When is the time to die? and Will there be an autopsy?

ethnic groups   See RACE/ETHNICITY.

ethnicity   See RACE/ETHNICITY.

etiology   The cause(s) or origin(s) of diseases; the study of the factors that cause disease.

etoposide   An antineoplastic drug; a semisynthetic derivative of podophyllotoxin, administered intravenously and used to prevent the development, growth, or proliferation of malignant cells.

etretinate   An antipsoriasis drug used in the treatment of severe recalcitrant psoriasis. Trade name Tegison.

eustachian dysfunction   Abnormal or impaired functioning of the auditory tube (eustachian tube) that extends from the middle ear to the pharynx. When the passage is blocked, OTITIS media may develop.

exclusion criteria In a clinical or research trial plan, the standards by which decisions are made not to include certain potential participants. These are generally health factors whose presence in a test subject would be undesirable or inappropriate. Often these are established for reasons of safety. For instance, doctors may know or fear that a new drug may cause people with a certain illness to get sicker. It would thus be wrong to allow them to participate in the clinical trial or study and take that risk.

exempt assets Assets that are not considered or counted in determining eligibility under benefit programs such as the SSI and VA pension programs.

exercise Bodily or mental exertion, especially for the sake of maintaining fitness, training, or improvement. Exercise is a time-proved method for coping with problems of all kinds. Today, virtually all cultures recognize the importance of regularly moving all parts of the body. In India, yogic exercise has played an important role in Ayurvedic medicine for more than 6,000 years. Similarly, in China, exercise has been practiced for 2,500 years using martial arts such as tai chi. Many studies have shown that people who exercise have fewer illnesses than sedentary persons. Vigorous exercise benefits the body both directly and indirectly by stimulating the immune system and enabling people to cope with a variety of stressors and toxins. The psychological benefits are equally as important, and exercise has been successfully used to treat disorders such as depression. Regular exercise is usually part of any holistic medical program because, next to diet, it most effectively produces total body health. Additionally, the healing process works at its best when the body is relaxed and energy is concentrated inward. A part of being able to relax and allow that to happen is exercise and meditation, which not only enhance general well-being but also aid in the overall health of the immune system.

The amount, type, and frequency of exercise to take in order to develop and maintain a state of fitness is an individual matter.

exhibitionism Sexual interest in exposing one's genitals. Slang term is flash.

exocervix The outer CERVIX.

exon The coding segment of a DNA strand.

exonuclease VII A cellular enzyme that degrades single strands of DNA. Most exonucleases also degrade cellular RNA, which is always single-stranded and orchestrates cellular metabolism. Destroying too much RNA is fatal to most cells. Exonuclease VII, in contrast, only targets single strands of the usually double-stranded DNA. Exonuclease VII is also large for such an enzyme, too large to pass through the pores of the nuclear membrane or MITOCHONDRIA, where the host cell's DNA is located. Exonuclease VII can chew up only single strands of foreign DNA, including HIV's, that it encounters in the cytoplasm outside the nucleus. HIV DNA exists temporarily in the cytoplasm as a single-stranded molecule. This occurs while it is being constructed by REVERSE TRANSCRIPTASE from the genes in an invading HIV particle, which are in RNA form.

Research has found that when exonuclease VII is introduced enclosed within a LIPOSOME, it blocks HIV infection in cell culture without harming the cells. Such liposomes isolate the enzyme until they contact one of the immune cells serving as reservoirs for HIV.

exotoxins Toxin released by a microorganism into surrounding growth medium or tissue during growth phase of infection. Generally inactivated by heat and easily neutralized by a specific antibody. It is produced mainly by GRAM-POSITIVE bacteria, such as the agents of botulism, diphtheria, Shigella dysentery, and tetanus.

expanded access Refers to any of the United States FOOD AND DRUG ADMINISTRATION procedures allowing patients who are failing on current treatments for their condition, who are unable to participate in ongoing clinical trials, and who meet certain criteria to take an experimental drug not yet approved for general use. In the program, doctors monitor patient's responses and report the data to the pharmaceutical company sponsoring the drug. Specific types of expanded access mechanisms include parallel track, compassionate use, and treatment IND. Also called *open-label study*.

expedited process Under a plan implemented by the Food and Drug Administration (FDA) early in 1989, Phases I and II of the U.S. DRUG APPROVAL PROCESS may be combined to shave two or three years from the development process for medicines that show sufficient promise in early testing and are targeted against serious and life-threatening diseases. Phase I clinical trials consist of tests that take about 1 year and involve about 20 to 80 normal, healthy volunteers. The tests study a drug's safety profile, including the safe dosage range. The studies also determine how a drug is absorbed, distributed, metabolized, and excreted and the duration of its action. In Phase II clinical trials, controlled studies of approximately 100 to 300 volunteer patients assess the drug's effectiveness. Phase II clinical trials generally take about two years.

experimental drug A drug that has not been approved for use as a treatment for a particular condition.

experimental group In experimental design, a group of subjects exposed to an independent variable in order to examine the causal effect of that variable on a dependent variable.

experimenter bias See EXPERIMENTER EFFECTS.

experimenter effects Biasing effects on the results of an experiment caused by expectations or preconceptions on the part of the experimenter.

explosive chain of lethal transmission The extremely rapid spread of a lethal infectious agent through a population, killing a large percentage. Also known as *burning*. This phenomenon has been likened to a biological meltdown.

exposed According to the provisions of the Public Health Service's HIV Health Care Services Program, the term *exposed* with respect to HIV disease or any other infectious disease means to be in circumstances in which there is a significant risk of becoming infected with the etiologic agent for the disease involved.

extracerebral toxoplasmosis   TOXOPLASMOSIS that occurs outside the brain in a disseminated form, with parasites found in the eyes, lungs, blood, bone marrow, muscles, bladder, and heart.

extrahepatic disease   A pathological condition occurring outside of or unrelated to the liver.

eyewear, protective   Safety glasses. See PROTECTIVE EQUIPMENT.

fab (fragment antigen binding)   A part of the antibody molecule that contains the antigen-binding site. It is obtained by enzymatic hydrolysis of the antibody.

facilitated DNA inoculation   A means of delivering (non-infectious) HIV genes into a patient's blood by direct injection into a muscle, along with an agent that promotes uptake of the genes into the host cells. The rationale behind this strategy is to induce production of HIV proteins by the patient's own cells, which in turn may prompt his or her immune system to produce antibodies and killer T CELLS to fight HIV. The vaccine includes a segment of HIV DNA comprising the *env* and *rev* genes, which code for a viral envelope protein and an essential regulatory protein, respectively. This is incorporated into a plasmid construct, which provides the regulatory elements required to express the HIV genes.

factor   Any substance or activity required to produce a result; a contributing cause in any action; a gene (hereditary factor).

factor VIII   A naturally occurring protein in plasma necessary for normal blood coagulation. A congenital deficiency in factor VIII results in the bleeding disorder known as HEMO-PHILIA. Also called antihemophilic globulin (AHG) and anti-hemophilic factor A.

factor IX   A naturally occurring protein essential for normal blood coagulation; it is deficient in patients with HEMO-PHILIA type B.

fag   Male homosexual, especially one considered effeminate. Fag may also be an abbreviation for faggot. In the 1973 Gay Activists Alliance and National Gay Task Force guidelines on homosexuality, *fag* and *faggot* were listed as terms of abuse. Other terms included *queer, homo, fairy, mary, pansy,* and *sissy.*

faggot   A 20th-century derogatory term for a male homosexual. Usually meant to be insulting, demeaning, and provocative. Gay men, however, have used it of themselves in an ironic fashion.

failure to thrive   Condition in which infants and children not only fail to gain weight but may also lose it. The organic causes may include almost any severe chronic condition. Non-organic causes include starvation, emotional deprivation, and social disruption.

fair hearing   A semi-judicial proceeding before a state welfare officer at which an applicant for or recipient of almost any state-administered benefit can present claims of error, unfairness, misapplication of rules, or other grievances in an attempt to reverse or modify an unfavorable decision.

Fair Housing Act   The Fair Housing Act, adopted by Congress in 1968, prohibits discrimination in the sale or rental of housing and in advertising, financing, and brokerage services. Congress amended the law in 1988 to prohibit discrimination because of "handicap." The Fair Housing Act defines "handicap" as a "physical or mental impairment which substantially limits . . . major life activities." People are also protected if they are *perceived* as having a handicap, even if they do not. This definition was taken from Section 504 of the Rehabilitation Act of 1973, which courts have unanimously interpreted to include HIV. The DEPARTMENT OF HOUSING AND URBAN DEVELOPMENT (HUD), which drafted the regulations for administering the act, has concluded that congress chose the Section 504 definition with the intention of including people with HIV as handicapped people protected by the Fair Housing Act. People subjected to discrimination in violation of the Fair Housing Act may file a complaint with HUD and may bring a lawsuit in a federal court. The attorney general may also bring actions in court to prohibit "a pattern or practice" that violates the Fair Housing Act. See FAIR HOUSING AMENDMENTS ACT.

Fair Housing Amendments Act   This act, adopted in 1988, is an outgrowth of the Fair Housing Act of 1968, which was amended numerous times in the 1970s and 1980s. The Fair Housing Amendments Act was designed to ban housing discrimination based on disability (including any stage of HIV illness) and covers most real estate transactions (financing, rental, sale). The act provides limited exemptions for religious organizations and private clubs,

97

owners of fewer than three units who do not use real estate agents, and owner-occupied buildings with fewer than four units. Under the act, no landlord may evict, refuse to rent to, refuse to renew the lease of, or legally harm in any way anyone with an HIV illness. If it does, an individual has the same right to file a discrimination complaint with a state or city agency as he or she has in a case of employment discrimination, or to sue in federal court.

During the 1970s and early 1980s, most states passed laws prohibiting disability discrimination in employment, housing, and public accommodations. These laws differ widely, however, in their interpretation and application.

fairy   Male homosexual, especially an effeminate one. This 20th-century derogatory term is not as pejorative as fag.

fallopian tubes   Delicate tubes that extend from the ovaries to the upper uterus, through which an egg passes to be fertilized.

false negative   A blood test result that indicates falsely that the sample under analysis doesn't contain enough antibodies or antigens to be characterized as positive. This result implies that the person tested is not infected with a virus even though he or she really is.

false positive   A blood test result that indicates falsely that the sample under analysis has enough antibodies or antigens present to be considered positive. This result implies that the person tested is infected with a virus even though he or she is really not.

famciclovir   A synthetic chemical that mimics one of the building blocks of DNA. Inside the body, famciclovir is converted to the antiviral agent penciclovir. In cells infected with the VARICELLA ZOSTER VIRUS, the drug slows down the replication of viral DNA. It has especially high bioavailability and is an approved therapy for shingles. Like other antiviral drugs, it does not rid the body of a virus but acts to reduce the severity and slow the growth of infection.

Famciclovir was developed as an alternative to ACYCLOVIR. Acyclovir has a long history of safety and efficacy and is still the drug of choice for shingles, but viral resistance to it is becoming more common. However, both acyclovir and famciclovir become activated by the same enzymatic pathway, and this pathway accounts for most resistance to acyclovir. Consequently, if a virus is resistant to acyclovir, it is often also resistant to famciclovir; many physicians use FOSCARNET as an alternative. Famciclovir has not been extensively tested in people with HIV. It has not been tested for long periods in any group, and it has not been tested for prevention of herpes virus diseases. However, in test-tube studies, famciclovir was effective in treating cells infected with HERPES SIMPLEX VIRUS; this effectiveness has been confirmed in humans. In limited experience, famciclovir appears to have few side effects. It is available in tablet form under the trade name Famvir.

family-centered care   Health and social-service care that recognizes and respects the crucial role of families in the lives of their members. It supports families in their natural caregiving roles, promotes normal patterns of living, and ensures family collaboration and choice in the provision of services to family members who are sick.

family law   Family law is the name now more commonly used for what was previously called domestic relations law. It encompasses prenuptial agreements, marriages, annulments, divorces, child custody and visitation rights, and other family issues. The American Bar Association's Policy on AIDS makes clear that the organization feels HIV status should not generally be deemed admissible evidence in a family law proceeding, and that when it is it should be considered only in the same manner as other medical conditions. The ABA believes that HIV status should not be deemed admissible evidence for the purpose of determining a party's sexual orientation.

family planning   At one time synonymous with "birth control," family planning is a concept whose purpose is to allow parents to determine the size of families through the spacing or prevention of pregnancies. Numerous social service agencies and voluntary organizations have programs of counseling and assistance in all aspects of family planning. Generally clinicians or counselors offer a supportive discussion of sexuality, safe sex, contraception, and the desire for children. They offer assistance and support for their clients' contraceptive and family planning needs, preferences, and choices, whether the client is HIV-positive or -negative.

When pregnancy is diagnosed and a woman or a couple seeks such assistance, an agency offers nondirective counseling and usually referrals as requested for abortion or prenatal care and information regarding disease transmission and risk to the mother and fetus. For a woman or a couple contemplating pregnancy, it is often important to initiate a discussion regarding feelings and ability to care for an ill child, and the willingness and ability of family members to provide support and assistance in the event of the illness of a parent. In a couple in which one partner is HIV-positive and the other is HIV-negative, further discussion is useful. Is the couple willing to consider options such as artificial insemination or adoption? Is the couple able to limit exposure to HIV during sex by learning fertility awareness techniques and having only limited unprotected sex?

Contraceptive choices for HIV-positive women include oral contraceptives, condoms with supermicides, diaphragms with spermicides or cervical caps, other barriers (creams, gels, suppositories, foams, sponges), intrauterine devices, surgical sterilization, progesterone implants, or intramuscular progesterone. The pros and cons of each choice should be evaluated before selection. See also CONTRACEPTIVES.

fatigue   Fatigue, generally measured by patients' responses to questions concerning reductions in daily activity, is one of the most prevalent and most undertreated problems experienced by persons with HIV infection and AIDS. Despite the fact that HIV/AIDS-related fatigue impacts significantly the psychological well-being and quality of life of patients with HIV/AIDS, many physicians tend to ignore it and do not consider it to be a complaint requiring clinical intervention. The bottom line, however, is that fatigue can be as debilitating as pain.

HIV/AIDS-related fatigue is multidimensional. It has no single cause, but rather a constellation of interactive causes of which psychological distress and depression are just one aspect. Physical symptoms, drug side effects, sleep disturbances, malnutrition and wasting, AIDS dementia, hormonal insufficiency (due to low adrenal gland output, for example), and muscular weakness (HIV- or AZT-related myopathy) all contribute to fatigue. Researchers have also noted a small but statistically significant association between fatigue and anemia (low oxygen transport by the blood).

Pneumocystis carinii pneumonia (PCP) and cytomegalovirus and other active opportunistic conditions directly trigger fatigue. Part of this fatigue results from the increase in inflammatory cytokines as the immune system responds to the opportunistic infections, but PCP lowers oxygen levels in the blood by interfering with lung absorption, and CMV can reduce hormonal levels by infecting the adrenal glands.

Addressing the medical causes of fatigue, which may be as simple as switching patients to alternative drugs, can have a rapid, positive effect. A better diet and special nutritional supplementation to combat malabsorption or the special needs of those with chronic infection can be useful in combating fatigue. Raising hemoglobin levels by administering blood transfusions, recombinant erythropoietin, or nutritional therapy also gives people improved energy levels and greater functional capacity. Red blood cell transfusions are a "quick fix" for treatment-associated anemia, but they carry a small risk of immune reactions and transmission of blood-borne infections. Recombinant erythropoietin has the advantage of being free of significant side effects. It requires three weeks to elevate hemoglobin levels, though, and occasional blood transfusions may still be required. Researchers are currently studying the ability of two commercially available psychostimulants (Ritalin and Cylert) to reduce fatigue in ambulatory HIV-positive individuals. Stimulants are considered an umbrella kind of therapy that help individuals deal with fatigue of any cause; however, they also can interfere with sleep and cause loss of appetite, both of which might further fatigue in the long run.

Physicians suggest that individuals should be encouraged to develop their own methods of coping with fatigue, including pacing their daily lives, altering activity/rest patterns, taking frequent rest breaks, and delegating activities to others. Working out at the gym or jogging is a form of natural psychological and physical stimulation, but more moderate exercise like walking can be helpful too. People have found such meditative exercise forms as yoga, tai chi, or chi gong to be very restorative even when their physical capacity is limited by disease. Massage, therapeutic touch, acupuncture, and other alternative therapies that claim to restore the body's "energy balance" also may have a role to play, if only for their meditative aspects that relieve mental tension and depression. Finally, psychosocial counseling and support groups can be important for helping the individual to cope with emotional stress or anxiety. Occupational therapy can also be a valuable strategy for distracting an individual from focusing on his or her disease, symptoms, and emotions.

Antidepressant medication can be used in cases of recalcitrant depression.

Fc fragment   Small pieces of immunoglobulins (antibodies) used by macrophages in their processing and presenting of foreign antigens to T lymphocytes.

Fc receptor   A receptor present on monocytes and macrophages that bind FC FRAGMENTS of immunoglobulins G and E.

FDA   See FOOD AND DRUG ADMINISTRATION.

FDC   See FOLLICULAR DENDRITIC CELLS.

fear of AIDS   The exploitation of irrational fears has often resulted in attacks on, or stigmatization of, gays and other heavily affected groups. Media scares have served and continue to serve to fuel both rational and irrational fear of AIDS. The very considerable medical evidence that transmission cannot occur through casual contact seems not to have been registered by large numbers of people. The high level of fear in so many in spite of the small number of cases and deaths so far, relative to the total population, supports the observation that there is no simple correlation between risk and fear.

fecal matter   See FECES.

feces   Solid body waste consisting of food residue, bacteria, exfoliated cells, and mucus, discharged from the intestines by way of the anus. Also called stool, excreta, dejecta, and excrement. The color, form, consistency, and odor of feces vary with disease and diet, and may be indicative of various disorders.

Federal Rehabilitation Act   See REHABILITATION ACT OF 1973.

feline leukemia virus (FeLV)   A virus that causes leukemia in cats. FeLV was discovered in the 1970s by a Scotsman and a veterinary-trained researcher named William Jarrett.

fellatio   The sexual act of stimulating a penis orally. Colloquially called a blow job, but the action is more sucking than blowing. See ORAL SEX.

female condom   A protective plastic (or natural membrane) sheath that fits into the vagina and provides a contraceptive and disease-prevention barrier for women that is at least as safe and effective as the male condom. The female condom keeps bodily fluids, such as semen, from entering the vagina.

The plastic female condom was first designed in the mid-1980s by a Danish gynecologist and his wife and developed by an international group of researchers and physicians. Combining features of a male condom and a diaphragm, it consists of soft polyurethane rings. The smaller ring lies inside the closed end of the sheath. It is inserted into the vagina and anchors the condom behind the pubic bone. The larger, outer ring lines the open end of the sheath and, after insertion, hangs outside the vagina.

A woman can insert the female condom as she would a diaphragm. Unlike the diaphragm, however, the inner ring of the condom comes in only one size and need not fit snugly over the CERVIX. The sheath lines the vaginal canal. During intercourse, the external outer end and ring cover the LABIA, preventing skin-to-skin contact with the base of the penis. The inner lining of the sheath is coated with a silicon-based lubricant. Women may add oil- or water-based lubricants on the outside of the sheath to facilitate insertion and on the inside to promote a natural feel during intercourse.

The benefits and advantages of a female condom are similar to those associated with a male condom. It provides adequate but not complete protection against pregnancy and STDS. The female condom, like the male condom, is a safe and practical alternative to other forms of birth control, and it need be used only during sex. There are no health risks to either partner. It is safe to use, with no vaginal side effects except infrequent labial itching and irritation. No prescription or medical exam is needed for purchase. It can be obtained in clinics and pharmacies without a prescription or fitting from a health care professional. Both oil- and water-based lubricants may be used, a distinct advantage of polyurethane over latex condoms. And, best of all, it gives women control over their own protection.

Problems and disadvantages include the fact that unlike male condoms, which can be bought in many places (drugstores, clinics, adult bookstores, vending machines in public restrooms, large supermarkets) and are given away in others (health clinics, doctors' offices, retail stores featuring sexual materials, gay bars), female condoms are as yet less easy to obtain and, therefore, to have handy. Female condoms, like male condoms, can also be used incorrectly and thus ineffectively. On rare occasions, the woman or man might be allergic to the material. Finally, like its male counterpart and other female barrier methods, it will not appeal to everyone. Cost is a major problem for many potential users. Initially, the plastic female condom sold for about three times the local price of male condoms. Even at half the retail price, the female condom is too expensive for women in developing countries without substantial government and other agency subsidies. Faced with limited budgets, agencies may have to choose between expanding supplies of male condoms and providing female condoms. And availability does not ensure use. As a relatively new product, the female condom may not be accepted easily by women or by health care providers who need information to promote the new method and to advise women accurately. Women need culturally-specific instructions and information to understand its benefits, allay concerns about potential side effects, and ensure correct use. They also need advice on convincing men to accept the product. Given the design, the cost, and the objections of men, many women are likely to use the female condom primarily to prevent STDs and only then as a back-up method to the male condom.

The plastic condom is the first vaginal barrier method designed specifically to prevent HIV transmission. Modifications are needed to make it more practical and more acceptable to all women, especially to those at highest risk of HIV infection. To reach potential users, the female condom will have to be promoted and widely distributed through the same channels as the male condom. Ensuring availability to women at high risk of sexually transmitted disease is particularly important. Many of the social marketing programs for condoms aimed specifically at AIDS prevention are setting up commercial outlets in places where high-risk behavior is likely to occur, such as hotels, truck stops, and bars. Such outlets ought to sell the female condom as well.

female homosexual　See LESBIAN.

female-to-female transmission　See TRANSMISSION.

female-to-male transmission　See TRANSMISSION.

feminine hygiene products　Vaginal douches, deodorants, and sprays that can encourage infection by destroying the normal balance in the vagina.

fertility　The quality of being productive or fertile; capable of conceiving a bady.

fetish　Object capable of pathologically arousing sexual excitement. This term is an extension of the belief among tribal communities that a specific object carries magical powers.

fetus　The unborn offspring of a human or an animal while in the uterus or within an egg during the latter stages of development. In humans, this period is considered to be from two or three months after conception until birth. Prior to this period, the fertilized egg is called an embryo.

fetus, transmission to　See TRANSMISSION.

fever　Elevation of body temperature above normal. The normal temperature taken orally is 98.6 degrees F (37 degrees C). From one degree above or two degrees below this value is considered within the range of normal. Rectal temperature is 0.5 degree to one degrees higher than oral temperature.

fimbria　The flared end of the fallopian tube, where it meets the ovary. It draws out and delivers the egg from the ovary into the FALLOPIAN TUBES.

financial counselor　A hospital employee who assists indigents in applying for MEDICAID, HILL-BURTON, GMS, or in-house charity care.

financial planning　Because AIDS is a progressive, debilitating disease, and the longer a person has it, the more likely he or she will become incapable of dealing with routine business, dealing with financial matters is an important part of the practical preparations for future illness and possible death. Responsible financial planning ensures that an individual will not have to deal with financial problems in a crisis. Financial planning involves consideration of disability payments and other benefits to which one may be entitled, such as food stamps, welfare, and MEDICAID, as well as medical insurance. It may involve exploring sources of financial help other than public programs.

finger cot   Generally made of latex and sometimes of plastic or metal, often found in first-aid kits, finger cots are worn to protect fingers from trauma while healing from injuries. For safe sex, they are used to encase a digit for FINGER FUCKING. They can be bought at most medical suppliers and pharmacies.

finger fucking   Moving a finger in and out of the vagina, anus, or mouth in a manner similar to that of a penis during intercourse. See also DIGITAL-ANAL SEX.

fist-fucking   This term is generally used to describe hand-anus contact but can be used to describe hand-vagina contact. See ANOMANUAL INTERCOURSE; BRACHIOPROCTIC EROTICISM; VAGINAL-MANUAL INTERCOURSE.

fisting   The insertion of an entire hand into someone's vagina or anus.

Fitz-Hugh–Curtis syndrome   A complication of gonorrhea and chlamydia in women that attacks the liver.

5-fluorouracil collagen matrix (5-FU)   A cancer chemotherapy drug. Collagen is a structural component of the skin and connective tissue. The collagen matrix was developed to keep the chemotherapy agent in the lesion longer. The drug was tested for use in HIV-negative people with anal or genital warts.

5-FU collagen matrix   See 5-FLUOROURACIL COLLAGEN MATRIX.

flaccid   Soft, nonerect.

flagellation   The striking of oneself or someone else with an object or one's bare hand(s). Flagellation can also include being struck by someone else. Objects include both short implements, such as paddles, riding crops, or doubled-up belts, and more flexible implements, such as cat-of-nine tails, canes, or blacksnakes. Flagellants may be sexually aroused and gratified by either being threatened with pain or having pain administered, or by threatening or inflicting pain. Within the context of HIV/AIDS it is noted that anytime the skin is broken there is risk of disease transmission and infection. This can be minimized by cleaning the area and one's hands and by using sterile objects. A bloodied object should never be reused on another person unless it is sterilized.

flash   See EXHIBITIONISM.

floater   A drifting dark spot within the field of vision. Floaters can be caused by CMV RETINITIS, but may also appear as a normal part of the aging process. An HIV-knowledgeable eye doctor can make a correct diagnosis.

FLT   See 3'=DEOXY = 3'FLUOROTHIMIDINE.

fluax   See INFLUENZA VACCINE.

fluconazole (Diflucan)   An antifungal drug that is approved for fungal infections, primarily those caused by CANDIDA ALBICANS (thrush or candidal esophagitis) and CRYPTOCOCCUS NEOFORMANS (cryptococcal meningitis), a severe complication of HIV infection. Fluconazole can be taken by mouth or vein. Side effects are unusual. Occasional problems are abdominal discomfort, nausea, rash or signs of liver damage. Fluconazole has many drug-drug interactions with a wide variety of agents, including those frequently taken concurrently by people with HIV. Four examples follow. RIFAMPIN has been shown to decrease the half-life of fluconazole. Fluconazole may also increase the blood levels of Dilantin, resulting in greater toxic effects for this drug. Levels of drugs used to control blood sugar are increased when fluconazole is given. Using fluconazole in conjunction with such drugs as chlorpropamide, cipizide, glyburide, and tolbutamide can result in hypoglycemia (low blood sugar). Additionally, the metabolism of the common anticoagulant Coumadin is decreased by fluconazole so that taking both drugs together may prolong Coumadin's effect. Finally, blood levels of various drugs (AZT, cyclosporine, Dilantin, and rifabutin) may increase when taken along with fluconazole. This may exacerbate their side effects.

While it is still under study for VAGINAL CANDIDIASIS and other fungal infections, recent trials have shown that weekly doses of fluconazole safely prevented certain common yeast infections, including mucosal candidiasis, the most common fungal infection affecting women with HIV, and was not associated with adverse events or drug resistance.

flucytosine   An antifungal drug, appearing as a whitish, crystalline powder, administered orally to treat yeast and fungal infections (including those caused by CANDIDA and/or CRYPTOCOCCUS, such as endocarditis, septicemia, and urinary tract infections.) Flucytosine is thought to work by inhibiting DNA and RNA synthesis in fungal cells. The result is unbalanced growth that causes the death of the fungus. The drug readily penetrates the BLOOD-BRAIN BARRIER and is an effective treatment for infections of the CENTRAL NERVOUS SYSTEM. For treatment of CRYPTOCOCCAL MENINGITIS, flucytosine is often combined with AMPHOTERICIN B, because test-tube studies show the two to have a synergistic effect against cryptococcus. Studies of its use in people have had mixed results, but the combination may be superior in effectiveness to amphotericin B alone. Steroids may be added to the combination for people with high cranial pressure. After treatment of acute infection, some type of maintenance therapy must be used for life to prevent the recurrence of cryptococcal disease. Amphotericin B is used occasionally as maintenance therapy, but fluconazole is generally the drug of choice because it is effective, has fewer side effects, and can be taken orally. Flucytosine should not be used by anyone with a known allergy to it. The drug should also be used with extreme caution in people with reduced kidney function, because of the increased risk of serious side effects. Similarly, the drug should be used with caution by people with bone-marrow suppression. The most common side effects are weakness, malaise, inflammation of the liver, yellowing of the eyes or the skin, abdominal pain, diarrhea, loss of appetite, nausea, vomiting, skin rashes, redness, itching, sore throat, bruising, or unusual bleeding. Also known as 5-FC and 5-fluorocytosine, it is sold under the trade name Ancobon.

fluid retention   Failure to eliminate fluid from the body because of renal, cardiac, or metabolic disorders, or a combination of these. A low-sodium diet is indicated in cases of fluid retention, since it is caused by excess salt in the body, which causes retention of water to maintain the proper chemical and physical properties of body fluids.

Fluogen   See INFLUENZA VACCINE.

fluorescent treponemal antibody absorption test (FTA-ABS)   A test of the treponemal variety (looking for *Treponema pallidum*, the corkscrew-shaped organisms that cause syphilis) of serological (blood) tests. The FTA-ABS test has been found to be more sensitive for syphilis than the Treponema pallidum immobilization test (TPI), another test of the treponemal variety. It is easier to perform, and therefore, used more often, but one patient out of 10 with very early syphilis will still be missed (have a false-negative reaction). False-positive reactions may occur when the patient's serum contains antinuclear factors, rheumatoid factor, or increased globulins. Blood from a vein is tested. Spinal fluid is also tested to detect latent syphilis and to follow the progress of treatment.

fluorouracil   An antimetabolite used in treating certain forms of cancer. Trade names are Efudex and Fluoroplex.

fluoxetine hydrochloride   An antidepressant that is approved for treatment of major forms of depression. Other (unlabeled) generally accepted uses include: refractory bulimia; refractory diabetic neuropathy; help in controlling kleptomania; help in treating obesity, especially when obesity is accompanied by depression; eases symptoms of panic attacks; may be given only during the premenstrual period to treat premenstrual syndrome (PMS); used to treat seasonal affective disorder. Fluoxetine works by slowly restoring normal levels of a nerve transmitter (serotonin). Possible side effects are decreased appetite and weight loss. Possible risks include serious allergic reactions and conversion of depression to mania in manic-depressive (bipolar) disorders (rare). Brand name is Prozac.

In 1990, it was reported that six patients being treated with fluoxetine experienced the onset of intense and violent suicidal preoccupation. All six had severe depression that had not responded to the use of fluoxetine for 2 to 7 weeks. For most of them, suicidal mentality persisted for 2 to 3 months after discontinuation of the drug. The resultant adverse publicity suggested that this experience may be somewhat characteristic of fluoxetine in contrast to other antidepressant drugs. A review of relevant literature on this subject reveals that development or intensification of suicidal thoughts during treatment (regardless of the severity of depression) has been documented for many antidepressant drugs in wide use. Suicidal thinking may emerge during treatment with any

antidepressant. Recent reports establish that some patients who become suicidal while taking one antidepressant can be switched to fluoxetine and experience cessation of suicidal thinking and satisfactory relief of depression.

flush   A sudden redness of the skin that may be associated with any febrile disease.

foam barrier   A form of chemical contraceptive; a spermicide-containing foam that is placed in the vagina prior to intercourse. It may be used alone but is most effective in combination with a another contraceptive method or device.

folic acid   A member of the VITAMIN B complex necessary for various metabolic reactions and used in the treatment of sprue. Inadequate amounts of folic acid cause megaloblastic anemia. Folic acid is found naturally in green plant tissue, liver, and yeast. Also called *Lactobacillus casei* factor, liver *Lactobacillus casei* factor, pteroylglutamic acid, and vitamin M.

folinic acid   A derivative of folic acid used to counteract the effects of folic acid antagonists and to treat anemia caused by a deficiency of folic acid. Also called citrovorum factor, leucovorin, and calcium folinate.

follicle   A small sac or cavity for excretion or secretion.

follicle-stimulating hormone (FSH)   A hormone produced by the anterior pituitary. It stimulates growth of the follicle in the ovary and spermatogenesis in the testes.

follicular dendritic cell (FDC)   A dendritic cell found in lymphoid follicles. It has threadlike tentacles and is found within hot spots of immune activity called GERMINAL CENTERS.

Recent research focusing on the activity of this specialized cell may have revealed one of the secrets of HIV infection, specifically, why HIV continues to thrive even after the immune system has mounted a powerful attempt to stop the spread of the disease. Shaped like miniature octopi FDCs reside in secondary lymphoid tissue such as the lymph nodes, spleen, and tonsils. They normally help the body ward off viral and bacterial infection by trapping individual pathogens and holding them in the germinal centers until B CELLS come along and initiate an immune response. HIV, however, remains infectious, even in the presence of a vigorous immune response. Close on the heels of B cells are CD4+ t cells, which respond to the call for help from the secondary lymphoid tissue and rush to the HIV-laden FDCs. CD4+ T CELLS are the primary targets of HIV. Coming in to boost the work of antibody cells, these cells may become infected as they enter the germinal center and encounter HIV trapped on follicular dendritic cells. Once infected, CD4+ T cells leave the germinal center and may infect many other CD4+ T cells that congregate in the region of the lymph node surrounding the germinal center.

It is known that HIV, when attached to the external surface of follicular dendritic cells infected CD4+ T cells even in the presence of a vast excess of neutralizing antibodies. In the absence of follicular dendritic cells, similar quantities of neutralizing antibodies blocked the infectivity of the virus. This findings confirms that the lymphoid organs are central to the pathogenesis of HIV disease.

FDCs are like flypaper in terms of their capacity to attract HIV. That the virus remains infectious on them is surprising because they are covered with antibody and other protective proteins that would normally be expected to neutralize virus infectivity. The process of infection within secondary lymphoid tissue continues over a period of years until the tissue is destroyed. This work is quietly accomplished with few symptoms. HIV-positive people may feel healthy, and unless tested for the virus, might not suspect anything is wrong. Until a couple of years ago, this stage of HIV infection was misnamed a "latent" period. It is anything but that. The research findings noted above will allow researchers to focus on the site where a devastating process of HIV infection occurs. The information will also help devise better vaccination and treatment strategies.

folliculitis   Inflammation of a follicle or follicles.

Food and Drug Act of 1906   The original legislation giving the federal government regulatory control over food and drugs. It is the basis for federal regulation of testing AIDS drugs. The act prohibited interstate commerce in misbranded and adulterated foods, drinks, and drugs. The power to administer the law was placed in the Agriculture Department's Bureau of Chemistry. Today, the FOOD AND DRUG ADMINISTRATION (FDA) administers a broad range of legislation, including the Public Health Service Act (1944), the Federal Hazardous Substances Act (1960), the Fair Packaging and Labeling Act (1966), the Radiation Control for Health and Safety Act (1968), the Drug Listing Act of 1972, the Infant Formula Act of 1980, the Orphan Drug Act of 1983 and its amendments of 1985 and 1988, the Federal Anti-Tampering Act (1983), the Drug Price Competition and Patent Term Restoration Act (1984), the Prescription Drug Marketing Act of 1987, the Health Omnibus Programs Extension of 1988, the Nutrition Labeling and Education Act (1990), the FDA Revitalization Act (1990), the Safe Medical Devices Act of 1990, the Generic Drug Enforcement Act of 1992, the Mammography Quality Standards Act of 1992, the Prescription Drug User Fee Act of 1992, the Dietary Supplement Act of 1992, and the Dietary Supplement Health and Education Act of 1994. See also FOOD, DRUG AND COSMETIC ACT (FDC) OF 1938.

Food and Drug Administration   An agency of the United States DEPARTMENT OF HEALTH AND HUMAN SERVICES that regulates the testing, sale, and promotion of pharmaceutical drugs and food products. The agency also approves new medical procedures for marketing based on evidence of safety and efficacy. Early in the AIDS crisis, when the epidemic's disastrous scope could not yet be imagined, AIDS activists pressed the FDA for a faster and more humane response to this public health emergency. In response, the FDA established accelerated approval and expanded access programs. For example, SAQUINAVIR, the first of the new generation of PROTEASE INHIBITOR drugs, was approved in a record three months, the fastest AIDS drug approval ever.

After the Republican victory in the 1994 congressional elections, the new Congress immediately took up the cause of FDA reform as one of its highest priorities. Instead of focusing on management problems at the FDA, the Republican Congress set its sights on the Food, Drug and Cosmetic Act (FDC) itself. The FDC gives the federal government the duty to ensure that drugs, biological products, and medical devices are safe and effective for the treatment of specific health conditions and that evidence of that safety and efficacy is accurately presented to the American people. The act fosters an environment in which medical innovation grows out of solid clinical research. People with AIDS, as well as those with other life-threatening diseases, need this research more than anyone to point the way to effective treatments. By seeking to amend fundamental government authority over drug regulation, Congress has focused not on problems at the FDA but on reducing the role of the federal government in medical, pharmaceutical, and clinical research. FDA-regulated industries, which would benefit financially from such reform, initiated a major lobbying and public relations campaign within a month of the 1994 election. In the summer of 1995, patient advocacy groups also joined together in the Patients' Coalition, which includes over 80 leading national organizations. Perhaps as a result, FDA reform legislation has taken longer to move through Congress than many had predicted. Despite numerous hearings held on FDA reform issues in both the House and the Senate during the 104th Congress, legislation has been very slow to emerge. In fact, there is no consensus on FDA reform.

Food, Drug and Cosmetic Act of 1938   A major overhaul of the basic food and drug legislation occurred in 1938 with the passage of the Food, Drug and Cosmetic (FDC) Act of 1938. Signed by President Franklin D. Roosevelt on June 25, 1938, this act broadened the original legislation by extending the regulatory power of the Food and Drug Administration (FDA) to cover cosmetics and medical devices; requiring predistribution approval of new drugs; requiring that tolerance levels be set for unavoidable poisonous substances; authorizing standards of identity, quality, and fill levels for containers for foods; authorizing inspections of factories where regulated products are manufactured; and adding court injunctions to FDA enforcement powers. The FDC has been amended several times since its passage. Examples include the Humphrey Amendment signed in 1951, the Food Additives Amendment signed in 1958, the Color Additive Amendments of 1960, the Drug Amendments of 1962, the Drug Abuse Control Amendments of 1965, the Vitamins and Minerals Amendments of 1976, the Medical Device Amendments of 1976.

food stamp program   A federally financed, state-run welfare program that gives low-income persons vouchers (food stamps) with which to purchase food.

foreplay   Activities a couple enjoys before sexual intercourse. For many couples these erotic activities are extremely exciting, stimulating, and fulfilling in themselves and are not simply a prelude to intercourse.

fornication   Voluntary sexual intercourse between two persons not married to each other.

foscarnet   A broad-spectrum antiviral (trisodium phosphonoformate) effective against CYTOMEGALOVIRUS in the retina and elsewhere in the body. It also has activity against HERPES SIMPLEX virus, including ACYCLOVIR-resistant strains. Possible adverse side effects include kidney toxicity, seizures, skin rashes, reduced blood levels of calcium and phosphorous, anemia, and nausea. Foscarnet should not be taken with other kidney-damaging drugs, aminoglycoside antibiotics, AMPHOTERICIN-B, and PENTAMIDINE. If any of these drugs is prescribed concomitantly with foscarnet, then patients must undergo hydration with INTRAVENOUS fluid (usually saline). Hydration may also prevent the formation of the penile ulcers occasionally noted with foscarnet, which are due to the local irritant effect of the drug in the urine. Another observed interaction is with pentamidine; together these drugs can lower blood calcium levels, a condition that can lead to seizures and spasms.

At the Nineteenth International Congress on Chemotherapy in Montreal in 1995, findings were presented from experiments with liposomal foscarnet in mice. These fat globules dramatically increase foscarnet's plasma half-life as well as its uptake into microphages and lymphoid organs. More importantly, the liposomes substantially lower accumulation of the drug in the kidneys, whose functioning foscarnet greatly impairs. Administration of liposomal foscarnet may therefore increase the drug's effect while decreasing its toxicity. Although liposomes are generally too large to cross the barriers between the blood and the brain and the retina, which is necessary in order to treat CMV encephalitis or retinitis, free drug concentrations in the brain and retina were higher in the mice injected with the liposomal drug than in the mice administered the nonliposomal product. This was possibly due to foscarnet's increased half-life. Researchers also reported that liposomal encapsulation can also increase foscarnet's antiviral activity against both CMV and HIV. Brand name: Foscavir.

foster care   Care of an orphaned, abandoned, abused, or neglected child by adults or facilities acting in place of the children's parents, supervised by welfare caseworkers.

free radicals   A highly reactive molecular fragment that bears one or more unpaired electrons. For some time, it has been known that foods contain more substances than just vitamins and minerals and energy-giving nutrients. There are known nutrient antioxidants like vitamins E and C and selenium, and there are the new nonnutrient antioxidants like the carotenoids, the phytochemicals, and the polyphenols. These substances aid in removing molecules that attack healthy cells in the body and leave it vulnerable to cancer.

The oxygen we breathe and cannot live without can become one of our worst enemies. Excess oxidation is damaging and destructive to the body. Four destructive forms of oxygen have been identified: hydroxyl radical and superoxide radical (the two real free radicals) and the "nonradical reactive species" oxygen singlet and hydrogen peroxide.

Destructive oxygen reactions have been linked to at least 50 diseases, including AIDS.

Oxygen reactions take place when an oxidant or free radical is created that has lost one electron and is no longer stable. In its search for stability, the radical grabs electrons from other healthy cells causing the creation of more radicals. When radicals attack fatty molecules, rancidity results, and the stage is set for deterioration and eventual disease. When these free radicals attack DNA molecules and begin to mutate them, conditions become positive for cancer and also for other degenerative conditions including aging. In order for the body to defend itself against free radicals, it produces free-radical scavengers, or endogenous ANTIOXIDANTS. These agents are made by the body and catch and destroy extra free radicals and keep them from creating greater damage. Exercise contributes oxygen to the system and can increase free radicals in the body. A selenium supplement (50 to 100 micrograms) is also thought to be beneficial, as it strengthens GSH (an antioxidant that counters hydrogen peroxide). Studies continue on the benefit of the coenzyme Q10 for those who exercise extensively. A physician should be consulted before any vitamin therapy is begun since side effects occur at large doses.

freebase   A form of cocaine used by addicts in which the hydrochloride salt is alkalinized, extracted with an organic solvent (e.g., ether), and then heated to 90 degrees C. After inhalation, the drug is absorbed rapidly through the lungs.

freebasing   The inhalation of a form of cocaine known as freebase.

freedom of speech   The right of people to express their opinions openly has come under attack, particularly in the area of AIDS education. Numerous attempts have been made at the local, state, and federal levels to control the content of specific AIDS educational materials. There have also been challenges to teachers' resources, such as curriculum guides and textbooks. In some states police have gone so far as to infiltrate AIDS activist organizations to keep them from demonstrating at public events; several lawsuits are pending.

French kiss   A kiss that includes tongue contact and exchange of saliva. Also called a *wet kiss*.

fruit   A derogatory 20th-century term for a male homosexual. Often used for humor or irony by gays.

FS   See FOOD STAMP PROGRAM.

FTA   See FLUORESCENT TREPONEMAL ANTIBODY ABSORPTION TEST.

fuck   To have sexual intercourse. "Fuck" is *the* four-letter word, by far the most widely used term for this activity in the English language. In its adjectival form it is also used almost universally as an intensifier, with no particular sexual connection although this usage is considered quite vulgar. See also COITUS.

funduscopy   Visual examination of the retina with an ophthalmoscope.

funerals   Funerals have often been turned into occasions of political protest during the AIDS epidemic, and many political protests have taken the form of mock funerals (for example, plans to scatter human ashes on the White House lawn as a protest of the Reagan Administration's management of AIDS education and treatment research). The obvious reason for this is to demonstrate the nature of the AIDS epidemic and to instill a sense of urgency by showing the consequences of delay, mismanagement, neglect, or callousness by those making and executing public health policy. This tactic has been controversial and has been attacked as tasteless or worse, but those activists who support it say that the direness of the crisis justifies it.

fungal encephalitis   Inflammation of the brain resulting from invasion by a PATHOGENIC FUNGUS.

fungal infection   The state or condition in which the body, or a part of it, is invaded by a PATHOGENIC FUNGUS. Toenail fungal infections are very common in HIV-positive persons and may be the first sign of an impaired immune system. Terbinafine, an allylamine antifungal agent, has been shown to be effective in treating HIV-positive patients with nail fungal infections. CANDIDIASIS, CRYPTOCOCCOSIS, and HISTOPLASMOSIS are examples of AIDS-related fungal infections.

Fungicidin   See NYSTATIN.

fungus   One of a group of plants, lacking chlorophyll, that includes yeast, molds, mildew, and mushrooms. Fungi exist parasitically on organic matter and are generally simple in structure and form. Some fungi are single-celled but differ from bacteria in that they have a distinct nucleus and other cellular structures. AIDS patients are especially vulnerable to infection by fungi because of their compromised immune systems. Recently, powerful antifungal agents have been developed for treatment.

furuncle   A painful, deep-seated nodule formed in the skin by circumscribed inflammation, enclosing a central core. Furuncles are contrasted with CYSTS. Also called BOIL and FURUNCULUS.

furunculosis   The persistent simultaneous occurrence of FURUNCLEs.

furunculus   See FURUNCLE.

future Medicare eligibility date   Two years after the first date of eligibility for SSDI benefits.

G

GAA See GEOGRAPHIC AREAS OF AFFINITY.

gallbladder disease The gallbladder is a pear-shaped organ on the interior surface of the liver. It acts as a reservoir for bile. Gallbladder disease without stones (also known as acalculous cholecystitis) is commonly associated with HIV infection. It can cause enlarged bile ducts, thus blocking the flow of bile between the liver and the intestine and resulting in jaundice and pain. It is not known definitively why HIV-related gallbladder disease occurs, but the condition is frequently associated with such opportunistic infections as CMV or CRYPTOSPORIDIOSIS (and to a lesser extent MAC, HISTO-PLASMOSIS, and other organisms) or with direct HIV infection of the GASTROINTESTINAL system. Symptoms of HIV-related gallbladder and bile duct disease include severe right-side abdominal pain with fever, vomiting, progressive weight loss, intermittent fevers, swollen glands, jaundice, and diarrhea. The vagueness of these symptoms makes it easy to misdiagnose this disease.

Although gallbladder disease was once assumed to occur only in severely ill patients, it has now been shown that it can also be the first manifestation of AIDS. The possibility of gallbladder disease without stones must be considered in patients with abdominal pain, especially in the presence of elevated serum alkaline phosphatase and the absence of jaundice. Ultrasound and CT SCANS are effective for evaluating the presence of bile duct disease. Due to the nature of these infections, actual tissue specimens may be necessary in order to make the diagnosis. ERCP (an endoscopic procedure in which dye is injected into the biliary ducts), removal of the infected gallbladder, and liver biopsy may all be required to identify the infectious agent positively and begin appropriate treatment.

If specific organisms can be identified, antibiotic therapy may be necessary. Further treatment, such as the surgical removal of the gallbladder or opening of the obstructed bile duct entrance, may be required to eliminate the infectious agent. Removal of the bile duct can help remove reservoirs of infection.

GALT (gut-associated lymphoid tissue) The accumulations of lymphoid tissue associated with the GASTROINTESTI-NAL tract.

gamma globulin A serum protein (formed in the blood) with gamma mobility. This type of protein makes up the majority of immunoglobulins and antibodies. The ability to resist infection is related to concentration of such proteins.

gamma interferon A protein formed by human cells that limits the production of some viruses.

ganciclovir A synthetic antiviral drug used to treat infections caused by CYTOMEGALOVIRUS RETINITIS in immuno-compromised patients and occasionally infections caused by HERPES SIMPLEX and other viruses. Licensed by the FOOD AND DRUG ADMINISTRATION in 1989, it was initially available only for INTRAVENOUS administration. An oral form is currently available and has been found to reduce the risk of developing CMV by half in people with advanced AIDS. It also delays the progression of existing disease, although not to the same extent as the intravenous formulation does. (It is obviously easier to administer as well. Patients receiving intravenous ganciclovir must have a central venous line inserted [usually a Hickman catheter], and receive infusions every day for the rest of their lives—an extremely burdensome and time-consuming—and expensive—procedure.)

The most important side effect is a low blood count, especially NEUTROPENIA, which predisposes to bacterial infections. If neutropenia is severe enough, the dose should be reduced or the drug temporarily stopped. Drugs with similar effects on the bone marrow should not in general be prescribed at the same time unless the benefits are felt to outweigh the risks; these include adriamycin, AMPHO-TERICIN, AZT, BACTRIM, DAPSONE, FLUCYTOSINE, imipenem-cilastatin, PENTAMIDINE, VINBLASTINE, and VINCRISTINE. However, the advent of agents like G-CSF (Neupogen) that help increase white blood cell production has made it possible to administer ganciclovir together with many of these drugs without running the risk of BONE MARROW SUPPRESSION. Another drug interaction is seen with imipenen-cilastatin, an antibiotic used to treat severe bacterial infections; this results in seizures. Oral ganciclovir has been reported to be associated with an increased risk of pancreatitis if administered in association with ddI. Ganciclovir is sold under the trade name Cytovene.

ganglion A mass of nervous tissue located outside the brain or spinal cord; also, a benign cystic tumor developing on a tendon or aponeurosis, sometimes occurring in the back of the wrist or dorsum of the foot; a knotlike mass.

Gantrisin See SULFISOXAZOLE.

Gardnerella A bacteria that causes at least half of all cases of VAGINITIS; it can be caught by having intercourse with an infected man.

garlic Garlic is a member of the lily family and has been given the distinction of being called the "wonder drug." It is the world's second oldest medicine, with ephedra being the first. It is made up of sulfur compounds; amino acids; minerals such as germanium, selenium, and zinc; and vitamins A, B, and C. Allicin, a sulfur-containing compound, is believed to be primarily responsible for most of garlic's suggested health benefits—along with its unique color.

Garlic has been used for many medicinal purposes in folk and holistic treatment. Raw garlic is said to work against bacteria, parasites and viruses. It has been said to be effective against heart disease and stroke as well as colds and diarrhea. It also contains compounds, including antioxidants, that are thought to be cancer preventatives. Garlic boosts immunity, acts as an antispasmodic, lowers cholesterol and blood pressure, and works as an anti-inflammatory. It helps relieve gas, is estrogenic and works as an antidepressant. It is effective raw and cooked.

Today, clinical and basic studies suggest a broad spectrum of potential uses. Some have postulated that garlic works as an ANTIOXIDANT against FREE RADICALS because of its germanium and selenium content. Claims of garlic's effectiveness against AIDS-related opportunistic infections are based on test tube studies that have shown garlic to be an anti-bacterial and anti-fungal agent. There have been no studies to date that have looked at garlic closely for its uses with IMMUNODULATION, but protocols are constantly being written and submitted by community researchers and activists.

Eating to much raw garlic, or taking too many garlic pills, can have toxic effects. The high sulfur content can cause dermatitis and can also cause colitis by an overkill of the normal flora of the intestines. In high doses, garlic may inhibit blood clotting and interfere with proper thyroid function.

gastric anacidity See ACHLORHYDRIA.

gastritis The stomach is susceptible to the same disease processes as the esophagus, including infection with CMV. Cytomegalovirus gastritis, or inflammation of the stomach, may be asymptomatic, but often results in severe continuous upper abdominal pain, fever, hemorrhage, or obstruction. CMV infection of the small intestine may result in similar symptoms as well as weight loss and diarrhea. While CMV may infect any part of the small intestine, it rarely does so without involvement of other gastrointestinal organs.

gastroenteritis Inflammation of the stomach and intestinal tract, which can cause abdominal pain and diarrhea.

gastrointestinal Pertaining to organs of the digestive system, also called the GASTROINTESTINAL TRACT.

gastrointestinal dysfunction Abnormal, impaired, or inadequate functioning of the stomach and intestines.

gastrointestinal exams X-ray examinations of the gastrointestinal (GI) tract are used in the diagnosis of a number of complications associated with HIV and AIDS. There are three basic GI tract exams: the upper GI exam focuses on the esophagus and stomach, the lower GI exam on the small intestine, and the barium enema exam on the large intestine and colon. All GI exams require the use of a contrast agent that blocks X rays and thereby silhouettes the body parts of interest, allowing visual interpretation.

Contrast agents used for the GI tract are usually composed of a barium sulfate liquid suspension, but iodine- and noniodine-based contrast agents are also used. The barium mixture has a thick milky consistency and is either swallowed or introduced into the rectum by an enema while the X rays are taken. The contrast agent and not the X rays generally cause any complications arising from the exam. Constipation, rectal bleeding, faintness, weakness, abdominal pain, inability to pass gas, polyuria (excessive urination), nocturia (excessive urination at night), and abdominal distention (extension of the abdomen with pressure) are examples of complications that may arise. Allergic reaction is also a major consideration when using any contrast agent. These are rare, and usually mild (itching, rash, hives, and sometimes nausea), but reactions can be severe enough to cause death if not stopped in time.

gastrointestinal (GI) tract The organs that absorb and digest food, including the mouth, esophagus, stomach, small and large intestines, colon, and rectum.

gay A term denoting sexual attraction to people of the same sex. As a noun, a woman or man who is sexually attracted to others of the same sex and defines herself or himself, or is defined by others, in terms of sexual orientation. Generally refers to male homosexuals, but may also include homosexual women. See also LESBIAN.

gay bowel syndrome A general term used to denote a constellation of intestinal diseases among gay men including proctitis, proctocolitis, and enteritis. The term was widely used in the 1970s with the dramatic increase in enteric diseases within the gay community, like AMEBIASIS and GIARDIASIS. Enteric diseases are caused by organisms that lodge themselves in the intestinal tract. It was postulated that gay men's infection with these parasites was a likely effect of anal intercourse, which was likely to put a man in contact with his partner's fecal matter and was virtually a certainty through the then-popular practice of rimming, which medical journals politely called ORAL-ANAL intercourse.

gay lymph-node syndrome A now obsolete term applied to generalized LYMPHADENOPATHY (with benign reactive changes shown in biopsy) prior to 1981, when the CENTERS

FOR DISEASE CONTROL AND PREVENTION published the first description of persistent generalized lymphadenopathy.

Gay Men's Health Crisis (GMHC)   An AIDS service organization (ASO), one of the first, in New York City. In the United States, as in other countries, privately organized prevention programs started before official government programs. In New York City, the threat of HIV was recognized by a small group of men, who, in September 1981, gathered in the apartment of the writer Larry Kramer in order to do something about the new epidemic in their midst. That day they created the Gay Men's Health Crisis (GMHC). In the following two years, after its example, similar organizations were formed in other major United States cities. Today, the GMHC is recognized not only as one of the premier ASOs, but also as a major nongovernmental HIV/AIDS prevention and care organization.

GMHC, like its counterparts elsewhere, has helped and continues to help thousands of homosexual men overcome the isolation and fear associated with a diagnosis of AIDS. Due in large measure to GMHC's work, large-scale behavior changes among gay men occurred in New York City and San Francisco (the San Francisco AIDS Foundation) in the early 1980s. GMHC has succeeded in responding with equal compassion to the needs of other groups besides gay men with a high incidence of HIV infection—persons of color, injection drug users, and women. GMHC's program is evolving in parallel to the evolving AIDS pandemic.

gay plague   In the early years of the epidemic, this term was often used to denote the acquired immunodeficiency syndrome, since gay men were the first infected and for some time constituted the greatest number of reported cases in the United States.

gay pneumonia   A term used in the early years of the epidemic to denote PNEUMOCYSTIS CARINII PNEUMONIA. See GAY PLAGUE.

gay-related immune deficiency (GRID)   One of a group of names initially used to denote the acquired immunodeficiency syndrome; now obsolete. See also ACQUIRED IMMUNODEFICIENCY SYNDROME, COMMUNITY ACQUIRED IMMUNE DEFICIENCY SYNDROME, and GAY-RELATED IMMUNODEFICIENCY DISEASE.

gay-related immunodeficiency disease   An obsolete term for AIDS. See GAY-RELATED IMMUNE DEFICIENCY.

G-CSF   See GRANULOCYTE COLONY STIMULATING FACTOR.

gel   A colloid or jellylike substance. Barrier contraceptives are available in gel form and work like foams and vaginal suppositories. Gels, as other contraceptives, are most effective in combination with condoms.

gender differences   Early in the AIDS epidemic, the number of men with HIV in developing countries vastly exceeded the number of women with HIV. Their relative lack of numbers limited women's participation in early clinical research. This unintended underrepresentation of women in clinical studies has contributed to a less complete understanding of HIV infection in women than in men. Nonetheless, today we do know that women have some manifestations of HIV infection that are different from those of men. These include, among others, VAGINAL CANDIDIASIS, GENITAL PAPILLOMAVIRUS INFECTIONS, and PELVIC INFLAMMATORY DISEASE, a painful condition of the genital tract that may be caused by a number of different microorganisms. The incidence of some malignancies differs in women and men. KAPOSI'S SARCOMA, a cancer affecting skin and lymph nodes, is relatively infrequent in HIV-infected women; abnormalities of the cervical tissue, including a greatly increased incidence of precancerous lesions, are fairly common in HIV-infected women. To date, there is little information concerning differences between women and men in the effects of various therapies directed at HIV infection.

Women also face a number of issues specific to them as women: rape and AIDS, pregnancy, artificial insemination, prostitution, and the incidence of HIV/AIDS in African women. Talking to children about HIV/AIDS is not a gender-specific issue, strictly speaking but it is a burden that falls on women disproportionately.

gender-specific issues   See GENDER DIFFERENCES.

gene   The basic unit in which is encoded the form and function of a cell or an organism. Chains of genes in ordered sequences make up the DNA of a cell. Genes function either to specify the formation of a protein or part of a protein or regulate or repress the operation of other genes. The complete human genome contains between 50,000 and 100,000 genes.

gene therapy   A distinct and emerging form of treatment in which new, manufactured genes are inserted into patients to fight disease or correct disorders of genetic origin by compensating for other deficient proteins, inhibiting abnormal cellular functioning, or regulating the expression of other genes.

HIV, like all viruses, can be described as an acquired genetic disease. HIV integrates itself into human DNA to transform cells into factories for creating copies of itself. HIV-infected cells produce viral proteins and then assemble them into new viruses. Ultimately, viral infection and replication destroy the host cell.

Scientists have identified many of the proteins that play a part in the replication of HIV, including enzymes such as REVERSE TRANSCRIPTASE, PROTEASE, and TAT. Anti-HIV drugs function by attacking these proteins. For example, drugs like AZT, ddI, and ddC are aimed at the reverse transcriptase enzyme; the protease inhibitor is aimed at the protease enzyme. The great disadvantage of this approach is that it does not halt the production of these malignant proteins at their source. A drug must be given in high doses to disable every copy of the protein and must be given for the lifetime of the patient. Gene therapy, on the other hand, acts against the origin of the disease, the malignant HIV genome.

Many strategies are being considered to fight HIV at the genetic level. Some scientists seek to engineer genes that protect a cell from infection; others create genes that regulate

HIV into harmlessness. Initial test tube models were encouraging, but none of these approaches has yet been tested in humans.

Theoretically, gene therapy has at least one great advantage over current therapies: the implanted mechanism for fighting disease within our genetic code would last as long as the host cell. There is great hope for the future that, if researchers can manage to implant therapeutic genes into stem cells (the progenitor cells of all blood cells), every blood cell could be immunized against HIV infection.

gene transfer therapy A form of GENE THERAPY that has been shown to prolong the survival of critical immune system cells, such as CD4+ T CELLS, that are typically depleted during the course of HIV disease.

General Assistance (GA) A generic term used for state-local welfare programs for poor persons who are not coverable by the federal SSI and AFDC programs.

General Medical Assistance (GMA) State and local programs to provide health care to poor persons who are not coverable by the federal MEDICAID program.

general paresis A progressive form of mental illness caused by neurosyphilis and characterized by gross confusion.

general population surveys Large-scale, population-based national HIV seroprevalence surveys have been conducted in only a few countries, including Uganda, Rwanda, Côte d'Ivoire, and the former Soviet Union. These surveys are distinct from the population-based sample surveys undertaken in a number of nonnational geographic settings. Data from a national survey provides, to some extent, a more complete picture of the epidemic in a country. However, it has become increasingly recognized that such surveys leave many important questions unanswered.

genetic engineering The synthesis, alteration, replacement, or repair of an organism's basic genetic material by synthetic means.

genetic material Material found in the cells of living things that is used in reproduction. In regard to AIDS, this is the material in a cell that determines what kind of cell will be created through transcription.

genetic mutation A change in the character of a gene that is perpetuated in subsequent divisions of the cell in which it occurs. See GENETIC ENGINEERING.

genetic predisposition Higher-than-normal susceptibility to a condition or disease by virtue of genetic endowment (i.e., heredity).

genetic research The study and examination of reproduction and heredity and its variance.

genetic variability The differences in genetic sequence between individual organisms of the same type.

The genetic structures of HIV-1 and HIV-2 are similar. However, in HIV-2, the vpu gene is absent and another gene, called vpx, is present. Precise comparative analysis of each genetic element of HIV-1 and HIV-2 has revealed important differences between these two HIV viruses, especially in the env gene. Genetic diversity is one characteristic of this family of viruses. Thus, differences in genetic sequence can be observed between variants of the same type of HIV-1 (or HIV-2) found in a given patient. Recent data have shown that these strain variations occur in a patient during the course of HIV infection, as early as five days after infections and several months after exposures. HIV mutates as it is submitted to selection by the host's immune system. This mutation may be the way the virus avoids destruction by the host's immune defenses. Persistent infections observed in patients may be a consequence of this viral escape mechanism. This variability is not a property of the entire genome. Gag, pol, vif, and vpr genes are usually genetically stable. Tat and rev genes vary, but to a lesser degree than do nef and env genes.

HIV virus's envelope proteins have many biological and immunological roles. The envelope's genetic variability therefore leads to differences between HIV variants in terms of biology as well as immunology. These differences affect the physiopathology of HIV infection, the development of efficacious drugs and vaccines, and the diagnosis of HIV infection. In the coming years as the HIV/AIDS pandemic continues to grow, the emergence of many variants of HIV should be expected. The diagnostic and therapeutic problems created will become increasingly complex. The efficacy of vaccines will depend on their capacity to cover an increasingly broad spectrum of variants.

genital herpes See HERPES GENITALIS.

genital intercourse Sexual intercourse involving penis-vagina contact.

genital secretions Body fluids produced by the genitals, including cervical and vaginal secretions. Examples of other fluids of the body include bile, chyle, chyme, gastric juice, intestinal juice, lymph, menstrual fluids, pancreatic juice, perspiration, saliva, and urine. These secretions can be external (if the material flows out through a duct) or internal (if it is returned to the blood or lymph). The particles of HIV circulate freely in the blood but mostly live in lymphocytes, which are present in most body fluids, like semen, blood, cervical and vaginal secretions, saliva, even urine and tears. Any activity or behavior that results in the sharing of bodily fluids in which the virus is found can transmit HIV. How likely one is to get the disease depends on the particular fluid and other factors. A sufficient quantity of the virus must be present and the virus must penetrate through the skin and into the body. Blood, semen, and vaginal and cervical secretions carry the highest concentrations of the virus, although saliva, tears, and urine carry minuscule amounts or no HIV. The virus can also be present in male pre-cum, the clear liquid found on the penis before ejaculation.

genital ulcer An ulcerative lesion on the genitals, usually caused by a sexually transmitted disease such as HERPES,

SYPHILIS, or CHANCROID. The presence of genital ulcers may increase the risk of transmitting HIV.

genital wart   A clusterlike growth on the VULVA, the vaginal wall, or the CERVIX in women and on the corona of the GLANS penis or immediately behind the glans in men. Genital warts result from a sexually transmitted disease caused by the HUMAN PAPILLOMA VIRUS. In immunocompromised women, the external warts—on the vulva, perineum, and ANAL areas—may become florid and respond inadequately to treatment. Warts may lead to more serious diseases, such as CERVICAL CANCER in women or cancer of the anus in men and women. In all cases of genital warts in women, a PAP SMEAR and follow-up for human papillomavirus infection (HPV) infection of the cervix must be conducted.

genitalia   The reproductive organs. Female genitalia consist of the vagina, clitoris, vulva, uterus, ovaries, fallopian tubes, and related structures. Male genitalia include the penis, testes and related structures, prostate, seminal vesicles, and bulbourethral glands.

genitourinary tract   The system involved in reproduction and elimination of urine. In women this consists of the kidneys, ureters, bladder, urethra, uterus, fallopian tubes, ovaries, and vagina. In men it is the kidneys, ureters, bladder, urethra, testicles, prostate gland, vas deferens, and seminal vesicles. The genital and the urinary systems are distinct, but they are so closely related developmentally and functionally that they are often studied and treated together.

genome   The total genetic material within a cell or individual, depending upon context. Specifically, the haploid chromosome complement (the complete set of chromosomes) and thus the total genetic information present in a cell.

Retroviral genomes are composed of at least three genes, designated gag, pol, and env. These genes provide genetic coding for the HIV NUCLEOSIDE antigens, REVERSE TRANSCRIPTASE, and surface proteins, respectively. A similar DNA sequence of varying length can be found at each end of the proviral DNA. This sequence contains elements that can promote proviral gene integration in the host cell's genome and expression of these genes. See also GENETIC VARIABILITY.

Genontech GP120   gp120 and GP160 are thought to be key proteins on the surface of HIV viral particles. The vaccines to them do not carry viral RNA, but they do stimulate the immune system to produce antibodies to HIV viral particles. To date, no data suggest that gp120 or gp160 prevent HIV infection. See also gp120 and gp160.

genotype   The genetic material inherited from parents; not all of it is necessarily expressed in the individual.

gentamicin   A broad-spectrum antibiotic of the aminoglycoside class that is derived from the fungi of the genus Micromonospora. Gentamicin is used to treat bacterial infections of the blood, central nervous system (meningitis), urinary tract, respiratory tract, digestive system, skin, bone, and soft tissue. In women living with HIV, gentamicin is used to treat PELVIC INFLAMMATORY DISEASE, a condition that develops when sexually transmitted infections such as CHLAMYDIA or GONORRHEA are left untreated.

Gentamicin is available in a variety of forms, including topical cream, eye drops, ointment, and injectable solution.

Gentamicin works by interfering with production of proteins in bacteria, which ultimately kills them. It is relatively toxic compared to other antibiotics used for similar conditions, and is used primarily when less toxic antibiotics are not effective or cannot be tolerated. Gentamicin works best when combined with drugs from other antibiotic classes. Standard gentamicin may be injected intravenously or into a large muscle; intravenous injection is used for severe infections of the blood or when an individual is in shock. The most serious side effects are kidney toxicity and damage to the eighth cranial nerve, which controls hearing. The risk of these side effects is low in people with normal kidney function using recommended doses, but they occur more frequently in people who take high doses for extended periods and those who have a preexisting kidney impairment.

A form of gentamicin in which the active drug is encoded in tiny fatty bubbles called liposomes is being tested in clinical trials for the treatment of MYCOBACTERIUM AVIUM COMPLEX (MAC). MAC is difficult to treat because macrophages, cells of the immune system that "eat" bacteria, do not effectively destroy those that cause MAC in people with HIV. Mycobacteria are ingested by macrophages, but they survive and multiply inside the cells. In theory, using gentamicin encapsulated with liposomes should increase the concentration of the active drug in macrophages without increasing the concentration in the blood or other healthy tissues. The liposomal version of gentamycin must be injected intravenously.

Gentamicin is also known as gentamycin and TLC G-65 (the latter is liposomal gentamicin); trade names are Garamyciun and G-myticin.

gentamicin sulfate   An antibiotic obtained from the actinomycete Micromonospora purpurea. Trade names Garamycin and Genoptic Liquifilm.

genus   In biology, the taxonomic division between the species and the family.

geographic areas of affinity (GAA)   A framework to facilitate tracking of the HIV/AIDS pandemic, analyze its impact, and monitor the response to it. The world has been divided into 10 Geographic Areas of Affinity (GAAs). The diversity of these areas is large enough to accommodate variability in modes of transmission of HIV, yet small enough to facilitate analysis. These GAAs are based on two major factors: evolving HIV epidemiology and the operational and programmatic characteristics of the response to the HIV epidemic. The degree of societal vulnerability to the further spread of HIV is an important underlying element. The 10 GAAs include North America, Western Europe, Oceania, Latin America, sub-Saharan Africa, the Caribbean, Eastern Europe, southeastern Mediterranean, Northeast Africa and Southeast Asia.

Despite its utility, it is important to note that the GAA system is still based on generalizations and assumptions. The present delineation of the 10 GAAs is therefore only intended as an interim classification. The Global AIDS Policy Coalition (a coalition and committed to tracking the evolving HIV/AIDS pandemic, critically analyzing the global response and encouraging policy analysis and advocacy activities) is commissioning work to develop a more sophisticated classification system which will seek to take into account an even broader range of relevant factors. Their goal is to understand the local, national, and regional features of the pandemic, information critical for generating a more robust and focused global response.

geographic distribution   HIV/AIDS has reached every part of the world. Its extensive spread started in the mid- to late 1970s, and in less than two decades—during the first of which it was unknown and unsuspected—HIV became the first modern pandemic.

geographic variation   Variation in levels of HIV infection, both between and within countries. Seroprevalence surveys have tended to highlight the trends in particular groups and focus on the differentials among populations at different levels of risk. Today we know that HIV is geographically highly clustered. We know, too, that even with adjustments for underreporting and delays in reporting, striking disparities exist in, for example, AIDS mortality among different geographic areas of affinity. To date, the geographical distribution of AIDS has reflected the progression of the pandemic to the developing world. Projections of AIDS to the year 2000 and beyond continue this trend—geographic variations are important. The range of proportional increases varies significantly by geographic area of affinity.

germanium   Discovered in 1886, the mineral germanium, with an atomic weight of thirty-two on the periodic table of elements, is not known to be essential to human health. Yet in the early 1990s considerable research into its therapeutic effects on the immune system was carried out in several countries, including the United States and Japan.

A number of claims have been made for this naturally occurring and apparently safe substance. Germanium was reported to be at the same time a profound immunostimulant, an oxygen facilitator, and a blocker of free radicals of oxygen. Organic Germanium is said to be a dramatic immune modulator with antitumor effects and interferon-inducing activities. Additionally, it has been reported to restore immune function in immunodepressed animals. Researchers also believe germanium induces the production of tumor necrosis factor-alpha, which would help explain its antitumor properties. It is also believed to increase production of these immunologic substances by direct stimulation of the monocyte/macrophage system. Germanium is known to increase the numbers and activity of natural killer cells and researchers have speculated that it has some direct antiviral activity. Germanium may normalize the function of T LYMPHOCYTES, B LYMPHOCYTES, and antibody-dependent cellular cytotoxicity. Germanium also decreases food intolerances, has analgesic properties, and helps regulate all body systems in postsurgical cases and keeps white blood counts within normal ranges.

Germanium is available in powdered form at better health food retailers or buyers' clubs. To date, no certain immunomodulating dose is recommended. Toxic side effects such as renal impairment have been attributed to the use of germanium in nonstabilized form, and some people have reported that the use of germanium stimulates the CENTRAL NERVOUS SYSTEM and recommend that it be taken in the morning so as not to interfere with sleep.

germinal centers   A collection of metabolically active lymphoblasts, macrophages, and plasma cells appearing within the primary follicle of lymphoid tissues following antigenic stimulation. Germinal centers are the sites of antibody production and are populated mostly by B CELLS but include a few T CELLS and MACROPHAGES. As HIV infection progresses, the germinal centers gradually decay.

giant cells   Large multinucleated cells sometimes seen in granulomatous reactions and thought to result from the fusion of macrophages. They are found in both kinds of marrow, especially red marrow, and spleen; also in tissues that are healing, around foreign bodies, and in the inflammatory reaction to tuberculosis.

giardia   An intestinal parasite, once common among homosexual men, which can cause severe diarrhea.

giardia intestinalis   See GIARDIA LAMBLIA.

Giardia lamblia   A species of *Giardia* found in humans, that may cause GIARDIASIS. They are transmitted by ingestion of cysts in fecally contaminated matter (water or food) and are found worldwide. The most frequently observed symptoms of infection with *G. lamblia* are diarrhea, fever, cramps, anorexia, nausea, weakness, weight loss, abdominal distension, flatulence, greasy stools, belching, and vomiting. Onset of symptoms begins about two weeks after exposure, and the disease may persist for up to two or three months. There is no known chemoprophylaxis for giardiasis, but treatment with metronidazole, tinidazole, or quinacrine is highly effective. Also called *Giardia intestinalis* and *Lamblia intestinalis*.

giardiasis   A common infection with the flagellate protozoan *Giardia lamblia*. Infection is spread through contaminated food or water. Most cases are asymptomatic. When present, symptoms include anorexia, cramps, diarrhea, fever, nausea, weakness, weight loss, and vomiting. Also called lambliasis.

ginseng   Ginseng root is an herb that has been used extensively throughout Southeast Asia and China for treatment of various disorders. There are three different families of ginseng: the Oriental and American ginsengs (*Panax schinseng*), the Siberian ginseng (*Eleutherococcus senticosus*) and the desert ginseng (*Rumex hymenosepalus*). For thousands of years, ginseng has been the most prized of herbal remedies, with a host of alleged benefits, including relief of fatigue, relief of stress, and other systemic benefits.

It has been suggested that *Panax* ginseng may increase natural killer cell activity. *Panax* and *Eleutherococcus* can produce insomnia, diarrhea, nervousness, depression, and skin rash. Ginseng can amplify the effect of certain antidepressant medications and, due to the small amount of estrogens in the plant, can affect menstruation in women.

gland   A group of cells that removes materials from the blood, alters them to produce a specialized substance (such as a hormone), and then releases that substance back into the bloodstream to act in the body.

glans   The head of the penis, the area covered by the foreskin in uncircumcised men.

glial cells   Non-conducting nerve cells, performing supportive and protective roles for neurones, including astrocytes, oligodendrocyte, Schwann cells, microglia and ependyma cells.

glory hole   A hole in a wall or partition through which a man sticks his penis. The person on the other side then anonymously fellates, masturbates, or otherwise stimulates the penis. This activity takes place at gay sex clubs.

glove   In medical care gloves are used to prevent the contamination of an operative site with organisms from the person wearing the glove and to prevent pathogens from the patient contaminating the health care worker. These factors are particularly important when the patient has a disease such as HEPATITIS B or AIDS. Medical gloves are generally made of latex.

GLQ-223   A drug derived from the Chinese cucumber. In phase I clinical trials it has been shown to be effective against the human immunodeficiency virus in vitro by selectively destroying infected cells. The drug is now being tested in phase II trials.

glucose-6-phosphate dehydrogenase   An enzyme that dehydrogenates glucose-6-phosphate to form 6-phosphoglucon. This is the initial step in the pentose phosphate pathway of glucose catabolism.

glucose-6-phosphate dehydrogenase (G6PD) deficiency   An inherited enzyme deficiency that can lead to HEMOLYSIS of red blood cells when an affected individual is exposed to drugs with oxidant properties.

glucosidase   An enzyme that catalyzes the hydrolysis of a glucoside.

glutathione   A key antioxidant compound required for the smooth functioning of all cells. It is composed of three amino acids: cysteine, glutamine, and glycine. Besides acting as an antioxidant, glutathione is involved in protein synthesis, amino acid transport, and in the recycling of other antioxidants, such as vitamin C. Glutathione, like other antioxidants, may or may not, play a role in slowing HIV disease progression. Study results are often conflicting; the findings that follow illustrate some of the claims made for this antioxidant. A deficiency of glutathione has been linked with

shortened survival in HIV-infected individuals who have CD4 counts below 200. In fact, researchers have found that glutathione levels in CD4 cells closely correlate with CD4 count. Researchers have also postulated the use of glutathione replacement therapy in the treatment of HIV infection to enhance the immune system. Other research has shown that NAC, or N-acetylcysteine, is essential for the synthesis of glutathione, and studies have indicated that oral administration of NAC can replenish glutathione stores in people with HIV. Some researchers have inferred that NAC itself may be useful in prolonging survival.

glycoprotein   Any of a class of compounds in which a carbohydrate group is combined with a protein; any of a class of compounds (including the mucins, the mucoids, and the chondronproteins) consisting of a carbohydrate and a protein. In decomposition, glycoprotains yield a substance frequently capable of reducing alkaline solutions of cupric oxide.

glycyrrhiza   The dried root of *Glycyrrhiza glabra*, known commercially as Spanish licorice. Used as an ingredient of glycyrrhiza fluid extract and glycrrhiza syrup, both of which are used as flavoring agents in compounding medicine. This substance has a weak cortisone-like action.

glycyrrhizin (licorice root)   Glycyrrhizin is a substance isolated from the root of the licorice plant (*Glycyrrhiza radix*). It is widely used in Japan and is reported to have benefits in the treatment of chronic HEPATITIS B. Some studies suggest that glycyrrhizin may have anti-HIV properties and may enhance the production of natural killer cells and INTERFERON. There are reports of glycyrrhizin causing high blood pressure, water retention, and possibly heart complications when taken in very high doses. Other possible adverse side effects include low potassium levels.

GM-CSF   See GRANULOCYTE-MACROPHAGE COLONY STIMULATING FACTOR.

GMHC   See GAY MEN'S HEALTH CRISIS.

go both ways   See BISEXUAL.

golden shower   Urination on a sex partner, or being urinated on, for sexual pleasure. See UROPHILIA.

gonad   A gland or organ that produces reproductive cells in animals; a general term for a gamete-producing gland, including both the female ovary and male testis.

gonorrhea   A sexually transmitted, or venereal, disease (STD or VD) caused by the bacterium *Neisseria gonorrhea*. It is transmitted when a mucous membrane or warm, moist part of a carrier's body comes into contact with similar tissue on another's. Symptoms include a puslike discharge from the penis in men or the cervix in women, and lower abdominal pain and fever in women. Other parts of the body (heart, throat, joints, rectum, and skin) may also be affected. If not treated, gonorrhea can cause severe infection and sterility.

Penicillin, orally or by injection, is standard treatment for gonorrhea. Tetracyclines and cephalosporins are also used. Slang terms include the *clap,* a *dose,* and the *drip.*

gossypol   A toxic chemical that is yellowish in appearance and found in cottonseed. It is detoxified by heating. Gossypol is used as a contraceptive agent in China. It has anti-HIV activity in test tubes and has been investigated as a potential viricide (like nonoxynol-9) that may reduce the risk of HIV transmission during sexual intercourse.

gp41   A GLYCOPROTEIN ("sugar-covered" protein) on HIV's outside envelope that complexes with GP120 to form the mechanism enabling HIV to latch onto and enter cells.

gp120   A protein on HIV's envelope that binds to the CD4 site on the T4 LYMPHOCYTE. Free gp120 in the body may be toxic to cells on its own, causing CD4 cell depletion through APOPTOSIS in the immune system and neurological damage leading to AIDS DEMENTIA COMPLEX. gp120 is the foundation for several of the older approaches to developing an HIV vaccine.

gp160   A glycoprotein ("sugar-covered" protein) made from HIV RNA. After synthesis, it is cleaved into GP120 and GP41, two glycoproteins inserted in or on the HIV envelope.

graft-versus-host (gvh) reaction   The clinical and pathologic sequelae of the reactions of immunocompetent cells in a graft against the cells of the histoincompatible and immunodeficient recipient.

Gram-negative   See GRAM'S STAIN.

Gram-negative bacteria   See GRAM'S STAIN.

Gram-positive   See GRAM'S STAIN.

Gram-positive bacteria   See GRAM'S STAIN.

Gram's stain   A differential method of staining bacteria for classification purposes, in which the specimen is first placed in aniline water–gentian violet or carbolic gentian violet, rinsed in water and immersed in an iodine solution, rinsed in water again and placed in strong alcohol for several minutes and rinsed again, and dipped in a dilute eosin solution. Gram-negative bacteria decolorize and assume the counterstain; Gram-positive bacteria stain a dark violet. This artificial coloring of bacteria is used to facilitate examination under the microscope. Some Gram-negative bacteria include bordetella, brucella, escherichia, hemophilus, klebsiella, legionella, neisseria, proteus, pseudomonas, salmonella, shigella, vibrio, and yersinia. The chief Gram-positive bacteria are bacillus, clostridium, corynebacterium, diplococcus, gardnerella, sarcina, staphylococcus, and streptococcus.

granulocyte colony stimulating factor (G-CSF)   A synthetic hormone that stimulates growth of granulocytes, a specific type of WHITE BLOOD CELL. It is used to alleviate the NEUTROPENIA caused by certain drugs and conditions.

granulocyte-macrophage colony stimulating factor (GM-CSF)   A naturally occurring CYTOKINE GLYCOPROTEIN that stimulates production of NEUTROPHILS, MONOCYTES, and MACROPHAGES. It is effective in treating BONE MARROW deficiency following chemotherapy or bone marrow transplantation. GM-CSF's generic name is sargamostim. (Trade names Leukine and Prokine).

granuloma   A granular tumor or growth, usually of lymphoid and epithelial cells. It occurs in various infectious diseases such as leprosy, cutaneous leishmaniasis, yaws, and SYPHILIS. Granuloma is treated with by streptomycin, chloramphenicol, trimethoprim/sulfamethoxazole, or tetracyclines. When treatment is completed, the patient should be followed for six months to determine if syphilis was contracted along with the granuloma.

granuloma inguinale   A sexually transmitted disease most often affecting the groin, genitals, or perianal area. It less commonly affects the CERVIX, UTERUS, BLADDER, and RECTUM in females. The infection is caused by a microbacillus known as *Donovania granulomatis,* and the condition is also known as donovanosis. First symptoms occur about one to four weeks after exposure and include swelling, usually in the groin. The swollen area ruptures, and chronic painful ulcers with an unpleasant odor form. New lesions continue to appear, and the disease may eventually cover the reproductive organs, lower abdomen, and buttocks. Massive swelling of the genitals (ELEPHANTIASIS) is a possible complication. Treatment includes ANTIBIOTICS such as streptomycin, and improvements are usually noted within a few weeks. Recurrences are common.

gray area   The intermediate area or room between a HOT ZONE, an a area that contains lethal, infectious organisms, and the normal world; a place where the two worlds meet. Also called gray zone.

green barley leaf extract (GBLE)   The dried leaves of young barley, widely used in Japan and other countries as a nutritional supplement. Green barley leaf extract is reported to contain high levels of superoxide dismutase, a potent ANTIOXIDANT. Studies of GBLE, almost all of which have been conducted in Japan, suggest possible in vitro anti-inflammatory and antileukemic activity, and reduced healing time of ulcerous lesions in rats. Other studies have reported antioxidative, anti-inflammatory, antiallergic, anticarcinogenic, antiulcer, and antiviral properties. It has been suggested that GBLE may increase production of INTERLEUKIN-2 when added to cell cultures. Il-2 is a protein, produced by the body, that may have immune-boosting properties and seems to decrease with progression to AIDS. Some researchers have suggested that there may be an anti-HIV substance in green barley leaf extract.

green juices   Barley extracts and other "green juices" are used by many HIV-positive individuals as nutritional supplements.

GRID   See GAY-RELATED IMMUNE DISEASE.

grief   Grief is an involuntary, complicated, emotional, and psychological response to loss or extreme TRAUMA. It is a process of movement through the pain of loss and simultaneously of healing and learning. Grief is the process that allows us to let go of intense emotional attachments and carry on with our lives.

The experience of grief is personal and subjective. With regard to AIDS, those who have HIV or AIDS will frequently be experiencing loss of health, jobs, homes, friends, finances, and independence and are having to face in the near future the loss of their lives. Their family members will be grieving for them and for the loss of their own future expectations. Medical personnel grieve their loss as well, along with the failure of *their* expectations of themselves—their inability to cure, "letting another person die."

Grief produces both emotional and physical manifestations. The initial reaction may include somatic symptoms such as easy fatigability, hollow or empty feeling in the chest and abdomen, sighing, hyperventilation, anorexia, insomnia, and the feeling of having a lump in the throat, and psychological symptoms beginning with shock and disbelief and an awareness of mental discomfort, sorrow, and regret, followed by tears, sobbing, and other more active expressions of pain. Duration of this initial reaction varies, but in the longer run the process generally includes these stages: denial, anger, bargaining, depression, acceptance, and hope. However, stages do not generally occur in neat, orderly progression. They are confused, frequently happening several at a time, repeated, and over time, assimilated. When the process becomes mired or interrupted, it is referred to as "complicated grief." If the process is not allowed to follow its normal course, it will go underground, so to speak, and fester, causing a variety of psychosomatic illnesses and more misery than the original loss.

Helping a person through grief requires receptiveness, physical presence, tolerance, and permissive listening, as well as a resolve to help him or her keep contact with the ordinary, mundane details of daily life.

Anticipatory grief makes the final grieving less intense and helps toward a more rapid healing. It is healthy and should not be met by family, friends, or providers with condemnation, but with encouragement and understanding. Anticipatory grief helps bring eventual closure. By giving us the chance to project into the future and see the loss before the fact, we are granted time to be "real" with the dying person, to say the things we always meant to and, perhaps, to share on a deeper level than previously.

grief work   Helping a person through GRIEF, which, while largely an individual experience, often needs social facilitation and accommodation by others who can provide a nurturing, safe atmosphere. In general, the people near a person in grief play a passive supportive role in the process. With a terminal patient, though, one active moment is often required of the rest of us at some existential point: giving the patient permission to die. Without that permission, it is extremely difficult for the person with AIDS to make it to the stages of acceptance and hope.

griseofulvin   An antibiotic commonly used to treat superficial fungal infections.

Group I infection   In 1986, to improve communication about the broad spectrum of HIV-related illnesses, the CENTERS FOR DISEASE CONTROL developed two hierarchical classification systems—one for adults and the other for children with HIV infection. The system for adults includes Group I–IV. (Centers for Disease Control, "Classification System for Human T-Lymphotropic Virus Type III/Lymphadenopathy-Associated Virus Infections," *Morbidity and Mortality Weekly Report*, 35 (1986), 334–339.) Group I infection is acute infection. One of the first signs of HIV-1 infection in some patients is an acute mononucleosislike or flulike disease. The condition lasts from a few days to several weeks and is associated with fever, sweats, exhaustion, loss of appetite, nausea, headaches, sore throat, diarrhea, swollen glands, and a rash on the trunk. The acute syndrome was first described by physicians monitoring the health of almost 1,000 homosexual and bisexual men in Sydney, Australia. Some of the symptoms of the acute illness may result from HIV-1 invasion of the central nervous system.

Group II infection   According to the CDC's HIV infection classification system (see GROUP I INFECTION), Group II infection is ASYMPTOMATIC infection. Patients in Groups II and III may be subclassified on the basis of a laboratory evaluation.

Group III infection   According to the CDC's HIV infection classification system (see GROUP I INFECTION), Group III infection is PERSISTENT GENERALIZED LYMPHADENOPATHY. Patients in Group II and III may be subclassified on the basis of a laboratory evaluation. Soon after AIDS was identified as a new disease, physicians noticed that a large group of previously healthy homosexual men were seeking treatment for persistent swollen glands not explained by specific illnesses or drug use. The epidemiologic characteristics of this population were identical with those of the population of AIDS patients. As the epidemic progressed, similar findings were reported among intravenous drug users, hemophiliacs, and the heterosexual partners of some persons with AIDS. When the blood test for HIV-1 antibodies became available, researchers demonstrated that lymphadenopathy was a frequent consequence of infection with the virus. Initially it was believed that people who developed persistent lymphadenopathy were more likely to progress to AIDS than infected patients whose glands remained normal. It was later determined that, in the absence of other symptoms, persistently swollen glands are not indicative of a declining immune system.

Group IV infection   According to the CDC's HIV infection classification system (see GROUP I INFECTION), Group IV is "Other Disease," and includes Subgroup A constitutional disease (HIV WASTING SYNDROME); Subgroup B, neurologic disease (acute aseptic MENINGITIS, subacute encephalitis—or AIDS DEMENTIA complex, VACUOLAR MYELOPATHY, abnormalities of the peripheral nervous system, etc.); Subgroup C, secondary infectious diseases (opportunistic infections such as PNEUMOCYSTIS CARINII PNEUMONIA, CANDIDA ALBICANS, CRYPTOSPORIDIUM, CYTOMEGALOVIRUS, HERPES ZOSTER, TOXOPLASMA GONDII,

TUBERCULOSIS and other MYCOBACTERIAL INFECTIONS); Subgroup D, secondary cancers (KAPOSI'S SARCOMA, LYMPHOMAS, and other miscellaneous cancers); and Subgroup E, other conditions.

group O   A rare genetic variant of HIV-1 that is not reliably detected by FDA approved tests. Plans to improve commercial tests so that they will be able to detect the unusual variant are underway. As of mid-1996, fewer than 100 cases of group O infection had been definitively diagnosed worldwide, and almost all of those were in Central and West Africa, where an estimated 6 percent of all AIDS cases were believed to be group O.

group sex   Sexual activities by a group of people, either heterosexual, homosexual, or a combination of the two, at the same place, involving exchange of partners, variations of types of sexual intercourse, and observation of each other.

group-specific complement   Any of a series of enzymatic proteins in normal serum that, in the presence of a sensitizer (a substance that makes the susceptible individual react to the same or other irritants) specific for a given group, destroys bacteria and other cells. The complement is important in maintaining a normal state of health.

group therapy   A form of psychotherapy involving two or more patients and one or more psychotherapists for the purpose of treating each patient simultaneously through group discussion and interaction.

growth factor   One of many intercellular regulatory molecules that regulate cell proliferation (rapid and repeated reproduction), function, and differentiation. Different growth factors elicit different responses from different cell types, such as stimulating growth, enhancing survival, initiating migration, and stimulating the secretion of tissue-specific hormones.

guanine   An organic compound that occurs as a natural constituent of animal and vegetable nucleic acids. It is abundant in the liver, in muscle, in glandular tissue such as the pancreas, and in seeds.

guanosine   The nucleoside formed from GUANINE and RIBOSOME. It is a major constituent of RNA and DNA. Two guanosine nucleoside analogs that received particular attention are Glaxco Wellcome's 1592U89 succinate and Bristol-Myers Squibb's lobucavir, formerly known as cyclobut G. It has been reported that "1592" is absorbed well when taken orally, and also has significant (18 percent) central nervous system penetration. Since it is not metabolized by the liver, "1592" should not have serious drug-drug interactions with PROTEASE INHIBITORS. The good news presented about lobucavir is that it appears that the compound has activity against most viruses in the herpes family and hepatitis B and is a potent inhibitor of HIV as well.

guardian   See SURROGATE.

guardianship   See SURROGACY.

guerilla clinic   Any of a group of for-profit facilities established during the AIDS epidemic for the purpose of dispensing black-market drugs or providing treatments or therapies not approved in traditional medical channels.

guided imagery   One of many visualization therapies that uses a variety of visual techniques to treat disease. Visualization therapies are based on inducing relaxation in patients and having them visualize their medical problems, literally willing them away. Positive results have been documented with patients suffering loss due to disease, altered body image, or the threat of death. Positive results have also been documented when a total cure may be out of the question. Guided imagery exercises also are used to help patients cope with stress. In these therapies, people imagine themselves in an environment they associate with relaxing—a peaceful beach, a lake, or a favorite mountain. Closing their eyes and taking a few deep, easy breaths, they remember the details of the setting—the sights, smells, and sounds—and focus on feeling peaceful and relaxed.

guidelines   In medical cases clinical practice recommendations formulated by experts or based on a literature review by a panel of experts and consumers. Their purpose is to educate health care providers, improve the care provided to individuals with specified conditions, and, when possible, enhance the cost-effectiveness of health care. Guidelines are distinct from "standards of care," which providers are required to meet.

gummatous syphilis   Late benign SYPHILIS.

GVH reaction   See GRAFT-VERSUS-HOST REACTION.

gynecological disorder   A disturbance in any of the female reproductive organs, including the BREASTS.
   Gynecological problems are common early symptoms of immunocompromise in HIV-positive women. These may include gynecological infections (most commonly VAGINAL CANDIDIASIS, BACTERIAL VAGINOSIS, TRICHOMONIASIS), as well as GENITAL ULCERS, VAGINITIS, simple urinary tract infections, POSTPARTUM endometritis, and PELVIC INFLAMMATORY DISEASE and cervical neoplasia. These problems may become chronic, less responsive to conventional therapies, and tend to progress as immunocompromise worsens. Specific protocols are needed for the treatment of gynecological problems in HIV-positive women that are appropriate to the degree of immunocompromise. Women who receive gynecological services in the same primary care clinics where they receive care for HIV infection are less likely to be lost to follow-up, and treatment plans can be initiated earlier.
   Sexually transmitted infections and genital lesions are likely to facilitate viral transmission. These include GENITAL ULCER diseases (GUD), SYPHILITIC CHANCRES, HERPES GENITALIS, CHANCROID, and, rarely, LYMPHOGRANULOMA VENEREUM (LVG), and GRANULOMA INGUINALE (donovanosis). Other genital lesions that may accompany HIV infection

include GENITAL WARTS and MOLLUSCUM CONTAGIOSUM. Chronic vaginitis may predispose women to HIV transmission and to other STDs.

Considerations for the management of gynecological infections include taking an appropriate sexual history, asking about symptoms, performing a speculum and bimanual examination, and obtaining relevant laboratory specimens. It is also important to consider the woman's overall state of health and the degree of immunocompromise. Clients with lowered T4 CELL COUNTS are often pancytopenic, increasing their susceptibility to infection and complicating response to treatment. These women may not mount an elevated white blood count in response to systemic infection, rendering an important diagnostic test less useful. ERYTHROCYTE SEDIMENTATION RATES (ESR) are often elevated in chronic illness and thus become a less useful clue in the diagnostic workup for acute infection. It has been observed that immunocompromised women with acute pelvic inflammatory disease (PID) are less symptomatic than their immunocompetent counterparts, even with marked disease. Consideration of the stage of HIV illness is a useful tool in planning follow-up. All sexually transmitted diseases must be treated by CDC guidelines, and tests of cures obtained. Treatment of sexual partners, where appropriate, should be arranged.

gynecological services Medical examination, care (including preventive care), and treatment for GYNECOLOGICAL DISORDERS. Gynecological services include taking comprehensive menstrual, sexual, and reproductive histories; performing comprehensive gynecological examinations and evaluations; referrals to prenatal and obstetric care and abortion services; regular screening and other services. Gynecological histories often bring up difficult and unpredictable topics such as early sexual abuse, current domestic violence, sexually transmitted infections, or concerns about sexual functioning. In HIV-positive women, concerns about fertility, menstrual problems, pelvic pain, and unprotected sex often surface during such an interview. (Gynecological examination often poses the risk of some blood exposure to the examiner, as do so many other simple medical procedures. Universal precautions include wearing gloves and disinfecting spills.)

HIV-positive women who are essentially asymptomatic, with CD4 counts greater than 400, who are not sexually active and who have no new gynecological complaints can be followed with gynecological screening and PAP SMEARS annually. Symptomatic women, women with AIDS, and sexually active women should be scheduled for gynecological evaluations, Pap smears, and STD screening every six months. Interval assessment should occur whenever a woman presents with low abdominal pain; vaginal or rectal discharge; abdominal bloating; genital sores; new onset of swollen or painful inguinal nodes; dysuria, hesitancy, frequency, or urgency; new onset amenorrhea; intermenstrual bleeding or any change in menstrual pattern; dyspareunia; or bleeding following sexual activity. Periodic assessments generally include an interval sexual history, careful inspection of external genitalia, speculum examination, GONORRHEA and chlamydia cultures, bimanual pelvic examination, microscopic wet mount, and VDRL. Tests are ordered as needed. Appropriate treatment plans are developed as needed. Client education is geared to the reasons for particular visits, but safe sex counseling should be reintroduced each time.

gynecology The study of the female reproductive organs, including the BREASTS; the branch of medicine concerned with GYNECOLOGICAL DISORDERS.

Gyne-Lotrimin See CLOTRIMAZOLE.

H

hair pie   Slang term for VULVA, with reference to CUNNILINGUS. See ORAL SEX.

hairy leukoplakia   A white lesion seen in the oral cavity of HIV-infected individuals, most commonly on the lateral margins of the tongue. It may be flat or raised with vertical corrugations and is not removable. Acyclovir is an antimicrobial, artiviral agent used to treat hairy leukoplakia as well as Herpes simplex virus, Varicella-zoster virus, and Epstein-Barr virus. Brand name is Zovirax.

half-life   In biology and pharmacology, the time required by the body tissue or organ to metabolize, inactivate, and eliminate half the amount of a substance (such as a drug) taken in.

hand job   Slang term for MASTURBATION, especially of a partner.

handshake   See TRANSMISSION.

haploid number   Half the usual number of chromosomes found in the cells of a species. Characteristic of the gametes of the species (human = 23).

haplotype   A haploid genotype. Pertaining to a single set of chromosomes, haploids are an organism or group of cells having only one complete set of chromosomes—ordinarily half the normal diploid number.

hapten   A small molecule that is incapable of inducing an antibody response by itself but can, when bound to a protein carrier, act as an epitope. DINITROCHLOROBENZENE molecules are haptens.

harm reduction   The harm reduction model of public health action against contagion was developed in Merseyside, England, during the mid-1980s as a specific response to HIV/AIDS and the increasingly harmful consequences caused by the use of prohibited drugs. Fundamental principles underlying this approach are that HIV/AIDS prevention takes priority over prevention of drug use because it presents a greater threat to drug users, public health, and the national economy; that abstinence from drug use should not be the only objective of services to drug users because it excludes those who will not or cannot abstain; that those who will not or cannot abstain from drug use may still be helped by minimizing the harmful consequences of their behavior, for them, the community, and society as a whole; that the quality of the lives of drug users can be improved and enhanced while they still use drugs; and that HIV infection is not inevitable for drug users. Harm reduction emphasizes needle exchange programs, safer drug use, proper injection techniques, alternative ways of taking drugs, and drug maintenance.

hashish   A more or less purified extract prepared from the flowers, stalks, and leaves of the hemp plant *Cannibis sativa*. The gummy substance is smoked or chewed for its euphoric effects.

Hassal's corpuscles   Spherical or oval bodies present in the medulla of the thymus, consisting of central areas of degenerated cells surrounded by concentrically arranged flattened or polygonal cells.

Haitian link   Early in the epidemic, the high incidence of AIDS in Haitians living in the United States and in parts of Haiti puzzled clinicians. Haitians were first thought to comprise a group at special risk for HIV infection. A variety of proposed theories attempted to implicate Haitians in the introduction of HIV to the United States. Additional study of HIV infection in Haiti, however, found that the pattern of infection there closely paralleled that found in the heterosexual population in the United States. Although the high incidence of AIDS in Haiti seemed to hold leads for the origin of AIDS, the opposite circumstances seemed more plausible. Instead of Haitians introducing HIV into the United States, it was more likely that vacationing Americans or Haitians returning from Central America had carried HIV to Haiti.

The clustering of AIDS cases around the Carrefour district of Port-au-Prince, the major locale for male and female prostitution in Haiti, supported well-established risk factors as the explanation for HIV infection in Haiti. As the epidemic spread, the mode of transmission of HIV remained associated with heterosexual contact.

HBV   Hepatitis B virus. See HEPATITIS.

HCW   See HEALTH CARE WORKER.

healing touch   Healing touch is believed by some to accelerate wound healing, relieve pain, promote relaxation, prevent illness, and ease the dying process. The practitioner uses light touch or works with his or her hands near the client's body in an effort to restore the client's energy system.

health advocate   A person trained in assisting patients to resolve complaints about and problems with health care services. Health advocacy is concerned with the description, trends, patterns, analysis, causes, and resolutions of patient and client complaints and problems. Health legislation specialists, client advocates, and patient representatives are all health advocates and practitioners of health advocacy.

health care   Treatment of disease or disability; the provision of services to promote or restore mental and physical well-being. The quality, amount, and expense of available health care varies according to numerous factors—social class, income, eligibility for public programs, amount and type of insurance, type of service required, geography, public funding levels, and of course intangible differences among individual providers and institutions. Anyone seeking health care is well advised to be as well informed as possible, actively willing to make choices and protect his or her interests. This is even more crucial for HIV-infected patients than it is for others.

health care facility   A place where HEALTH CARE is provided, usually operated by an institution or small organization. The settings in which health care is provided are, in broad terms, two: outpatient facilities and inpatient facilities. Outpatient facilities are individual physicians' offices, clinics staffed by physicians who practice as a group, HEALTH MAINTENANCE ORGANIZATIONS, and public health department clinics. Inpatient facilities, primarily hospitals and nursing homes, are generally used by persons who need more intensive care.

health care professional   An individual who has received special training or education in a health-related discipline concerned with the direct provision of care (medicine, dentistry, medical technology, dental hygiene, physical therapy, and occupational therapy), health care administration, or ancillary services and who is licensed, certified, or registered by a professional organization or government agency to provide health services in his or her field. A health care professional may be an independent practitioner or an employee in a health facility or program.

health care provider   One who treats the sick and disabled or provides services to promote or restore mental and physical well-being. The category includes physicians, physicians' assistants, and nurses as well as others who are not licensed professional medical personnel. See also HEALTH CARE WORKER.

health care proxy   A legal document that authorizes one person to make medical decisions for another in the event he or she cannot make them him- or herself. This document also gives the person named visitation rights in the hospital and access to the patient's medical records. Under normal circumstances, an individual's next-of-kin would have these powers automatically. A health care proxy is suggested if a nonfamily member is preferred. People are generally advised to sign a medical directive in conjunction with a health care proxy as the best guarantee of realizing their wishes for treatment under particular circumstances. See also MEDICAL DIRECTIVE.

health care worker (HCW)   Anyone employed in the treatment of illness or disability or the provision of services to promote or restore mental and physical well-being. The category includes medical professionals, laboratory personnel, technicians, physical facility staff, and others. See also HEALTH CARE PROVIDER.

health insurance   A generic term for all forms of insurance and prepayment plans that reimburse (in whole or in part) an individual or organization for the costs of hospital and medical care. Health insurance plans may also reimburse an individual, again in whole or in part, against loss from disease or accidental bodily injury. Health insurance is usually divided into two types: individual (individually purchased) and group (purchased through employment or by reason of association with a defined group or organization).

Health insurance is available under such names as accident and health insurance, accident insurance, sickness insurance, disability insurance, service benefit plan, prepaid health plan, preferred provider plan, health maintenance plan, foundation medical plan, hospital insurance, and dental plan.

health maintenance organization (HMO)   An organization that provides comprehensive health care services to members for a nominal fee in addition to an annual charge. A component of MANAGED CARE, an HMO is an alternative to traditional fee-for-service care based on a relationship with an individual doctor.

HMOs provide comprehensive services for a fixed, prepaid fee. When you join a group plan offered by an HMO, you pay a flat fee for all your health care bills, regardless of how much health care you actually get. HMOs finance nearly all medical care. Unlike commercial insurance companies, HMOs allow little choice in physicians and hospitals. Because competition among HMOs for employer contracts is fierce, costs must be kept low. Consequently, the HMO must carefully regulate hospital admissions, expensive drugs, and expensive procedures and must preapprove any consultation or procedure done outside the resources of the HMO.

Health Omnibus Programs Extension of 1988   The Public Health Services Act required development of research and education programs, counseling, testing, and health care for AIDS patients. It also required the FDA to develop a registry of experimental AIDS drugs.

heartburn   A burning sensation in the substernal area due to reflux of acid contents of the stomach in the lower esophagus.

heat cautery   The use of heat to destroy tissue, especially for curative purposes. Method used for removing genital warts.

helminthic infestation   Infestation with intestinal parasites or worms. Helminths are wormlike animals.

Helms Amendment   In 1987 Congress enacted a law, commonly known after its Senate sponsor as the Helms Amendment, requiring the exclusion from the United States of HIV-infected aliens as carriers of a "dangerous contagious disease." As a result of this classification, all immigrants were tested for HIV, and those who tested positive were refused entry, including applicants seeking adjustment of status to permanent residency, applicants for amnesty, and refugees. Although the United States has not routinely tested nonimmigrants such as tourists, students, and other travelers to the United States, those whom immigration officials learned were HIV-positive were subject to exclusion as well. The Helms Amendment provoked a torrent of criticism from scientific and human rights authorities. The restriction placed on international travel and temporary residency sparked particularly vehement opposition. Critics were quick to point out that the United States is much more an exporter than an importer of HIV and that casual, everyday contact with HIV-positive travelers posed no public health threat to U.S. residents. The virtually unanimous outcry by public health and human rights authorities against the HIV exclusion led Congress to repeal the Helms Amendment in 1990. As part of the Immigration Act of 1990, Congress directed the secretary of HEALTH AND HUMAN SERVICES to draw up a new list of diseases that would be grounds for excluding aliens. Seeking to remove politics and prejudice from the selection process, Congress specifically admonished Health and Human Services that the list should contain only "communicable disease[s] of public health significance."

helper cells   Differentiated T LYMPHOCYTES whose cooperation is necessary for the production of antibodies against most ANTIGENS. Helper cells are marked by the T4 antigen in humans.

helper-suppressor-T-cell ratio   The ratio of the number of helper T cells to the number of suppressor T cells. It is normally two to one in a healthy person but reversed in AIDS-infected persons.

helper T cells   Term used for a subpopulation of T LYMPHOCYTES that secrete INTERLEUKIN-2 and play a major role in directing the specific immune response.

helper (Th) cells   A functional subclass of T CELLS that can help to generate CYTOTOXIC T cells and cooperate with B CELLS in production of antibody response. Helper cells recognize ANTIGEN in association with class II MHC molecules.

helper T-lymphocyte   A lymphocyte that bears the CD4 molecule on its surface and is the primary target of HIV infection; also called CD4 lymphocyte.

hematocrit   The volume of red blood cells expressed as a percentage of the total volume of blood. The volume of red blood cells is obtained by separating the cells from other blood components by means of a centrifuge.

hematopoietic system   All tissues responsible for production of the cellular elements of peripheral blood. This term usually excludes strictly lymphocytopoietic tissue such as LYMPH NODES.

hematuria   Red blood cells in the urine.

hemiparesis   Paralysis on one side of the body.

hemodialysis   A method for artificially performing the function of the kidneys (removing wastes or toxins from the blood) by circulating the blood through a series of tubes made of semipermeable membranes that are bathed in solutions that selectively remove undesirable elements.

hemodialyzer   An apparatus used in performing HEMODIALYSIS.

hemoglobin   The oxygen-carrying pigment of the red blood cells; the iron-containing pigment of the ERYTHROCYTES. It is formed by the developing erythrocyte in BONE MARROW and serves to transport oxygen from the lungs to the tissues.

hemolysis   The destruction of red blood cells (RBCs) by the action of drugs, serum protein (complement), infectious agents, or turbulent blood flow.

hemophilia   A hereditary bleeding disorder caused by a deficiency or abnormality of a protein known as FACTOR VIII, which is essential to blood coagulation. The blood fails to clot and hemorrhage occurs. Hemophilia is inherited through the mother and mainly affects men. HEMOPHILIACs bleed easily, even with a minor cut. Many have severe hemorrhaging into the joints and eventually get joint disease. Hemophilia has two forms, hemophilia A and hemophilia B. Each form lacks a different clotting protein, called a clotting factor. Hemophilia A (classic hemophilia), results from factor VIII deficiency and hemophilia B, from FACTOR IX deficiency.

Hemophilia is treated by lifelong injections of a synthetic version of the clotting factor the blood lacks. The commercial clotting factor is extracted chemically from blood donated by hundreds or thousands of people. As a result, hemophiliacs are exposed to the blood of thousands of blood donors. Between 1978 and 1985 at least 80 percent of the hemophiliacs in the United States who repeatedly infused factor VIII concentrates became infected with HIV. During that period, the internal bleeding that occurs in persons with hemophilia was treated with pooled blood products that contained impurities, including HIV.

In 1985, heat-treated intermediate-purity factor concentrates became generally available. These products were free of HIV but contained other viruses and proteins. In 1989, a new generation of high-purity concentrates was approved by the FDA. These products are purified using MONOCLONAL ANTIBODIES and contain substantially fewer contaminants. In December 1992, the FDA approved a second type of high-purity product, which is manufactured through recombinant technology. The higher-purity products are significantly more expensive than the earlier concentrates.

Since 1985, the risk of being exposed to HIV through clotting factors has dropped to practically nil. One reason is that donated blood is now screened for HIV. Another reason is that clotting factors are heated and purified by detergents and biochemicals that kill HIV. The CENTERS FOR DISEASE CONTROL found that between 1985 and 1988, only 18 hemophiliacs acquired HIV, an annual rate of under one per thousand.

hemophiliac   One afflicted with HEMOPHILIA.

hemophiliac sexual partners   Men with HEMOPHILIA and HIV are faced with a double challenge: the treatment and management of both hemophilia and HIV/AIDS. They and their partners have to deal with medical and social problems that others do not have to face. Living with hemophilia means spending time and energy negotiating the health care system as well as identifying specialized resources and sources of support. Living with hemophilia and HIV means spending more time and energy doing both.

hemoptysis   The coughing up of blood from the lungs; may be a symptom of TUBERCULOSIS.

hemorrhage   Abnormal, severe internal or external discharge of blood. May be venous, arterial, or capillary, from blood vessels into tissues, into or from the body. Venous blood is dark red and the flow is continuous. Arterial blood is bright red and flows in spurts. Capillary blood is of a reddish color and exudes from tissue. Very small hemorrhages are classified as *petechiae*, those up to one centimeter as PURPURA, and larger ones as *ecchymoses*.

hemorrhagic   Pertaining to or marked by HEMORRHAGE.

heparin   See HEPARIN SODIUM.

heparin sodium   An anticoagulant drug; polysaccharide that has been isolated from the liver, lung, and other tissues. It is produced by the mast cells of the liver and by BASOPHIL LEUKOCYTES. It inhibits coagulation by preventing conversion of prothrombin to thrombin by forming an antithrombin and by preventing liberation of thromboplastin from PLATELETS. Heparin is usually administered by IV or subcutaneous injection. The action of heparin requires the presence in the blood of a cofactor found in serum albumin of the plasma. Trade names are Hep-Lock, Lipo-Hepin, and Liquaemin Sodium.

hepatitis   Inflammation of the liver. It may be caused by a variety of agents, including viral infections, bacterial invasion, and physical or chemical agents. Clinically it is usually accompanied by systemic signs including fever, jaundice, and an enlarged liver. There are three different types of hepatitis: hepatitis A, B, and C. Comparing the types of hepatitis reveals differences in transmission, severity, prevention, and treatment.

Hepatitis A is a self-limiting virus-induced liver disease spread through contact with fecal matter containing the hepatitis A virus. Contact can happen during eating, drinking, or sexual activity. Two groups cited as having high risk for hepatitis A are also at high risk for HIV: gay men and injection drug users. The traditional therapy, gamma globulin shots rich in hepatitis A antibodies, provides most people with temporary protection against the disease. In 1995, the Food and Drug Administration approved a hepatitis A vaccine sold under the trade name Havrix. The efficacy of vaccine in people with HIV still needs clarification.

Hepatitis B is caused primarily by the hepatitis B virus. It is endemic worldwide and transmitted primarily by parenteral routes (blood transfusions, sharing of needles), intimate personal contact (sexual activity), and perinatally from mother to fetus. In the initial stage, there may be anorexia, fever, malaise, nausea, and vomiting. These decline with the onset of clinical jaundice, arthritis, and angioedema.

Infection may be acute and cause serious symptoms that last up to a few weeks. It may be chronic with occasional symptoms and abnormal liver tests that last for months or years, or it may cause no symptoms at all and may show up only on a blood test. In about 10 percent of cases, hepatitis B is chronic and life threatening. About 5–10 percent of those infected become chronic carriers of hepatitis B virus. They continue to carry and can transmit it to others for years. The hepatitis B virus is transmitted the same way HIV is, by sexual contact or blood-to-blood transmission. Hepatitis B is transmitted far more efficiently than HIV so that a person exposed by a needlestick accident involving a person with both infections is about 20 times more likely to develop infection with the hepatitis virus than with HIV. The blood supply used for transfusions is screened for the hepatitis B virus and is therefore an unlikely source of this infection.

There is no evidence that hepatitis B is any different in people with HIV infection than in people without HIV infection. However, the presence of liver damage or ongoing inflammation may complicate the use of certain drugs that (like AZT) require the liver to metabolize or that (like AZT and pentamidine) may occasionally cause further liver damage.

Once infection takes place, no treatment will eradicate the hepatitis B virus. Infection may be prevented, however, by a vaccine. The vaccine is recommended for people most at risk for this infection: those who share needles to inject drugs, those who practice unsafe sex with gay men, family members of infected people who live in the same household, sex partners of people known to be hepatitis B carriers, and health care workers.

Hepatitis C appears to be more common among heterosexuals and injection drug users than hepatitis B. It is the most common post-transfusion hepatitis in the United States. Clinically and epidemiologically, it resembles hepatitis B.

hepatitis A See HEPATITIS.

hepatitis B See HEPATITIS.

hepatitis C See HEPATITIS.

hepatobiliary symptoms Any perceptible change in the liver, bile, or biliary ducts, including disease.

hepatoma A tumor of the liver.

hepatomegaly Enlargement of the liver.

hepatotoxicity Toxicity to the liver.

herbalism An ancient form of healing still widely used in much of the world, herbalism uses natural plants or plant-based substances to treat a range of illnesses and to enhance the functioning of the body's system. Though herbalism is not a licensed professional modality in the United States, herbs are "prescribed" by a range of practitioners, from holistic M.D.s to acupuncturists to naturopaths.

herbs A flowering plant whose stem above ground does not become woody and persistent. Today more and more facts are being reported in prestigious medical journals about their preventative and healing benefits. The exact reasons for the positive effect herbs exert on the human body is not always known. It is evident, however, that the nutrient and nonnutrient chemicals stored within a plant's cellular structure are in forms that are easily metabolized by the gastric juices, enzymes, and hormones of the body. The therapeutic action of herbs comes from alkaloids, organic nitrogenous compounds that cause certain chemical reactions within the body. Herbs also contain minerals, vitamins, and salts that help the body resist disease, strengthen tissues, and improve the nervous system. They also contain glycosides, which are important sugars for the proper functioning of the heart and bloodstream.

Herbs can be prepared in a variety of ways, including decoction, fomentation, infusion, oil, ointment, poultice, syrup, and tincture. In order to receive the full beneficial effects that can be obtained from herbs, most must be consumed regularly for long periods of time. However, there are several exceptions like goldenseal, which if taken too long can retrogress the illness. Instructions on the labels should be followed. Additionally, because of vast differences amongst individual metabolisms, if an herb is not agreeable or if adverse effects are experienced, usage of the herb should be discontinued and a more agreeable herb substituted. Herbs can be potent, and moderation is generally recommended. Adverse side effects are possible with many herbs when taken in excess. Medicinal amounts of any herb should not be taken without first consulting a physician. Herbs can be obtained from health food stores, herbalists, homeopathic pharmacies, and some food markets. They should be kept in airtight containers away from heat, light, and dampness to prevent deterioration of their active ingredients.

The use of herbs is often suggested as an additional aid in keeping HIV dormant. Herbal remedies should not be used as the only treatment for HIV or AIDS. One or more of the following may be chosen for a particular ailment: aloe vera (works like the drug AZT without the side effects), ASTRAGALUS (for the immune system), ECHINACEA (immuno-stimulant capability for infectious diseases), bee and flower pollen (boost immunity), capsicum (hot peppers for pain of peripheral neuropathies), goldenseal root, myrrh (to fight tooth decay and gum disease), ginseng, mistletoe (high blood pressure, cancer), St. John's wort, red seaweed like Irish moss, chamomile, slippery elm (overall soothing agent), spearmint, catnip, Chinese tonic herbs, schizandra, ligustrum, ganoderma, white atractylodes, godonopsis, and licorice.

heroin A narcotic morphine derivative that appears as a white crystalline powder. Because of its highly addictive nature, importation, sale, and use are illegal in the United States. Its chemical name is *diacetylmorphine*.

herpes A general term for viral infections of HERPES SIMPLEX I or II. These infections cause the eruption of painful blisters, usually in the oral or genital area, and can be sexually transmitted. All can be opportunistic infections of AIDS.

Herpes is a family of large viruses that contain a large amount of DNA. Besides HERPES SIMPLEX I (HSV-1) and HERPES SIMPLEX II (HSV-2), it contains CYTOMEGALOVIRUS (CMV), EPSTEIN-BARR VIRUS (EBV), VARICELLA ZOSTER VIRUS (VZV), and HUMAN HERPES VIRUS-6 (HHV-6).

herpes encephalitis Encephalitis due to infection with herpes simplex virus. Though rare, it is frequently fatal. It has been successfully treated with an antiviral agent.

herpes genitalis Infection of the genital and anorectal skin and mucosa with HERPES SIMPLEX VIRUS type 2. It is usually spread by sexual contact and is classed as a sexually transmitted disease. Itching and soreness are usually present before a small patch of erythema develops. Then a vesicle that erodes appears. These are usually painful and heal in about 10 days. They may occur in any part of the genitalia. Although genital herpes lesions usually occur in limited areas (such as the CERVIX), as HIV infection progresses, the herpes may involve more widespread anatomical areas and be resistant to topical therapy. ACYCLOVIR has been of considerable benefit in treating the initial infection.

Genital herpes is one of the gynecological problems that Social Security Disability Determination Service (DDS) specialists consider when assessing the degree to which the disease affects a woman's ability to function.

herpes simplex An acute disease caused by HERPES SIMPLEX VIRUSES, types I or II. Groups of watery blisters, often painful, form on the skin and mucous membranes, especially the borders of the lips (cold sores) or the mucous surface of the genitals. The cold sores usually heal themselves after a while. Type I infections generally do not involve genital areas of the body; type II infections do. ACYCLOVIR applied locally has been an effective form of treatment, with ANTIBIOTICS often used to treat secondary infections. In persons with AIDS, herpes simplex sores require the intervention of other drugs to heal. Herpes simplex virus persists indefinitely in the body after initial infection and reactivates unpredictably. There is no known cure.

Herpes simplex I, caused by the herpes simplex virus 1 (HIV-1), commonly produces oral herpes, characterized by cold sores or fever blisters on the lips, in the mouth, or around the eyes.

Herpes simplex II, caused by the herpes simplex virus 2 (HSV-2), is a sexually transmitted herpes virus that causes painful sores in the anus or the genital area. Lesions usually appear two to twelve days after infection. In people with weakened immune systems, lesions may persist for a long period, are more extensive, and can result in severe ulcerations. Physicians use acyclovir to treat outbreaks of HSV-2 and as preventive therapy for people with deficient immune systems. FOSCARNET has been used to treat people with acyclovir-resistant herpes simplex infection.

Herpes simplex genitalis, or herpes genitalis, lesions usually appear as painful multiple crops of vesicles, which are often unilateral with coexisting unilateral LYMPHADENOPATHY. Systemic symptoms, such as fever and malaise often accompany primary infection. Recurrences are typical and follow an exacerbated course in immunocompromised patients. Diagnosis is achieved by viral culture of a weeping lesion or tzanck smear of an open lesion. The treatment is acyclovir; in immunocompromised patients, the dosage often needs to be increased. If recurrences are frequent, or infections become chronic, oral or INTRAVENOUS acyclovir at doses sufficient to heal the lesions is initiated, followed by suppressive therapy indefinitely. Local therapy with acyclovir ointment is recommended only for initial outbreaks.

Genital herpes may be chronic and recurring, and no known cure exists. It has been associated with an increased risk of acquiring HIV. Case reports suggest that persons with immunodeficiency have a more severe clinical course of anogential herpes than do immunocompetent patients. Genital herpes can present as painful coalescing ulcerations requiring prophylactic maintenance therapy.

Genital ulcers should be considered in the differential diagnosis of any painful ulcerative genital lesion. Ulcerations from this disorder may increase the risk of transmission in women who are HIV-negative. Repeated or persistent treatment may be necessary to control symptoms; symptoms often recur when medication is discontinued.

Herpes simplex virus in the HIV-positive woman is often more persistent and requires higher doses of acyclovir than in the HIV-negative woman. Systematic acyclovir treatment provides partial control of the symptoms and signs of herpes episodes and accelerates healing. It does not eradicate the infection or affect the subsequent risk, frequency, or severity of recurrences after the drug is discontinued. Safety and efficacy have been documented among persons receiving daily acyclovir therapy for up to three years. Most episodes of recurrence do not benefit from therapy with acyclovir.

HIV infection should be considered a possibility in all women with recurrent or persistent herpes simplex. HIV-infected women have herpes simplex more often than women without HIV infection.

herpes simplex I (HSV-1)   See HERPES SIMPLEX.

herpes simplex II (HSV-2)   See HERPES SIMPLEX.

herpes simplex genitalis   See HERPES SIMPLEX.

herpes simplex virus   See HERPES SIMPLEX.

herpes varicella zoster (VZV)   See HERPES ZOSTER.

herpes virus   See HERPES.

herpes zoster   An acute infectious disease caused by the varicella zoster virus (VZV), characterized by inflammation of the sensory ganglia. Severe neuralgic pain and lesions, or vesicular eruptions on the skin (presented as patches of red spots), occur along the affected nerve. Herpes zoster generally affects or occurs on only one side and is self-limited. It is believed that herpes zoster represents reactivation of latent varicella zoster virus in individuals who have previously had chicken pox and were rendered partially immune. SHINGLES is the more common name for herpes zoster.

het   In the gay subculture, a pejorative term for heterosexual.

heterosexual   Pertaining to a sexual orientation to persons of the opposite sex; one having such sexual orientation. The opposite of homosexual. Often referred to as "straight."

heterosexual intercourse   See HETEROSEXUAL SEX.

heterosexual sex   Sexual activity that takes place between people of the opposite sex.

heterosexual transmission   See TRANSMISSION.

heterosexuality   Sexual orientation toward persons of the opposite sex.

HHV-8   Also known as KSHV or the KS Herpes Virus, HHV-8 was first identified by a Columbia University team of scientists who reported a link between the virus and KAPOSI'S SARCOMA in the *New England Journal of Medicine* (July 25, 1996; 335:233–41). It is believed that HHV-8 is sexually transmitted.

Hickman catheter   People who require long courses of drugs that must be regularly and slowly introduced into the body and cannot be taken orally will often have a flexible tube called a Hickman catheter, through which drugs can be injected, surgically inserted into a large vein in the chest and left in place for a long period of time. See also CATHETER.

high-grade squamous intraepithelial lesion (HSIL)   Abnormalities in the cells on the surface of the CERVIX. They cause an aberration that can be discovered by Pap tests. There is unanimous agreement that tissue classified as HSIL should be removed. See also ATYPICAL SQUAMOUS CELLS OF UNDETERMINED SIGNIFICANCE and LOW-GRADE SQUAMOUS INTRAEPITHELIAL LESION.

high risk In the context of AIDS, a term applied to patterns of behaviour that place individuals at risk of contracting the HIV virus; any behavior that puts the bloodstream in contact with any of the bodily fluids of another person that can transmit the AIDS virus. High-risk behavior includes sharing needles when injecting intravenous drugs and having unprotected vaginal, anal, or oral sex or sex with an IV drug user. The mode of transmission may influence the likelihood that an exposed individual will become infected. There appears to be a continuum of risk for HIV/AIDS. The risk of HIV infection has been categorized as no risk, low risk, medium risk, and high risk.

high-risk behavior See HIGH RISK.

high-risk group/population A group or population sharing a common behavior or characteristic placing it at high risk for HIV infection compared to the population as a whole. Our understanding of, and belief in, the existence of high-risk groups and populations has evolved since the beginning of the epidemic. In the earliest stages of the AIDS epidemic in both the United States and Europe, homosexual and bisexual men accounted for upward of 90 percent of all cases. INTRAVENOUS drug users were a small minority of all cases, limited to only a few geographic areas, and heterosexual cases were distinctly unusual outside of Africa. The epidemic in Africa, more widespread than elsewhere, was almost exclusively in heterosexuals.

Over the first decade of AIDS in the industrial world, it was believed that the virus moved across groups, gaining access to new groups where they overlap. HIV first appeared in the developed world in the male homosexual population and at one point was thought to be a disease exclusively of homosexuals. Bisexual men and male homosexual drug users, who could be categorized in more than one group, formed a ready bridge from this affected group to others. Female partners of bisexual men were exposed to HIV through these sexual relationships. Because of the common practice among intravenous drug users of sharing needles and syringes, infected homosexual users passed HIV on to nonhomosexual men and women with whom they shared them. A large portion of female prostitutes also inject drugs; they introduced HIV among men who neither injected drugs nor were homosexuals, and through them to their wives and other sex partners. Before 1985 anyone from a group at risk for HIV infection could donate blood for medical purposes; thus HIV-infected blood transmitted the virus to those not belonging to such groups. Anyone receiving a blood transfusion or any type of blood product before 1985 was at risk for infection regardless of behavior. Parents especially mothers exposed to HIV by any of these means, passed the virus to their children and fetuses.

Today, we know that HIV does not discriminate and that no group or population is immune to HIV/AIDS. Today, our focus has shifted from groups or populations to behaviors. We no longer ask why homosexual men form a large percentage of all AIDS cases or if HIV transmission by intravenous drug abusers can be reduced, but ask instead such questions as How is HIV transmitted by homosexual intercourse? How do intravenous drug figure in the transmission of HIV? Why are hemophiliacs at risk for HIV transmission? and Who should not donate blood?"

high-risk person A person who engages in HIGH-RISK behavior.

high-risk population See HIGH-RISK GROUP/POPULATION.

high-risk sex Unsafe sex practices with high risk of HIV transmission include having numerous sex partners; unprotected anal-receptive sex with an infected partner; unprotected anal penetration with the hand ("fisting"); anal douching in combination with anal sex; oral-anal contact; and vaginal intercourse without a condom with an infected partner.

highly active antiretroviral therapy (HAART) Specialized combination therapies. Potent HAART combination therapies have recently been shown to be of benefit even to people with advanced AIDS and with extensive past exposure to anti-HIV therapy. As of 1996, however, many people continue to fail on their current HIV medications, even if they are receiving one of the new triple combinations. Enthusiasm about HAART was further tempered by recent findings that HIV persists and can replicate in patients who have no detectable virus in their blood, as a result of combination antiretroviral therapy. These findings indicate that an inducible reservoir of HIV exists in infected patients despite prolonged treatment with HAART, and suggest that the time required for eradication of HIV from the body, if indeed possible, may be considerably longer than previously indicated. These results underscore the importance of developing more potent antiretroviral drugs, as well as treatment strategies that specifically target latently infected cells that serve as hiding places for the virus. It is generally agreed upon that although our current armamentarium of antiretroviral drugs has served many patients well, at least in the short-term, more progress must be made in the area of HIV therapeutics if we are to speak of a cure for HIV deisease. The quest to find a truly optimal combination of drugs, or at least provide options to switch to after failing whatever cocktail one is currently ingesting, continues.

Hill-Burton Reconstruction Act The Hill-Burton Reconstruction Act (Hospital Survey and Construction Act of 1946) was a postwar measure designed to create employment and provide better health care through hospital construction grants. In return for grant funds, the private hospitals were expected to provide services for some indigent patients. This quid pro quo was conveniently ignored by hospitals throughout the 1950s and 1960s. In the 1970s, however, litigation about the act developed a right to health care for indigent people at Hill-Burton facilities. In response to these cases, the Department of Health and Human Services promulgated new regulations requiring Hill-Burton hospitals to render a certain amount of uncompensated care to indigent patients each year.

Not all hospitals have Hill-Burton—only those which have received federal construction help are required to participate. However, all publicly owned or operated hospitals, even some private, noncharity hospitals, have some patients who meet income (and, sometimes, asset) guidelines. In addition, a variety of federal, state, local, and private philanthropic health agencies finance free or reduced-fee health clinics, which are typically run by local health departments or nonprofit agencies. Generally those with income below the federal poverty level are fully eligible, with partial bill reductions sometimes available on a sliding scale as income rises above that level. Income and asset levels vary from state to state, locality to locality, and even health program to health program. All Hill-Burton facilities give free care to those with incomes up to the poverty level; many, however, also take the federally offered option of also giving free care to those with incomes up to twice the poverty level. For those becoming eligible for Medicaid via a "spend down," Hill-Burton and hospital charity bill write-offs can cover the portion of a hospital's bill that would otherwise be the patient's liability. Services are available to all needy residents, not just to those found "disabled." Hill-Burton programs have no assets eligibility level and no income disregards; other programs' assets and income disregard policies vary. Hill-Burton hospital and charity programs, as well as many local low-income clinics, require an applicant to apply for and follow through on Medicaid or other public medical assistance: Eligibility is then granted only to those found ineligible for complete Medicaid coverage of their bills. Benefits vary from facility to facility, although all Hill-Burton hospitals and clinics must comply with certain Hill-Burton rules. Details pertaining to how and where to apply also vary from facility to facility.

histamine   A major vasoactive amine (released from mast cell and basophil granules) that exerts a pharmacological action when released from injured cells. Functions of histamine include increasing gastric secretion, dilation of capillaries, and contraction of bronchial smooth muscle responsible for itching/sneezing during allergy.

histocompatibility   The quality of living tissue of one individual of being immunologically compatible with the tissue of another. Histocompatible tissues have ANTIGENS of the same HUMAN LEUKOCYTE ANTIGEN (HLA) complex, and therefore will not cause an immunologic response and will continue to function following transplantation from one individual to another.

histocompatibility complex   The cluster or family of genes that control immune reactions, genes that contain the coding information necessary for the synthesis of ANTIGENS, the specific proteins found on the surface of cells. There is some evidence of an HLA-linked genetic factor in AIDS patients that is not present in non-AIDS individuals.

histocompatibility genes   The genes (comprising the HUMAN LEUKOCYTE ANTIGEN (HLA) complex) that determine the histocompatibility antigenic markers on all nucleated cells. These genes create the antigens by which the immune system recognizes "self" and, therefore, are important in determining the success of transplanted organs and tissues.

Many different forms of one particular histocompatibility gene are found at the seven sites on chromosome 6.

histoincompatibility   The quality of living tissue of one individual not being immunologically compatible with the tissue of another, and therefore unsuitable for transplantation. See HISTOCOMPATIBILITY.

histopathology   The study of the microscopic structure of diseased tissues.

histoplasma capsulatum   A fungus present in soil and dust, widespread in the south-central United States and in Latin America. It is the causative agent of HISTOPLASMOSIS.

histoplasmosis   *Histoplasma capsulatum* is a fungus endemic to the south-central United States and South America. It is found in soil in spore form. When contaminated soil is disturbed, the spores may be inhaled causing germination into yeast form which spreads via the blood throughout the body. It appears that after infection, some viable organisms remain intracellularly which in immunocompromised patients may result in reactivation infection. The symptoms of histoplasmosis are reflective of the diffuse invasive nature of the infection. Fever, weight loss, skin lesions, adenopathy, respiratory complaints, and cough are common. Meningitis and cerebritis are rarely seen. Identification of the fungus in tissue specimens or in culture provides the definitive diagnosis. Bone marrow, blood, lymph nodes, lungs, and skin are all commonly infected tissues that should be examined and biopsied. Serologic tests for histoplasmosis are available. Complement fixation tests are reliable when positive, but may be negative in up to 30 percent of infected people. A new radioimmunoassay for the detection of a histo polysaccharide antigen may be more sensitive. Maintenance or suppressive therapy is then required. Patients with disseminated histoplasmosis disease require intensive induction treatment with amphotericin. Good results have been found with itraconazole according to early studies.

historical control   A group of participants in a clinical trial that did not take the experimental drug being tested, used as a comparison in a later clinical trial.

history taking   Systematically recording past medical events as they relate to a person or group of people.

HIV   See HUMAN IMMUNODEFICIENCY VIRUS.

HIV-1b   A viral subtype of HIV that is most common in the United States.

HIV-1e   A viral subtype of HIV that is most common in parts of Asia and Africa, where 90 percent of HIV cases are attributed to heterosexual contact.

HIV-2   HUMAN IMMUNODEFICIENCY VIRUS type 2. HIV-2 is found mostly in western Africa. Like HIV-1, HIV-2 induces AIDS, albeit at a much slower rate, and with less transmissibility. Researchers have found that HIV-2 infection can protect individuals from subsequent infection with HIV-1. Investigators, supported by the National Institute of Allergy and Infectious Disease (NIAID), however, note that the use of HIV-2 as a live attenuated vaccine against HIV-1 infection probably has risks that far outweigh the potential benefits.

HIV antibody (HIV-Ab)   The antibody to HIV, which usually appears within six weeks after infection. Antibody testing early in the infection process may not produce accurate results, since some recently infected people have not yet begun producing antibodies and test negative even though they are infected. Thus, a single negative antibody test result is not a guarantee of freedom from infection. The change from HIV-negative to HIV-positive status is called SEROCONVERSION.

HIV antibody negativity   Absence of antibodies in the blood directed against HIV. The absence of these antibodies indicates either absence of infection or that infection is too recent to have generated detectable antibodies.

HIV antibody positivity   The presence of antibodies in the blood directed against HIV, detected by any of several diagnostic tests (see ELISA; WESTERN BLOT TEST). Synonymous with HIV infection.

HIV antibody test   A blood test that shows whether or not a person has antibodies to the virus that causes AIDS. The test indicates only whether a person has at some time been infected with HIV. It cannot determine if a person has AIDS or will develop AIDS in the future. See HIV ANTIBODY TESTING; ELISA; WESTERN BLOT TEST.

HIV antibody testing   HIV antibody testing is one of three means of diagnosing HIV infection. This method detects the presence of the virus through the body's response to it. The most common response is the production of antibodies. Tests that detect these antibodies are inexpensive and readily available to all medical laboratories. The other two methods to diagnose HIV infection are by the isolation of virus in the laboratory from blood or other infected fluids and tissues and to infer infection from the presence of characteristic symptoms. This last technique was used before the wide availability of antibody diagnostic kits, and it remains a frequent method of diagnosis where access to these kits is limited.

HIV-contaminated blood   HIV-contaminated blood contains blood from donors who have or had AIDS or who are or were HIV antibody positive, and are thus at high risk for AIDS. As of 1987, approximately half of the recipients of seropositive blood were seropositive, and significant percentages of these persons had developed symptoms of HIV infection or AIDS. Routine serological testing of donated blood did not begin until March 1985 in the United States. See also BLOOD SUPPLY PROTECTION.

HIV counseling   Information provided to an individual before and after HIV testing regarding the implications and impact of testing, HIV infection care, and prevention of HIV transmission. Pretest counseling may include questions and discussion about past sexual activity, drug use, and medical history. Individuals may also be asked if they think their test will be positive or how they will react if their test is positive. This enables counselors to identify people who need additional counseling or whose tests are more likely than those of others to be positive for HIV. The counselor will then give the individual the opportunity to ask any questions she or he may have about HIV, AIDS, or the test. Post-test counseling includes discussion of the test results (negative, positive, or inconclusive) and may introduce issues pertaining to living with AIDS (treatment, management, prevention).

HIV dementia   See AIDS DEMENTIA COMPLEX.

HIV encephalitis   See AIDS DEMENTIA COMPLEX.

HIV encephalopathy   See AIDS DEMENTIA COMPLEX.

HIV envelope protein gp120   An understanding of both viruses and the nuclear envelope is essential to understanding HIV envelope protein GP120. Viruses consist of a strand of either deoxyribonucleic acid (DNA) or ribonucleic acid (RNA), but not both, and are surrounded by a capsid, a covering of protein. There is no cell wall. The nuclear envelope is a double-membrane layer of lipids and proteins surrounding the nucleus of a cell. Eight amino acids which constitute part of the viral envelope called gp120 are thought by some scientists to be the key by which HIV gains entry through the CD4 receptor. It is theorized that HIV enters the CD4 receptor by mimicking a chemical produced by the body that uses the same receptor. Peptide T is an example of one treatment designed as a way of plugging all the body's CD4 "locks" with artificial "keys," and thereby preventing attachment of the virus to cells. See also PEPTIDE T for an outline of the complex.

HIV genome   The entire genetic information present in a cell. See also GENOME.

HIV guidelines   See UNIVERSAL PRECAUTIONS.

HIV incidence   See INCIDENCE.

HIV-infected   Infected with the human immunodeficiency virus. See HIV INFECTION.

HIV infection   Infection with the HUMAN IMMUNODEFICIENCY VIRUS, at any stage from the early asymptomatic to the late stages of AIDS.

HIV latency   See LATENCY.

HIV measurement   In 1995, two new tests for the measurement of HIV came into widespread use in sophisticated laboratories. Dr. David Ho, director of the Aaron Diamond AIDS Research Laboratory in Manhattan, pioneered their use in the analysis of HIV disease. These tests allow the rapid and easy measurement of the amount of HIV genetic code, or RNA, in a sample of blood. Until 1995, diagnostic tools to monitor levels of HIV in patients' blood were not precise enough to indicate which drugs might be the most useful for a patient.

Much has been learned about the virus's activities using these new tools. Every day in people infected with HIV, including individuals who are otherwise healthy, 10 billion copies of the virus circulate in the body. Every five hours and 45 minutes about one billion new copies enter the bloodstream, a million of which infect CD4 cells of the immune system. Those cells become factories for viral production, spewing out another 10 billion copies over the next 24 hours. In the process, the CD4 cells die but are rapidly replaced. One of the most urgent implications of these staggering numbers—orders of magnitude beyond that seen with any other chronic infectious disease—is that every drug is doomed to fail because with each round of reproduction, HIV mutates, which increases the chances that it will become resistant to the drug being used. With each cycle millions of millions of HIV variants are generated. They, in turn, initiate more mutations with which to cope. Ho argues that the key to HIV treatment has to involve dosing people immediately after they are infected with powerful combinations of drugs, including the then newly developed class of PROTEASE INHIBITORS. Many argue that the new tests should be the standard diagnostic tool, and that all decisions for HIV medical treatment should be based on them. However, it remains to be seen whether or not HEALTH MAINTENANCE ORGANIZATIONS and MANAGED CARE companies will pay the costs, which are considerable.

HIV-negative   Having no detectable HIV antibodies in the blood. A negative test result does not guarantee than an individual is virus-free or cannot transmit the virus to someone else. Case reports have shown that the period between initial HIV infection and the production of detectable antibodies (that is, between infection and SEROCONVERSION) is most often between one and six months. (Uncommon cases have occurred in which more than six months elapsed before antibody was produced. How often this occurs and how to find the virus when infection is suspected but tests are negative, are matters of controversy.) If an individual is tested during this period after being infected but before producing antibodies, the test result will be negative.

See HIV-POSITIVE; ELISA; WESTERN BLOT TEST.

HIV pathogenesis   The origin and development of HIV.

HIV-positive   Having HIV antibodies present in the blood. The presence of the antibodies confirms the presence of the HIV virus. Inaccurate test results are possible. Antibodies elicited by other substances in the blood may be similar to antibodies directed against HIV and may crossreact in the ELISA, the most commonly used test, falsely indicating the presence of HIV. In all cases of a positive test result, a second blood test must be performed to confirm the results of the first. The western blot is run as a confirmatory test.

Being HIV-positive means that at some point exposure to the virus and infection with HIV have occurred. It does not mean that an individual now has AIDS or will definitely develop AIDS in the future. Being HIV-positive does not

mean that an individual is immune to the virus. Being HIV-positive does not mean that an individual can no longer have sex. It does mean, however, a major change in the way an individual lives his or her life.

See HIV-NEGATIVE; WESTERN BLOT TEST.

HIV RNA   The genetic material of HIV. Many people believe that changes in the level of HIV RNA are good indicators of drug effectiveness; this has not been proved. A new technology that detects blood levels of HIV RNA has been suggested as a promising way for clinicians to gauge the effectiveness of therapy and predict when the disease might get worse. A National Institute of Allergy and Infectious Disease multicenter study began in 1995 to determine if monitoring levels of HIV in the blood can keep patients healthier longer by helping doctors make better treatment decisions.

See RNA.

HIV screening   Epidemiologic surveillance of HIV/AIDS in a given population. Such surveillance generally involves an assessment of the existing distribution and scope of infection and its likely spread in the population. Generally such surveillance is an important first step in responding to a disease. Screening is most often associated with compulsory and mass HIV testing, which targets either certain demographic or occupational groups or captive populations (aliens entering the country, military personnel, police officers, drug users, commercial sex workers, prisoners, people with hemophilia, and so forth). Prohibitive cost and complex logistics, as well as human rights considerations, lack of safeguards for confidentiality in testing, and for avoiding discrimination against persons who are found to be infected, have contributed to a decrease in the use and effectiveness of HIV screening programs.

HIV seroprevalence   The prevalence of HIV infection. HIV seroprevalence is an important indication of the scope of the disease and its related problems. With multiple seroprevalence surveys that are based on sample blood specimens, organizations like the CENTERS FOR DISEASE CONTROL AND PREVENTION collect data on HIV infection from several subpopulations. The data collected provide information on the prevalence and incidence of infection in selected populations, provide early warning of the emergence of infection in new populations, and target intervention programs and other resources.

HIV setpoint   The level at which an individual's viral load eventually plateaus. Several studies suggest that the HIV setpoint predicts the rate at which that person will progress to AIDS. If antiviral therapy can help to lower the viral load setpoint so that there is a more stable equilibrium with the immune system, it might slow disease progression.

HIV status   The term "HIV status" often connotes a division between HIV infected and uninfected people. The word "status" implies both a rigid social or moral hierarchy, like caste, and a state of being that is mutable, like a status report. HIV-positive individuals are often portrayed as threatening "others." HIV-negative status is often portrayed as better than—rather than merely different from—an HIV-positive status. When HIV-negative individuals think about the possibility of becoming HIV-positive, they realize their HIV status is something that can change. Their negative status is both precarious and valuable—something they want to protect.

HIV suppressors   A substance that halts the growth of HIV in cell cultures. See also CELL ACTIVATED FACTOR (CAF), IL-16 and CHEMOKINES.

HIV testing   The use of blood tests that detect the presence or absence of antibodies directed against HIV. The question of involuntary testing emerged early and forcefully in the AIDS pandemic, and testing remains at the center of controversies relating to AIDS prevention and control, including issues of privacy, selectiveness of testing, fear of stigmatization, notification of others, and nondiscrimination. See HIV SCREENING.

HIV transmission   See TRANSMISSION.

HIV wasting syndrome   See WASTING SYNDROME.

HL   See HAIRY LEUKEMIA.

HLA   See HUMAN LEUKOCYTE ANTIGEN.

ho   See PROSTITUTE.

Hodgkin's disease   A chronic progressive disease of unknown ETIOLOGY that is characterized by inflammatory enlargement of the LYMPH NODES, SPLEEN, and often LIVER and KIDNEYS. Other symptoms may include anemia, anorexia, fever, night sweats, severe itching, and weight loss. It may appear as acute, localized, or latent with relapsing fever or as lymphogranulomatosis and SPLENOMEGALY. Treatment includes radiation and CHEMOTHERAPY.

holistic (wholistic)   Various systems of health protection and restoration, both traditional and modern, that are based on the body's reputed "natural healing powers," the various ways the different tissues affect each other, and the influence of the external environment.

home- and community-based services   Under MEDICAID's 2176 waiver program, these are home health care, home chore aid, personal attendant, outpatient hospice, visiting nurse, and even board-and-care-home services, which are offered as an alternative to more expensive hospitalization or nursing home care.

home care   A continuum of outpatient and home- and community-based services given by family members, nurses (nurse practitioners, licensed practical nurses, RNs), health care providers, home care agencies, technicians, home attendants, social workers, and case managers. A physician is in overall charge of care, but the people who actually deliver the care are removed from his or her immediate supervision. Home care can be a more comfortable, patient-centered, flexible form of care that is also somewhat cheaper than hospital care, and the trend has been to extend it to sicker and sicker patients. But it can also be fragmented, erratic, poorly administered and supervised, and literally out of control. Successful home care must carry into the home setting the team approach that characterizes hospital care, in which case the family and other caregivers must be part of the team in a way that they are not in an institution.

home health care   See HOME CARE.

home health services   Health services, given to a patient in his own home, that can be provided only by a licensed professional such as a registered nurse or a physical, speech, or occupational therapist. Unskilled care such as housekeeping, feeding, and grooming assistance, comes under this heading only when it is necessary to accomplish the core health service rendered by a professional. Home health services are covered by MEDICARE, MEDICAID, and many private health insurance plans. See HOME CARE.

homeopathy   An approach to healing that is popular in Europe and has many followers in the United States. Its followers believe that a substance which produces a certain set of symptoms in a healthy person has the power to cure a sick person manifesting those same symptoms. Homeopathy has been used by people living with HIV because treatments are unlike conventional scientific medicine, which attacks disease head-on with drugs meant to kill specific bacteria. Homeopathic approaches try to treat "like with like." Once a homeopath has diagnosed a disorder in a patient, a diluted solution to treat the problem is prescribed. This is done by matching or "proving" symptoms with the one substance that most closely reproduces these symptoms in a normal person. Substances may include chemicals, minerals, plant extracts, dilute preparations of animal and insect venom, disease-causing germs, and some standard drugs. Matching the patient's symptoms with the substance that most closely reproduces them is crucial because homeopaths assert that a single dose of that substance, highly diluted and properly prepared, has the capacity to cure the ailing patient. Many people living with HIV report significant reduction of their symptoms using homeopathic remedies.

To date, there have not been an extensive number of controlled clinical studies evaluating the effectiveness of homeopathic treatments. The American Medical Association does not recognize homeopathic medicine because they believe the approach is not based on scientific principles. Currently, only several states license homeopaths. As a result, homeopathic practitioners are often licensed under other accepted forms of medicine, such as a medical doctor, acupuncturist, osteopath, or chiropractor.

homeostasis   The state in which the internal environment of the body remains relatively stable by responding appropriately to changes.

homing receptors   Cell surface molecules that direct the cell to specific locations in other organs or tissues.

homo   Derisive slang term for homosexual.

homophobia   The intense fear and/or hatred of homosexuals or of anything having to do with homosexuality. Although the term is of recent origin, homophobia (or heterosexism) as a component of our culture has long historical roots, going back at least to early Christian condemnation of sex except for procreation. Like all prejudices, it is based on social myths and stereotyping. Some of the common myths and stereotypes that perpetuate homophobia are that gays are easy to spot—gay men are "swishy," and lesbians are "butch"; that most gays are attracted to certain jobs, e.g., hairdressers, florists, decorators; that gay men are all promiscuous and prone to abuse children; that gay male and lesbian couples have rigid gender roles, with one being the "man" and one the "woman"; that gay men and lesbians have no parental instincts; and that gay parents or teachers can influence children to be gay or lesbian.

Homophobia is manifested in many ways. Gays and lesbians may legally be denied their civil rights jobs, housing, marriage, parenthood), be taunted and insulted publicly (antigay speech is still tolerated in a way that other prejudiced speech is not), and at times be physically assaulted and even murdered because of their sexual orientation. Homophobia as a response to the AIDS crisis is based entirely on prejudice and misrepresentation. It is inappropriate and destructive.

homosexual   Pertaining to same-sex sexual orientation; one sexually attracted to persons of the same sex. Generally, a homosexual woman is called a lesbian. Homosexual men and women are also called gay.

homosexual intercourse   See HOMOSEXUAL SEX.

homosexual sex   Sexual activity between members of the same sex.

homosexual transmission   See TRANSMISSION.

homosexual/bisexual transmission   See TRANSMISSION.

homosexuality   Sexual attraction toward persons of the same sex.

hooker   A slang term for a prostitute.

horizontal transmission   See TRANSMISSION.

hormone   An active chemical substance secreted by an organ or gland into the blood, which carries it to specific target cells/organs by whose response they bring about a specific and adaptive physiological response (e.g., stimulation or suppression of cell or tissue activity). Hormones tend to be either water-soluble peptides and proteins or lipid-soluble steroids, retinoids, thyroid hormones, and vitamin D3. Examples of hormones include adrenaline, ecdysone, gastrin, thyroxine, insulin, testosterone, and estrogen.

horny   Slang term for being sexually aroused.

hospice   A facility that provides palliative and supportive services for the terminally ill. Hospice care is an interdisciplinary approach to providing for the terminally ill. The hospice concept emphasizes alleviating a patient's discomfort and supporting the family in the grieving process. Supportive care may include financial, physical, social, and spiritual services. Covered by MEDICARE, MEDICAID, and some private health insurance plans, hospice care may be provided at a hospice facility, at a patient's home, or both. Care is generally provided by a team of health care professionals.

host   An organism on which another organism lives and from which the second organism derives nourishment.

host factors   Factors intrinsic to the HIV-infected individual that influence the rate at which HIV replicates in the person's body and how rapidly the patient will develop AIDS. These factors include the specific immune response to the virus, nonspecific factors, and the individual's genetic makeup. Such factors are as important, or in some cases even more important, to the HIV disease process than the intrinsic virulence of the virus itself. Host factors, together with viral factors, determine the pathogenesis of HIV disease, the complex events which lead to the destruction of an HIV-infected person's immune system.

hot   In sexual terms, slang for sexually arousing. It may be used of a person, image, activity, or thing.
In epidemiological terms, slang for actively infective.
"Hot" may also mean radioactive.

hot agent   Extremely lethal virus that is potentially airborne.

hot zone   An area that contains lethal, infectious organisms. Also hot area or hot side.

hot line   Telephone service providing crisis intervention to individuals experiencing severe problems. Hot lines are usually staffed continuously by paraprofessionals or professionals in the medical or social sciences. HIV/AIDS–related hot lines typically provide answers to questions about the disease and offer referrals to local service providers.

housebound   Incapacitated and unable to leave home, medical facility, or community residence without assistance. The term is sometimes used in MEDICAID and other social service programs. In military pension programs of the Department of Veterans Affairs, housebound disabled veterans are entitled to a higher pension income eligibility level.

housing   People with HIV/AIDS face difficulties in obtaining and maintaining housing. They may have difficulty renting or buying in the private market and may be evicted from current rental agreements. The Fair Housing Act, adopted by Congress in 1968, prohibits discrimination in the sale or rental of housing and in advertising, financing, and the provision of brokerage services. Congress amended the law in 1988 to prohibit discrimination because of "handicap." The Fair Housing Act defines "handicap" as a "physical or mental impairment which substantially limits . . . major life activities." This definition was taken from Section 504 of the Rehabilitation Act of 1973, which courts have unanimously interpreted to include HIV. People subjected to discrimination in violation of the Fair Housing Act may file a complaint with HUD and may bring a lawsuit to federal court. The attorney general may also bring actions in court to prohibit "a pattern or practice" that violates the Fair Housing Act. Today, many states have their own laws prohibiting discrimination in housing on the basis of handicap, some including HIV infection. Several cities have also adopted ordinances prohibiting discrimination in housing against people with HIV. State and local laws have also been used to oppose discrimination by landlords against agencies and professionals providing services to people with HIV/AIDS.

One of the realities people with HIV/AIDS may face is the possibility of losing their homes because of inability to make rent or mortgage payments. Some people with full-blown AIDS may need specialized care facilities or group housing. Many people with HIV become homeless and require housing assistance. The law provides very little support for general claims that the government must provide shelter to those who need it. But people with HIV have redress under the Fair Housing Act and local antidiscrimination laws when they are refused admission to or are evicted from group housing, such as homeless shelters and publicly owned housing, because of their condition.

In the long run, most litigation is likely to concern special-care facilities and group homes for people with HIV. Organized community opposition to group homes or care facilities is a common barrier. These facilities generally must meet state and local health and fire codes. Usually, efforts to prevent homes from opening focus on zoning restrictions. Discriminatory use of zoning restrictions is subject to challenge under both the United States Constitution and the Fair Housing Act. Some cases have also applied the equal protection clause of the federal Constitution to invalidate zoning restrictions and decisions that discrimination against group homes for special populations, such as people with HIV/AIDS.

While much has been done for people with HIV to eliminate discrimination in housing, much remains to be done in meeting their housing needs. People with HIV/AIDS must cope with pressing income as well as health needs. Funding for housing is crucial, a fact Congress recognized in the 1990 Cranston-Gonzalez National Affordable Housing Act, which includes a block grant program designed to encourage state and local governments to provide housing for people with HIV/AIDS. Additionally, the United States social welfare system offers a variety of financial and health care benefit programs for people, including SOCIAL SECURITY, welfare, MEDICAID, MEDICARE, FOOD STAMPS, drugs, and housing. With federal funding, many state, city, or county housing departments run a variety of housing programs for low-income persons, with special projects or units set aside for the aged and the disabled. Persons with HIV/AIDS who need access to housing must identify the programs that are available, find out what benefits are offered, and determine and assess their eligibility before applying and, if necessary, appealing.

HPA-23   See ANTIMONIOTUNGSTATE.

HPMPC   See CIDOFOVIR.

HPV   See HUMAN PAPILLOMAVIRUS.

HTLV   See HUMAN T CELL LYMPHOTROPIC VIRUS.

HTLV-II   See HUMAN T CELL LYMPHOTROPIC VIRUS.

HTLV-III   See HUMAN IMMUNODEFICIENCY (HIV) VIRUS.

HTLV-III/LAV   See HUMAN T-LYMPHOTROPIC VIRUS TYPE III.

HTLV-IV   See HUMAN T-LYMPHOTROPIC VIRUS TYPE IV.

HUD   See DEPARTMENT OF HOUSING AND URBAN DEVELOPMENT.

HUD voucher   A document that eligible low-income recipients can present to landlords in lieu of rent payment; landlords, in turn, redeem the vouchers for cash from HUD, in a housing counterpart to the food stamps program. Not all landlords participate in this program.

human chorionic gonadotropin (HCG)   A hormone that may have an anti-KS and anti-HIV effect. Produced in the placenta during pregnancy, HCG inhibits the mother's immune system from rejecting the fetus as "foreign tissue." It is an approved therapy for treating infertility in women and cryptorchidism (failure of the testicles to descend) in boys. In the first human trial with HCG, intralesional injection of a formulation of HCG was shown to reduce the size and occasionally lead to complete regression of the treated KS lesions. Investigators observed that the active material is not the normal HCG molecule, but something that accompanies it in the crude material, in the pregnant woman's urine. Investigators hypothesize both that the amount of this active component probably depends on what stage the urine is collected during pregnancy, and that there probably is more of it early in the course of pregnancy. Whatever the active component, it appears to induce apoptosis (a form of cell suicide) in the lesion. Investigators believe that this component probably acts as both a growth and rejection factor early in the growth of the fetus.

A number of companies have approval to market HCG. More is expected to be published on the anti-HIV activity of the HCG extract. Additional research may shed light on what HCG may do in immune-compromised individuals or how it may interact with other HIV therapies. Headache, irritability, aggressive behavior, and phallic or testicular enlargement are some of the side effects caused by injectable HCG.

human gene therapy   Treatment of human disease by gene transfer. Most approved gene therapy trials involve use of retroviral vectors for gene transfer into cultured human cells that would be administered to patients. Retroviral vectors are RETROVIRUSES lacking all functional viral genes, so no viral protein is produced in infected cells. Viral replication is achieved using "packaging cells" that produce all the viral proteins without the infective virus. This results in efficient and stable targeting of cells. The main drawback though, is the inability of the vectors to infect non-dividing cells. Proposals for human gene therapy have to pass several levels of review to ensure safety.

human growth hormone (HGH)   A peptide hormone, secreted by the anterior pituitary gland in the brain, that enhances tissue growth by stimulating protein formation. Made under the trade name Serostim.

Many people with AIDS lose protein from lean tissue mass in the course of their disease. WASTING SYNDROME, unlike malnutrition caused by a digestive problem, springs from a metabolic change during chronic HIV infection that causes the body to break down protein to meet its energy requirements rather than first using its stores of fat. This process is either acute and due to a specific gastrointestinal or other infection or chronic and nonspecific. During intermittent periods of relative health, the body may restore some of its weight, but this takes the form of new fat, not restored protein or lean tissue mass.

Possible contributors to wasting include low testosterone levels, which can be treated by testosterone replacement supplemented by anabolic steroids, or excessive production of such inflammatory compounds as TUMOR NECROSIS FACTOR ALPHA, which can be reversed with anti-inflammatory drugs such as thalidomide. (A number of clinical trials of thalidomide are ongoing. These include trials where the drug is being evaluated as an anti-HIV therapy, antiwasting therapy, and as a therapy for people with tuberculosis and HIV. Recent data suggest that thalidomide may interfere with the metabolism of oral contraceptives. Because of the risk of serious and severe birth defects, women who have sex with men should use two forms of birth control if using thalidomide.) HGH is thought to reorient the body's metabolism so that it focuses on rebuilding protein stores. HGH does not reverse the underlying metabolic defect; high doses of HGH just overwhelm it through other hormonal channels. HGH has proved that it is possible to replace lean tissue mass.

Under a FOOD AND DRUG ADMINISTRATION "Treatment Investigational New Drug" (TIND) protocol, people with AIDS-related wasting syndrome may receive human growth hormone. To be eligible, a person with HIV must have lost 10 percent of normal body weight without apparent cause (such as a weight-loss–inducing opportunistic infection like MYCOBACTERIUM AVIUM COMPLEX or CRYPTOSPORIDIUM). She or he must also have first tried Megace and Marinol, approved appetite stimulants that frequently fail (especially Megace).

HGH's manufacturer, Serono Laboratories, required patients (or their third party payers) in the TIND protocol to reimburse doctors for the data collection and paperwork involved and to pay for the drug itself, at an enormous price—$150 per day, or more than $1,000 per week. Although charging for the cost of the drug is allowed by the Food and Drug Administration, this had never been done before. Except for some in California, few insurance companies will compensate their subscribers for the cost of HGH, and no state MEDICAID or AIDS DRUG ASSISTANCE PROGRAM (which subsidizes people of moderate income) has agreed to cover the compound. Serono operated a very modest "indigent program" that provided free or discount HGH for people who could not purchase the drug any other way.

While the therapy's costliness threatens to undermine its rational use, the price issue is compounded by uncertainty over how and when to use the drug. Although growth hormone can have a very dramatic effect, there are many loose ends surrounding the use of human growth hormone therapy for AIDS-related wasting. It is still not clear what is the optimum dose or duration of treatment, and the timing of initial use of HGH has not been pinned down. Moreover, authorities on AIDS-related wasting syndrome caution that HGH is for the semistable, to improve their quality of life. For people with acute wasting, there is a need to treat the underlying condition. They note too that HGH without therapy only slows the weight loss and that, for therapy without HGH, recovery is low or nonexistent. HGH has not yet been approved by the FDA, and further data is required to resolve the uncertainties over this therapy.

Most people with wasting may have alternatives to HGH. A considerable number of doctors are prescribing an extremely inexpensive regimen of testosterone plus synthetic anabolic steroids to men, at least, and reporting very good results on an anecdotal basis.

human herpes virus-6 (HHV-6)   A type of herpes virus thought to be a cofactor in the progression of HIV disease.

human immune deficiency virus   See HUMAN IMMUNODEFICIENCY VIRUS.

human immunodeficiency virus (HIV)   One of a large group of IMMUNODEFICIENCY viruses (IVs) widely spread among primates and other mammals. SIMIAN IMMUNODEFICIENCY VIRUS (SIV) is the closest relative of HIV. HIV is believed to be the causative agent of AIDS in humans. HIV is not an oncogenic virus like HTLV-I (HUMAN T CELL LYMPHOTROPIC VIRUS TYPE I), but rather the first human LENTIVIRUS to be discovered. IVs form a subgroup of the RETROVIRUSES—whose life is shared with the genomic elements called retrotransposons. Each virion has a protein core surrounding the genome and an enclosed enzyme (REVERSE TRANSCRIPTASE), the whole encapsulated by a segment of host cell membrane in which viral glycoproteins are located. This GLYCOPROTEIN (GP120) recognizes and binds to the accessory molecule CD4, so HIV infects any CD4+ cell, including T-HELPER CELLS. Once bound, the membranes of HIV and the host cell fuse, releasing the infective virus core within the host cell.

HIV's genome comprises an RNA molecule, housing at least three genes (Gag, encoding core proteins; Pol-encoding viral enzymes; and env, encoding envelope GLYCOPROTEINS). On entry into the host cell, viral reverse transcriptase creates a DNA copy of the RNA genome, which is then converted into double-stranded DNA capable of inserting into the human genome and existing as a PROVIRUS for long periods. However, there is no evidence that HIV integrates into the germ line. Eventually, productive virus synthesis occurs and new HIV particles leave the host cell encapsulated in its modified membrane. T CELLS producing HIV no longer divide, and eventually die. Also, because of the gp120-CD4 binding, HIV-infected cells bind to uninfected CD4+ cells to produce syncytia, at which point the uninfected T cells lose their immune capacity and die. Immunodeficiency results.

There are numerous strains of HIV that cross-react minimally or not at all with neutralizing antibodies targeting other strains and it is not known how many strains would be needed in a vaccine providing broad anti-HIV protection.

human leukocyte antigens (HLA)   The major HISTOCOMPATIBILITY genetic region in humans. Specifically, they are the antigens on white blood cells that are representative of the antigens present on all the cells of the individual. Class I MHC are HLA-A, B, C, and the class II MHC are HLA-DP, DQ, DR.

human papilloma virus (HPV)   A member of the papova family of viruses, this virus has many different subtypes that cause venereal warts and warts on the skin.

Refractory and persistent lower genital tract disease in women may be a marker of HIV disease. There is also a strong association between HIV-positive status and abnormal PAP SMEARs. In addition, HIV infection may increase the risk of human papilloma virus infection; women with HIV infection appear to be at substantial risk for cervicovaginal squamous cell abnormalities. Exophytic genital and anal warts are caused by certain types (mostly types 6 and 11) of HPV. Other types found in the anogenital region (mostly types 16, 18, and 31) have been found to be strongly associated with genital dysplasia and carcinoma. For this reason, biopsy is needed in all instances of atypical, pigmented, or persistent, warts. All women with anogenital warts should have an annual Pap smear. Genital warts and disruption of the epithelian integrity as a result of HPV may facilitate inoculation and contribute to the spread of HIV infection.

HIV-infected women seem to be susceptible to unusually aggressive HPV disease. The clinical course of HPV and anogential neoplasia is accelerated in immunodeficient patients. HPV infection and neoplasia in HIV-infected women are often persistent and recurrent, extend to adjacent areas of skin and mucous membranes, resist conventional therapy, and frequently progress to invasive cancer. Whether women with both HIV and HPV infection will have an accelerated rate of progression to invasive genital tract cancer cannot be predicted. HIV-infected women have a significant increase in cervical abnormalities and a higher prevalence of cervical intraepithelia neoplasia (CIN) squamous cell abnormalities. Dysplasia and cancerous lesions occur at a younger age, are frequently multifocal, and occur at multiple sites.

Due to the increased risk of cervicovaginal squamous cell abnormalities in HIV-infected women, surveillance with frequent Pap smears, careful and frequent pelvic exams, and cervicovaginal smears is recommended. The same prompt gynecological follow-up care is urged for all women with genital tract abnormalities. Because colposcopy evaluation of abnormal Pap smears usually involves directed biopsy, and treatment may include cryotherapy, laser therapy, or local incision, patients may be unusually susceptible to HIV infection or transmission because of the exposed surfaces. Therefore women should avoid intercourse or use condoms during intercourse after BIOPSY and treatment. Patients with anogenital warts should be made aware that they are contagious to uninfected sex partners. The use of condoms is recommended to help reduce transmission.

No therapy has been shown to eradicate HPV. The effect of genital wart treatment on HPV transmission and the natural history of HPV is uncertain. Condylomata and other HPV-related/induced lesions are common and difficult to eradicate, often requiring prophylactic therapy because of their persistence and recurrence. Therefore, the goal of treatment is removal of exophytic warts and amelioration of signs and symptoms, not eradication of HPV. In most clinical situations, cryotherapy with liquid nitrogen or cryoprobe is the treatment of choice for external genital and perianal warts. For patients with cervical warts, dysplasia must be excluded before treatment is begun.

human rights   AIDS is the first worldwide epidemic to occur in the modern era of human rights. Public health practitioners face a dual standard in the design and implementation of public health programs in order to prevent HIV transmission. Programs must be effective in public health terms and must respect and respond to human rights norms. National and international attention to the human rights aspects of HIV/AIDS prevention and care have ebbed and flowed over the course of the epidemic, often in direct response to the rise of discrimination and a lack of protection of human rights and dignity.

The relationship between HIV/AIDS prevention and care and human rights can be considered in two ways. First, there are possible pressures and problems related to human rights that are created by the choice or manner of implementation of public health measures. This is the more traditional arena in which public health and human rights issues have been negotiated. Second, during the first decade of the epidemic it became clear that a discriminatory social environment was counterproductive for HIV information/education and prevention programs. Because societal discrimination in all its forms creates increased vulnerability to HIV infection, efforts to protect human rights and to promote human dignity are extremely important for protecting public health in the AIDS pandemic. As understanding of the pandemic evolved, the relationship between societal discrimination and the risk of becoming HIV infected became more evident. Being excluded from the mainstream of society, or being discriminated against on grounds of race/ethnicity, national origin, religion, gender, or sexual preference led to an increase in HIV infection. Thus, during the first decade of work against AIDS, the positive contribution that improving protection of human rights could have for public health became evident.

The ways in which many national authorities have responded to the AIDS epidemic have created a wide range of human rights problems by imposing coercive or restrictive AIDS control measures. Virtually every measure of disease control has human rights implications: public health surveillance may seek and record the personal identity of infected persons, and people identified as carriers may be subjected to isolation and quarantine. Even how a disease is classified may lead to compulsory medical examination or hospitalization, depending on local or national disease control legislation. Public health laws specify what individuals must do and what they must not do by defining offenses against public health (including the transmission of infectious diseases). Whether it is AIDS or any other epidemic, the bulk of public health measures identify affected groups and individuals and safeguard against further spread of disease.

To date, no worldwide review of AIDS-related human rights problems has yet been made to indicate what acts constitute human rights violations. Nonetheless, there are patterns of human rights problems. Problems have surfaced with regard to national laws, policies and practices, HIV testing, targets of mass testing, notification, counterproductiveness of compulsory testing, discrimination, and AIDS-related violence.

human T cell leukemia   The first human RETROVIRUS. In published reports of its finding in 1980, Robert C. Gallo of the National Cancer Institute labeled it as "human T-cell leukemia/lymphoma virus" (HTLV). The virus principally targets T4 helper cells.

human T cell leukemia virus   See HUMAN T CELL LYMPHOTROPIC VIRUS.

human T cell leukemia virus III (HTLV-III)   See HUMAN IMMUNODEFICIENCY VIRUS.

human T cell lymphotropic virus (HTLV)   A family of retroviruses that are lymphocytotropic and particularly partial to T lymphocytes of the inducer/helper subset. Also called human T cell leukemia virus. This is the family of viruses to which HIV belongs.

human T cell lymphotropic virus I (HTLV-I)   A virus associated with adult T cell leukemia. It is found more often in Japan than in the United States.

human T cell lymphotropic virus II (HTLV-II)   A virus associated with hairy cell leukemia.

human T cell lymphotropic virus III (HTLV-III)   A slow-acting virus that causes HUMAN IMMUNODEFICIENCY SYNDROME (AIDS). For a more complete discussion of the naming and renaming of the virus, see ACQUIRED IMMUNODEFICIENCY VIRUS.

human T cell lymphotropic virus variant III   Chronicles of the isolation and discovery of the AIDS virus invariably include discussion of the confusion over the virus's name. Luc Montagnier, head of the Viral Oncology Unit of the Institut Pasteur in Paris, and his colleagues first isolated the virus later shown to be the cause of AIDS in May 1983. They named the virus LYMPHADENOPATHY-ASSOCIATED VIRUS (LAV) because they had isolated it from one of the swollen lymph nodes of a patient with LYMPHADENOPATHY SYNDROME. A second isolate identified by the same group was called immunodeficiency-associated virus, or IDAV.

In May 1984, workers in Robert Gallo's laboratory at the National Cancer Institute (NCI) reported that they had identified a line of cancerous T CELLS that had two important characteristics: 1) susceptibility to infection with the new

virus, and 2) the ability to resist the killing effects that had destroyed other infected T-cell cultures. The NCI researchers reported that they had isolated the new virus, which they designated HTLV-III, from 48 patients. The meaning of HTLV was changed from "human T-cell leukemia/lymphoma virus" to "human T-cell lymphotropic virus" to reflect the fact that all known human retroviruses shared an attraction to T lymphocytes. Another virus isolate was described in August 1984 by Jay Levy and his coworkers from the University of California at San Francisco. They named their virus AIDS-ASSOCIATED RETROVIRUS OR ARV.

Scientific journals in the United States and Europe adopted one of two compound names, HTLV-III/LAV or LAV/HTLV-III. The compound names afforded recognition to the two principal groups involved in the discovery of the AIDS virus. But, the names were unwieldy and failed to address an issue even more important than who had discovered the virus: how the new virus related to other known human and animal retroviruses. Early studies showed that although the new human retrovirus resembled HTLV-I and HTLV-II in its preference for T-cells, it acted on these cells in a very different way: HTLV-I and HTLV-II caused uncontrolled proliferation of the T-cells, whereas the AIDS virus killed them. The two human T-cell leukemia viruses share many features with the animal ONCOVIRUSes, but the structure and function of the AIDS virus are more akin to those of the LENTIVIRUSes.

Several events in late 1985 and early 1986 increased the urgency of resolving the name issue. First, researchers identified a monkey virus that appeared very similar to the human AIDS virus. Researchers named this virus STLV-III (simian T-lymphotropic virus type III). Several months later, United States and French research teams announced that they had discovered two new human retroviruses in people in West Africa; the United States group called their virus HTLV-IV, while the French group called theirs LAV-2. Subsequent studies showed that the populations studied by the two groups were infected with variants of the same virus and that the new virus was more closely related to the monkey virus than to the original AIDS virus in humans.

Finally, in May 1984, a subcommittee of the International Committee on the Taxonomy of Viruses proposed a new system for naming all AIDS retroviruses in humans and subhuman primates. The human viruses were to be called HUMAN IMMUNODEFICIENCY VIRUSes (HIVs). The monkey virus was renamed SIMIAN IMMUNODEFICIENCY VIRUS, or SIV.

Today, HIV-1 is used to refer to all isolates of HTLV-III, LAV, and ARV. HIV-2 is the official designation for LAV-2 and all related isolates.

human t-lymphocyte virus type III (HTLV-III)   The organism believed to cause the body to lose its immunity. The name HTLV-III came about because the suspected virus is the third member of a family of viruses that are known to cause lymph disorders such as leukemia and other cancers of T lymphocyte cells. These are the same white blood cells that contribute to the body's immunity by producing antibodies against disease. Because the virus is thought to be of the RETROVIRUS family (different virus families have unique physical and growth characteristics), some doctors call the HTLV-III virus the AIDS-ASSOCIATED VIRUS. And yet another term for the virus is LYMPHADENOPATHY-ASSOCIATED VIRUS (LAV). Any one, or a combination, of these terms may be used for the AIDS antibody test. While there are some doctors who feel all three viruses may be identical, there are others who feel the African swine fever virus (a species from a different family of viruses called IRIDOVIRUSES) is the real cause of AIDS. Tests to reveal these antibodies are under investigation. There are also those who feel AIDS may come from several different viruses rather than just one as a means of explaining the variation of signs and symptoms in different patients.

human t-lymphotropic virus type III/lymphadenopathy-associated virus In medical literature, the virus responsible for AIDS is called by different names, including this one. The nomenclature of the virus continues to be debated. Human T cell lymphotropic virus-Type III and lymphadenopathy-associated virus are the same virus or closely similar. Members of the retrovirus family, they are considered a primary cause of AIDS. See HUMAN IMMUNODEFICIENCY VIRUS.

human t-lymphotropic virus type IV This variant was reported in mid-1986. It is believed to be closely related to SIMIAN T-CELL LYMPHOTROPIC VIRUS (STLV, SIV), which causes AIDS in certain species of monkeys in Africa but has not been linked with the disease in humans.

humoral Pertaining to molecules in solution in a body fluid, particularly antibody and complement.

humoral abnormality A deficiency or deviation from the norm in body fluids (the antibody limb of protection).

humoral immunity The human defense mechanism that is coordinated by the TH2 CELLS cells and involves the production of ANTIBODIES and associated molecules present in body fluids such as SERUM and LYMPH. It is now known that the production of antibodies enables viral and other microbial pathogens to flourish because it does not destroy the infected cells that are the source of infection, but only temporarily controls cell-free or cell-surface (extracellular, exogenous) pathogens. Flu, colds, and many common viral and other infections are controlled by humoral immunity. Humoral immunity is contrasted with CELLULAR IMMUNITY, which is critical in controlling and clearing the infectious agents that cause HIV and the opportunistic infections and neoplasms seen in AIDS, which are considered to be in the cells (intracellular, endogenous) and can only be controlled by cellular immunity initiated by DELAYED-TYPE HYPERSENSITIVITY.

hustler Slang for prostitute.

hydrocortisone The CORTICOSTEROID hormone produced by the adrenal cortex and produced synthetically. It is essential in maintaining life, sustaining blood pressure, and providing mineralocorticoid activity. Used in the treatment of various ailments, e.g., allergies, collagen abnormalities, inflammations, and certain neoplasms. Many people with advanced HIV disease have decreased adrenal gland function. Hydrocortisone is often used by them as replacement therapy to correct the low natural level. Hydrocortisone is available in a number of formulations. Skin creams containing 0.5 percent to 1.0 percent hydrocortisone are available over the counter. More concentrated preparations are available in various forms by prescription. For most uses, hydrocortisone is applied topically. The side effects of topically administered hydrocortisone are generally mild and may include burning, itching, irritation, dryness, thinning of the skin, slow growth of skin, or secondary infection. The side effects of oral or injectable forms of the drug include dizziness, increased appetite, increased sweating, restlessness, sleep disorders, or weight gain. Serious but rare, side effects include abdominal enlargement, acne, bone or muscle pain, blurred vision, black or tarry stools, convulsions, eye pain, fever, sore throat, headache, slow wound healing, mental depression, mood changes, muscle wasting, nightmares, unusual bleeding, and growth impairment in children.

hydrogen peroxide A colorless syrupy liquid with an irritating odor and acrid taste, which decomposes readily, liberating oxygen. Light is particularly effective in decomposing hydrogen peroxide, so it should be stored in tightly sealed glass jars in a dark place. Hydrogen peroxide is used as a commercial bleaching, oxidizing, and reducing agent. In a 3 percent aqueous solution, it is used as a mild antiseptic, germicide, and cleansing agent. A solution of hydrogen peroxide has value as a cleansing agent for suppurating wounds and inflamed mucous membranes.

hydroxyurea An approved oral chemotherapeutic agent for the treatment of some types of leukemia and other cancers in wide use for the last 30 years. More recently, it has been found to be effective in decreasing painful crises in patients with SICKLE-CELL ANEMIA. The most significant side effect of this drug is dose-related BONE MARROW SUPPRESSION.

Hydroxyurea's purported mechanism of action against HIV is radically different from the leading HIV drugs, which work by blocking or disrupting a viral enzyme, at present either REVERSE TRANSCRIPTASE or PROTEASE. Hydroxyurea acts as a free radical quencher and blocks the action of the cellular enzyme ribonucleotide reductase, which helps produce the nucleotides needed for DNA formation. With fewer natural DNA nucleotides present, HIV's reverse transcriptase enzyme may be more likely to incorporate NUCLEOSIDE ANALOG compounds such as AZT or ddI into the DNA it is creating from HIV's RNA gene template. These nucleoside analogs are defective versions of the natural building blocks and force the viral DNA chain under construction to terminate prematurely. Hydroxyurea has been found to be particularly synergistic with ddI in lab tests.

Hydroxyurea further inhibits cellular DNA synthesis during the S phase of the cell division, and it is believed to inhibit tumor cell growth through this mechanism. The use of hydroxyurea in the treatment of AIDS has recently received attention.

HIV reproduces more abundantly in rapidly dividing activated cells than in nondividing resting CD4 LYMPHOCYTES. But viral DNA synthesis in resting cells occurs as efficiently as in activated ones. Such synthesis creates HIV reservoirs that eventually serve as the source of new virus particle formation. It is therefore imperative that these resting cells be the target of antiretroviral therapy. Traditional anti-HIV therapy with nucleoside analogs like AZT has more of an effect on rapidly dividing cells because these drugs are preferentially absorbed by activated cells. Use of AZT and the other nucleoside analogs (ddI, ddC, etc.) also leads to the rapid emergence of drug resistant strains of HIV due to mutations in reverse transcriptase, the viral enzyme they block. One solution to these problems is to target drugs like hydroxyurea at the cellular enzymes that help HIV infect new cells and reproduce. Since hydroxyurea inhibits cellular enzymes and not HIV directly, it is not expected to lead to viral resistance, the major limiting factor of the conventional antiviral drugs. In addition, hydroxyurea can be taken for years because it is only mildly toxic and contributes to IMMUNOSUPPRESSION only at excessive doses and is reversible. (The myelosuppressive effects may be especially acute in patients with AIDS who have low bone marrow reserve. For this reason it is often recommended that people at any stage of infection who are taking the drug should have their white blood cell and platelet counts closely monitored by their doctors.) It may be temporarily interrupted without loss of its antiviral effects. Finally, hydroxyurea readily penetrates the CENTRAL NERVOUS SYSTEM and may have a role in treating neurological complications of AIDS. Such symptoms may be related to the HIV infection of brain MACROPHAGES.

Alternative experimental medications utilizing the same strategy as hydroxyurea are currently in line for more extensive testing.

hygiene   The practice of keeping the body clean and in conditions that promote health.

hymen   A membrane that partially covers the opening of the vagina. It is broken or greatly stretched after first coitus.

hypercapnia   The condition of having an excess amount of carbon dioxide in the blood.

hypergammaglobulinemia   Excessive amount of gamma globulin in the blood.

hyperglycemia   An increased amount of sugar in the blood resulting in a condition that may lower resistance to infection and may precede diabetic coma.

hypericin   A chemical extract from the St. John's wort plant, traditionally known to farmers as goatweed. It has a long history of use in Europe as an antidepressant medication. In August 1991 a form of hypericin was successfully synthesized and FDA-approved for testing in humans as an AIDS therapy. In test tube studies, hypericin hardens the outer surface of HIV, inhibiting the virus from infecting cells. Hypericin also inhibits the replication of cells already infected with HIV and is able to enter both lymphocytes and macrophages. These functions, if indeed they occur in the human body, could slow the progression of HIV disease. Researchers have also shown that correct concentrations of hypericin can inactivate lipid viruses, HERPES, and CYTOMEGALOVIRUS.

Hypericin should only be used as an alternative treatment for a specific condition and not on a regular basis for prophylaxis or as an HIV retroviral treatment. Not only does it result in a photosensitive condition that suppresses the cellular immune response and interferes with delayed-type sensitivity, but it is believed to activate the antibody system. The increased activation of antibodies has been known to suppress cellular immunity and, possibly, result in B-cell lymphomas.

hyperimmunoglobulinemia   Abnormally high levels of ANTIBODIES. One of the first abnormalities observed in HIV-POSITIVE people is hyperimmunoglobulinemia. Why B CELLS of HIV-positive people make abnormal amounts of antibodies is unknown. The cause may be an indirect signal from HIV, CYTOKINES such as IL–6, or a cofactor such as EPSTEIN-BARR VIRUS, which is known to infect B cells and spark antibody production. Whatever the cause, many different B cells (which recognize many different ANTIGENS) produce antibodies, as well as TNF and IL–6.

Several lines of evidence suggest that abnormal antibody levels may contribute to disease in AIDS. Some of the antibodies may be targeted against the body's own tissues, resulting in autoimmune reactions that are commonly found in HIV-positive people. High levels of antibodies that link to antigens and circulate in the blood, called CIRCULATING IMMUNE COMPLEXES (CICs), have also been found in people with AIDS-related conditions, and these levels correlate with decreasing CD4 counts. CICs can collect in certain tissues, causing inflammation that may lead to fevers and joint pain. CICs may also cause tissue damage and may be the source of AIDS-related THROMBOCYTOPENIA (low platelets), NEUROPATHY, or kidney damage.

Several drugs that inhibit activated LYMPHOCYTEs have been proposed for or have entered trials for use against HIV infection or AIDS. Given that the hyperactivation of the immune system is prevalent primarily early in HIV disease and that immune suppressive agents may exacerbate opportunistic infections when people become symptomatic, the effects of such treatment may depend upon the stage of disease.

hyperkalemia   Excessive amount of potassium in the blood, generally caused by defective renal excretion.

hyperkaliemia   See HYPERKALEMIA.

hyperplasia   Excessive proliferation of normal cells in a tissue or organ.

hyperreactivity   A state of increased reactivity to a provoking stimulus, for instance bronchial hyperreactivity in asthma. Specifically, a greater-than-normal magnitude of response to a given concentration of stimulus.

hypersensitivity   In immunology, synonymous with allergy.

hypertension   The condition of having higher blood pressure than normal or safe.

hyperthermia   Unusually high body temperature. Also an experimental procedure that involves temporarily raising a patient's body temperature to an abnormal height to treat HIV disease, on the theory that this temperature kills free HIV and HIV-containing cells. Public attention first focused on this therapy in 1990. At that time, Kenneth Alonso, M.D., and William Logan, M.D., of Atlanta, announced that they had at least temporarily cured a patient of AIDS-related KAPOSI'S SARCOMA (KS) while raising his CD4 count from 50 to 330, by elevating his body temperature to 42 degrees C (108 degrees F) for one hour.

Since then, "whole body hyperthermia" has had peaks of public attention from time to time, fed by Italian reports of successful treatment of people with HIV. Dr. Alonso and a team from Rome's European Hospital published the results of single hyperthermia treatments in 31 patients with disseminated KS, but these treatments by no means amounted to a carefully controlled study with precisely defined eligibility criteria.

One of the Italian group's patients, Chuck DeMarco, was so impressed by the results of his 1991 hyperthermia treatment—he recounted not only the disappearance of his KS lesions but eventual remission of his HIV infection as well—that he formed an organization known as HEAT INFO to promote further study of the therapy. Mr. DeMarco's major accomplishment was pressuring the FDA to allow a U.S. study of hyperthermia. This test was inconclusive, although it did indicate that the hyperthermia technique was safe.

In December 1994, the FDA allowed a larger trial. The data from this trial were much more rigorously collected than the essentially anecdotal information provided by Dr. Alonso and the Italian group. The trial took place with people who were on stable anti-HIV drug therapy, with an average CD4 count of 120. The results did not bear out previous claims.

If hyperthermia works, it would back up drug therapy and might delay the appearance of drug-resistant HIV strains. Many feel that, if it works at all, hyperthermia would have to be repeated at least weekly to have any lasting impact on the disease process, given the rapid dynamics of HIV replication. Lasting suppression of HIV will need constant treatment with extremely potent agents. Frequent application is hardly practical, especially considering that patients are heavily sedated during treatment to reduce the stress such heating poses for the heart. As of this writing, hyperthermia sessions might cost around $6,000 each. Many researchers and scientists feel that the potential effect from hyperthermia pales by comparison with the results of combinations of PROTEASE INHIBITORS and NUCLEOSIDE ANALOGS, which provide persistent 99 percent drops in many people's viral loads. Researchers and scientists advise individuals considering the pursuit of hyperthermia in the United States or abroad to investigate treatment with 3TC and protease inhibitors before embarking on what is still a relatively new treatment.

hypertrophy   The enlargement or growth of an organ or structure, not involving tumor formation, due to an increase in the size of its constituent cells.

hypnotherapy   A range of techniques that ostensibly allow practitioners to bypass the conscious mind and access the subconscious, where suppressed memories and repressed emotions may remain recorded. Hypnosis may facilitate behavioral, emotional, or attitudinal changes. Often used to help people lose weight or stop smoking, it is also used in the treatment of phobias, stress, and as an adjunct in the treatment of illness.

hypodermic   Under or inserted under the skin, as a hypodermic injection. It may be given subcutaneously (under the skin), intracutaneously (into the skin), intramuscularly (into a muscle), intraspinally (into the spinal canal), or intravascularly (into a vein or artery). It is given to secure prompt action of a drug when the drug cannot be taken by mouth, when it may not be readily absorbed in the stomach or intestines, when it might be changed by action of the gastric secretions, or to act as a local anesthetic.

hypogammaglobulinemia (agammaglobulinemia)   Decreased gammaglobulins in the blood, resulting in a state of immunodeficiency. Acquired hypogammaglobulinemia has its onset in early childhood. Congenital hypogammaglobulinemia is an inherited form of hypogammaglobulinemia in which all immunoglobulins are decreased; this usually manifests as immunodeficiency at six months of age, by which time the maternal immunoglobulins have disappeared.

hypoglycemia   Deficiency of sugar in the blood. This condition may result in shakiness, cold sweat, fatigue, hypothermia, headache, and malaise, accompanied by confusion, irritability, and weakness. Hypoglycemia may ultimately result in seizures, coma, and possibly death.

hypogonadism   Defective internal secretion of the gonads, resulting in slowed growth and sexual development or, in adults, impairment of normal sexual function.

hypokalemia   Extreme potassium depletion in the circulating blood, commonly resulting in episodes of muscular weakness or paralysis, tetany, postural hypotension, renal disease, and gastrointestinal dysfunction. Loss of potassium may occur through renal secretion or through expulsion via the gastrointestinal tract (diarrhea or vomiting).

hypopharynx   The lowermost portion of the pharynx, which leads to the larynx and esophagus.

hypotension   Decrease of systolic and diastolic blood pressure below normal. Hypotension occurs in shock, hemorrhages, infections, fevers, cancer, anemia, neurasthenia, Addison's disease, debilitating or wasting disease, and approaching death.

hypothermia   The condition of having a body temperature below normal. Also a technique of lowering body temperature, usually to between 78 and 90 degrees F, to reduce oxygen need during surgery and in hypoxia, to reduce blood pressure, and to alleviate hyperpyrexia.

hypovolemia   Diminished blood volume.

hypoxemia   Insufficient oxygenation of the blood.

hypoxia   Deficiency of oxygen in the blood; also decreased concentration of oxygen in inspired air.

I

IAS guidelines Antiretroviral treatment guidelines released at the XI International AIDS Conference in Vancouver, Canada, on July 6, 1996. The guidelines have significant shortcomings because they do not take into account either the rapid evolution in anti-HIV therapy or real-world limitations and complications practitioners will encounter in following these outdated recommendations. Recommendations included when to initiate therapy, what types of drugs to use for initial therapy, when to change therapy, and when to stop antiretroviral therapy.

iatrogenic Resulting from the activities of a physician.

ibuprofen A nonsteroidal anti-inflammatory agent available with or without a prescription. Trade names Advil, Motrin, and Nuprin.

ichthyosis A noninflammatory condition in which the skin is dry and scaly. Depending on the stage and degree of the condition, it has been described as alligator skin, crocodile skin, or fish skin. Ichthyosis is a hereditary disorder.

ICOD The proximate cause of death; one of two separate designations for the cause of death distinguished by autopsy pathologists.

icterus See JAUNDICE.

ICU See INTENSIVE CARE UNIT.

idiopathic inflammatory pulmonary disease A pathological condition of unknown origin causing inflammation of the lungs. It is not a result of any other disease.

idiopathic thrombocytopenia purpura (ITP) An autoimmune disorder characterized by a low platelet count that can result in symptoms from easy bruising to bleeding. ITP is unassociated with any definable systemic disease in which the blood platelet count is decreased. ITP is common in HIV-infected people and often manifests as bluish and purplish spots.

idiotype The molecular arrangement of amino acids unique to the antigen-binding site of a particular antibody.

IFN See INTERFERON.

Ig A, D, E, G, M See IMMUNOGLOBULIN.

IL See INTERLEUKIN.

IL-1, -2, -3, -4, -5, -6, -12 and -16 See INTERLEUKIN.

imagery One of a number of treatment techniques that are alternatives and/or adjuncts to traditional American medical therapeutics. Imagery is one of many mental disciplines which serves to direct our thoughts in order to utilize mental energies to augment the healing process and to combat the debilitating effects of stress. Others include biofeedback, color and sound, meditation, and yoga. The technique is easy and accessible. With eyes closed, one relaxes by envisioning a soothing image. For example, by visualizing walking down a shaded stairway, one might become more and more relaxed as he/she descends into comforting darkness. Once relaxed, an image is brought to mind that may represent a desired change. Some people simply see themselves as being completely healthy. Others imagine the healing white blood cells as white knights charging forth, conquering the invading infections and visualizing the "bad guys" in full retreat. For those who may have trouble focusing clearly on an image, it is suggested to draw the desired image on paper to give it more substance and reality. In addition to visual imagery there are other types of mental imagery. Mental imagery may also be auditory (mental image of sounds that can be recalled); odorous (mental concept of odor sensations previously experienced); tactile (mental image of the feeling of an object); or oral (mental concept of taste sensations previously experienced).

Tapes, books, and even classes on visualization and imagery are available through local metaphysical bookstores.

See VISUALIZATION.

immediate hypersensitivity An antibody-mediated immunological sensitivity that manifests itself in tissue reactions within minutes after an ANTIGEN combines with its appropriate ANTIBODY.

immigration   The act of coming to a country of which one is not a native, usually for permanent residence.

With the spread of AIDS during the past decade, countries all over the world have set up barriers against those with AIDS to "protect" their citizens from the spread of the disease, despite the constant admonitions of the World Health Organization (WHO). Some have imposed restrictions on all aliens who have tested positive for HIV, while other nations have imposed testing requirements as conditions of entry, denying entry to those who test positive for the virus. While the WHO stresses the importance of cooperation in fighting the pandemic, these countries, including the United States, continue to exclude immigrants and aliens who are infected with HIV. Many countries, however, have heeded the WHO. Some have altered their restrictive travel and immigration laws to allow the entry of HIV-positive aliens. Several countries require HIV testing, not as a condition for exclusion, but to alert domestic health care facilities or other caregivers within the country. Still others explicitly admit HIV-positive aliens within their borders, following WHO's spirit of global solidarity.

Despite internal opposition from the American public and external opposition from the WHO, the United States has continued to maintain restrictive policies toward HIV-positive aliens. These restrictions, although ratified by Congress, have been opposed by President Clinton and modified, in emergency situations, by the U.S. courts.

Before the Immigration Act of 1990, immigrants could be excluded on 33 grounds, including affliction "with a dangerous contagious disease." In June 1987 the Public Health Service (PHS) added Acquired Immune Deficiency Syndrome to the list of such diseases. Soon thereafter, despite considerable opposition from AIDS and immigration advocates, doctors, and public interest organizations, the PHS replaced AIDS on the list with Human Immunodeficiency Virus (HIV) infection, dramatically expanding the definition of persons considered to be afflicted with a contagious disease. On July 8, 1987, the Immigration and Naturalization Service (INS) and the State Department began testing aliens seeking admission to the United States for AIDS.

The Immigration Act of 1990 completely revised the grounds of exclusion. It also permitted, for the first time, a waiver of exclusions on health-related grounds for permanent resident and immigration visa applicants. Early in 1993, shortly after President Bill Clinton indicated that he was prepared to remove HIV from the exclusion list, the PHS drafted new regulations to that effect. In reaction, Congress passed the National Institutes of Health Revitalization Act of 1993, which specifically codified HIV-infection as a ground of exclusion. The United States, therefore, now has a statutory ban on the admission of aliens with HIV.

Aliens of 15 years of age or older are required to undergo serologic testing for HIV if they are applying for immigrant visas, nonimmigrant visas such as student or refugee, or to adjust their status. No testing is required if the alien is under age 15 unless there is "reason to suspect infection." Testing is done by a physician, called a "medical examiner," designated by the director of the CENTERS FOR DISEASE CONTROL AND PREVENTION. Once the requisite testing has been completed, the medical examiner must submit a document to INS certifying the presence or absence of HIV infection or any other "communicable disease of public health significance."

If an alien tests positive for HIV, he can request a reexamination from the director of the Centers for Disease Control. The board that reexamines the alien must be composed of "three medical officers, at least one of whom is experienced in the diagnosis and treatment of HIV infections." The majority decision of the board comprises the final report.

A formal reexamination includes a review of all records and laboratory studies. It may also include an independent physical examination performed by the board if the board so requires. The alien has the right to offer information and witnesses and may cross-examine any witnesses called by the examining board. He or she is also free to have an attorney or be assisted by the board in the presentation of his/her case. The board must report its findings to the INS and give prompt notice to the alien. The INS then makes the final decision as to admissibility based on the board's findings. The alien may request reconsideration only once in connection with the current application.

It remains to be seen how the United States will apply the current statutes. The United States has been divided on the issue of whether to allow or refuse entry to HIV-positive aliens.

immigration restrictions   See IMMIGRATION.

immune   See IMMUNITY.

immune activation   Activation of the immune system by stimuli such as parasites and other organisms as well as persistent infections. The normal activation of the immune system in response to microbes results in a transient increase in HIV replication, a phenomenon that researchers feel is important to the pathogenesis of HIV disease. It is thought that chronic immune activation (the cumulative effect of multiple episodes of immune activation and bursts of virus production) probably contributes to the progression of HIV disease. Therapies directed at the microbes that contribute to a state of chronic and persistent immune activation may have a role in the treatment of HIV-infected people, as may drugs that could be used at certain times to dampen immune activation.

immune-based therapies   Immune-based therapies are treatments intended to have their effect by enhancing the general activity of the immune system or by specifically modulating the activity of some of its components. They may be used to help restore a person's general immune responsiveness, suppress specific viral infections, or counteract the bone-marrow toxicity of some of the drugs used for HIV-related conditions. Drugs used in such therapies include preparations of antibodies and drugs that stimulate production of red and white blood cells, cytokines, and other immune modulators. Vaccines are also immune-therapy drugs. Specific drugs used in immune-based therapies include cyclosporine, cytomegalovirus immune globulin, erythropoietin, G-CSF, GM-CSF, immune globulin, and interleukin-2. Experimental immune therapies used to treat HIV-related conditions include NAC, procysteine, pentoxifylline, thalidomide, OPC-8212, TNF MoAb, sTNFr, Tenidap, THF gamma 2, thymopentin, thymosin alpha, thymodulin, thymostimulin, DEHSPM, DNCB, F105, HIVIG, IL-4, IL-12, gamma interferon, and MSL-109.

immune boosters   Medicines that strengthen the body's natural defensive response to infections or foreign particles. Some of these are ISOPRINOSINE, IMUTHIOL, Naltrexone, and ANTABUSE.

immune boosting   A drug treatment that repairs or reconstitutes an impaired immune system. See IMMUNE BOOSTERS.

immune complex   An aggregate of antibody and antigen that may induce a hypersensitivity response, often by stimulating the complement cascade. When antibodies bind to antigen nine, interacting serum proteins (beta globulins, C1–C9) are activated in a coordinated way. Complement activation causes an amplifying cascade of reactions as each complement protein is activated sequentially. Immune complexes circulate in the blood and may eventually attach to the walls of blood vessels, producing a local inflammatory response. Immune complexes form in type III hypersensitivity reactions and are involved in the development of glomerulonephritis, serum sickness, arthritis, and vasculitis.

immune deficiency   A breakdown or inability of certain parts of the immune system to function, thus making a person susceptible to certain diseases that they would not have contracted with a healthy immune system. Immune deficiencies may be temporary or permanent. In AIDS, the immune deficit is caused by infection with HIV.

immune globulin   A preparation used INTRAVENOUSLY in patients with IMMUNODEFICIENCY syndromes and in immunosuppressed recipients of BONE MARROW transplants.

immune modulators   Agents that restore certain immune responses that are diminished or lost in HIV infection. See INTERLEUKIN.

immune reconstitution   It is now obvious to researchers, doctors, and people with AIDS that antiretroviral therapies like AZT, ddI, and ddC may do little to repair immunity. Therapies that may restore immunity in people with damaged immune systems hold much interest. However, reconstitution of the immune system depends on a substantial understanding of the immune system and of immunology, the branch of medicine that studies the immune system, an infant science. While some progress has been made, little is actually known about the basic elements that regulate and control the normal functioning of the human immune system. See PROTEASE INHIBITORS; THYMUS.

immune response   The reaction of the body to foreign ANTIGENs so that they are neutralized or eliminated, preventing damage. It requires that the body recognize the antigen as "nonself" or foreign. There are four major types of immune response: cell-mediated immune response, humoral immune response, nonspecific immune response, and specific immune response.

Cell-mediated immune response involves the production of LYMPHOCYTEs by the thymus (T CELLS) in response to exposure to an antigen. This reaction is important in delayed hypersensitivity, rejection of tissue transplants, response to malignant growths, and in some infections.

Humoral immunity response involves production of plasma lymphocytes (B CELLS) in response to antigen exposure with subsequent antibody formulation. This response can produce immunity or hypersensitivity.

Nonspecific immune response is the response of the body's tissues and cells to injury from any source, e.g., trauma, organisms, chemicals, ischemia. The initial response of the immune system to any threat, it involves vascular, chemical, and white blood cell activities.

Specific immune response is required when inflammation is inadequate to cope with injury or invasion of an organism. It is directed and controlled by T and B lymphocytes.

"Cellular immunity" is used to refer to the T lymphocyte response. "Humoral immunity" is the term previously used to refer to the T lymphocyte response.

immune response genes   Genes that control the ability of LYMPHOCYTEs to respond to specific ANTIGENs.

immune suppression   See IMMUNOSUPPRESSION.

immune suppressive therapies   See IMMUNOSUPPRESSION.

immune surveillance   A theory that holds that the immune system destroys tumor cells, which are constantly arising during the life of an individual.

immune system   In the body, an elaborate internal defense network that includes different types of blood cells. It recognizes foreign agents or substances, neutralizes them, and recalls the response later when confronted with the same challenge. If weakened, the immune system has difficulty resisting diseases. If destroyed, it provides the body no defense against disease.

The immune system is composed of tissues, organs, and physiological processes. LYMPHOCYTEs and MACROPHAGEs are the primary cellular components. ANTIBODIEs and LYMPHOKINEs are the primary molecular components. GRANULOCYTEs and the complement system are involved in immune responses but are not necessarily considered part of the immune system.

The principal components of the immune system are cells called B LYMPHOCYTEs, NEUTROPHILs, and T LYMPHOCYTEs. B lymphocytes make antibodies, the proteins that attack bacteria and viruses. Neutrophils envelope and kill bacteria. T lymphocytes provide communication between the parts of the immune system. T4 lymphocytes, or "helper T cells," function to identify an intruder and authorize an attack on it. Although these three components are somewhat independent, each takes a primary responsibility for defense against certain types of microbes. For this reason, people deficient in different components are prone to infections with quite different microbes.

There are two aspects of the immune system's response to disease: innate and acquired. The innate part of the response is mobilized very quickly in response to infection and does not depend on recognizing specific proteins or antigens foreign to an individual's normal tissue. It includes complement, macrophages, dendritic cells, and granulocytes. The acquired, or learned, immune response arises when dendritic cells and macrophages present pieces of antigen to lymphocytes, which are genetically programmed to recognize very specific amino acid sequences. The ultimate result is the creation of cloned populations of antibody-producing B cells and CYTOTOXIC T-lymphocytes primed to respond to a unique population.

HIV has no life of its own—it is simply a protein capsule containing two short strands of genetic material (RNA) and a few enzymes. It uses human cells to perpetuate itself. After infecting someone, HIV may spend 10 years or more quietly ensconced within various tissues and organs. When activated, it turns certain immune cells into virus factories, which produce a flurry of new virus capsules and die. Other cells become infected in the process, and the immune system falls like a house of cards. The cell type that is primarily affected in people with HIV infection is a type of T lymphocyte called a CD4 cell. Every T4 cell has appendages called CD4 receptors, through which it exchanges information with other immune cells. It is through these CD4 receptors that HIV attacks. The outer shell of the HIV capsule (known as the envelope) is equipped with an appendage called GP120. This distinctive protein molecule fits the CD4 receptor as a plug fits a socket. When the two molecules connect, the contents of the viral capsule—the RNA and the enzymes—flow freely into the cell's interior.

Once inside, HIV becomes a permanent feature of the cell. First, an enzyme called REVERSE TRANSCRIPTASE uses information encoded in the RNA to manufacture a double strand of DNA. This DNA, known as the PROVIRUS, then integrates itself into the host cell's chromosomes. It represents just a tiny segment of the cell's genetic code. Once activated, however, it is the only segment that counts. When the provirus starts directing enzymes in the host cell to produce new strands of viral RNA, the rogue pieces of RNA serve as a blueprint from which other enzymes start producing raw material for new virus capsules. An enzyme called protease chops these raw materials into shorter pieces. Those pieces then clip together to form new HIV particles, which burst from the surface of the host cell and float off to infect others. The host cell is killed in the process.

The most common infections encountered in people with few CD4 cells are caused by PNEUMOCYSTIS CARINII, CYTOMEGALOVIRUS, MYCOBACTERIUM AVIUM-INTRACELLU-LARE, HERPES SIMPLEX VIRUS, HERPES ZOSTER, CANDIDA ALBICANS, TOXOPLASMA GONDII, CRYPTOSPORIDIUM, CRYP-TOCOCCUS, SALMONELLA, and the bacterium that causes TUBERCULOSIS. People with immune systems weakened by HIV are not only subject to high rates of infection with these organisms, but infections tend to be severe, prolonged, and recurrent. At the same time, many other microbes that commonly cause infections in everyone do not appear to be unusually common or severe in people

with HIV, presumably because the other components of the immune defenses remain relatively strong.

immune system abnormality   A deviation in the normal functioning of the immune system.

immune thrombocytopenia purpura (ITP)   A form of purpura occurring as a consequence of a disturbance in the immune system in which the platelet count is decreased. Common in people with HIV, ITP often resolves as immune deficiency worsens. HIV-related ITP usually does not have serious consequences. Its cause has not been definitively determined. Treatment with AZT frequently alleviates the condition.

immune tolerance   Acquired inability to react to particular self- or non-self-antigens. Both B cells and T cells display tolerance, generally to their specific antigen classes. The concentration of antigen required to induce tolerance in neonatal B cells is 100-fold less than for adult B cells.

immunity   The state of being resistant to or protected from a disease, especially an infectious disease. Immunity is usually induced by exposure to the antigenic marker on an organism that invades the body, or by administration of a vaccine that has the capability of stimulating production of specific antibodies (immunization). Immunity is also the response of the body and its tissues to a variety of antigens, including pollens, red cells, transplanted tissues, or the individual's own cells.

Acquired immunity results from the development of active or passive immunity. It is contrasted with natural or innate immunity, a more or less permanent immunity to disease with which an individual is born, the result of natural factors. Natural immunity may be due to the natural presence of immune bodies, but other factors such as diet, metabolism, temperature, or adaptive features of infectious organisms may be involved. Congenital immunity is present at birth, and may be natural or acquired, the latter resulting from antibodies received from the blood of the mother.

Active immunity results from the development within the body of antibodies or sensitized T lymphocytes that neutralize or destroy the infectious agent. This may result from the immune response to an invading organism or from inoculation with a vaccine containing antibodies. Passive immunity, on the other hand, is immunity acquired by the introduction of preformed antibodies into an unprotected individual. This can occur through injection or in utero from antibodies that pass from the mother to the fetus through the placenta or acquired by the newborn by ingesting its mother's milk.

Local immunity is limited to a given area or tissue of the body. Two other types of immunity are cell-mediated, resulting from activation of sensitized T lymphocytes, and humeral immunity, mediated by antibodies in body fluids such as PLASMA and LYMPH.

immunization   The process of creating immunity to a specific disease in an individual, usually by the administration of a vaccine consisting of antigenic components of an infectious agent (a weakened form of a disease that cannot cause sickness). These components, in turn, stimulate a protective response and induce the body to form antibodies against the disease. The immune response may be induced naturally or artificially.

The immunizations necessary for travelers with HIV vary according to the destination. Travel to developing nations generally requires immunizations. Some immunizations are considered safe for HIV-infected persons (vaccines for measles, cholera, rabies, influenza, pneumococcus, and hepatitis B, for example), others are generally not recommended for HIV-infected individuals (for instance the yellow fever vaccine), and still others are not appropriate for patients with HIV (the live oral polio and typhoid vaccines). See also VACCINATION.

immunoassay A test to measure the protein and protein-bound molecules that are concerned with the reaction of an ANTIGEN with its specific ANTIBODY.

immunocompetent Capable of developing a normal protective response when confronted with invading microbes or cancer.

immunocompromise The condition that exists when the body's immune system defenses are lowered and the ability to resist infections and tumors weakens.

immunodeficient See IMMUNODEFICIENCY.

immunodeficiency A breakdown or inability of certain parts of the immune system to function, rendering the body susceptible to certain diseases that it would ordinarily be able to resist. Immunodeficiency is classified as an antibody, cellular, combined deficiency, or phagocytic dysfunction disorder.

immunoenhancer Anything that increases the body's ability to fight off infection and disease.

immunofluorescence antibody (IFA) A serologic assay using antibody tagged by a fluorescent molecule. There is an HIV-specific IFA assay available to confirm the results of a positive HIV ELISA test.

immunogen A substance that, when introduced into an animal, stimulates the immune response. The term *immunogen* may also denote a substance that is capable of stimulating an immune response, in contrast to a substance that can only combine with antibody, that is, an ANTIGEN.

immunogenetics The study of genetics by use of immune responses. Investigations of IMMUNOGLOBULINs and HISTOCOMPATIBILITY ANTIGENs.

immunogenicity The quality of producing an effective or measurable immune response.

immunoglobulin (Ig) An ANTIBODY-rich preparation administered to reduce the likelihood of developing infec-

tion, following exposure to certain infectious agents. Specifically, IMMUNOGLOBULIN is a protein produced by plasma cells derived from B-LYMPHOCYTES and found in the blood and other body tissues. All antibodies are immunoglobulins, but researchers have not yet determined if all immunoglobulins have antibody functions. There are five classes: IgA, IgD, IgE, IgG, IgM. Increased levels of two types of immunoglobulins, IgA and IgG, are usually seen in patients with HIV infection and are related to the HIV-induced activation of B-lymphocytes. Immunoglobulin G is found in the serum and does not cross the placenta.

Immunoglobulin A (IgA): a class of antibodies, present in saliva, tears, and other secretions, that render viruses ineffective and prevent bacteria from attaching to mucous membranes.

Immunoglobulin D (IgD): antibodies, receptors on most cell surfaces, that remove foreign substances from the bloodstream and hold them for further destruction.

Immunoglobulin E (IgE): antibodies, abundant in tissue spaces, that activate histamines and leukotrienes as an allergic reaction to foreign particles.

Immunoglobulin G (IgG): class of antibodies, produced by memory cells and blood plasma cells, that circulate in the bloodstream and impart long-term immunity against previously encountered viruses, bacteria, etc.

Immunoglobulin M (IgM): antibodies that exist for a short time as aggregates of other antibody molecules. They seek out and attach themselves to viruses in the circulatory system and along the internal walls.

immunoglobulin class A subdivision of immunoglobulin molecules based on unique antigenic determinants in the Fc region of the H chains. In humans there are 5 classes of immunoglobulins designated IgA, IgD, IgE, IgG, and IgM.

immunoglobulin class switch The process in which a B-cell precursor expressing IgM and IgG receptors differentiates into a B-cell producing IgA, IgE, or IgG antibodies without change in specificity for the antigenic determinant.

immunoglobulin subclass A subdivision of the classes of immunoglobulins based on structural and antigenic differences in the H chains. For example, for human IgG (a class of monomeric immunoglobulin proteins), there are 4 subclasses IgGl-4, accounting for at least 70 percent of human immunoglobulin titre.

immunoglobulin superfamily A large GLYCOPROTEIN superfamily including antibodies and their membrane-bound isotypes; T cell receptors, lymphocyte Fc receptors, the CD2, CD4 and CD8 accessory molecules, and MHC molecules.

immunoglobulin supergene family A structurally related group of genes that encode immunoglobulins, T cell receptors, B2-microglobulin, and others.

immunologic markers Components of the immune system, including different types of cells, such as T4 and T8 cells, as well as proteins secreted by the immune system cells, like neopterin and beta-2 microglobulin. Immunologic markers are used as laboratory measurements of biological activity within the body that indirectly indicate the effect of treatment on disease state. See also SURROGATE MARKER.

immunological markers   See IMMUNOLOGIC MARKERS.

immunology   The branch of medical science dealing with the study of immunity.

immunomodulation   The effect of various chemical mediators, hormones, and drugs on the IMMUNE SYSTEM. Effects might include the restoration or the enhancement of the immune system.

immunomodulator   A substance capable of modifying one or more functions of the IMMUNE SYSTEM. Also called an immunostimulator or an immunoregulator. So far immunomodulators have not been found to be very effective in modifying the course of AIDS.

immunopathogenesis   A process in which the course of a disease is affected or altered by an immune response or by the products of an immune response.

immunopathology   The study of tissue alterations that result from immune or allergic reactions.

immunoregulator   See IMMUNOMODULATOR.

immunostimulant   See IMMUNOMODULATOR.

immunosuppression   The suppression of, or interference with, the body's IMMUNE SYSTEM and its ability to fight infection or disease, by means of drugs or or other medical techniques, or through infection or disease. Powerful immunosuppressive drugs can inhibit the production of white blood cells or interfere with their actions in the immune system. For example, STEROIDS suppress LYMPHOCYTE function, and the drug CYCLOSPORINE holds down the production of INTERLEUKIN-2, which is needed for T CELL growth. Immunosuppression may be used during organ or BONE MARROW transplantation to prevent the body's own immune system from rejecting the foreign organ or bone marrow. Until their immune systems are functioning normally, immunosuppressed persons are at a much higher risk of infections and developing LYMPHOMAS.

Immunosuppression results from HIV infection as well as from some antiviral or anticancer treatments, of which it is a side effect. In its earlier stages, though, HIV infection is associated with chronic stimulation of the immune system. Hyperactive immune responses in people with HIV include overproduction by B CELLS of ANTIBODIES (also called IMMUNOGLOBULINS or Igs); abnormal levels of CYTOKINES, such as TUMOR NECROSIS FACTOR (TNF) alpha and interferon alpha; and increased activation of T cells. Markers of this increased immune activity, such as elevated Igs, can predict CD4 cell count declines and progression of disease. Some scientists believe these overactive immune responses contribute to HIV reproduction, illness, wasting, or the loss of normal immune function. If so, some hypothesize, suppressing such responses early on might slow progression.

immunosuppressive   A drug that significantly impairs (suppresses) the functions of the body's immune system. In some cases, IMMUNOSUPPRESSION is an intended drug effect. In other cases, it is an unwanted side effect, as in the long term use of cortisone-like drugs suppressing the immune system sufficiently to permit reactivation of a dormant tuberculosis. Immunosuppressant drugs are being used to treat several chronic disorders that are thought to be autoimmune diseases.

immunosuppressive drugs   Drugs which induce IMMUNOSUPPRESSION.

immunotherapy   Treatment aimed at reconstituting an impaired immune system. Examples of experimental immunotherapies for AIDS include passive hyperimmune therapy (PHT), IL-2, and therapeutic vaccines. See also BIOLOGICAL THERAPY.

impairment   Damage or disability; in Social Security Administration parlance, a particular disease or condition that may render the afflicted patient too disabled to perform substantial gainful activity (SGA) and therefore possibly eligible for assistance. Patients can and do have multiple impairments.

impetigo   A contagious, inflammatory skin disease caused by direct inoculation of group A streptococci or staphylococcus aureus into superficial cutaneous abrasions or compromised skin. It is marked by isolated pustules that rupture to discharge an amber-colored fluid (composed of serum and pus) that dries to form a thick yellowish crust. The pustules may spread peripherally, but they are usually found around the nose and the mouth.

impotence   Weakness; the inability of the male to achieve or maintain an erection.

imreg   A natural LEUKOCYTE-derived, polypeptide IMMUNOMODULATOR that has been shown to enhance production of certain lymphokines in the laboratory.

Imreg 1 is an immune modulator to treat AIDS patients that is derived from natural substances produced by white blood cells. It enhances the production of IL–2 and gamma interferon by lymphocytes from patients with symptomatic HIV infection.

Imuran   See AZATHIOPRINE.

imuthiol   An organic compound that contains sulfur and facilitates the development of T lymphocytes (see T CELL). It has been shown to have anti-HIV activity in vitro.

in utero transmission   See TRANSMISSION.

in vitro   Literally, "in glass"; the phrase refers to a biological process or reaction that takes place in an artificial environment, usually a test tube or culture plate in a laboratory, rather than in the body. In vitro studies are usually the first step in the development of new treatments of diseases.

in vitro cultivation   The propagation of living organisms in an artificial environment such as a Petri dish or test tube.

in vitro fertilization   A procedure in which an egg is fertilized outside the womb, in a test tube or Petri dish. The fertilized egg is then surgically implanted in the prospective mother's, or a surrogate mother's, uterus—not necessarily the biological mother. The technique is most often used to help women who cannot conceive naturally.

in vivo   Literally, within a living body. The term refers to experiments or testing in animals or humans in a living, natural environment. In AIDS research, in vivo studies are conducted in clinical trials.

inactivation   The rendering ineffective of an agent or substance, such as the HIV virus, through the destruction or negation of its activity or effects.

inactivation agent   An agent used to destroy biological activity, as of an enzyme, microorganism, or virus.

incapacitated parent   See INCAPACITY.

incapacity   An incompetence or inability to function. In social services jargon, disability, which can be less severe or less long lasting than that required for SSDI/SSI, used to qualify a parent and thus (even in a two-parent family) an entire low-income family, for AFDC and MEDICAID; sometimes used in GENERAL ASSISTANCE programs, too.

incidence   The frequency of a phenomenon; in epidemiology, the frequency of occurrence of a disease over a period of time in relation to the population within which it occurs. Incidence is usually reported in terms of the number of cases per 100,000 population per year.

HIV/AIDS are now found on every inhabited continent. The epidemology of AIDS is, today, a specialty in its own right. The rate of rise in reported AIDS cases varies from country to country, and different patterns of infection are found throughout the world. The World Health Organization (WHO) of the United Nations maintains the most complete statistics of HIV infection outside the United States. The exact incidence of AIDS throughout the world, however, is unknown, largely because the accuracy of reporting varies greatly from country to country, for many reasons. Additionally, most developing countries lack the means to screen large numbers of people for the presence of antibodies against HIV. In the absence of this kind of testing, asymptomatic carriers go undetected.

incidence rate   See INCIDENCE.

inclusion criteria   In a clinical trial or research study, the health factors whose presence is required in all participants. Because each person who takes part will have the same factors, researchers can compare like with like.

income level   Amount specified in needs-based programs, usually on a monthly basis, to determine eligibility for benefits; those with income below the level are eligible, but those with income above it are not.

income maintenance   A generic term for welfare, including GA, AFDC, and SSPS; used in New York and several other states.

inconclusive   Not determinable definitely one way or another. In medicine, the term usually refers to test results, for instance, a blood test from whose results the presence of the AIDS virus cannot be inferred.

incontinence   The inability to control excretory functions (defecation and urination). Also, generally, the absence of restraint; habitual immoderation or excess.

incubation   1. The interval between exposure to a pathogen and the appearance of the first clinical symptom in the development of an infectious disease. See INCUBATION PERIOD. 2. The development of bacteria culture under controlled conditions. 3. The development of a fertilized egg. 4. The care of a premature infant in a controlled environment to promote development and survival.

incubation period   The interval between initial infection with a microbe and appearance of the first symptom or sign of disease. For influenza and the common cold, the incubation period is usually several days; for measles, chickenpox, mumps, and infections caused by many other viruses, the incubation period is two to three weeks. An unusual feature of HIV infection is that the first symptoms of a weakened immune system usually do not occur until several years after the infection takes place. The incubation period for AIDS is at present unknown but has been estimated to be between 3 to 34 months.

IND   See INVESTIGATIONAL NEW DRUG.

independent variable   See VARIABLE.

index case   The initial individual whose condition led to an investigation of a hereditary disorder.

indication   The purpose for which a drug is prescribed. FOOD AND DRUG ADMINISTRATION–approved indications for a drug appear on a printed insert in the drug's packaging.

indicator disease   One of a group of infections and diseases, established by the CENTERS FOR DISEASE CONTROL AND PREVENTION, whose presence indicates HIV infection. These diseases are among the criteria used to diagnose a person as having full-blown AIDS.

indigent   Impoverished; poor and without resources. In hospital jargon, a poor person without HEALTH CARE coverage.

indigent care coordinator   Financial counselor who works with indigent care programs (state, local, or hospital free medical care programs for the poor). They are increasingly used for public subsidies or rate allowances to compensate hospitals for bad debts of indigents, rather than for a patient-oriented entitlement program.

indigent care program Any free state, local, or hospital medical care program for the poor. The term increasingly designates a program of public subsidies or rate allowances to reimburse hospitals for indigent care, rather than a patient-oriented entitlement program.

Individuals with Disabilities Education Act (IDEA) Originally entitled the Education for All Handicapped Children Act, this federal legislation sets out requirements for the public education of children with disabilites including AIDS, and allocates federal money to states that meet these requirements. Prior to the act's passage by Congress in 1975, half of the more than 8 million children with disabilities in the United States did not receive appropriate educational services. One million were entirely excluded from the public school systems. State and local authorities generally rationalized this situation as being due to a lack of funding for special programs. As a result, wealthy parents often paid out of pocket for special services that allowed their children to benefit educationally. The children of those who could not afford to pay were left out. Congress stepped in and passed the IDEA to ensure that disabled children would have access to a free, appropriate education and related services designed to meet their special needs. The act applies to children with a variety of disabilities, including mental retardation; impaired hearing, sight, or speech; serious emotional disturbances; impairments that prevent physical movement; and other chronic health problems that negatively affect a child's strength, vitality, or alertness.

individual treatment IND A program established by the FOOD AND DRUG ADMINISTRATION in which a patient may receive an experimental drug free of charge from the pharmaceutical manufacturer, with the assistance of his or her personal physician. Admission to this program is granted on an individual basis by the Food and Drug Administration. See also INVESTIGATIONAL NEW DRUG.

induced immunosuppression The prevention or diminution of an immune response by artificial means. See IMMUNOSUPPRESSION.

indurate To harden. For example, pressure and heat indurate the rock. Induration may also be an abnormal hardening of an area of the body.

infant A child from birth through one year of age. See also NEONATE.

infected blood Blood contaminated by a virus, which can be passed to anyone whose bloodstream it enters, as in a transfusion.

infection The state or condition in which the body or part of it is invaded by MICROORGANISMS. The microorganisms will multiply under conditions favorable to them, producing injurious results. If the body's defense mechanisms are effective, the infection will remain localized. If the body's defense mechanisms are not capable of staving off the invasion and multiplication, the local infection may persist and spread. Infections occur more readily when the BONE MARROW's ability to produce white blood cells is decreased and the IMMUNE SYSTEM response is lowered. Symptoms of an infection include fever, chills, sweating (especially at night), loose bowels, a burning feeling when urinating, a severe cough, and/or a sore throat. An infection with bacteria that invade the bloodstream is referred to as bacteremia. Bacteria that release byproducts into the bloodstream may cause septicemia, which may progress to shock. Infection with viruses in the bloodstream is known as viremia. Fungus in the blood is known as fungemia.

Today it is recognized that viral and most opportunistic infections in AIDS are intracellular. Intracellular and extracellular pathogens have different means of expressing their presence, leading to the interpretation that CD8+ and CD4+ T CELLS have a division of tasks: CD8+ CYTOTOXIC T cells (CTL) control intracellular pathogens, and CD4+ helper T cells help to eradicate extracellular PATHOGENS by cooperation with B cells and by release of cytotoxins.

infectious Pertaining to a disease due to a MICROORGANISM; capable of being transmitted with or without contact; producing infection. See CONTAGIOUS.

infectious agent An organism that produces infection or is capable of being transmitted with or without contact.

infectious disease Any disease caused by growth of PATHOGENIC MICROORGANISMS in the body. An infectious disease may or may not be contagious.

infectious mononucleosis An acute infectious disease that primarily affects lymphoid tissue and is characterized by enlarged LYMPH NODEs and SPLEEN with an increase in abnormal mononuclear LEUKOCYTES in the blood. An abnormal functioning liver will be found in about 90 percent of cases. Clinical manifestations are highly variable. The disease is caused by the Epstein-Barr virus, a herpes virus. Incubation period may be as long as four to seven weeks. There is no specific treatment, but for serious complications (for example hemolytic anemia, pharyngeal swelling interfering with swallowing), cortisone is used.

infertility Inability to become pregnant or bear children.

infibulation The process of fastening, as in the joining of lips of wounds by clasps; also the sewing together of the labia of females or the foreskin of males to prevent sexual intercourse.

inflammation The body's response to tissue injury or infection that occurs in the affected tissue and adjacent blood vessels. The blood vessels' permeability is increased, and the area becomes heavily populated with white blood cells. Signs of inflammation are redness, swelling, pain, and sometimes loss of function. Not all of these signs are necessarily present in any given case.

inflammatory bowel disease   A general term that denotes inflammatory bowel diseases of unknown origin. Ulcerative colitis, Crohn's disease, and regional enteritis are examples of such diseases.

inflammatory neuropathy   Inflammation of the PERIPHERAL NERVOUS SYSTEM, causing abnormal function.

influenza vaccine   A sterile suspension of killed influenza virus types A and B, either individually or combined. Commonly known as a "flu shot." Trade names Fluax and Fluogen.

The influenza vaccine varies in its effectiveness, depending on whether the strain of the virus in the vaccine is related to the virus that is causing the influenza. The effectiveness of the vaccine changes annually with every flu season, since the prevalent types of flu are different each year. In most years, however, the vaccine probably prevents illness in about 70 percent of the people who receive it, and those who become infected despite having been vaccinated usually have less severe symptoms. Influenza does not seem to be unusually common or severe in people with HIV infection. The only problem specific to people with HIV infection is that the symptoms of influenza can be confused with the symptoms of other disorders, such as PNEUMOCYSTIS PNEUMONIA. The CENTERS FOR DISEASE CONTROL AND PREVENTION's Advisory Committee on Immunization Practices recommends that people with HIV infection be vaccinated every year.

information campaign   Advertising program that is limited to the provision of information. For example, the Centers for Disease Control and Prevention's "America Responds to AIDS" information campaign produced and distributed a brochure to assist parents in discussing HIV and AIDS-related issues with their children. Effective information campaigns are composed of culturally and linguistically appropriate messages; are targeted towards a particular population, such as adolescents, blood donors, IV drug users; and choose persons who maintain credibility with the targeted population to deliver their messages. While print-based materials are an integral component of more effective information campaigns, print information alone cannot be relied on to produce behavioral change. Audiovisuals and multimedia can also be used to disseminate information and promote ideas, as can lectures and discussions; skills training; individual and group counseling education; peer- and professionally-led counseling groups; and empowerment messages.

informed consent   Consent given for a course of treatment, surgical procedure, or diagnostic test after being informed fully about its possible benefits and risks. Consent is a legal requirement, and a patient must be given enough information so that he or she can make an informed decision. In an investigational drug trial, individuals considering participation must be informed of the risks and possible benefits of the proposed experimental treatment. A participant must sign a written document attesting that he or she understands the nature, purposes, and risks of the study. Specifically, the consent form contains an explanation of why the research is being done; what researchers want to accomplish; what will be done and for how long; what risks are involved; what benefits can be expected; other treatments available; and a statement confirming a participant's right to leave the trial at any time.

Generally, an HIV test requires a patient to sign an informed consent form.

infuse-a-port   A small device containing a thin CATHETER that is surgically implanted under the skin for long-term administration of anti-AIDS drugs as well as other substances, including blood transfusions, nutrients, bone marrow, and medications. A blood sample may also be taken from a patient by drawing it from the infuse-a-port reservoir. The infuse-a-port eliminates the constant need to search for a "good" vein, which can be a vexing problem, sometimes stressful and painful as well for a patient receiving regular treatments intravenously. Barring infection, it can remain in the body for months.

infusion   The introduction of a fluid other than blood into a vein. Infusions are often used when the digestive system does not absorb appreciable quantities of a drug that is also too bulky or too toxic to be given by quick INJECTION.

inguinal lymph nodes   Small round masses of tissue located in the groin that drain fluids from the body.

inhalant   A volatile drug, chemical, or other substance inhaled for the effect of its vapor. The apparatus or device used in this procedure is called an inhaler; it usually nebulizes the substance with an aerosol or other spray mechanism. Dry or moist air, vapor, or gases such as oxygen, carbon dioxide, or helium, aromatic spirits of ammonia, or anesthetics are among the substances introduced into the lungs for therapeutic purposes.

Inhalants are also subject to abuse. In the context of AIDS, the word *inhalants* generally means "poppers," nitrite inhalants which have been used in the gay community as a sexual aid. See also POPPERS.

inhibitor   A chemical or other substance that inhibits or blocks a biological process in the body from taking place.

injection drug users   Drug users who inject drugs into their veins or under the skin. Abbreviated IDUs.

innate immunity   Various host defenses that are present from birth and do not depend on immunologic memory.

inoculation   The introduction of an ANTIGEN or antiserum into humans and other animals to confer immunity.

inoculum size   The number of MICROBEs necessary to cause an INFECTION. In HIV infection, the number is not known. What is known is that the probability of transmitting

HIV with the transfusion of one unit (or 500 milliliters) of infected blood is 80 to 90 percent. The probability of transmitting HIV with a needlestick injury, which injects only a fraction of a milliliter of blood, is 0.4 percent. This difference in the probabilities of transmission is most likely due to inoculum size.

inoculum threshold　The minimum dose of a substance introduced by inoculation (generally an ANTIGEN, antiserum, or antitoxin injected to produce immunity to a specific disease) that will produce an effect on a patient.

insect bites　There is no evidence that HIV is spread in any way other than exposure through blood, blood products, perinatal contact between mother and child, or sexual contact. These types of exposure may occur without knowledge that an exposure is taking place. Biting insects may seem like likely candidates to transmit HIV, but if that were so, household AIDS cases that are unrelated to known transmission routes would appear. In addition, young children, other than those in risk groups, are frequently bitten by insects and some should be infected if transmission takes place in this way. There are no reported cases that clearly fit either of these situations.

Researchers have created laboratory circumstances to determine if insects carry HIV. They have isolated HIV genetic material from bedbugs and mosquitoes one hour after feeding the insects blood contaminated with HIV, but the isolated virus did not grow in the insects' cells. The very low levels of HIV in blood, the tiny volumes ingested by insects, and the absence of field data implicating spread of HIV by insects makes this form of transmission highly unlikely, if not impossible.

insertive anal intercourse　See ANAL INTERCOURSE.

insomnia　The inability to sleep, or to get enough sleep. The difficulty may be either in falling asleep or remaining asleep, or both. This sleep disorder may be primary or secondary to some other illness, condition, or circumstance. Primary insomnia exists when there are no signs or symptoms of a mental or physical condition that would account for the disorder. Secondary insomnia is usually readily explained by the existence of a condition that causes anxiety, stress, or pain or by the use of a drug that interferes with sleep. The causes of insomnia may be mental or physical. A great variety of drugs are available for primary insomnia, including over-the-counter medications. Their use on a short-term basis might be advisable, but all prescription drugs may have undesired side effects, such as overdose, habituation, tolerance, addiction, daytime drowsiness, lethargy, or amnesia. In secondary insomnia, treatment consists of determining the condition causing the insomnia and then treating that disorder. Self-help measures are also recommended to induce sleep.

institutional (or internal) review board (IRB)　A regulating committee (composed of internal staff, hospital affiliates, and community members) that reviews and approves all human trials conducted within a particular hospital or research center. The IRB ensures that a trial is conducted in an ethical manner, with proper protection of human subjects.

insurance　The act, system, or business of insuring property, life, one's person, etc., against loss or harm arising from specified contingencies, in return for payment. As the insurance industry grew increasingly aware of the financial consequences of the AIDS phenomenon, it sought ways to escape from responsibility for health care costs; as affected populations and political decision makers became increasingly aware of the potential for costs that neither was prepared to bear, insurance soared in importance as a legal issue.

In the earliest stages of the AIDS chronology, insurers rather freely admitted to trying to screen out applications from single men in the nation's largest cities, as approximately 80 percent of the AIDS cases at that time occurred in this group. They were also denying life insurance coverage to those already diagnosed with AIDS. Denying coverage to those already diagnosed with a preexisting condition that was then considered to be a terminal illness is a different thing from denying coverage to those who were considered at high risk for the disease. The insurers, however, seemed unable—or unwilling—to see the difference.

Since those early days, the insurance industry's practices relating to HIV disease have come under increasing government regulation. Lawyers and others who work with AIDS patients have long asserted that insurance companies across the country are using unfair and devious tactics to avoid paying claims for AIDS-related medical problems. Suits are being filed about insurers' testing applicants without their consent. Other cases have focused on the possibility of a preexisting condition. An objection sometimes raised by insurers is that treatments performed or sought are experimental—many health policies do not cover experimental treatments. There is a continuing series of cases in which discrimination is the issue. And there is increasing attention being paid to employers' practice of trying to limit their expenses by changing their coverage from outside insurers to self-insured plans, especially once one or more employees file HIV-related claims. Self-insured plans are allowed under the federal Employee Retirement Income Security Act, known as ERISA. Because they are authorized by federal law, these plans generally escape regulation by states, whose laws and regulations are often those most heavily relied on by employees with HIV disease.

Nationally, the way was paved for a more responsible and sensible direction on AIDS and insurance issues by the National Association of Insurance Commissioners (NAIC) in December 1986, when it adopted guidelines recommended by its Advisory Committee on AIDS. These guidelines include the prohibition of discrimination on the basis of sexual orientation. NAIC, however, is merely an association of state insurance regulators, and it has no authority to issue actual regulations in any jurisdiction.

intake　The administrative and assessment process for admitting a person to a health care program or facility.

integrase　HIV integrase is the virus's third enzyme (the other two are REVERSE TRANSCRIPTASE and PROTEASE). It binds to HIV DNA, which is created by the reverse transcriptase enzyme, and integrates DNA into the host cell's chromosomes. The first integrase inhibitor, Aronex Pharmaceuticals' AR-177, does not inhibit this integrating activity but rather appears to keep the enzyme from binding to the newly processed DNA in the first place. Inhibition of HIV integrase is an attractive therapeutic strategy, since it would potentially protect healthy cells from infection, thereby helping to bolster the immune system.

AR-177 is an oligonucleotide (string of nucleotides—the building blocks of DNA). Most oligonucleotides cannot be administered systemically, because they break down and rapidly pass from the body. But AR-177 is unique—formed by 17 nucleotides (mostly guanine), it is a stable structure less prone to destruction in the blood. In animal studies, it was not easily metabolized and was excreted very slowly. Some drug remained in the animals' bodies a week after a single dose.

So far AR-177 is in injectable form only. Its manufacturer hopes that the compound's half-life will be long enough to allow for infrequent dosing. Preliminary data in rodents show that the drug does have some oral bioavailability. The company is now studying an oral formulation in primates.

Integrase as a therapeutic target does have several possible pitfalls. While HIV reverse transcriptase and protease are required to act for a significant period of time during the viral life-cycle, integrase acts for only one brief step during infection of the cell. This reduces the chances that a drug will interfere with integration. Conversely, however, the intracellular levels of integrase may be extremely small, and this scarcity works in favor of an integrase inhibitor. Also, interfering with the integration step would not affect the yield of viable virus from infected cells. Since HIV seems to produce many mutations throughout its genes, inhibition of existing HIV integrase may merely cause the rise of drug-resistant mutant versions. The hope is that a combination of therapies targeting different enzymes, including integrase, will convey lasting benefit to the infected person by reducing HIV's replication rate, and therefore the emergence of mutant strains.

integrase inhibitor   Drugs that inhibit integrase catalytic activity.

A common problem with many of the integrase inhibitors is lack of activity in cell culture. Either the compounds do not effectively get into the cell, or doses that inhibit HIV become lethal to cells that the drug is meant to protect. The one integrase inhibitor to reach human studies (as of early fall 1996) is Aronex Pharmaceuticals' AR-177, which sports the name Zinetvir. This compound does not inhibit the "active" part of the integrase enzyme. Instead, it keeps integrase from binding to the HIV genetic material.

intensive care   Service provided by skilled medical personnel to seriously ill patients with life-threatening conditions requiring special equipment, complex treatment and constant care, and/or monitoring. It is usually provided in a specialized area of a care facility known as an INTENSIVE CARE UNIT (ICU).

Some intensive care units, such as those for coronary, surgical, or newborn intensive care, limit their services to certain types of patients.

intensive care unit (ICU)   See INTENSIVE CARE.

interaction   See DRUG INTERACTION.

intercourse   Interaction; the most common euphemism for coitus (SEXUAL INTERCOURSE). The term covers both heterosexual and homosexual coitus. Types of intercourse include ANAL INTERCOURSE (both insertive and receptive anal intercourse) and VAGINAL INTERCOURSE.

interfemoral   Between the thighs; e.g., interfemoral intercourse (rubbing the penis between a partner's thighs).

interferon   One of a number of antiviral proteins that modulate the immune response. Interferons serve multiple roles as antiviral, antitumor, and immune stimulating agents. Studied since the 1960s, interferon was the first cytokine discovered. Interferons are obtained in two ways: they are made naturally by the body when cells are stimulated by a virus as well as by several other agents; or they are produced by genetically engineered microorganisms. The two brands are Roferon-a and Intron a. In November 1989, the United States Food and Drug Administration approved a "natural" interferon (produced by cultured human cells deliberately infected with a virus) to treat genital warts. This product, Alferon N Injection, contains at least 14 variations of the interferon molecule, whereas each of the recombinant (genetically engineered) products contains only one. Some experts doubt whether it makes a difference if it is natural or recombinant, thus illustrating that there is much confusion and disagreement among experts about interferons in general.

There are three major groups of interferons—alpha interferon, beta interferon, and gamma interferon. These major classes have been synthesized and each is being studied in various applications for the treatment of HIV and AIDS. Alpha and beta interferons appear to be made by virtually all white blood cells, whereas gamma interferon is made only by T cells and large granulocytes. Gamma interferon is much more potent in its effect on the immune system than alpha or beta interferon. Interferons are important in immune function, have antitumor activity, and can repress the growth of nonviral parasites within the cells.

In November of 1988, the United States Food and Drug Administration approved interferon as a treatment for Kaposi's sarcoma; it had previously been used to treat hairy cell leukemia, and genital warts. The drug is normally given by injection because it is believed that digestion, if taken orally, would destroy it.

Interferon alpha (IFNα) is secreted by a virally infected cell and strengthens the defenses of nearby uninfected cells. Alpha interferon has been available as a prescription drug in the United States since 1986. A manufactured version of interferon alpha is a Food and Drug Administration–approved treatment for KS, hepatitis B virus, and hepatitis C virus. Trade names: Roferon, Intron A.

In early 1990, startling claims, press reports, and rumors turned a proposed AIDS treatment into the latest "miracle" cure. On February 7 of that year, researchers in Kenya reported success in treating AIDS with "Kemron," their name for a treatment consisting of very low doses of a kind of alpha interferon, held in the mouth but not swallowed. Claims that AIDS patients treated with Kemron had all their AIDS symptoms disappear within several weeks and that several patients serodeconverted (changed from HIV-positive to HIV-negative) after four to six weeks of treatment surfaced and were greeted by questions, doubts, and trials.

Interferon alpha-2 (IFNα-2) is a variation of alpha interferon that with beta interferon has been used as an experimental treatment for progressive multifocal leukoencephalopathy (PML).

Interferon beta (IFNβ) is an antiviral which may work like alpha interferon but have fewer side effects. Early clinical trials tested beta interferon and low-dose AZT on patients who could not tolerate full-dose AZT. Beta interferon with interferon alpha-2 has been used as an experimental treatment for PROGRESSIVE MULTIFOCAL LEUKOENCEPHALOPATHY (PML).

Interferon gamma (IFNγ) is synthesized by immune system cells (NK CELLS and CD4 CELLS). It activates MACROPHAGES and helps orient the immune system to a mode that promotes cellular immunity (TH1 response).

interim analysis   An intermediary analysis of clinical trial data, performed at a point at which enough data have been gathered to derive preliminary, but not necessarily complete, conclusions. Interim analyses are performed to see whether continuation of a clinical trial is warranted.

interleukin (IL)   Interleukin-1 (IL-1 or hematopoietin-1) is a protein produced by a variety of cells in the body, including the natural KILLER CELLS, T CELLS, and B CELLS. IL-1 triggers a range of processes involved in inflammation, a localized immune reaction. It activates T cells and stimulates BONE MARROW growth.

Interleukin-2 (IL-2) is a protein produced by activated T cells in the body. It plays a central role in the regulation of immune responses against infection or cancerous cells. In people living with HIV, IL-2 levels are abnormally low. It is thought that this deficiency contributes to the overall deterioration of the immune system in HIV disease. IL-2 was discovered in 1976 at the National Cancer Institute and was originally called T cell growth factor. IL-2 stimulates the growth and activities of a range of cells, including CYTOTOXIC T LYMPHOCYTEs (CTL), LYMPHOKINE-activated killer cells (LAK cells) and tumor-infiltrating lymphocytes (TIL cells).

As HIV disease progresses, levels of IL-2 are reduced. Like alpha interferon, IL-2 has been synthesized and is approved for treatment of kidney cancer in several countries. In addition, it is under development as a treatment for other diseases, including HIV/AIDS. It is known that IL-2 induces the multiplication of CD4 (T-helper) cells in the test tube; if the same effect can be achieved in the human body, CD4 cells destroyed by HIV could be replaced, and the immune system perhaps reconstituted.

There is also evidence suggesting that HIV is controlled in the body during the early period of infection by a strong response by the cell-mediated arm of the immune system (chiefly suppressor and cytotoxic CD8 T cells activated by IL-2 released by CD4 cells). The cells involved in this response gradually lose their ability to respond effectively to HIV and other pathogens, possibly owing to a decline in IL-2 production by CD4 cells. Although IL-2 trials in the past have found that the positive influence on CD4 cell numbers disappeared after a few weeks on continuous infusion therapy, more recent studies have found substantial and prolonged IL-2 induced CD4 cell increases. These recent studies employed a unique cyclical dosing regimen (intermittent continuous infusion) rather than steady weekly schedule. However, the recent studies indicate that benefits are less likely to be seen in patients with AIDS or with low numbers of circulating CD4s. IL-2 does not appear to increase CD4 cells in patients with low CD4 counts (fewer than 100). In fact, these patients are far more likely to get an *increase* in HIV levels. The evidence suggests that patients with over 200 CD4 cells have a good chance of receiving a CD4 boost from IL-2 therapy.

IL-2 has serious dose-limiting toxicities. Debilitating side effects that historically have accompanied high-dose IL-2 therapy (3–18 million IU/day) include fever, severe flulike symptoms, capillary leakage, lung congestion and swelling, liver, kidney, and gallbladder disorders, neutropenia, thrombocytopenia (low platelets), glucose intolerance, and irritating dermatological problems such as psoriasis flare-ups. The side effects have been found to be less severe under a regimen of intermittent continuous infusion.

There has also been a grave concern that IL-2 stimulates HIV along with T cells. The virus reproduces in infected, activated CD4 cells, and HIV-free activated CD4 cells are especially vulnerable to infection. Studies suggest that IL-2 boosts both CD4 counts and viral levels and that IL-2's treatment effect may be determined by the balance between IL-2's stimulation of CD4 cells and the increased amounts of HIV's destruction of CD4 cells. In other words, the benefit of boosting CD4+ cells must be weighed against the potential for stimulating production of the virus. Because of this potential the drug should only be given to people receiving antiretroviral therapy.

It has also been suggested that IL-2 stimulates CD8 suppressor cells, which block HIV replication within infected cells. These suppressor cells are lost in advanced disease, which may help explain the different responses to IL-2 in the high and low CD4 cell groups. Increased HIV levels often go back to baseline in a matter of days or weeks, but nevertheless it is generally recommended that all patients given IL-2 remain on antiretroviral therapy, and that the therapy should include at least one new agent to which the patient's virus is not resistant. Furthermore, new antiviral drugs should not be started at the same time as IL-2, since it may be impossible to distinguish between side effects from IL-2 and the new drug. The HIV-promoting nature of IL-2 is probably worse among patients in whom HIV has developed resistance to the antiretroviral drugs they are taking.

Researchers have presumed that a boost in CD4 cells is a good sign. There is, however, no way of knowing yet if an

IL-2 induced CD4 count of 1,000 is as good as a naturally occurring CD4 count of 1,000. IL-2 may boost or preserve CD4 numbers without necessarily making those cells competent. Alternatively, IL-2 may simply cause a "retrafficking" of CD4 cells, in which cells enter the blood from the lymph system, where 95 percent of them are concentrated. Researchers caution that it cannot be assumed that IL-2 induced CD4 increases will translate into any clinical benefits, such as delayed disease progression or prolonged survival.

There have been reports that people with HIV and their doctors are obtaining commercial IL-2 (trade name Proleukin), which is approved for the treatment of renal cell carcinoma, and trying to mimic various protocols. Some of these doctors are giving patients injected IL-2, while others are offering intermittent continuous infusion of IL-2. However, there is still no indication that IL-2 can yield any clinical benefit to people with HIV.

Interleukin-3 (IL-3 or multicolony stimulating factor) is another powerful interleukin that stimulates the growth of many precursor bone marrow cells. They are early cells with the potential to develop into mature blood cells.

Interleukin-4 (IL-4 or B-cell stimulatory factor-1) is another immune-system messenger naturally present in the body and has been tested as an anti-KS treatment. Synthetic versions are produced in the laboratory by genetic engineering. Early results of the IL-4 study showed the drug had no apparent effect on KS progression but appeared to have some anti-HIV activity. IL-4 enhances B cell growth and antibody production and stimulates the production of other immune system cells.

Interleukin-5 (IL-5 or eosinophil colony stimulating factor) stimulates the growth of the blood cells known as eosinophils, which kill bacteria.

interleukin-6 (IL-6 or B-cell stimulatory factor-2) stimulates B cell growth.

Interleukin-12 (IL-12) triggers the maturation of Th1 CD4 cells, specific cytotoxic T-lymphocyte responses, and an increase in the activity of NK cells. It is under study as an immunotherapy in HIV infection, since it stimulates production of the very cells that AIDS destroys, thereby boosting immune cells directly.

Researchers first tried giving high doses of the substance to try to counteract the damage the AIDS virus was doing. It didn't work very well. A new regimen was tried: the drug was given for a few days at a time, then the body was allowed to rest for several weeks before the next dose. This tactic resulted in large CD4 increases. The treatment works best in those starting out with fairly high CD4 counts to begin with. Those who are sickest, with the lowest counts, do poorly on it, perhaps because their immune systems have already been irreparably damaged. Side effects include a very severe flu-like syndrome lasting several days, with shaking, chills, and high fevers. Not all patients respond to interleukin-12, but most of those who do have shown a sustained increase in CD4 counts. How and when interleukin-2 should be used have yet to be determined.

IL-12 has been synthesized and, unlike many other experimental AIDS drugs, is already on the market for another purpose, treating a certain kind of kidney cancer.

That means doctors can legally prescribe it, although insurance companies may refuse to pay.

Interleukin-16 (IL-16) is another naturally occurring variety of interleukin. How it works is unknown, but it does bind to the CD4 receptor and may inhibit CD4 cell activation. Investigators have found that a factor isolated from the CD8 cells of African green monkeys that suppresses SIV, the monkey virus similar to HIV, is virtually identical to human IL-16, but has a more dramatic HIV-suppressive than pure IL-16. Other scientists suggest that IL-16 may be working together with other suppressive factors. At the doses used by the investigators, IL-16 was not toxic to cells and so perhaps has some therapeutic potential. However, like other cytokines that have shown anti-HIV activity in the lab, it may also concurrently stimulate the production of inflammatory cytokines when administered in people, undermining whatever direct anti-HIV activity it might have. And generally, administration of the HIV-suppressor cytokines have been associated with severe side effects.

See also CHEMOKINEs and HIV-SUPPRESSORS.

intermammary   Between the breasts; e.g., intermammary intercourse or rubbing the penis between a partner's breasts.

intermediate care facility (ICF)   A facility that provides health-related care and services to individuals who do not require the degree of care and treatment standard nursing facilities (SNFs) provide. The bulk of nursing home patients need ICF- rather than SNF-level care. MEDICAID and cash payments are the sole sources of financing for this level of care. It is not covered by MEDICARE or HEALTH INSURANCE.

interstitial pneumonia   See INTERSTITIAL PNEUMONITIS.

interstitial pneumonitis   A localized acute inflammation of the lung. A definite diagnosis of interstitial pneumonia in a child under 13 years of age is indicative of AIDS unless another cause is identified or tests for HIV are negative.

intertriginous infection   An inflammation or superficial dermatitis occurring in the folds of the skin, such as the creases in the neck, between the toes, or in the groin. It is characterized by redness, maceration, burning, itching, and occasionally ulceration and erosion.

intertrigo labialis   See PERLECHE.

intervention   In health care economics and clinical practice, intervention refers to an action that interrupts or changes events in progress; in behavior modification research, to those techniques or devices by which one behavior is interrupted and another, presumably healthier, behavior is instituted. Within the context of HIV/AIDS, many intervention efforts of the first decade were designed and implemented quickly in response to a new health problem that in some areas took on characteristics of a crisis. Today, many researchers and program planners believe that the time has come to view behavioral intervention from a more long-term perspective. Today's challenge is to develop effective intervention strategies that sustain healthy behavioral patterns in individuals who are not currently at risk and facilitate change among individuals who are at risk. Efforts of the first decade bear witness to the fact that, to be effective, intervention efforts must be well-designed, carefully implemented, and thoughtfully evaluated.

Intervention models vary considerably, ranging from individual intervention efforts to community-level intervention efforts that are designed to reach a critical mass of individuals with information, motivation, and skills training. There are information interventions that utilize lectures, videotapes, and support groups; social interventions, such as safer sex parties; and media interventions, such as the multimedia public service campaign utilized in the second year of the Centers for Disease Control and Prevention's "America Responds to AIDS" media campaign. This latter campaign included television and radio announcements, print advertisements, and public transit posters.

intestinal malabsorption   A condition in which nutrients found in food are not properly absorbed by the body and can lead to malnutrition and weight loss at a result.

intolerance   In medicine, inability to take a drug, or a food substance, because of an extreme sensitivity—an allergic reaction or side effect.

intracranial disorder   Any pathological condition within the skull.

intrahepatic disease   Any pathological liver condition that produces a group of clinical symptoms peculiar to it and that sets it apart as abnormal.

intralesional   Inside or into a lesion; e.g., an intralesional injection.

intramuscular   Inside or into muscle; e.g., an intramuscular injection.

intraocular   Inside or into the eye; e.g., an intraocular injection.

intraocular implant   A tiny device (about half the size of a peppercorn) surgically placed directly into the eye. It is designed to deliver a steady, concentrated dose of a drug directly to the infected area for an extended period of time. Intraocular implants are used to deliver GANCICLOVIR to the area of the eye infected by CMV.

intrapartum   During childbirth or delivery.

intrapartum transmission   Transmission that occurs during childbirth or delivery. It more commonly occurs than IN UTERO TRANSMISSION, which occurs during pregnancy. To date, there are few data concerning the impact of certain obstetrical practices on the transmission of HIV. It is thought that events during delivery that expose the baby to maternal blood or cervicovaginal secretions might promote transmission. Minimal use of invasive procedures involving the fetus may decrease the risk of transmission, but optimal treatment of the fetus should take priority. Delivery by cesarean section has not been proved to protect the fetus better than normal spontaneous delivery. Allowing women to deliver in a more comfortable position does not compromise the use of UNIVERSAL PRECAUTIONS for blood and body fluids.

Intrapartum care includes the use of universal precautions; managing labor to optimize outcomes for both mother and infant; utilizing the method of delivery indicated by obstetrical conditions. HIV infection is not currently a contraindication to the use of any analgesia or method of anesthesia.

See TRANSMISSION; ANTEPARTUM PERIOD; POSTPARTUM PERIOD.

intrathecal   In or into the fluid surrounding the spinal cord.

intrathoracic adenopathy   Swelling of the glands or lymph nodes within the chest.

intrauterine device (IUD)   Any of several small plastic devices that may be fitted into a woman's uterus as a barrier to prevent pregnancy. The use of an IUD is considered an effective method of contraception; the failure rate is said to be about 3 percent. For almost 100 percent effectiveness, the simultaneous use of contraceptive cream, jelly or foam, and condoms, is recommended. Using IUDs increases a woman's chances of developing PELVIC INFLAMMATORY DISEASE (PID) and consequent infertility, and are a poor choice for woman at risk of developing a SEXUALLY TRANSMITTED DISEASE (STD). IUDs alone offer no protection against STDs, including HIV.

intravenous (IV)   In or into a vein; e.g., an intravenous injection or feeding tube.

intravenous drug abuser (IVDA)   See INTRAVENOUS DRUG USER.

intravenous drugs   Drugs, such as heroin, that are administered by injection into a vein, directly into the bloodstream.

intravenous drug user (IVDU)   A person who uses a hypodermic needle to inject drugs, including illegal drugs such as heroin or cocaine, into his or her body, for a purpose that deviates from the drug's intended use. IV drug users frequently share such drug paraphernalia as needles and syringes thereby providing opportunities to transmit viruses via their infected contents. Viruses are transmitted through blood that remains in the needle or syringe after injection, not through the injected drug itself. Intravenous drug users are a crucial link in the spread of HIV to ever wider circles of the population.

intravenous immunoglobulin (IVIG)   A sterile solution of concentrated antibodies extracted from the blood of healthy people, injected into a vein or muscle to prevent bacterial infections in people with low or inappropriate ANTIBODY production.

intravitreal   In or into the eye's vitreous humor, between the lens and the retina.

intromission   The introduction of the penis into a partner's body; i.e., vaginal intromission, anal intromission, or oral intromission.

introns   Noncoding regions of DNA interspersed among the EXONS.

intubation   The insertion of a tube into a body canal or into any hollow organ, such as the trachea or larynx, to permit the entrance of air; to dilate a structure. Endotracheal intubation refers to the insertion of a tube through the nose or mouth into the trachea. Nasotracheal intubation refers to insertion of a tube through the nose into the trachea.

invasive nutritional substitute   Any nutrient administered intravenously as an alternative to solid food ingested orally.

invasive procedure   Any technique involving the insertion of foreign matter into the body. The term covers procedures ranging from simple injection to intubation to major surgery.

investigational new drug (IND)   An experimental drug approved for use in the INVESTIGATIONAL NEW DRUG (IND) PROGRAM. Treatment IND is a Food and Drug Administration-approved program that allows a physician to procure an experimental or investigational drug that appears to be safe, and may be effective, for seriously ill patients who have no other treatment options in exchange for data on the safety and perhaps the effectiveness of the drug. The purpose of the program is to facilitate availability of promising new drugs as early in the drug development process as possible. Treatment IND status is granted after researchers have concluded that the drug is safe and very likely effective, but before completion and approval of the final paperwork that accompanies drug approval.

investigational new drug (IND) program   A FOOD AND DRUG ADMINISTRATION program that allows drugs still under investigation to be approved for use by some patients for whom there is no other treatment available. Drugs given IND status may be made available by the manufacturers to patients even though the drugs' safety, effectiveness, and side effects are not fully known. Not all investigational new drugs are available for such "compassionate release."

iodoquinol   An antiamebic agent appearing as a yellowish-to-tan crystalline powder used in the treatment of AMEBIASIS and TRICHOMONAS HOMINIS infection of the intestine and trichomonas vaginalis vaginitis. It is administered orally in the treatment of intestinal disorders and intravaginally for VAGINITIS. Also called DIIODOHYDROXYQUIN. Trade name Yodoxin.

IPV   See POLIOVIRUS VACCINE INACTIVATED.

IRB   See INSTITUTIONAL REVIEW BOARD.

irrevocable beneficiary   A beneficiary designation on a life insurance policy that cannot be changed without the beneficiary's consent.

Iscador   See MISTLETOE.

ischemia   Local deficiency of blood supply due to functional constriction or actual obstruction of a blood vessel.

Ischemic   Pertaining to or affected with ISCHEMIA.

isobutyl nitrite inhaler   Also known as "poppers." Nitrite inhalants, originally made for treating certain heart conditions, which came to be used as sexual stimulants in the gay community. Following research reports that these chemicals might be contributing to immune problems in AIDS or to the development of KAPOSI'S SARCOMA, they were banned in the United States in 1988. Section 8 of the Consumer Product Safety Act bans the manufacture for sale, distribution in commerce, or importation of various forms of "butyl nitrite." In 1990, Congress amended the law to also ban "volatile alkyl nitrites that can be used for inhaling or otherwise introducing volatile alkyl nitrites into the human body for euphoric or physical effects." The amendment specifies a broader class of nitrites, not just the chemical named in the 1988 law. But manufacturers found a way around the ban by substituting different kinds of nitrites. These chemicals were then sold in adult bookstores, sex clubs, and bars. The result was that, unknown chemicals, never tested for human consumption, came into widespread use with no regulatory or public-health oversight. It is noted that the issue of poppers in the gay community first surfaced in 1981. Some observers suspected that poppers themselves might cause AIDS. Later, those theories were largely dismissed, but confusion occurred because some people thought the issue was finished. Remaining concerns are that poppers might be a cofactor in the development of AIDS, could lead to relapses to unsafe sex, may make HIV infection more likely by causing changes in blood vessels, or could possibly cause poisoning if unknown chemicals are substituted in an effort to evade the law. Additionally, some of the chemicals are known to degrade over time allowing harmful byproducts. Some researchers also suspect that the body may metabolize the nitrites into the strongly carcinogenic nitrosamines While there are many medical journal articles on poppers, most of them reporting evidence of health risks, poppers have not been conclusively proven to be harmful. It is generally felt that we may never fully understand the health hazards of poppers. Evidence does strongly suggest that poppers are certainly not safe and probably do cause damage to health, especially to persons with HIV.

isolation   In medical institutions, procedure that keeps patients with contagious infections separated from others who are sick but do not have the same disease. Specifically, it is the limitation of movement and social contacts of a patient suffering from or who is a known carrier of a communicable disease. Quarantine contrastingly, limits the movements only of exposed or contact persons. The value of isolating AIDS patients is questionable, since the HIV virus associated with AIDS is not airborne or spread by casual contact. UNIVERSAL PRECAUTIONS suggest blood and body fluid precautions and a private room if personal hygiene habits are poor.

isoniazid (INH)   An ANTIBIOTIC that has activity against M. tuberculosis, the MICROORGANISM that causes TUBERCULOSIS. Isoniazid is an odorless antibacterial compound appearing as colorless or white crystals or as a white crystalline powder. Isoniazid is usually recommended for persons with HIV infection who have tuberculosis or have had a positive tuberculosis skin test. It may be administered orally or intramuscularly. The most important side effect is hepatitis, with jaundice (yellowish skin and eyes), dark urine, nausea, and abdominal pain. This side effect is more likely in older people and in those people who already have liver damage for other reasons. Anyone taking isoniazid and having these symptoms should stop taking the drug immediately and call his or her physician.

Aluminum-containing antacids can decrease the absorption of INH and reduce its effect. On the other hand, INH can inhibit liver enzymes that metabolize certain drugs, leading to increased blood levels of such medications as Coumadin, Dilantin, Tegretol, theophylline, and the bensodiazepines (Ativan, Valium). Isoniazid is sold under the trade names Cotinazin, Dinacrin, and Nydrazid.

isoprinosine   An IMMUNOMODULATOR that enhances certain cell-mediated immune functions. It has been shown to have anti-HIV activity in vitro. The drug is available without prescription in several countries, including Mexico. Although it has been popular for self-treatment, isoprino-sine's antiviral effects have not consistently correlated with clinical improvement.

Isospora belli   A species of coccidian protozoa that occasionally cause disease of the small intestine and colon in humans. See COCCIDIOSIS.

isosporiasis   Infection by any member of the protozoan family isospora. See COCCIDIOSIS.

itch   Any irritation of the skin, inducing the desire to scratch; any of a variety of skin disorders characterized by itching; scabies.

ITP   See IMMUNE THROMBOCYTOPENIA PURPURA.

itraconazole   An oral antifungal drug used for a number of AIDS-related fungal infections. Itraconazole concentrates in the skin and is particularly effective for skin conditions. Possible side effects include digestive upset, loss of potassium, and headache. Trade name Sporanox.

IUD   see INTRAUTERINE DEVICE.

IV   See INTRAVENOUS.

IVDU   See INTRAVENOUS DRUG USER.

jack-off party   A group sex event in which people masturbate either themselves or each other. It can be a safe-sex technique.

jaundice   A condition characterized by yellowness of skin, whites of eyes, mucous membranes, and body fluids due to deposition of bile pigment resulting from excess bilirubin in the blood. It may be caused by obstruction of bile passageways, excess destruction of red blood cells, or disturbances in functioning of liver cells. Jaundice is a symptom that may indicate a benign and curable disease. Noninvasive procedures such as ultrasonography and computed tomography, as well as clinical laboratory studies, may be used to determine the cause of jaundice. Invasive studies may be used, including cholangiography (radiographic examination of the bile ducts) or endoscopic retrograde cholangiopancreatography (a procedure used to test pancreatic secretions and pancreatic cells directly). Percutaneous transhepatic cholangiography is also employed. It is a procedure used when it is impossible to tell whether jaundice is caused by bile stones or by liver damage. It involves the insertion of a needle into the liver through the skin and the injection of dye into a bile duct.

jilling off   A women's slang term for female masturbation.

jockstrap   A piece of underwear that holds and supports a man's penis and scrotum.

john   Slang for a prostitute's customer.

joint   See PENIS. Also a slang term for marijuana cigarette.

judgment-proof   Beyond the legal reach of creditors; immune from legal compulsion to pay debt. A person with no assets and no income (except from public entitlements) may be said to be judgment proof.

junkie   A slang term for a heroin addict.

K

K cell A type of nonspecific LYMPHOCYTE that seeks out and kills any cells coated with any ANTIBODY. The cells become coated because they are infected with virus and contain viral proteins on their surface membranes.

Kaposi's sarcoma (KS) A blood vessel cancer rare in almost every group of people except male homosexuals with AIDS. The latest research seems to indicate that KS is caused by a virus. This finding supports the widely held suspicion that KS is an infectious disease and helps explain its mysterious clustering in only one segment of the diverse population of AIDS patients. The microbe itself, has yet to be isolated. Kaposi's sarcoma is rarely life threatening in non-HIV patients; in HIV-infected patients it is an AIDS-defining illness.

The appearance of several cases of KS among gay men in New York in 1981, and an outbreak of a rare pneumonia among gay men in San Francisco, together led to the first recognition of the AIDS epidemic. KS, however, rarely appeared in women or heterosexual drug users, leading epidemiologists to suspect that gay men had some particular risk factor for the disease. Research from London in 1990 and 1991 showed convincingly that oral-anal sexual practices greatly increased a man's risk of developing the disease, further bolstering the hypothesis that some causal agent was circulating among gay men.

The symptoms of Kaposi's sarcoma are purplish nodules, a quarter of an inch to an inch in diameter, anywhere on the skin. The nodules will grow in size and number. They sometimes occur on internal organs like the lung, brain, and gastrointestinal tract, though they often cause no specific symptoms at these sites. Some nodules are painful. The face and legs may swell if the lymph channels nearby are blocked. If Kaposi's sarcoma becomes extensive, there may be fever, weight loss, and severe fatigue.

Diagnosis can be established by a biopsy of the nodules. Biopsies are easy to do with nodules on the skin, but more difficult when the nodules are on internal organs. The main reason to do the biopsy is that the nodules might possibly turn out to be something other than Kaposi's sarcoma. Therapy is controversial. Treatment is neither easy nor universally effective. If the nodules are painful, disfiguring, or complicated by swelling, they can be treated with radiation

or interferon. If the nodules have spread widely over the skin or into internal organs, causing symptoms, they can be treated with the same drugs given to people with cancer.

In about 50 percent of people with AIDS-related KS, lesions form in the lungs and gastrointestinal tract. KS in the lungs is most life-threatening, causing pulmonary fluid buildup, obstruction of airways, bleeding with resultant coughing, and difficult breathing. Wherever, and whenever KS occurs, it can be compounded by inflammation, ulceration and secondary infections of the surrounding tissues. KS involvement of the lymph tissues leads to a particularly poor prognosis as the disease rapidly spreads to other organs.

AIDS-related KS is much more aggressive than other subtypes, such as classical KS. In AIDS, KS lesions are characterized by an abnormally fast growth of spindle-shaped cells, whose origins are still a mystery. Lesions form when capillaries (fine threadlike vessels that carry blood) begin to grow irregularly and rapidly. The capillaries become leaky, resulting in accumulation of red blood cells that give the lesions their reddish purple color. In black or dark-skinned people, lesions can appear as dark spots that are often mistaken for other skin disorders. These lesions are usually not painful or tender.

At its earliest stage, AIDS-related KS does not require therapy, except to clear up disfiguring lesions, usually accomplished by exposing the site of the lesion to an antitumor therapy. Radiation has been a common type of local therapy, although intralesional injections have been moderately effective. Local radiation has been reported to be effective as a therapy to reduce pain and swelling. It has been used as well to clear up lesions on the skin, in the mouth and the lining of the eyelids. Freezing lesions with liquid nitrogen, a procedure known as "cryotherapy," and laser surgery are also local treatments for lesions. Lesions that appear in the lymph system may need more immediate, aggressive treatment, depending on the stage of the disease. At an early stage, KS of the lymph nodes can cause swelling in the limbs that can be painful and severely limit mobility, in which case local radiation may be administered.

Alpha interferon is a drug for KS which is sometimes used to treat individual KS lesions and sometimes to treat the whole body (systemic treatment). Interferons are natural proteins occurring in the body that can prevent or fight cell infection. They have been synthesized into an injectable drug that can be used to treat many different diseases. Interferon seems to work best against KS when the immune system is still fairly functional. The main side effect of the drug is a flulike illness.

Disseminated (also known as widespread or advanced) KS may be said to occur when the disease appears with one of the following circumstances: 25 or more lesions; a formation of 10 new lesions per month; disease when T4 counts are under 200; or spread of lesions to the lungs or stomach. Chemotherapy is currently the closest to a standard treatment for disseminated KS. For example, paclitaxel (brand name Taxol) is a chemotherapeutic drug used widely for the treatment of solid tumors. It works by inhibiting cell division. In vitro studies have recently shown that Taxol is cytotoxic to spindle cells from Kaposi's sarcoma lesions.

In the past, chemo regimens often used single agents. Drawbacks to standard chemotherapy include possible suppression of the bone marrow, nausea, vomiting, fever, diarrhea and hair loss. To keep the immune system protected, COLONY-STIMULATING FACTOR drugs may be prescribed. These drugs, synthesized versions of naturally occurring hormones that are known to stimulate the bone marrow, increase the number of white blood cells. There has been some controversy about the actual value of these drugs. Liposomal technology may be the answer to some of the problems associated with chemotherapy and its side effects. A liposome is a fatty substance that can be used to encapsulate a drug. The process makes the chemotherapeutic drug less toxic and more target-specific to cancer cells, while causing it to bypass the healthy ones. Examples of new KS therapies include antiangiogenesis agents and immune modulating devices. Angiogenesis (new blood formation), necessary for the growth and metastasis of tumors, refers to a normal body process that can be abnormally stimulated. Cancer tumors in general seem to secrete factors that can switch on the body's angiogenesis function, so that a tumor can induce the growth of capillaries that will then sustain it with a supply of blood. Inhibiting angiogenesis, some theorize, may inhibit the growth of tumors. Fumagillin, SP-PG, and Platelet 4 factor are antiangiogenic drugs that have recently attracted attention.

Remission from KS after shark-cartilage treatments has also been documented. Shark cartilage contains an agent that inhibits the growth of new blood vessels that make solid tumors. Retinoic acid (trade name Retin-A) a derivative of vitamin A, is a common antiacne ointment that has also been investigated for use in AIDS-associated KS.

To date, there is an absence of guidelines on what treatments should be used and when. Much of the published clinical information on KS is often inconsistent and confusing. Doctors are further challenged by the fact that people with KS often have different types of lesions that progress at different rates with concurrent opportunistic infections and different states of immune dysfunction.

One of the biggest mysteries of the AIDS epidemic has yet to be clarified; scientists have been perplexed over why KS suddenly turned from a rare nuisance to a common killer in gay men with AIDS. Before the epidemic was recognized in 1981, Kaposi's sarcoma was known primarily as a benign disorder affecting a few hundred older Jewish men and men of Mediterranean descent in the United States each year, and many people who took immunosuppressant drugs to prevent rejection of transplanted organs. It also affected many Africans. Now it is a highly aggressive cancer that contributes to the death of thousands of young gay men with AIDS each year. Kaposi's sarcoma is 20,000 times more common in people with AIDS than in those without it. Among those with AIDS, it is far more prevalent among gay and bisexual men. The epidemiology of KS in women is filled with conflicting reports, but one thing is clear: Women develop KS far less frequently than men. Women with AIDS are more likely to have Kaposi's sarcoma if they were infected by bisexual men than by intravenous drug users. The introduction of a previously unknown virus that coincided with the advent of the epidemic of AIDS could explain such a phenomenon. A number of efforts have been made to link known infectious agents with KS, but none has succeeded.

Central Africa contains the other population in which KS is relatively common. Before the AIDS epidemic, KS was the third most common cancer in Uganda. With the arrival of AIDS, it is now the most common cancer there.

In the early 1990s, researchers speculated that KS may not be a true, or spontaneous, cancer at all. Several claims were made that certain CYTOKINES (naturally occurring proteins) induce the growth of AIDS-associated KS in the test tube. These have included interleukin-6 (IL-6), the HIV protein called TAT, interleukin-1B (IL-1B), TUMOR NECROSIS FACTOR (TNF) alpha, gamma interferon, and platelet factor 4. Some say the disease is caused by an infectious agent—CYTOME-GALOVIRUS (CMV) has been named as a suspect, as has the HUMAN PAPILLOMA VIRUS (HPV). Other data suggest that contact with feces in anal-oral sex may be a primary mode of transmission, if KS is indeed caused by an infectious agent. Others have found evidence that a natural body protein called Ocostatin M may be a growth factor in the development of KS cells. Finally, some researchers have suggested that a new herpes virus, popularly known as KSHV, plays a role in the development of KS. They believe that they have fulfilled the epidemiological criteria for establishing KSHV as the cause of KS because (1) the virus is found in KS lesions of all subtypes; (2) the virus is not found in other tumors, except for BCL; (3) there is a biological gradient since virus is found in a KS lesion and in tissues close to the lesion but not in tissues farther away; 4) there is a temporal association—the virus appears in the white blood cells of some patients before they develop lesions; (5) these findings have been reproduced in several labs; and (6) there is a biological plausibility, since the virus belongs to a family of organisms that is thought to cause cancers. Other researchers are unconvinced that KSHV8 is the cause of KS. Many have found the virus in a number of different neoplasms and prefer to call the virus human herpes virus 8 (HHV8) instead of KSHV.

If KS is indeed caused by a herpes virus, there is a possibility that an antiviral drug may have a therapeutic effect. FOSCARNET may be the available treatment with the greatest potential, as it has activity against all known herpes viruses. The KS virus controversy is a long way from being resolved; in the meantime, trials and studies on the effect of foscarnet on KS can be expected.

A study published by a Columbia University research team in 1994 found DNA that was clearly of nonhuman origin in about 90 percent of KS tumors taken from a sample of gay men with AIDS. The molecular sequence of the DNA—its "fingerprint"—bears a resemblance to members of the large family of herpes viruses, suggesting an undiscovered herpes virus causes Kaposi's sarcoma. It is possible, however, that the microbe was merely an opportunistic invader that showed up in KS tumors after they were growing and when patients' immune defenses were down because of advanced AIDS.

Starting with the hypothesis that any infectious agent causing KS is present in the cancers but not in normal skin, the Columbia team sought a new way to identify a virus that might have escaped a detection through other methods. Using a technique known as representational difference analysis (RNA), developed by scientists at the Cold Spring Harbor Laboratory on Long Island, they took tissue with and without KS from the same patient to try to identify extra DNA that would have come from an infectious agent. Using other standard methods, the team tested tissue taken from biopsies from 27 people who had died of AIDS and found that 25 had the unique DNA sequences. The sequences were not found in 85 non-KS tissues from people without AIDS. More recently the team looked for the viral DNA fragments in a more diverse group of Kaposi patients: homosexuals infected with HIV, homosexuals not infected with HIV, and heterosexuals not infected with HIV. They used the presumed viral fragments isolated from the earlier experiments as "probes" to study the contents of cells from the new subjects. The fragments, known as sequences of DNA, are unique and seem to place the agent in the herpes virus family. The sequences closely resemble those of the EPSTEIN-BARR VIRUS, which causes INFECTIOUS MONONUCLEOSIS and has been linked to two cancers in humans. The agent also resembles the saimiri virus, a member of the herpes family that causes lymphoma in New World monkeys. The team found the telltale DNA fragments in virtually all the KS patients.

The scientists did not isolate and determine the complete structure of the virus, and even if it turns out to be a previously unknown virus they have not proved that it was the cancer's cause. The possibility exists that the virus is present in KS only after the tumor develops. Nevertheless, it is the first clear evidence that strongly implicates a specific type of virus in development of KS. The finding holds promise for a test for the disease and could lead to effective therapies for it. Some drugs are effective against herpes viruses, and although KS patients have been treated with various antimicrobial drugs case by case, there have been no systematic studies of such therapy for KS and herpes virus.

As explained earlier not all scientists agree about whether KS is a true cancer or merely a skin growth in reaction to infection by an unknown agent. Cancers are generally characterized by one type of cell that mutates and begins to proliferate without control. Although many of the cells that compose a KS lesion are spindle shaped like fibroblasts (a cell that contributes to the formation of connective tissue fibers), they are derived at first from various cell types. But as the lesion advances, one cell line might become dominant, making the KS growth resemble a cancerous tumor.

Whatever the initial cause, everyone agrees that cytokines and other growth factors play a primary role in the development, growth, and spread of KS. The list of these growth factors is quite long, and besides bFGH and TAT, includes a host of other fibroblast growth factors: PDGF (platelet-derived growth factor), IL-1, IL-6, TNF-alpha, onconstatin-M, scatter factor, and others. Inhibitors of any of these factors may hold potential as treatments for KS. The future treatment of KS will probably rely on combination approaches that address all the various factors that contribute to the development of KS. It is safe to say that the focus is shifting from the standard anticancer chemotherapies.

Karnofsky index (or scale)   Clinical estimate of a patient's physical state, performance, and prognosis. The scale is from 100 (perfectly well) to O (dead). It is used in studying cancer and chronic illness.

Kegels   A series of exercises to strengthen the pubococcygeal (P.C.) muscles, which aid in the enjoyment of sex and ease in reaching orgasm. Kegel exercises also help women prepare for childbirth. Also called elevator exercises.

kemron   Kemron is an oral form of ALPHA-INTERFERON given in doses of more than 100,000 times lower than in conventional subcutaneous administration. At one point Kenyan researchers reported dramatic improvements, including "HIV-seroreversions" (that is, HIV-POSITIVE to HIV-negative), with the drug. Subsequent studies have failed both to replicate these results and to find any benefit to kemron.

Kennedy-Cranston Amendment   In 1987, Senator Jesse Helms sponsored legislation forbidding the use of federal funds to "promote or encourage, directly, homosexual sexual activities," and requiring instead that all sex education materials "emphasize" sexual abstinence outside of heterosexual marriage and complete abstinence from drug use. The Helms Amendment was replaced, after one year in effect, by a compromise engineered by Senators Edward M. Kennedy and Alan Cranston. The Kennedy-Cranston Amendment forbade use of federal funds only for materials "designed to promote or encourage, directly" IV drug abuse or homosexual or heterosexual activity. When it passed the Kennedy-Cranston Amendment in 1988, Congress also stipulated that federally funded HIV education "contain material, and be presented in a manner, that is specifically directed toward the group for which such materials are intended." It ordered that the prohibition on promoting or encouraging homosexuality and drug abuse "may not be continued to restrict . . . accurate information about various means to reduce an individual's risk . . . provided that any informational materials used are not obscene." This satisfied proponents of HIV education, who took the position that even the most explicit messages were "designed to promote" risk reduction.

ketoconazole   An antifungal medication, available in pill and liquid form, that is effective against a variety of fungal infections such as oral, vaginal, and esophageal thrush and CRYPTOCOCCOSIS. Ketoconazole requires acid in the stomach to be absorbed into the system. Other medicines that neutralize stomach acids should therefore not be taken until at least two hours after taking ketoconazole. Ketoconazole may also alter the blood levels of either Dilantin or fluconazole, and taking these drugs together is generally not recommended. Also not recommended is the use of the antihistamines Hismanal and Seldane along with ketoconazole, since the combination may cause arrhythmias and cardiac toxicity. Possible side effects include nausea, vomiting, hormonal problems (menstrual problems and reduced sex drive), rash, headaches, and liver damage. Brand name is Nizoral.

ketotifen   An antihistamine approved in Europe, ketotifen is also a TUMOR NECROSIS FACTOR alpha inhibitor that may be useful in the treatment of AIDS-related wasting. Studies report that the drug has potent anti-inflammatory activity and reduces edema, rashes, and allergy-associated dermatitis. It may have activity against ulcerative colitis. A study of ketotifen for EOSINOPHILIC gastroenteritis, a wasting syndrome of unknown cause, reported substantial weight gains. A number of studies note that the drug's chief side effects are appetite stimulation and weight gain.

kidneys   The organs that remove poisons and other harmful waste from the body in the form of urine. They are located in the small of the back on each side of the spine.

killer cell   A general name for immune cells that kill cancerous and virus-infected cells. Among the killer cells are killer T CELLs (cytotoxic T-lymphocytes), NK (natural killer) cells, and K CELLs.

kinins   A group of vasoactive mediators formed in body tissues and produced following tissue injury. Kinins are capable of influencing smooth muscle contraction, inducing hypotension, increasing the blood flow and permeability of small blood capillaries, and inciting pain.

kinky   In slang, pertaining to any unconventional sexual behavior or desire.

kiss   A touch or contact with the lips. Kisses may be light and gentle or passionate, dry ("social" kisses) or wet (French kisses). They may be tokens of affection, greeting, or reverence.

kissing   French kissing is considered to be a practice with a low risk of HIV transmission and dry kissing is considered to have almost no risk of HIV transmission. Given that the AIDS virus has been found in saliva, although only in low concentrations, French kissing, also called deep kissing or tongue kissing, cannot be considered completely safe. An infection through very long and intimate deep kisses is, however, not very likely. If one of the partners carries the virus and the other suffers from bleeding gums or other, even slight, injuries inside the mouth, there could be danger. Dry kissing, and social kissing, on the other hand, do not involve an exchange of saliva or any other body fluid. This is also true of kissing any other part of the body, except, of course, the anus, the vaginal opening and the tip of the penis. Any other part of the body may be kissed without any fear of infection as long as the skin is intact.

Klebsiella   Bacteria found in the feces that can cause cystitis.

knowledge and ignorance   The literature on AIDS has attempted, and attempts, to teach us the "facts" about this disease, or to provide a narrative account of scientific discovery and developing public health policy. In addition to precipitating a crisis that is medical, political, financial, and social, AIDS has precipitated a crisis of signification. The "meaning" of AIDS continues to be hotly contested. That there is a powerful cultural narrative surrounding AIDS (as there is around every cultural phenomenon) goes without saying; analysis of this narrative reveals that AIDS has given rise to a semantic as well as a pathological epidemic.

An analysis of AIDS discourse by author Paula Treichler reveals that "no clear line can be drawn between the facticity of scientific and nonscientific (mis)conceptions." Treichler observes that AIDS is both a material and a linguistic reality and notes that in speaking, writing, and thinking about AIDS, "the facts" change less often than the way in which they are used to construct the AIDS "text," or cultural narrative, and the meanings we are allowed, or able, to read from that text. Treichler focuses on one particular aspect of this linguistic reality—that it is constructed around a series of discursive oppositions fundamental and apparently natural. "Knowledge and ignorance" is one of these. In terms of this opposition, cultural analysts ask us to question: What is knowledge and what is ignorance? Is science knowledge and not-science ignorance? Who has access to knowledge and who is denied access to knowledge? Are scientists and other health care providers privy to knowledge that is "off-limits," or otherwise unaccessible to persons with HIV/AIDS? Cultural analysts and activists advise us to resist the luxury of listening to the thousands of language tapes playing in our heads that tell us in plain English, in black and white, what AIDS "really means." Within the context of this example, each of us is encouraged to use what science (or knowledge) offers us in ways that are selective, self-conscious, and pragmatic. Each of us is also encouraged to question whether, or to what extent, scientific discourse can be privileged.

Other discursive oppositions are: self and not-self; homosexual and heterosexual; active and passive; guilty and innocent; perpetrator and victim; vice and virtue; us and them; anus and vagina; sins of the parent and innocence of the child; love and death; sex and death; sex and money; death and money; science and not-science; doctor and patient; expert and patient; doctor and expert; addiction and abstention; contamination and cleanliness; life and death; injection and reception; instrument and receptacle; normal and abnormal; natural and alien; prostitute and paragon; whore and wife; safe sex and bad sex; safe sex and good sex. If we are to understand the AIDS text, to (re)read or (re)write the narrative more clearly and perceptively, then we must see how these discursive oppositions structure our thinking. We must *deconstruct* the text, in other words, so we can evaluate what goes into it and revise our thinking with less unrecognized conceptual bias.

kombucha   The kombucha (or Manchurian) "mushroom," a substance that is said to have anti-AIDS effects, is one of a number of organic "miracle" treatments that come and go with the seasons. The distributor of the kombucha states that according to "folklore," the kombucha is a super immune booster that can fight a list of ailments including AIDS, cancer, arthritis, constipation, hemorrhoids, stress, chronic fatigue syndrome, indigestion, gall- and kidney stones, high cholesterol, acne, diabetes, multiple sclerosis, memory loss, wrinkles, weight problems, gout, impotence, and hair loss. The kombucha is not really a mushroom at all—it is a yeast culture. It is not eaten, but placed in a large glass bowl with a solution of water, tea, and sugar. The culture grows there at room temperature for seven to ten days. During this time, the solution ferments to produce a "tonic" or tea which is drunk for its therapeutic properties.

There are safety concerns with kombucha, focusing on the storage of the mushroom and the fermentation process. The seven- to ten-day period in which the solution ferments may permit the contamination and growth of other organisms. Since it purportedly contains naturally occurring antibiotics, the chronic use of this substance raises concerns about developing bacterial strains that can resist standard, approved antibiotic drugs. Furthermore, nothing is known about how the ingredients may interact with other drugs. References to kombucha in the standard medical literature are, to date, few. Most of what has been written has appeared in articles in health food and alternative medicine newsletters and magazines.

KS   See KAPOSI'S SARCOMA.

KS-OI   Kaposi's sarcoma and opportunistic infections, an early designation for AIDS used by CDC officials when it was first reported in 1981.

kuru disease   A rapidly progressive neurological disease that is invariably fatal. The disease affects mostly adult women and children of both sexes of members of the Fore tribe of New Guinea. The disease is transmitted by the practice of ingesting tissue from a victim who has died and rubbing infected tissues over the body of women and children kin to the victim. Kuru disease is probably due to a transmissible slow infection rather than a slow virus.

K-Y   The brand name of a water-based lubricant. Unlike petroleum-based lubricants like Vaseline, it does not degrade latex and is therefore suitable for use with gloves in medical examinations and with condoms.

K-Y jelly   See K-Y.

L

L. acidophilus   See LACTOBACILLUS ACIDOPHILUS.

L. bulgaricus   See LACTOBACILLUS BULGARICUS.

labeled uses   Uses of a drug currently included in Food and Drug Administration approved labeling.

labia   Scientific term for lips of the vagina, usually used to denote the genital labia minora and labia majora.

labia majora   Large folds of skin-covered fatty tissue protecting the vagina and urethral openings.

labia minora   Small folds of mucous membrane inside the labia majora.

laboratory testing   Testing that is done in a room or building equipped for scientific experimentation, research, testing, or clinical studies of materials, fluids, or tissues obtained from patients.

labyrinthitis   Inflammation of the labyrinth (the internal ear consisting of osseous and membranous labyrinths). It can cause loss of balance or dizziness. It is caused by primary infection, trauma, complication of influenza, otitis media, or meningitis.

lactic acid   A mixture of lactic acid and lactic acid lactate, equivalent to a total 85 to 90 percent, by weight, of $C_3H_6O_3$. A colorless syrupy liquid formed in milk, sauerkraut, and in certain types of pickles by the fermentation of the sugars by microorganisms. It is also formed during muscular activity by the breakdown of glycogen.

lactobacillus   Any of a group of bacteria that create LACTIC ACID in the body. Plural is *lactobacilli*.

Lactobacillus acidophilus   The best-known type of acidophilus bacteria (bacteria attracted to acid), *Lactobacillus acidophilus* (*L. acidophilus*) produces lactic acid by fermenting sugars in milk. Found in milk, feces of infants fed by bottle, and in teeth and saliva. In the vagina it helps protect against infection. *L. acidophilus* is a beneficial or "friendly"

bacteria that performs an important function in the body. *Lactobacillus acidophilus* produces lactic acid by fermenting the sugars in milk. Live cultures of *L. acidophilus* can be found in yogurt or acidophilus milk and in the form of powders, capsules, tablets, and liquids available in health food stores. *L. acidophilus* is measured by the amount of viable bacteria per dosage (in the millions). Test tube studies have shown that *L. acidophilus* can inhibit the growth of CANDIDA ALBICANS (CANDIDIASIS), the fungus associated with "thrush" in the mouth, esophagus, or vagina. Varying levels of success have been reported using yogurt and *L. acidophilus* as a treatment for vaginal candidiasis. It has been suggested that *L. acidophilus* may be used to reimplant friendly bacteria in the gastrointestinal system, when they have been reduced by antibiotics, for instance. Finally, it has been suggested, also based on test tube studies, that *L. acidophilus* may have potential antibiotic effects of its own. There have been no reports of *L. acidophilus*–related toxicities; it is unknown whether the compound has any effects on the absorption of antibiotic medication.

Lactobacillus bulgaricus   A bacillus found in fermented milk. Milk fermented with this organism is known as Bulgarian milk.

Lactobacillus casei factor   See FOLIC ACID.

lactose intolerance   The inability to digest milk products owing to the absence or low activity of the enzyme lactase, which breaks down milk sugar.

Lambda Legal Defense and Education Fund   National organization committed to achieving full recognition of the civil rights of lesbians, gay men, and people with HIV/AIDS through impact litigation, education, and public policy work. Founded in 1973, Lambda is not-for-profit and tax-exempt. *The Lambda Update* is the tri-annual newsletter of the Lambda Legal Defense and Education Fund. It contains docket listings and articles about crucial cases and legal issues of relevance to lesbians, gay men, and people with HIV/AIDS. The *Update* includes an AIDS docket. Lambda has addressed a broad spectrum of AIDS-related challenges, cases, and issues in areas such as employment, standards of care, prisons/confidentiality and the right to privacy, and criminal and family law.

Lamblia intestinalis   See GIARDIA LAMBLIA.

lambliasis   See GIARDIASIS.

lamivudine   See 3TC.

Langerhans cells   Antigen-presenting cells, found primarily in the epidermis, that emigrate to local LYMPH NODES to become DENDRITIC CELLS; they are very active in presenting antigen to T CELLS.

laparoscopy   A procedure in which a lighted tube is inserted into the body below the navel so that the pelvic organs can be closely examined.

large granular lymphocytes (LGLs)   A group of morphologically defined LYMPHOCYTEs containing the majority of K CELL and NK CELL activity. They have both lymphocyte and MONOCYTE/MACROPHAGE markers.

large simple trial (LST)   A type of expanded access mechanism allowing patients to take an experimental drug, or drug combination, not yet approved by the United States Food and Drug Administration and available for general prescription use. Large simple trials are used to measure with certainty whether a particular treatment has an effect on survival. The "simple" in large simple trial refers to simplifying the study design so that researchers do not have to collect much information. Additionally, the paper work required to enroll a patient in these trials is greatly reduced. The methodology for these trials was developed by Dr. Richard Peto of Oxford University.

In the mid-1990s, the LST approach was proposed by New York's Treatment Action Group (TAG) to answer questions pertaining to PROTEASE INHIBITORS, such as How are we to determine when and how well they work? and How easily can HIV evolve to overcome this new therapeutic challenge? TAG proposed a large two-year clinical efficacy trial comparing various protease inhibitors to a placebo in a sample of approximately 18,000 people with HIV. As proposed, this LST would go beyond previous parallel track or expanded access programs that have allowed people failing standard therapies to receive experimental drugs even before FDA approval. It was proposed that the phase II/III LST efficacy trial commence immediately after the preliminary phase I safety trials were completed. The trial would be open to nearly anyone with HIV, and participants could take any drugs they desired in addition to the protease inhibitor.

The proposed trial would offer access to the experimental protease inhibitor, one-third of the trial participants would receive placebo rather than protease inhibitor in blinded fashion, i.e., neither the doctors nor participants would know who was in the placebo arm. But TAG also proposed a nonplacebo trial comparing different doses of protease inhibitors for people who have CD4 counts of less than 50, who cannot tolerate any of the NUCLEOSIDE ANALOGS, or who have reached advanced disease in the large simple trial.

As proposed, the large simple trial concept is one that has a number of attractive features. The data collected in the LST would be much more extensive than that previously gathered from expanded access participants. The information on clinical outcome (incidence of opportunistic infections, death, etc.) would be recorded by people's usual physicians and would reflect the effects that a certain drug or combination of drugs has during actual use by the public. Finally, LSTs lend themselves to subset analysis, in which particular subgroups are monitored for the predictive power of laboratory tests, drug-drug interactions, and specific toxic reactions that might normally go unobserved.

The LST concept also has a number of immediate drawbacks. Conducting a large trial as proposed would consume huge amounts of resources in terms of research dollars, risk to human beings exposed to an experimental drug, and attention diverted from other potential therapies inching their way through the pipeline. Additionally, cooperation between industry, government agencies, patients from diverse communities, and primary care providers, essential in completing these trials, does not have a long history. One often-heard criticism of LST designs is the belief that participants might have to remain on one treatment, excluding all others for the duration of the trial. The criticism is countered by the argument that, if that were the case, then a lot of the polemics about "body counts" determining trials analysis would have more validity. Those in favor of LSTs believe that treatment restrictions are not only unnecessary, they are undesirable.

LAS   See LYMPHADENOPATHY SYNDROME.

laser surgery   See LASER THERAPY.

laser therapy   The use of extremely narrow, intense and controlled light beams in the diagnosis and treatment of some forms of cancer. A laser beam can sever, fuse, or eliminate body tissue. The first working laser (light amplification by stimulated emission of radiation) was developed in 1960. Lasers were first medically used in 1961 to treat skin discoloration and to repair detached retinas. Laser therapy has several advantages over traditional surgical treatment: It is more precise than a scalpel; the heat produced by the laser sterilizes the surgery site; there is less chance for infection; less operating time may be required; healing time is frequently reduced; there is less bleeding, swelling, and scarring; and more procedures can be done on an outpatient basis. The major disadvantages associated with laser treatment are the relatively small number of trained surgeons, the high cost of the equipment, and the fact that strict safety precautions must be observed.

Lassa fever   A viral disease with a relatively high mortality rate in Africa. Lassa fever is caused by an arenavirus. The common carrier is a native African rat species. Acute high fever, abdominal and chest pain, headache, dizziness, cough, nausea, diarrhea, and vomiting are among the symptoms. The skin and membranes may begin to hemorrhage.

latency   The period between the initiation of a stimulus, or contracting of a disease, and the response or clinical manifestation of the disease.

Clinical latency is an asymptomatic period in the early years of HIV infection. The period of latency is characterized in the peripheral blood by near-normal CD4 counts and HIV levels. Cellular latency is the period after HIV has integrated its GENOME into a cell's DNA but has not yet begun to replicate.

One of several widely held myths about AIDS in conventional medicine before 1992 was that HIV remains dormant, or latent, for up to 10 years before initiating immune damage. Findings presented that year by Dr. Anthony Fauci and associates indicate that much of the damage done to the immune system occurs during this evidently asymptomatic stage. Although the clinical course of HIV infection is characterized by a prolonged period of latency after primary infection, HIV replication continues at high levels in the lymphoid organs during this period. Since the lymphoid organs are the major reservoirs of virus and sites of viral replication, peripheral blood measurements (measurements of P24 ANTIGEN, NEOPTERIN levels and CD4 cells) do not accurately reflect the total body burden of HIV infection. By the time of the onset of symptoms, the lymphoid organs will have become massive generators of the vectors of disease. These findings suggest the importance of the widespread use of the POLYMERASE TECHNOLOGY that measures total body viral load.

Latency may also refer to the state of being concealed, hidden, inactive, or inapparent; for example, a MICROBE is said to be latent when it is in the body but not actively reproducing, invading tissues, or causing symptoms. Once in the body, these microbes remain in the body. PNEUMOCYSTIS CARINII, TOXOPLASMA GONDII, HERPES SIMPLEX VIRUS, and CYTOMEGALOVIRUS are microbes that are latent or dormant in most healthy people. They remain so until something disorders the immune system and permits them to become active.

latent period (reaction time)   Time between application of a stimulus and first detectable response in an irritable tissue.

See LATENCY.

latex   A natural or synthetic rubbery substance used to make flexible, sterile nonporous barrier materials like condoms and surgical gloves.

latex agglutination test   A medical test to see if antigens of a known condition have already caused a defensive (antibody) reaction against that condition. If antibodies are present and clump with the known antigen, the test response is positive. In a latex agglutination test, antigens are exposed to latex particles (antigens clump better when exposed to latex particles). Agglutination occurs as a reaction against various diseases, primarily infections. Whenever the body is exposed to bacteria, viruses, fung, or toxins containing antigens, the body reacts by producing antibodies. These antibodies then attempt to fight off the specific organism that has invaded the body. Antibodies found in the patient's blood indicate that the patient has already been exposed to a particular infection. The exposure may have occurred many years previously, or it may be of very recent origin.

latex allergy   Allergy to the fluid or sap produced by some plants. People with this allergy could be allergic to such simple things as balloons, doctors' gloves or condoms made out of latex. This is a potential problem for doctors, fast-food workers, toll takers, janitors, police officers, and especially health care workers who routinely wear latex gloves as protection against AIDS. Mild sensitivity can produce a skin rash. Extreme sensitivity can include symptoms similar to hay fever or asthma. Severe allergic reactions to latex can include anaphylactic shock and death. Medical and dental personnel should ask every patient about the possibility of latex allergy, especially those scheduled for surgery. Patients who have had multiple surgeries are at high risk. Also at high risk are those allergic to bananas, chestnuts, avocados, and some tropical fruits. Potential sexual partners should also be queried about latex allergy. The government has yet to set standards on safer alternatives.

LAV   See LYMPHADENOPATHY-ASSOCIATED VIRUS.

L-carnitine   A naturally occurring cell constituent that modulates fat metabolism, in particular the mitochondrial intake of lipid derivatives. L-carnitine has been proposed as a treatment for AIDS-related wasting and the myopathy associated with AZT.

LD-50   Median lethal dose of a substance that will kill 50 percent of the animals receiving that dosage. Dosage is usually calculated on amount of material given per gram or kilogram of body weight or the amount per unit of body surface area.

lecithin   A fatty substance of the group called phospholipids (phosphoglycerides), found in blood, bile, brain, egg yolk, nerves, and other animal tissues. It yields stearic acid, glycerol, phosphoric acid, and choline on hydrolysis.

lectin   One of several plant proteins that stimulate lymphocytes to proliferate. Lectins are commonly MITOGENS as well.

Legionella pneumophila   A species of GRAM-NEGATIVE bacterium that causes Legionnaires' disease and Pontiac fever. *Legionella* has been isolated from numerous locations including tap water, soil, cooling tower water, aerosolized droplets from heat-exchange systems, human lung tissue, respiratory secretions, and blood.

lentivirus   A subfamily of RETROVIRUSES that until recently was known to include only the VISNA viruses in sheep, the equine infectious anemia virus in horses, and the caprine arthritis-encephalitis virus in goats. Newly recognized members of the family include the HUMAN IMMUNODEFICIENCY VIRUS (HIV), the SIMIAN IMMUNODEFICIENCY VIRUS (SIV), the feline immunodeficiency virus (FIV), and the bovine immunodeficiency virus (BIV). The original ungulate lentiviruses produce chronic diseases in their natural hosts. Visna viruses cause a chronic interstitial pneumonitis similar to that seen in AIDS and young children. All cause ENCEPHALITIS. The diseases are characterized by erratic relapses and remissions. The chronic carrier state, in which infected animals themselves do not get sick but can transmit the virus to other animals, is common.

Lentiviruses persist in the body by evading natural defense mechanisms. Lentiviruses can cross the blood-brain barrier, destroy brain tissue, and remain in the body in a chronic subclinical state (period before appearance of typical symptoms of a disease) for long periods. HIV is a lentivirus that causes forms of mental incapacity in an estimated 70 to 80 percent of patients and end-stage dementia in many.

leprosy   A chronic infectious disease caused by MYCOBAC-TERIUM LEPRAE. It progresses slowly and may manifest itself in various clinical forms. The two principal, or polar, forms are lepromatous and tuberculoid. The lepromatous form is characterized by the development of lesions in the skin and symmetrical involvement of the peripheral nerves, yielding skin anesthesia, muscle weakness, and paralysis. The lepromatous form tends to involve the skin, respiratory tract, and testes. In the tuberculoid forms, skin anesthesia occurs early and the nerve lesions are symmetrical; this form is usually benign. Lepromatous leprosy is much more contagious and malignant. Two other types of leprosy include borderline and indeterminant leprosy. Borderline leprosy possesses clinical and bacteriological features representing a combination of the two polar forms. Indeterminant types of leprosy present fewer skin lesions and less abundant bacteria in the lesions.

lesbian   A woman sexually and emotionally attracted predominantly to other women and who identifies herself voluntarily as such.

The myths that lesbians are at low risk for AIDS, that lesbians don't and can't get AIDS, that AIDS has nothing to do with lesbians, persisted well into the first decade of the epidemic. That lesbians suffered through the negligence and bias of HIV researchers early in the epidemic and beyond is unquestionable. The lack of research or documentation on female-to-female TRANSMISSION clearly helped fuel the myths, as did the CENTERS FOR DISEASE CONTROL AND PREVENTION's initial "stance" that there was no female-to-female transmission.

Today, however, cases of AIDS transmitted between lesbians have been reported. The following factors are also likely to put lesbians at higher risk: sharing needles or other IV drug paraphernalia; having or having had repeated vaginal or anal intercourse with men who have been actively gay or bisexual since 1979, with people whose sexual history is unknown, with women who use IV drugs, or with HEMO-PHILIACS or others who received blood transfusions between 1979 and 1985; having received blood transfusions or blood products between 1979 and 1985; and having used semen for donor insemination from a donor in a high-risk group who is known to be ANTIBODY-POSITIVE, or whose risk status is unknown. Another potential risk is the unsafe use of needles for piercing and tattooing.

Another myth about lesbians is that if they are not exposed to high-risk factors or high-risk groups, they do not have to be concerned about AIDS. Although they are likely to be at lower risk for AIDS medically, lesbians are still at high risk for discrimination by virtue of their HOMOSEXUAL-ITY. The public often perceives lesbians to be in the same high-risk category as gay men, and as a result vulnerable to the same discrimination and hostility and the same AIDS hysteria as their gay male counterparts. Fear of AIDS has become synonymous with fear of homosexuality, a phenomenon that potentially threatens the rights of gay men and lesbians relevant to employment, housing, and freedom to travel. Legislative measures generated during the AIDS crisis affect lesbians as well as their gay male counterparts, and discriminatory practices by insurance companies affect gay males and lesbians and heterosexuals as well.

Many lesbians have been personally affected by AIDS-related deaths or illnesses of people close to them. The AIDS epidemic raises the need to address problems of substance abuse, and especially IV drug abuse, in the lesbian community. Insemination choices and coparenting options have been limited by AIDS. Many lesbians are involved in AIDS-related work as volunteers and paid workers. Lesbian contributions have strengthened and enriched the entire gay and lesbian community and furthered the fight against AIDS.

For lesbians who would like to make sex safer—if they are unsure of their own or their partners' HIV/STD status, or if they or their partners are HIV-POSITIVE—several guidelines are suggested to reduce the risk of transmission. Avoid contact where either partner's blood or vaginal fluids can get into the other partner's body through the mouth, vagina, anus, or a cut in the skin. Use non-powdered surgical gloves for digital penetration and fisting. Surgical gloves can be found at most drugstores. Finger cots can also be used for digital penetration. Change gloves between vaginal and anal insertion, or use one hand for vaginal and the other for anal sex. Use latex or plastic barriers for oral sex and rimming. Special care should be taken if either partner is menstruating. Several products can be used as barriers, such as unlubricated latex condoms (which can be cut into flat barriers by cutting off the tips and cutting through one edge before unrolling), dental dams, or plastic wrap.

Other guidelines advise the use of water-based lubricant, which makes safe sex not only more comfortable and enjoyable but safer. Activities to avoid include sharing sex toys without putting a fresh condom on between uses or washing thoroughly with soap and warm water; S&M activities that draw blood when the blood may get in eyes or open cuts; and sharing IV needles without cleaning them with bleach.

Today there are lesbian-sensitive AIDS-related resources; there are services for lesbian inmates and ex-offenders who are HIV-positive. There are programs that affirm the lives of lesbians living with AIDS by recognizing and responding to the fact that lesbians with HIV are in many ways a unique group. Their clinical symptoms can differ from those of men and they have different psychosocial concerns and needs than their heterosexual or bisexual female peers. Data are being collected about lesbians and are being used to shape service delivery, education, prevention, and transmission messages.

lesbianism   Homosexual practice between women.

lesion   Any pathological or traumatic damage to tissue, which may cause a loss of function of the affected or surrounding tissue.

lesser AIDS   See AIDS-RELATED CONDITION.

leucovorin   A vitamin, also called FOLINIC ACID or citrovorum factor, long used to counteract the effects of the anticancer drug METHOTREXATE. While that is still its primary use, it is now also used by people with HIV to counteract the toxicity of drugs used for opportunistic infections. These drugs include PYRIMETHAMINE, SULFADIAZINE, CLINDAMYCIN, and TRIMETREXATE.
FOLIC ACID is a B vitamin essential for a wide variety of biochemical reactions in the body, including the synthesis of components of proteins, DNA, and RNA. A number of ANTIBIOTICS and anticancer drugs, called folic-acid antagonists, interfere with the body's ability to use folic acid. When that happens, serious side effects, including life-threatening anemia, can occur. Leucovorin is a water-soluble B vitamin that counteracts the effects of folic-acid antagonists. It is available in tablet form or as a sterile powder for intravenous or intramuscular injection. The injectable form is used primarily when the digestive tract is not functioning well enough to absorb the oral drug, a condition that often occurs during anticancer chemotherapy. Leucovorin may increase the toxicity of the anticancer drug FLUOROURACIL. Deaths from severe digestive tract disease have been reported in elderly people receiving leucovorin and fluorouracil. Leucovorin in high doses may counteract the antiseizure effect of epilepsy drugs and increase the frequency of seizures in children. The trade name is Wellcovorin.

leukemia   A chronic or acute disorder of the blood-forming elements characterized by the unrestrained growth of LEUKOCYTES and their precursors in the blood and BONE MARROW. Types of leukemia are classified on the basis of the dominant cell type involved.

leukocyte   A white blood cell essential to the body's defenses against infection. Leukocytes may be classified into two main groups: granulocytes and agranulocytes (nongranular). Granulocytes possess granules in their cytoplasm and include neutrophils (cells that gobble up microbes), eosinophils, and basophils. Agranulocytes do not possess granules in their cytoplasm and include monocytes and LYMPHOCYTES (cells that recognize foreign material). The normal leukocyte count is 4,000 to 8,000 per milliliter of blood. In people with certain infections, especially bacterial infections, leukocyte count is high (this condition is called *leukocytosis*). In people with viral infections, including HIV infection, leukocyte count is low (*leukopenia*).
See also LYMPHOCYTE; LYMPHOPENIA; NEUTROPENIA.

leukocyte functional antigen (LFA)   One of a group of three molecules that mediate intercellular adhesion between LEUKOCYTES and other cells in an ANTIGEN-nonspecific fashion.

leukocytosis   A condition of the blood in which there is an abnormally large number of LEUKOCYTES (white blood cells), a condition that may occur in acute infection.

leukoencephalopathy   Any of a group of diseases affecting the white matter of the brain.

leukopenia   A condition of the blood in which there is an abnormally a low number of LEUKOCYTES (white blood cells). The condition may occur in viral infections, including HIV infection. Leukopenia may also be caused by drugs or BONE MARROW failure.

leukoplakia   Formation of white spots or patches on the MUCOUS MEMBRANE of the tongue or cheek. The spots are smooth, irregular in size and shape, hard, and occasionally fissured. The lesions may become malignant.

leukotrienes   A collection of metabolites of arachidonic acid, which have powerful pharmacological effects.

levamisole hydrochloride   An anthelminthic drug used originally in veterinary medicine. It is now used as adjuvant therapy in treating metastatic colorectal cancer. The trade name is Tramisol.

LFA   See LEUKOCYTE FUNCTIONAL ANTIGEN.

LGV   See LYMPHOGRANULOMA VENEREUM.

libido   In psychoanalysis, a Freudian term for sexual instinct, drive, or psychic energy.

licorice   A dried root of the licorice plant, glycyrrhiza glabra, used as a flavoring agent, demulcent, and mild expectorant. Ingestion of large amounts of licorice can cause salt retention, excess potassium loss in the urine, and elevated blood pressure.

lidocaine   A local anesthetic drug. Its trade name is Xylocaine.

life and death   One of the oppositions that structures and determines the discourse of AIDS. Author Paula A. Treichler notes that AIDS is no different from other linguistic constructions thought to transmit preexisting ideas and represent real-world entities but, in fact, do neither. Oppositions such as "life and death" help construct the disease and make it intelligible. We can think about AIDS in terms of life or death, as the possible loss of life, in terms of our mortality, and as a life-and-death struggle.

life cycle   The series of changes in form undergone by any developing organism from its earliest stage to the recurrence of that same stage in the subsequent generation.

life expectancy   The expected remaining average number of years of life for a group of persons of a given age according to a mortality table. The data from which such tables are constructed may be obtained as much as two decades or more prior to their date of publication. This is particularly true for data used for insurance purposes.

life insurance Insurance that provides for the payment of a specific amount to a designated beneficiary in the event of the death of the insured. Illinois-based Guarantee Trust Life Insurance was the first company in the nation to offer life insurance to people infected with the HIV virus. The company, which specializes in insuring high-risk individuals, announced that it would test-market the coverage in 1997. (Guarantee Trust Life Insurance believes that many otherwise healthy HIV-positive individuals are more appropriately viewed as having a treatable chronic illness rather than a terminal disease.) Other companies that do not share these beliefs have said they have no plans to offer similar coverage to HIV-positive individuals. These companies contend that the underlying principle is the same for anyone with any other serious, life-threatening disease.

lipopolysaccharide See ENDOTOXIN.

liposomal amphotericin B Liposomal amphotericins are "high-tech" versions of standard amphotericin (used to treat such life-threatening fungal infections as CRYPTOCOCCAL MENINGITIS as well as other fungal infections that are resistant to other antifungal drugs), in which the drug is encapsulated in tiny fat globules known as liposomes. Liposomal amphotericin must be administered through INTRAVENOUS infusion like the standard drug, but it is hypothesized that the liposomes will be preferentially absorbed at the sites of infection and avoid most of amphotericin's side effects. Toxic effects of amphotericin can include fever, chills, muscle pain, phlebitis, vomiting, potassium loss, kidney dysfunction, and anemia. Approval of liposomal versions of amphotericin B in the United States has been delayed because of a number of factors, including the size and lack of experience of the companies behind the products and other problems peculiar to liposomes. For example, although lipsomal encapsulation does in fact markedly reduce the incidence of adverse effects, improved EFFICACY is not a certainty. The amphotericin must be released from the liposome to be active, and depending on the packaging, this may not occur readily. Also, laboratory comparisons have shown that to be effective, doses of liposomal amphotericin B need to be significantly higher than doses of the standard amphotericin. Unless the liposomal drug's bioavailability and its uptake by infected cells is significantly higher, using liposomal amphotericin may just be a very elaborate and expensive way to lower the dosage of AMPHOTERICIN B a patient is receiving. The jury is still out as to whether the drugs will only be a rarely used last resort or whether they represent a significant advance in the treatment of systemic fungal infections. Trade names are AmBisome, Amphocil, and ABLC.

liposomal chemotherapy Liposomal chemotherapy involves the use of chemotherapeutic agents encapsulated within LIPOSOMES (tiny fat globules that regulate the passage of the entrapped drug from the blood stream to specific sites). These agents have been successfully used in patients with AIDS-related KS. Liposomal chemotherapy drugs include liposomal daunorubicin and liposomal doxorubicin.

liposome The sealed concentric shell formed by certain lipid substances in an aqueous solution. As it forms, the liposome entraps a portion of the solution in the shell. Liposomes may be found inside a cell or in the bloodstream. Liposomes may be manufactured and filled with a variety of medications. These have been used to deliver substances to particular organs. These drugs may be more effective and less toxic than drugs given by other means.

lipoxgenase See LIPOXIDASE.

lipoxidase An enzyme that catalyzes the oxidation of the double bonds of an unsaturated fatty acid.

liquid nitrogen A substance used in the process of removing genital warts.

Listeria monocytogene A type of GRAM-POSITIVE BACTERIA. In humans, it produces such disorders as MENINGITIS and perinatal septicemia. Also called *Corynebacterium infantisepticum* and *Corynebacterium parvulum*.

listing of impairments A comprehensive listing, in SSDI and SSI regulations, of the most common diseases and medical conditions, including standards of diagnosis, medical proof, and evaluation to determine disability.

lithium carbonate A drug that is particularly useful in treating the manic phase of manic-depressive illness. Trade names are Eskalith, Lithane, Lithonate, and Litho-tabs. Given orally, it is readily absorbed and eliminated at a fast rate for five to six hours and eliminated at a much slower rate over the next 24 hours. It is essential to monitor the blood level of the drug in patients on this therapy. Side effects including fatigue, weakness, fine tremor of the hands, nausea and vomiting, thirst, and polyuria (the passing of an excessive quantity of urine) may be noticed in the first week of therapy. If these are mild, most will disappear, but the thirst, polyuria, and tremor tend to persist.

live-attenuated vaccine A vaccine composed of a live virus chemically or procedurally weakened so that it is incapable of causing disease.

lived-in home A residence owned and actually dwelled in by an applicant for or recipient of assistance; generally, it is the only kind of real estate whose ownership is permitted by welfare programs.

liver The largest organ in the body, situated on right side beneath the diaphragm, the liver secretes bile and is the site of a great many metabolic functions (see LIVER FUNCTION). Disorders of the liver and the associated bile ducts and gallbladder can have serious complications involving many organs in the body, all of which depend on the liver's products to support their activity.

Liver problems are frequent causes of illness and death in people with HIV infection, even in those previously considered healthy. Both physicians and patients should be aware of the symptoms, methods of diagnosis, and available treatments (and drug toxicities) for HIV-related liver conditions. Symptoms such as pain on the right side of the stomach, enlarged liver (hepatomegaly), jaundice (yellowing of eyes or skin), fever of unknown origin, fatigue, malaise, itching, and abnormal liver function tests (LFTs) deserve early and complete evaluation.

The majority of liver diseases in patients with HIV are caused by viruses (especially HEPATITIS B and HEPATITIS C) or opportunistic infections (MAC, CRYPTOSPORIDIOSIS, CMV). As early as 1990, studies suggested that the liver is an important site of HIV replication, too. There have been well-documented cases of liver inflammation during primary HIV infection, the initial flulike syndrome that often precedes SEROCONVERSION, and this is a strong indication that HIV attacks liver cells directly.

Cancers most commonly found in the liver of AIDS patients are NON-HODGKIN'S B cell LYMPHOMA and KAPOSI'S SARCOMA (KS). Up to one third of people with KS will have some involvement in the liver, but this generally remains asymptomatic, being found only at autopsy. In lymphoma, the GASTROINTESTINAL TRACT and liver are the most common sites of involvement outside of the lymph nodes. For non-Hodgkin's lymphoma, treatment with intensive chemotherapy can be beneficial.

Since the liver processes toxic compounds absorbed by the body, its cells are particularly sensitive to the side effects of medications. Many drugs used in AIDS therapy induce changes in liver enzymes or cause other impairments of liver function. Most drug-related toxicities can be reversed when the drug is discontinued or the dose lowered. But effect of drugs taken alone does not necessarily predict the combined effect of several drugs taken together.

Certain therapies commonly used for HIV or AIDS-related purposes are known to be particularly damaging to the liver. These include CLARITHROMYCIN, DAPSONE, dilantin, FLUCONAZOLE, FLUCYTOSINE, ISONIAZID, KETOCONAZOLE, RIFABUTIN, RIFAMPIN, and TMP/SMX (bactrim or septra). AZT, ddI and ddC do not seem to cause significant liver toxicity in most people with HIV. Physicians nonetheless must carefully monitor patients on NUCLEOSIDE ANALOG THERAPY who have progressively worsening liver function tests and evidence of enlarged livers. There is also concern that in some people with HIV and HEPATITIS C, the use of nucleoside analogs like AZT, ddI or ddC may cause additional liver damage.

Selective experimental and alternative therapies for liver disease include RIBAVIRIN (a nucleoside analog that has shown little efficacy against HIV, but which may be useful against chronic hepatitis); lamivudine (3TC; a nucleoside analog active against both HIV and hepatitis B in the test tube); alpha thymosin (a synthesized thymic peptide that has shown promise in phase I trials for chronic hepatitis B as well as HIV); thymic humoral factor (THF; another thymic hormone that has been investigated as a treatment for HIV); N-acetyl cysteine (NAC; a derivative of cysteine, essential for the production of the antioxidant glutathione in the body,

which has been studied as a treatment for HIV and is used to treat acetaminophen poisoning, which damages the liver); beta interferon (a second type of the interferon that has shown promise in small studies for treatment of chronic and acute hepatitis C); astragalus (an herb used in China reportedly for the purpose of boosting the immune system and preventing chemotherapy-related BONE MARROW SUPPRESSION and nausea); glycyrrhizin (a substance isolated from the root of the licorice plant and widely used in Japan against infectious diseases); milk thistle (specifically the seeds of "milk thistle" considered useful for such problems as cirrhosis, jaundice, hepatitis, diarrhea, and drug, alcohol, and chemical toxicity); and thiocitic acid (a synthetic version of a natural compound found in the liver and other tissues and also known as lipoic acid or alpha lipoic acid).

liver function   The liver has many critical functions, including filtering blood, eliminating toxins, secreting bile (a fluid that helps absorb and digest fat), and making clotting factors. It also converts sugar into triglycerides (lipids) and glycogen (a carbohydrate) to be stored for energy and, between meals, converts triglycerides, glycogen, and amino acids into blood sugar to meet the body's immediate energy needs. The work of the liver is particularly critical to the brain and central nervous system. These tissues receive their energy supply only from sugar, and so are extremely vulnerable to liver failure.

Various tests are available for liver disorders. These include tests for liver function and viral hepatitis. COMPUTERIZED AXIAL TOMOGRAPHY (the familiar CAT, or CT, scan) and ultrasound sonograms may also frequently be useful. Liver chemistry tests are an initial means for measuring the liver's condition. High blood levels of two common liver enzymes involved in amino acid breakdown (AST and ALT, also designated as SGOT and SGOT in lab reports) are a sign of acute liver cell injury. Such damage to cell integrity allows these chemicals to escape from the cells and is associated with viral hepatitis and the toxic effects of drugs and poisons.

Some specialists recommend a liver BIOPSY for HIV-positive patients with unexplained fever or abnormal liver tests. In this procedure, a segment of tissue is removed with a needle inserted through the skin. The tissue is then examined microscopically.

liver function test (LFT)   A blood test that measures the levels of specific enzymes and proteins produced by the liver. An elevated liver function is a sign of possible liver damage. Sometimes referred to as AST, ALT, SGOT, or SGPT.

liver Lactobacillus casei factor   See FOLIC ACID.

living will   A document detailing a person's wishes regarding artificial life support in the event of impending death. Living wills are not legally binding in all states. See also POWER OF ATTORNEY, MEDICAL DIRECTIVE, and NO CODE.

locus   A location or a place. In genetics, the specific site of a gene on a chromosome.

long-term asymptomatics Generally, HIV-positive persons who have remained asymptomatic for at least seven years. Why some HIV-infected people can remain asymptomatic for an unusually long time is not understood. Speculation focuses on these questions: Is long-term asymptomatic HIV infection associated with high levels of antibodies to HIV core proteins? Is it associated with the absence of HEPATITIS B markers? Is there an association between unsafe sex practices, the use of recreational drugs, and long-term lack of symptoms? Is there an association between the level of psychological coping skills and slower disease progression in long-term asymptomatics?

long-term care Care, usually for more than 30 days, in a mental hospital, specialized rehabilitative hospital, skilled nursing facility, intermediate care facility, board-and-care home, or, sometimes, hospice.

long-term nonprogressor See LONG-TERM SURVIVOR.

long-term survivor An individual infected with HIV for at least seven to twelve years (different researchers and authors use different time spans) who yet retains a CD4 CELL count within normal range. It has been found that the good health of long-term survivors probably is due to multiple factors, which may vary from individual to individual. Multiple immune system factors, genetic and other host factors, and viral factors contribute to the clinical profiles of these patients, who usually have preserved immune function and low levels of HIV in their bodies.

Recently there was some speculation that heterozygosity for a defective gene for CC chemokine receptor 5 (CCR5) is the sole determinant for the immunologic and virologic phenotype of HIV-infected long-term survivors. However, investigators found that long-term survivors with one copy of the mutant CCR5 gene were indistinguishable from long-term survivors with two normal copies of the gene with regard to all immunolgic and virologic parameters they measured, including CD4+ T cell counts and viral load in the bloodstream and lymph nodes. Investigators reported that although an HIV-infected individual who carries one copy of the mutant CCR5 gene has an increased chance of becoming a long-term survivor, other factors in the complex interaction between HIV and the body allow individuals with normal copies of the gene to maintain similar immunologic status. The epidemiological data that show that many people with the CCR5 gene mutation in cohorts of long-term survivors is explained as follows. Around the time of initial infection with HIV, people with the specific mutation in the CCR5 gene have lower levels of virus in their blood and a smaller initial decline in CD4+ T cells, as compared to other patients. The lower "set point" probably has an important influence on the subsequent rate of disease progression.

Studies of long-term survivors have contributed greatly to our understsnading of the HIV disease process, and provide perhaps the best evidence that protective immunity may exist in HIV infection. Also called a long-term nonprogressor.

long terminal repeat (LTR) The genetic material at each end of the HIV GENOME. When the HIV genome is integrated into a cell's own genome, the LTR interacts with cellular and viral factors to trigger the transcription of the integrated HIV DNA genes into an RNA form that is packaged in new virus particles. Activation of the LTR is a major step in triggering HIV replication.

longitudinal study A research design in which the same sample of subjects is examined repeatedly over an extended span of time, typically to investigate problems of developmental psychology.

look-back program In HIV/AIDS terminology, a program that attempts to identify recipients of blood from a donor who is later found to be HIV ANTIBODY positive.

loop See INTRAUTERINE DEVICE.

loperamide A drug used to treat the symptoms of diarrhea. In people with HIV, it is often used to treat diarrhea caused by intestinal infections or that is a side effect of other drugs. Loperamide is available by prescription and over the counter as a liquid and in tablet form for oral administration. The prescription form of the drug should be used only under the guidance of a physician. At over-the-counter and prescribed doses, loperamide is generally well tolerated. Reported side effects include allergic reactions, abdominal pain or discomfort, nausea, vomiting, constipation, tiredness, drowsiness or dizziness, and dry mouth.

lotrimin See CLOTRIMAZOLE.

love and death One of the oppositions that structures the discourse of AIDS. See KNOWLEDGE AND IGNORANCE.

loviride A non-nucleoside REVERSE TRANSCRIPTASE inhibitor that has recently been shown to be effective in combination therapy. The results of a preliminary trial (the CAESAR trial) of the three-drug combination of loviride, lamivudine (3TC), and zidovudine indicate that this combination regimen is safe and well-tolerated, according to a multi-center European team. Nevirapine is the first non-nucleoside drug to be approved by the Food and Drug Administration; research continues with loviride and delavirdine.

low-dose oral alpha interferon (LDAI) Low-dose alpha interferon, including Kemron and other similar products, attracted a great deal of attention in the late 1980s and early 1990s when Dr. Davy Koech of Kenya announced a stunning reversal of the AIDS disease process in patients who let lozenges containing the substance dissolve in their mouths. Dr. Koech also claimed a series of controversial "serodeconversions," in which HIV-POSITIVE patients became HIV ANTIBODY-NEGATIVE after Kemron therapy. These results received widespread publicity, creating a significant demand. In 1992, however, the National Institute of Allergy and Infectious Diseases reviewed thirteen different LDAI studies in the United States and abroad and concluded that the initial claims made on behalf of Kemron have not been confirmed. In 1993 a study sponsored by the World Health Organization found no difference between

Kemron and a placebo. There was no evidence of any effect on CD4 CELLS, viral load, disease progression, survival, or "quality-of-life" indicators. And more recent scientific evidence also shows that LDAI products give no benefit in fighting HIV or in improving the immune system of persons with HIV infection.

Nonetheless, LDAI keeps reappearing, as evidenced by calls for more trials. Many observers have reported that LDAI is being kept alive by political pressure, especially from medical clinics connected with the Nation of Islam, which has helped popularize LDAI in the African-American community. But LDAI has also received support from the National Medical Association, the well-established organization of African-American physicians in the United States. Other observers note that LDAI keeps reappearing precisely because the medical establishment has nothing really effective to offer people with HIV, especially those in disenfranchised and poor communities, who have the least access to care and promising therapies.

low-grade squamous intraepithelial lesion (LSIL)   Abnormalities in the cells on the surface of the cervix; an aberration that turns up on Pap tests. LSILs have a slightly higher degree of abnormality than do atypical cells of undetermined significance (ASCUS). Three approaches to managing this abnormality include colposcopy (a procedure in which the clinician examines the cervix through a lighted, binocular-like magnifying instrument and biopsies abnormal areas), "watchful waiting" (repeating the Pap test every six months), and testing the cells in the smear for the strains of human papilloma virus (HPV). See also HIGH-GRADE SQUAMOUS INTRAEPITHELIAL LESION and ATYPICAL SQUAMOUS CELLS OF UNDETERMINED SIGNIFICANCE.

low-risk group/individual   A group or individual whose behavior does not put them at risk for exposure to the virus that causes AIDS. AIDS research to date indicates that low-risk groups include those who have not used intravenous drugs, those who have not been sexual partners of IV drug users or individuals who had or later developed AIDS, those with only one sex partner, those who have not received blood transfusions, and lesbians.

low-risk sex   Low-risk practices with some risk of HIV transmission include ANAL or VAGINAL SEX with proper use of an intact CONDOM; WET KISSING; and FELLATIO interruptus (contact with male genitals without ejaculation).

LPS   See LYPOPOLYSACCHARIDE.

lube   See LUBRICANT.

lubricant   An agent, either artificial or natural, that reduces friction between parts that brush against each other as they move. In sexual activity, lubricants are used to lessen friction and add moisture during intercourse. Lubrication aids the insertion of penis, dildo, or fingers into an orifice.

Lubricants may be oil based or water based, and may or may not be made for the specific purpose. Oil-based lubricants include petroleum jelly, mineral oil, most hand creams, massage oil, baby oil, butter, and Crisco. Oil-based lubricants weaken latex and natural membrane fibers, so should not be used with condoms. (Many condoms come with their own lubricant, a water-based gel or silicone, along with a spermicide.) The most common water-based lubricant is K-Y Jelly. Vegetable-based lubricants are oil based.

lumbar puncture   A procedure in which a needle is inserted into the lumbar region of the spinal canal to obtain a sample of CEREBROSPINAL FLUID for examination. Also known as a SPINAL TAP.

lumbosacral polyradiculopathy   Any of a group of diseases affecting the nerve roots in the lumbar vertebrae and the sacrum (low back region).

lung inflammation   Pneumonia.

lupus anticoagulant   An acquired coagulation inhibitor first noticed in patients with systemic lupus erythematosus, but since found in association with other immune disorders, neoplastic disorders, myeloproliferative disorders, and pregnancy and which is secondary to the administration of certain drugs.

luteinizing hormone   A hormone, secreted by the anterior lobe of the hypophysis (the pituitary gland), that stimulates the development of the corpus luteum (the temporary endocrine gland formed from an ovarian follicle that has released an ovum; secretes progesterone and estrogen).

lymph   A clear fluid containing LYMPHOCYTES, or white blood cells (including CD4 CELLS), that are a part of the immune system. It differs from blood in that red blood corpuscles are absent and the protein content is lower. Osmotic pressure is slightly higher than in blood plasma; viscosity slightly less. Lymph may vary considerably in different parts of the body. Lymph is manufactured in the LYMPH GLANDs.

lymph gland   A clump of lymphatic tissue. Lymph glands are distributed widely throughout the body and are responsible for manufacturing lymph. Lymph glands near the surface of the skin can be felt as bumps below the skin's surface. The back of the neck, below the jaw, under the armpits, and the groin are the usual locations where lymph glands can be felt. Many infections involve the lymph glands, which are commonly swollen and sometimes painful and tender when infected. In HIV infection, swollen lymph glands are likely to occur in three circumstances: with persistent generalized LYMPHADENOPATHY, in which many lymph glands are swollen for months; with infection of the lymph glands by certain opportunistic diseases; and with LYMPHOMAS, which are tumors of the lymphatic system seen more frequently in people with HIV infection than in the general population. Swollen lymph glands may require diagnostic tests. The usual test is a biopsy of the lymph gland or removal of the whole gland to permit microscopic examination of the lymphatic tissue. See also LYMPH NODE.

lymph node Small mass of lymphatic tissue located along the pathway of a lymph vessel; produces lymphocytes and monocytes and destroys pathogens in the lymph.

Recent findings have shown that HIV, when attached to the external surfaces of lymph node cells, called FOLLICULAR DENDRITIC CELLS, infected CD4+ T CELLS even in the presence of a vast excess of neutralizing antibodies. Ensnared viruses may infect critical immune cells that migrate through the lymph node, a scenario that provides a possible explanation for the large quantities of HIV and HIV-infected cells found in the lymph nodes of people with HIV disease, many of whom have abundant anti-HIV antibodies. In the absence of follicular dendritic cells, similar quantities of neutralizing antibodies blocked the infectiviy of the virus. These findings build on previous data that demonstrate that the lymphoid organs are central to the pathogenesis of HIV disease. See also LYMPH GLAND.

lymph nodule A small, compact, densely staining mass of cells, each containing a lighter-staining central area in which lymphocytes are formed. They constitute the structural unit of lymphatic tissue. May occur singly, in groups (as in Peyer's patches) or in encapsulated organs as lymph nodes.

lymphadenopathy A chronic condition of the LYMPH NODEs and glands due to infection or cancer, in which the nodes enlarge, grow, and swell and may be palpable or visible from outside the body. Swollen LYMPH GLANDs, most common at the back of the neck, along the jaw, in the armpits, and in the groin, may feel like rubbery, discrete pea-sized nodules that are rarely tender to touch. Swollen glands occur in everyone, in conditions unrelated to HIV infection. However, lymphadenopathy is sometimes thought to be an early sign of infection with the virus associated with AIDS. If lymph glands are swollen to abnormal size for longer than a month in at least two different areas, they constitute persistent generalized lymphadenopathy.

lymphadenopathy-associated virus (LAV) The name given by French researchers to the first reported isolate of the RETROVIRUS now known to cause AIDS. This retrovirus was recovered from a person with LYMPHADENOPATHY (enlarged lymph nodes) who also was in a group at high risk for AIDS.

The French classified LAV as a lentivirus, a subgroup of slow-acting viruses that cause disease in horses, goats, and sheep but was not previously known to cause disease in humans and other primates.

See HIV.

lymphadenopathy syndrome (LAS) Also known as generalized lymphadenopathy syndrome, a condition characterized by persistent, generalized, enlarged LYMPH NODEs (sometimes accompanied by signs of minor illness, such as fever and weight loss) and that apparently represents a milder reaction to infection with HTLV-III than full-blown AIDS. BIOPSY reveals nonspecific lymphoid hyperplasia. Some patients with LAS have gone on to develop full-blown AIDS. In others, LAS represents the height of clinical illness in reaction to infection with HTLV-III.

lymphatic system A circulatory system of vessels, spaces, and LYMPH NODEs that fight infection.

lymphatic vessel One of a bodywide network of channels, similar to the blood vessels, that transports LYMPH to the LYMPHOID TISSUE and into the bloodstream.

lymphoblast An immature cell that gives rise to a LYMPHOCYTE.

lymphocyte A white blood cell that matures and resides in the lymphoid organs and is responsible for the acquired immune response. The two major types of lymphocytes are T CELLS and B CELLS. The acquired immune response is achieved by means of HUMORAL IMMUNITY produced by B cells and CELL-MEDIATED IMMUNITY produced by T cells. Lymphocytes originate in the BONE MARROW, pass through the bloodstream and enter other organs, where they become modified to B or T lymphocytes. During infections B lymphocytes (bursa dependent) are transformed into plasma cells that produce antibodies to specific pathogens. This transformation occurs through interactions with various types of T cells and other components of the immune system. T lymphocytes (thymus dependent) are derived from the thymus and participate in a variety of cell-mediated immune reactions. Three fundamentally different types of T cells are recognized: helper, killer, and suppressor.

lymphocytic interstitial pneumonitis (LIP) An inflammation within the lungs that develops gradually and is characterized by infiltration of the lungs by LYMPHOCYTEs, LYMPHOBLASTs, and PLASMA CELLS. LIP affects 35 to 40 percent of children with AIDS and causes hardening of the lung membranes involved in absorbing oxygen. LIP is an AIDS-defining illness in children. The cause is unknown, but it is often associated with a compromised immune system. Also called LYMPHOID INTERSTITIAL PNEUMONIA.

lymphogranuloma venereum (LGV) A tropical STD caused by the chlamydia trachomatis bacterium. Its most common presentation is inguinal lymphadenopathy.

lymphoid interstitial pneumonia See LYMPHOCYTIC INTERSTITIAL PNEUMONITIS.

lymphoid tissue The organs of the lymph system throughout the body, including the BONE MARROW, THYMUS, LYMPH NODEs, SPLEEN, tonsils, PEYER'S PATCHES, and the lymphocyte aggregates on mucosal surfaces.

lymphokine One of a number of substances that act as mediators of cellular immunity, released by sensitized LYMPHOCYTEs when they contact specific ANTIGENS. Lymphokines help to produce cellular immunity by stimulating MACROPHAGEs and MONOCYTEs. Included in this group of materials are INTERLEUKINS 1, 2, and 3; INTERFERON-GAMMA; TUMOR NECROSIS FACTOR; COLONY STIMULATING FACTOR; B-CELL growth factor; LYMPHOTOXIN; migration inhibition factor; leukocyte migration inhibition factor; macrophage chemotactic factor; macrophage activating factor; lymphocyte mitogenic factor; soluble immune response suppressor; and T-CELL replacement factor.

lymphoma   A cancer of the cells responsible for normal immune function. Lymphoma occurs most frequently in people without HIV infection, but people with weakened immune systems, including those with HIV infection, have lymphomas about 40 times more frequently than normal. About one to three percent of people with AIDS have lymphomas, which are classified as opportunistic tumors. There are many types of lymphomas. Some progress extremely slowly, cause few symptoms, and require minimal treatment. Some are more severe, and symptoms may include LYMPH NODE swelling, weight loss, and fever. People with AIDS generally have lymphomas called NON-HODGKIN'S LYMPHOMAS, of B CELL origin. These lymphomas tend to be severe, and they also tend to involve unusual areas of the body like the brain, intestines, kidneys, and lungs. The diagnosis is usually established with a biopsy. Treatment is variable and often requires chemotherapy or radiation.

lymphopenia   Deficiency of LYMPHOCYTEs in the blood.

lymphoproliferative disease   See LYMPHOPROLIFERATIVE DISORDER.

lymphoproliferative disorder   Any of a group of malignant neoplasms that involve LYMPHORETICULAR CELLS. Hodgkin's disease, lymphocytic lymphomas, multiple myeloma, and the histiocytic, lymphocytic, and monocytic lymphomas are included. Also called *lymphoproliferative disease* and *lymphoproliferative syndrome.*

lymphoproliferative response   A specific immune response that entails rapid T CELL replication. Standard ANTIGENS, such as tetanus toxoid, that elicit this response are used in lab tests of immune competence.

lymphoproliferative syndrome   See LYMPHOPROLIFERATIVE DISORDER.

lymphoreticular cell   Any reticuloendothelial cell of the lymph node.

lymphotoxin (LT or TNF-B)   A LYMPHOKINE that causes direct cytoloysis following its release from stimulated LYMPHOCYTEs.

lymphotrophic   Having an affinity for lymphatic tissue. HUMAN IMMUNODEFICIENCY VIRUS and human T CELL leukemia virus are lymphotropic for CD4+ LYMPHOCYTEs and EPSTEIN-BARR VIRUS is lymphotropic for B LYMPHOCYTES.

lypopolysaccharide (LPS)   A product of some GRAM-NEGATIVE bacterial cell walls, which can act as a polyclonal B-CELL mitogen.

lysine   An amino acid that is a hydrolytic cleavage product of digested protein. It is essential for growth and repair of tissues.

lysis   The splitting and dissolution of cellular or viral material by chemical action.

M

MA   See MEDICAL ASSISTANCE.

MAC   See MYCOBACTERIUM AVIUM COMPLEX.

MAC disease   See MYCOBACTERIUM AVIUM COMPLEX.

macrobiotics   A way of life according to the macroscopic, or largest possible, view. Translated literally, *macro* is Greek for "large" or "great," and *bios* is the word for "life." The practice of macrobiotics involves understanding and applying this universal order of change to one's lifestyle, including the selection, preparation, and manner of eating food. The first principle in the selection and preparation of food is to eat unrefined cereal grains and cooked vegetables as the main foods. A second principle is to eat in accordance with the immediate environment, specifically the climatic conditions in which one lives. Within a particular climate, various seasonal changes are experienced, and diet should vary accordingly, primarily using foods that are either naturally available during a particular season or can be naturally stored. The fourth principle of macrobiotic eating is modifying the diet to suit individual differences.

A macrobiotic diet is also based on the belief that there is a yin/yang quality of all foods. For example, it is believed that animal foods exert a yang, or contractive, influence and vegetables produce a more yin, or expansive, influence. External factors, such as pressure, fire, salt, and time (aging), produce a more contractive influence, whereas less pressure, water, oil, and freshness (less time) result in expansion. For example, within the vegetable kingdom, a vegetable's size, direction of growth, color, juiciness, firmness, and chemical composition affect its yin/yang. Indeed, all foods, not only vegetables, can be classified into yin/yang. In order to reflect the over-all order of biological evolution in eating, as well as to maintain a proper yin/yang balance, the macrobiotic diet calls for approximately 50 percent of one's daily food to be unrefined cereal grains. In fact, following the macrobiotic regime to its highest level has been interpreted to mean eating a 100-percent cereal diet.

A macrobiotic diet is a radical departure from the dietary customs of the Western world. Proponents of this lifestyle argue that such a diet of natural foods, cooked in accordance with macrobiotic principles, can promote health and minimize disease. Some supporters claim that a macrobiotic diet is an effective primary treatment for cancer. Others claim that it can be effective when combined with other forms of treatment. Critics caution that macrobiotic diets are hazardous because they are both nutritionally unbalanced and restrictive, excluding nearly everything but grains. The American Medical Association, the Food and Drug Administration, and many nutrition experts say that a macrobiotic diet can be harmful. The National Cancer Institute and the American Cancer Society believe that strict adherence to it poses a serious health hazard and that it is not effective in preventing or treating cancer. They further claim that there is no scientific evidence supporting its use, either alone or combined with standard cancer treatment.

macrophage   A phagocyte cell of vertebrate connective tissue but not typically of the blood itself. Included here are the wandering macrophages derived from monocytes and more static macrophages dispersed throughout connective tissue but capable of migrating towards a site of infection. Phagocytes of the reticuloendothelial system are more specialized macrophages, but all are important as antigen-presenting cells, capable of collecting immune intelligence about pathogens and activating a sensitized helper T CELL.

Macrophages reside in the liver, brain, spleen, LYMPH NODES, BONE MARROW, thymus, nerves, lungs, bones, and elsewhere in the body and are critical to normal immune functioning in these areas. Macrophages fight infection by attacking and ingesting invading pathogens. They have the ability to recognize and ingest all foreign antigens through receptors on the surface of their cell membranes; they act by surrounding a foreign particle, virus, or bacterial cell and destroying it. T lymphocytes "present" antigen to macrophages. There is evidence that macrophages activate lymphocytes as well by producing factors that affect lymphocyte function. Macrophages also secrete various chemical mediators that are involved in the body's defenses, including coagulation proteins, complement compounds, enzymes, ERYTHROPOIETIN, INTERFERON, INTERLEUKIN-1, and PROSTAGLANDINS.

MACS   See MULTICENTER AIDS COHORT STUDY.

macula   The pigmented central area or "yellow spot" of the retina, adjacent to the optic nerve. It is the most sensitive area of the retina and contains the fovea, the region responsible for detailed central vision.

magic bullet   A hypothetical, hoped-for single drug that can knock out a particular malignancy or other disorder without toxicity.

magnetic resonance imaging (MRI)   A noninvasive, non–X-ray diagnostic technique that produces images of the interior of the body using powerful electromagnets, radio waves, and a computer; formerly known as nuclear magnetic resonance, MRI is used, along with other procedures, in the diagnosis and evaluation of disease and disorder and to monitor for their recurrence. MRI may be done in conjunction with a CT SCAN and/or ultrasound. It can produce clear three-dimensional images of blood vessels, blood flow, cartilage, BONE MARROW, muscles, ligaments, cerebrospinal fluid and the spinal cord. MRI is somewhat different from a CT (computerized tomography) scan. The person undergoing MRI is placed inside a large tubular structure and remains motionless for a lengthy period of time (approximately 30 minutes to an hour). During that time, her body is bathed in a magnetic field, which causes the atoms in different tissues to give off tiny radio signals. The signals are different depending on the kind of tissue.

An MRI is better than a CT scan at detecting diseases of the brain and spinal cord. An expensive technique, MRI is painless, harmless, and does not involve exposure to ionizing radiation. Nor is there a need, as in radiological (X-ray) imaging, to inject a radiopaque contrast medium such as barium sulfate to provide a visual contrast between the tissue or organ being filmed and the surrounding tissue. MRI may not be suitable for people with heart pacemakers, joint pins, surgical metal clips, artificial heart valves, IUDs, shrapnel, or any other electronic or metal implants.

MAI   See MYCOBACTERIUM AVIUM COMPLEX.

MAI infections   See MYCOBACTERIUM AVIUM COMPLEX.

mail-order pharmacies   A source for filling prescriptions by mail to reduce costs. Mail-order pharmacies are high-volume operations which can locate where costs are low and can negotiate good prices from suppliers. They compete with each other primarily on price because location doesn't matter, whereas traditional corner drugstores have a captive market. They usually, but not always, have the lowest prices available. Shopping around is therefore recommended. Patients can get price and other information over the phone.

If patients can pay by credit card or if the prescription is fully paid by insurance, physicians usually can call in the prescriptions, avoiding the need to wait for the mail. Most drugs are sent by two-day express, unless overnight delivery is necessary. Drugs which need to be refrigerated are shipped overnight in insulated containers. Delivery can be to a separate address, so that nobody needs to stay home to receive the medicines. The pharmacies generally bill insurance directly and handle the paperwork. Some mail-order pharmacies require full payment from the patient, with the insurance company reimbursing the patient for the percentage it pays—a process which can take months. Filling prescriptions is usually a solitary or personal activity, one which patients seldom talk about. For some people, ordering prescriptions by mail meets important needs of privacy and convenience. Local pharmacies, unlike mail-order pharmacies, provide both a place where individuals can develop a working relationship with their pharmacist or physician, and a place for in-person discussion of drugs and drug interactions.

Mail-order pharmacies exist serving both regional and national audiences. Some mail-order pharmacies specialize in serving HIV-infected people and offer supplementary educational materials. Some accept 80 percent payment from insurers as "payment in full" and sell other products at a discount.

maintenance therapy   Extended drug therapy, usually at a diminished dose, administered after a disease has been brought under control; also called *continuation therapy*. Maintenance therapy is utilized when a complete cure is not possible and the disease is likely to recur if therapy is halted. Maintenance therapy is generally given for a fixed amount of time and then stopped.

major histocompatibility complex (MHC)   A group of genes that code for Human Leukocyte Antigens (HLA) (markers on the surface of cells for the differentiation of self from nonself). MHC consists of either of two classes of molecules on cell surfaces. MHC class I molecules exist on all cells and hold and present foreign ANTIGENS to CD8 CYTOTOXIC T-LYMPHOCYTES if the cell is infected by a virus or other microbe. MHC class II molecules are found on the immune system's antigen presenting cells and display antigen to activate CD4 T-HELPER CELLS.

major medical insurance   Insurance that covers expenses for most serious medical conditions, up to a maximum limit, usually after deductible and coinsurance provisions have been met. These policies usually complement hospital-medical-surgical coverages.

malabsorption   Faulty or incomplete absorption of nutrients in the intestines.

Cells in the gastrointestinal (GI) tract are particularly prone to damage during HIV infection, and this results in reduced absorption of nutrients. The HIV virus itself, intestinal parasites, and COLITIS induced by CYTOMEGALOVIRUS (CMV) are the main sources of tissue damage. The diarrhea connected with these conditions may also result in malabsorption. Fat, carbohydrate, protein, and micronutrient (vitamin and mineral) malabsorption can occur. Malabsorption may also be present before infection with HIV. Infection by intestinal parasites triggers diarrhea and malabsorption in persons with AIDS by causing atrophy of the villi, the small threadlike projections (on the interior of the small intestines) that absorb nutrients when working properly. The protozoan CRYPTOSPORIDIUM *parvum*, the most commonly identified parasite in people with AIDS, causes massive secretory diarrhea. MICROSPORIDIA (*Enterocytozoon bieneusi* or *Septata intestinalis*) is a second common GI parasite in people with AIDS. Infection can cause diarrhea and decreased intestinal absorption.

malabsorption syndrome   Decreased intestinal absorption resulting in loss of appetite, muscle pain, and weight loss.

malaise   A vague feeling of discomfort or uneasiness, often the result of infection or a drug's side effects.

malaria   One of the most widespread infectious diseases in the world, malaria is an acute and sometimes chronic disorder caused by the presence of protozoan parasites within the red blood cells. Malaria is transmitted to the human by the bite of an infected female *Anopheles* mosquito. The mosquito becomes infected by ingesting the blood of a human infected with malaria. Chloroquine and mefloquine, the medications that prevent malaria, do not interact with medications commonly prescribed for HIV-related indications. Despite prophylaxis, certain forms of malaria can occur weeks to months after leaving a malaria-infested area. Fever is the prominent symptom, and a simple blood test determines the diagnosis.

Chloroquine phosphate is prescribed in all types of malaria except those due to drug-resistant *Plasmodium falciparum* or *P. falciparum*. In drug-resistant *P. falciparum,* treatment with combinations of quinine, pyrimethamine, and a sulfonamide is indicated. Malaria due to other species should be treated with both chloroquine and primaquine. Severe malaria due to *P. falciparum* with evidence of cerebral involvement may be treated with continous infusion of quinidine gluconate and exchange transfusion.

male homosexual   A man whose primary erotic and emotional interests are in other men.

male-to-female transmission   See TRANSMISSION.

male-to-male transmission   See TRANSMISSION.

malignancy   A cancerous tumor or neoplasm.

malignant   Evil, malicious; in medicine, life-threatening. When used in a medical setting, it means "cancerous" and commonly refers to a cancerous tumor, as distinct from a benign tumor. The main characteristic of a malignant tumor is that it is likely to penetrate the tissues or organ in which it originated as well as move to other sites (metastasize), eventually causing death.

malnutrition   Any disorder of nutrition; specifically, either the deficit of efficient or substantive food substances in the body or the inability of the body to properly absorb food substances. Physical signs of malnutrition and deficiency state in adolescents and adults include nasolabial sebaceous plugs; sores at the corners of the mouth; Vincent's angina; red, swollen lingual papillae; glossitis; papillary atrophy of tongue; stomatitis; spongy, bleeding gums; muscle tenderness in extremities; poor muscle tone; loss of vibratory sensation; increase or decrease of tendon reflexes; hyperesthesia of skin; bilateral symmetrical dermatitis; purpura; dermatitis; thickening and pigmentation of skin over bony

prominences; nonspecific vaginitis; follicular hyperkeratosis of extensor surfaces of extremities; rachitic chest deformity; anemia not responding to iron; fatigue of visual accommodation; vascularization of cornea; and conjunctival changes.

The word *malnutrition* often conjures up images of emaciated people who do not have regular meals. However, the medical application of the word is more subtle. Most people with HIV disease do not know they are malnourished, since malnutrition is specific to the absence of vitamins and minerals essential to healthy body function. Research has shown that nutrient deficiencies begin very early in HIV infection and have a significant influence on how well the immune system functions and how quickly HIV disease progresses.

Malnutrition in AIDS can result from many different factors. Inability to take in a proper amount of nutrients can be the result of impaired swallowing and taste due to infections in the mouth or the esophagus, AIDS medications that have anorexia, nausea, and vomiting as side effects, or limited financial resources that make three meals a day difficult to manage. Diarrhea and changes in absorption caused by bacteria, viruses, or parasites may impair nutritional intake. Some medications, particularly antibiotics, may change the normal bacterial composition of the intestine and interfere with breakdown of food. Finally, an increase in metabolism often occurs in many people with HIV and leads to an increased need for nutrients. The presence of HIV itself as well as some of its associated infections can increase the metabolic rate. These three factors—diminished intake, malabsorption, and hypermetabolism—usually occur simultaneously to deplete the body of nutrients.

In addition to a balanced diet, vitamin therapy and vitamin and mineral megadosing have been used to treat malnutrition. Multivitamins are generally preferred over individual vitamins because of lower cost and lower risk of toxicity, and because single-nutrient deficiencies are unusual. Despite the high cost and time involved, megadosing has been effective for many people; studies have demonstrated heightened immune function when supplements are given at several times the United States Recommended Daily Allowance (RDA). Caution should be exercised since toxic effects are possible when vitamins and minerals are used improperly. Generally, people with HIV/AIDS are advised to consult with a trained professional and a doctor before changing treatment regimens and to inform all health care providers when making significant alterations in their diets. It is also important to note that not all trained nutritionists subscribe to various regimens.

malpractice   Incorrect or negligent treatment of a patient by professionals responsible for health care, such as dentists, nurses, or physicians.

MALT   See MUCOSA-ASSOCIATED LYMPHOID TISSUE.

mammography   The use of radiography to diagnose breast cancer. This technique has increased the rate of early detection. Mammography is capable of detecting 85 to 90 percent of existing breast cancers.

The American Cancer Society (ACS) and the National Cancer Institute (NCI) delivered their recommendations on mammography for women in their 40s, even though the

National Institutes of Health Consensus Development Panel abstained from doing so. Both advise regular mammograms for women in this age group (the ACS, annually; the NCI, every 1–2 years). Women who are in this age group and who have decided to have regular mammograms are advised to have an annual screening. Breast cancer tends to develop more rapidly in younger women, and having a mammography every year increases the likelihood of catching early-stage tumors. Use of mammography as a diagnostic tool does not mean that careful, periodic clinical (physical) examinations should be omitted. Similarly, use of mammography as a diagnostic tool does not mean that self-examination should be omitted. The benefits to the self exam include its convenience, cost (it is free) and the fact that it is without physical risk. There is another benefit to the self exam. A women is likely to have more time for a careful examination than her clinician does. Given the limitations of the office visit under MANAGED CARE, many clinicians simply cannot devote several minutes to a routine breast examination. A woman who has examined her own breasts for years is likely to have a better idea of what is abnormal for her as each monthly exam gives her more information about the structure of her breasts.

managed care   The goal of containing costs by coordinating care through a gatekeeper, or general practitioner who decides on all referrals. Employers increasingly are choosing managed care plans to cut costs even though such plans have traditionally been reluctant to cover "high risk" groups such as people with HIV. HIV-positive beneficiaries should educate themselves on the services provided by each plan. Some features that are left out may be important in managing HIV infection, including mental health and substance abuse coverage. It is also advisable to ascertain which medications, nutritional supports, and alternative treatments are in the plan's formulary, as some therapies have been "carved out" from the program, and to determine the HIV expertise of the network or health maintenance organization physicians. A plan's complaint and grievance procedures also are important should needed services be denied.

Patients insured under the MEDICAID or MEDICARE programs also are experiencing a growing shift toward mandatory managed care plans, although many state Medicaid programs have little experience providing HIV care under this new type of system. Managed care presents particular problems for both HIV specialists and HIV/AIDS care. First, most persons with HIV/AIDS, even if they are treated initially by a primary care physician, eventually become the patients of an AIDS specialist. Studies have demonstrated that experience of primary care physicians in the management of AIDS is significantly associated with survival of their patients. One of the hallmarks of managed care is the gatekeeping function of the primary care physician; referrals to specialists are closely monitored and often reluctantly granted. The supply of primary care physicians is inadequate, and many of those already in practice are not trained in state-of-the-art HIV/AIDS management. Limiting the choice of primary health care providers to doctors who have agreed with health maintenance organizations to charge less but who have little or no experience treating AIDS patients may decrease quality of care. Furthermore, state-of-the-art AIDS care must include the treatment to many different groups of people, types of conditions, and co-morbidities, such as substance abuse, tuberculosis, sexually transmitted diseases, and others.

A second issue, somewhat related to the first, is that the HIV specialist is being squeezed by managed care. Often, the HIV specialist is not considered as primary care so that patients can be kept out of health plans. HIV specialists have long recognized that delivering comprehensive, coordinated high-quality care costs more up front but saves on big ticket items, including hospitals and emergency room services.

A third issue arises in the access to investigational protocols or alternative therapies, including natural and alternative medicines. Payer constraints severely and adversely influence what treatments are possible for their patients. Managed care organizations are not the ideal environments to support or accept either investigational protocols or alternative therapies. They are not even ideally suited to adapt rapidly to changing standards of care, which happen frequently in AIDS care. Yet, there are forms of care that are important to patients and physicians. The earliest gains in speeding up the drug approval process and in broadening the inclusion criteria for clinical trials may have little effect in a managed care setting that reacts slowly and cautiously to change, especially to financial change.

Fourth, managed care plans may limit, contractually or in practice, access to beneficial but expensive treatments, or to such relatively routine decisions as emergency hospital admission. The appeal process may be slow or unresponsive, while the patient's needs are urgent. Providers may have financial disincentives to offer such care, and real incentives, such as bonuses, to deny it.

Fifth, and in a related vein, managed care plans may limit, contractually or in practice, reimbursement for "off-label" prescriptions. Managed care has prior authorization and restricted formularies. HIV/AIDS specialists often prescribe drugs for indications that are not officially approved, mostly for treatment and prevention of opportunistic infections. Although such usage frequently reflects the standard of care, third-party payers often deny reimbursement for these prescriptions. When faced with such obstacles, many patients will receive less effective, albeit covered, therapies or be hospitalized to gain access to the preferred therapy.

management trials   Part of the drug development process that integrates multiple trials, such as the MAPS (Master Antiretroviral Protocol Strategy) proposal from the COMMUNITY PROGRAMS FOR CLINICAL RESEARCH ON AIDS (CPCRA) or the SMART (Standardized Master Antirrovial Trial) concept from the American Foundation for Aids Research. In contrast to the prevailing trial methods, with restraints on eligibility, concomitant medications, and clinical management, management trials cultivate diversity of clinical management. Management trials incorporate the heterogeneity of the HIV population and ask "What is the effect of starting this treatment now, rather than another time—or never?" They do not presume that people can be assigned to a treatment or placebo and remain on it like lab rats.

man-to-man transmission   See TRANSMISSION.

man-to-woman transmission   See TRANSMISSION.

mandatory reporting   A legal requirement for a physician to inform health authorities when a specified illness is diagnosed. Reporting of AIDS is mandatory in all 50 states, and it has been proposed that the requirement be extended to HIV infection.

mandatory testing   Medical testing that is legally required. In the case of AIDS, some government agencies do have mandatory testing policies. For example, before enrollment in the Job Corps, the Peace Corps, or the military, applicants are required to take a blood test. The Immigration and Naturalization Service, which regulates immigration and the entry of noncitizens into the United States, requires all potential immigrants to take a blood test. An infected person wishing to visit the United States may receive a waiver that allows him or her to travel here for 30 days.

mange   A skin disease in mammals characterized by itching, lesions, scabs, and loss of hair caused by parasitic mites. Mange is a communicable disease occurring in various animals, including dogs, cats, cattle, horses, sheep, rabbits, rats, and some birds. The causative agent is any of several mange mites, including *Chorioptes, Demodex, Psoroptes,* and *Sarcoptes.* In humans, this condition is known as scabies.

mange mite   Any of the various mites that cause mange.

mania   Mental disorder characterized by excessive excitement; a form of psychosis characterized by exalted feelings, delusions of grandeur, elevation of mood, psycho-motor overactivity, and overproduction of ideas.

manicure   A cosmetic treatment of the hands or fingernails, especially the cleaning, trimming, and polishing of the nails and the removal of cuticle. Because HIV is transmitted via blood, manicurists and their clients constitute a group at potential risk for HIV infection. Exposure to small cuts and abrasions that may develop during a manicure, or that existed before, may lead to HIV infection. However, the risk is not considered high.
See TRANSMISSION.

manifestation   An outward sign that an illness is present—a symptom or condition.

Mantoux method   A test for tuberculosis (after Charles Mantoux, a French physician, 1877–1947); also called the Mantoux test. It consists of an intracutaneous injection of one-tenth ml of intermediate strength PURIFIED PROTEIN DERIVATIVE (PPD). Within 24 to 72 hours the injected area becomes hard (indurated) and grows to 10 mm in diameter if either an active or inactive tuberculous infection is present. Induration of 5 to 10 mm is doubtful, and a reaction of less than 5 mm is considered to be negative.

manual-vaginal intercourse   See VAGINAL-MANUAL INTERCOURSE.

MAO inhibitors   See MONAMINE OXIDASE INHIBITORS.

MAOI   See MONAMINE OXIDASE INHIBITORS.

MAP-30   See BITTER MELON.

Marburg virus   A disease caused by a virus classed as a member of the family Filoviridae. Clinically, it is identical to that caused by the EBOLA VIRUS.

marijuana   The dried flowering tops and leaves of the hemp plant (*Cannabis sativa*). Smoked, it is an intoxicant—possibly the most widely used, after alcohol—and an illegal drug. Marijuana and its constituents or derivatives may be useful in the treatment of acute glaucoma and to control the severe nausea and vomiting caused by cancer chemotherapy. The psychoactive constituent of marijuana is DELTA-9-TETRAHYDROCANNABINOL (THC). Synthetic THC, DRONABINOL, is approved for use as an antiemetic in treating cancer. Many people with AIDS contend that smoking marijuana is more convenient and useful than swallowing dronabinol. In addition, studies have reported that cannabidiol, one of the nonpsychoactive components of marijuana, reduces blood levels of the immune modulators TNF and IL-1, and that this may moderate the basic wasting process.

Marinol   See DRONABINOL

masochism   The deriving of pleasure from receiving physical and/or psychological pain.

mass media disease   Many hold that AIDS is the first international mass media disease. Throughout the world, more people have learned about AIDS from radio, television, and the press than from personal contacts with health professionals. Although there has been considerable criticism of the media's coverage of AIDS, virtually every treatment of AIDS in the mass media has in fact been a first. Although other sexually transmitted diseases remain relatively taboo as mass media topics, AIDS has been discussed extensively.

News coverage of AIDS has concentrated on new information released by scientists, on human interest stories, and on controversies rather than prevention. Journalists tend to focus on coverage that attracts large audiences. As different media compete to release information that appears to be new or controversial, relatively little press and broadcast space is devoted to detailed analysis or to the natural history of the disease, and even less on education and prevention specific strategies. Many countries have organized national information/education campaigns on AIDS, because efforts to curb the epidemic cannot rely solely on news media, whose coverage of AIDS has been slow, erratic, and focused on new and unusual events. Today it is safe to say that the mass media are gradually becoming more effective channels for AIDS education. At the same time, however, government resources and political motivation for mass media education campaigns are becoming constrained.

massage   Manipulation, methodical pressure, friction, and kneading of the body. Types of massage include introductory (massage consisting of centripetal strokings around the affected part), local (massage confined to particular parts), tremolo (a type of mechanical massage), vapor (treatment of a cavity by a medicated and nebulized vapor under interrupted pressure), or vibratory (massage by rapidly repeated tapping of the affected surface by means of a vibrating hammer or sound). Caressing and stroking of the body may also be done for sensual enjoyment or relaxation. Touching, massaging, hugging, and stroking are considered to be practices with probably no risk of HIV transmission.

massage therapy   This is a general term for a range of therapeutic approaches with roots in both Eastern and Western cultures. It involves the practice of kneading or otherwise manipulating a person's muscles and other soft tissue with the intent of improving a person's well-being or health.

mast cell   A cell resident in connective tissue just below epithelial surfaces, serous cavities, and around blood vessels, including those in bone marrow. They synthesize and store histamines. When stimulated, they release mediators of inflammation. They are also important in producing the signs and symptoms of immediate hypersensitivity reactions (e.g., drug anaphylaxis, urticaria, insect stings, allergic reactions, and certain forms of asthma).

mastitis   Inflammation or infection of the breast or mammary gland. It is most common in women during lactation but may occur at any age.

mastoiditis   Inflammation or infection of the air cells of the nipple-shaped portion of the temporal bone (mastoid process), located behind the ear.

masturbation   The purposeful stimulation of one's genitals, or other erogenous zones, to produce sexual pleasure, sexual excitement, and/or orgasm. It is usually thought of as an activity one practices alone, but it can be done to a partner or to oneself in the presence of others. Self-masturbation and masturbation of a partner (if there are no cuts on the hands of either partner) are considered to be practices with probably no risk of HIV transmission. Slang terms include *beating off, beating your meat, jacking off, jerking off,* JILLING OFF, *frigging,* and *diddling.*

maternofetal transmission   See TRANSMISSION.

measles   A highly communicable disease caused by the rubeola virus and characterized by fever, general malaise, sneezing, nasal congestion, brassy cough, conjunctivitis, spots on the buccal mucosa, and a maculopapular eruption over the entire body. It is most common in school-age children. An attack of measles almost invariably confers permanent immunity. Active immunization can be produced by administration of measles vaccine. Passive immunization is afforded by administration of GAMMA GLOBULIN. Pregnant women who are not immune to German measles are advised to avoid exposure. If they are exposed in the first 16 weeks of pregnancy and if they get the disease, chances are high that the fetus will have problems. At this point, they will have to make a decision about whether or not to continue their pregnancy. A blood test will determine if they have or have had German measles.

mechanical ventilation   The process of exchanging air between the lungs and surrounding atmosphere by artificial, extrinsic means (i.e., a respirator).

Medicaid   Medicaid, one of our country's two major government-run health insurance programs (the other is MEDICARE), is a federally aided but state-operated and -administered program that provides medical benefits to eligible low-income persons. Authorized by TITLE XIX of the SOCIAL SECURITY ACT OF 1965, it is basically for the poor, but it doesn't cover all of the poor. Rather, Medicaid is only for those who are members of one of the categories of people who may also be covered under welfare cash payment programs—the aged, blind, disabled, and members of individual families and dependent children in which one parent is absent, incapacitated, or unemployed.

Medicaid is operated by state health or welfare agencies under the rules of the Health Care Financing Administration of the United States DEPARTMENT OF HEALTH AND HUMAN SERVICES. Subject to broad federal guidelines, states determine eligibility, coverage, rates of payment for providers, and methods of administration. Eligibility varies from state to state, but generally, persons whose incomes and assets are below state-set poverty levels, or (in most states) whose incomes fall to those poverty levels through incurred (but not necessarily paid) medical expenses are eligible. In most states, Social Security's decision that an individual is eligible for SSI also makes them eligible for Medicaid coverage. Others covered are those in AFDC-eligible families, those who meet the SSI/SSDI medical definition of blindness or disability, pregnant women, those under age seven or over age 65, and some or all persons (depending on the state) between ages seven and 21.

Programs vary widely from state to state, but Medicaid generally covers these services: care in skilled and intermediate nursing homes; inpatient hospital services; outpatient hospital services; clinic health services; laboratory and X-ray services; hospice services (in about half the states); home health services of registered nurses or other medical professionals; physician services; M.D. psychiatrist services (some states also cover services of licensed psychologists and psychiatric social workers); premiums, coinsurance, and deductibles for poor, disabled, and aged people also on Medicare; ambulance service; mass-transit charges, taxi vouchers, and handicapped van services to get to medical care (in some states); outpatient prescription drugs (with some exceptions); personal home care attendants when ordered in writing by a doctor; and home- and community-based services. Medicaid recipients are also eligible for social services such as counseling, "meals on wheels," home chore aid, and transportation through the "adult services" sections of the state welfare agencies. There is a broad right of appeal for unfavorable agency decisions.

Medicaid recipients are given plastic or paper cards with which to purchase covered services from participating providers. Cards are used similarly to credit cards. However, cash outlays by patients are never reimbursed.

Information about Medicaid can be obtained from local welfare offices or Medicaid agencies. How and where to apply varies slightly from state to state.

The Clinton administration currently is exploring ways to provide free health insurance coverage to large groups of poor Americans who have HIV but have not yet developed full-blown AIDS. By expanding the eligibility requirements of Medicaid, the administration argues that it can save both lives and money because individuals infected with HIV could receive new drug therapies that would postpone their need for costly hospital care. AIDS patients must now be disabled before they can qualify for Medicaid. By making new drugs and other therapies available much earlier, the government would attempt to prevent them from developing full-blown AIDS.

medical assistance (MA) A generic term for MEDICAID, GENERAL MEDICAL ASSISTANCE (GMA), and other health care programs for the poor.

medical care The range of services provided by physicians for the maintenance of health, the prevention of illness, and the treatment of illness and injury.

medical consultation A physician's review of a patient's history, examination of a patient, or recommendations for treatment, given to another physician at the request of the first.

medical directive A document detailing a patient's wishes concerning kinds of treatment he or she does not wish to have administered under particular circumstances in the future. A patient can request, for example, that he or she not be kept alive on a respirator if his or her medical condition is irreversible. Individuals have a much better chance of realizing their wishes if they express them in writing in advance. The best guarantee is to sign a medical directive in conjunction with a HEALTH CARE PROXY in which a sympathetic person is named as a health care agent. See also CODE STATUS, POWER OF ATTORNEY, LIVING WILL, and NO CODE.

medical history The portion of a patient's life history that is important in diagnosing and caring for the medical or surgical condition or conditions present. Ancestry and social, occupational, and medical information are all components of a complete medical history. This information is recorded in the patient's permanent record.

medical waste Infectious or physically dangerous medical or biological waste material, including discarded blood and blood products; pathology lab waste; contaminated animal carcasses and body parts; contaminated bedding; sharps (medical articles such as hypodermic needles that may cause punctures or cuts to those handling them); and discarded preparations made from genetically altered living organisms and their products. In 1985, the CENTERS FOR DISEASE CONTROL AND PREVENTION (CDC) developed the strategy of "universal blood and body fluid precautions" to address concerns regarding transmission of HIV and other infectious illnesses in the health care setting. See UNIVERSAL PRECAUTIONS.

medically needy In MEDICAID parlance, persons who share qualifications with AFDC or SSI recipients, but who have incomes above AFDC, SSI or SSI/SSP eligibility levels. At state option, medically needy people can receive Medicaid when their income is below (or falls below through "spend-down") a state-set level between the AFDC level and an amount one-third higher.

Medicare One of our country's two major government-run health insurance programs (the other is MEDICAID), Medicare is a nationwide health insurance program for people aged 65 years and over, persons eligible for Social Security disability payments for at least two years, and certain workers who need kidney transplantation or dialysis. Medical health insurance protection is available to eligible persons without regard to their income. Medicare consists of two separate programs: hospital insurance (Part A) and supplementary medical insurance (Part B). The programs are financed from payroll taxes and premiums paid by beneficiaries. Medicare monies are deposited in special trust funds for use in meeting the expenses incurred by the insured. The program was enacted on July 30, 1965, as TITLE XVIII of the SOCIAL SECURITY ACT, "Health Insurance for the Aged," and became effective on July 1, 1966.

Eligibility for Medicare is fairly straightforward—anyone who has been entitled to SOCIAL SECURITY DISABILITY INSURANCE (SSDI) benefits for two years, or who is over 65, or who experiences permanent kidney failure, is eligible. Allowable benefits vary, depending on whether an individual has hospital or medical insurance. There are certain charges and services Medicare will not cover, such as charges billed at amounts above those in the Medicare allowable fee schedule; services provided by organizations or individuals not Medicare-approved and participating; intermediate nursing home care; custodial care in any setting; care that is not reasonable or necessary; and services or supplies not generally accepted. Hospice benefits have no deductibles and cover inpatient care, home health care, "significant other" counseling and support services, and almost all charges for drugs.

The Hospital Insurance Program, Part A, is compulsory for everyone. Part A automatically enrolls all persons aged 65 and over who are entitled to benefits under the Old Age, Survivors, Disability and Health Insurance Program or the railroad retirement program; persons under age 65 who have been eligible for disability for more than two years; and insured workers (and their dependents) requiring renal dialysis or kidney transplantation. The Supplementary Medical Insurance Program, Part B, is the voluntary portion of Medicare. It covers physician and other individual provider services for all persons entitled to Part A who enroll and pay a monthly premium.

Those receiving Social Security Disability Insurance benefits will automatically be enrolled when the two-year waiting period is over. Others may apply at the local Social Security office. A fairly broad range of appeal rights exists.

medication   Treatment with (drug) remedies; administration of medicine.

meditation   According to Dr. Bernie Siegel it is "an active process of focusing the mind into a state of relaxed awareness. There are many ways of doing this. Some teachers recommend focusing attention on a symbolic sound or word (a mantra) or on a single image, such as a candle flame or mandala. Others teach people to focus on the sound and flowing of the breath. The result of all meditation methods is ultimately the same: to induce a restful trance which strengthens the mind by freeing it from its accustomed turmoil." In the last 25+ years, a considerable body of research has demonstrated how meditation benefits health. For example, blood chemistry reports have shown a lessening of lactate in the blood. Also, electroencephalograms have shown an increase in alpha brain wave activity. Meditation tends to lower or normalize blood pressure, pulse rate, and the levels of stress hormones in the blood. It also lowers abnormally high cholesterol levels and reduces mild hypertension. There is also evidence that with regular practice over a period of time, meditation may increase concentration, memory, intelligence, and creativity.

medroxyprogesterone   Female sex hormones; progestins used to initiate and regulate menstruation and to correct abnormal patterns of menstrual bleeding caused by hormonal imbalance. Medroxyprogesterone works by inducing and maintaining a lining in the uterus that resembles pregnancy. This drug can prevent uterine bleeding until it is withdrawn. By suppressing the release of the pituitary gland hormone that induces ovulation and by stimulating the secretion of mucus by the uterine cervix, this drug can prevent pregnancy. Possible risks include thrombophlebitis (rare), pulmonary embolism (rare), liver reaction with jaundice (rare), and drug-induced birth defects.

medulla   The inner portion of an organ.

Megace   See MEGESTROL ACETATE.

megadose   A very large dose of a nontoxic substance, usually a vitamin.

megaloblast   An abnormally large red blood corpuscle, oval and slightly irregular in shape, from 11 to 20 microns in diameter. Megaloblasts are classified as basophilic, orthochromatic, and polychromatic, and are found in the blood in cases of pernicious anemia.

megaloblastic anemia   Anemia characterized by the presence of MEGALOBLASTs in the blood and BONE MARROW.

megestrol acetate   An antiestrogen drug which is a progesterone. These drugs often induce an early and sometimes permanent menopause. Some doctors include these drugs as part of chemotherapy. Its trade name is Megace.

melanin   The dark, protective pigment of the skin. Exposure to sunlight stimulates melanin production. It can be prepared chemically. MELANOMA, the most serious type of skin cancer, originates in the cells that produce melanin.

melanoma   A malignant, darkly pigmented mole or tumor of the skin.

membrane   A thin sheet or layer of pliable tissue serving as a covering.

membrane attack complex (MAC)   The terminal complement components that, when activated, cause lysis of target cells.

membrane fluidizers   Nutritional substances made from egg and soy lecithin, believed to extract cholesterol from the cell walls of viral lipid coatings and the cell membranes of T CELLS. It was theorized that the cholesterol produces structural rigidity essential for binding of a virus to the target host cells, so that causing a fluidity of interaction between virus and host would reduce infectivity. Prior to the advent of reverse transcriptase-inhibiting drugs, many people reported some degree of success using these products as a treatment for HIV.

memory   The mental registration, retention, and recall of past experience, knowledge, ideas, sensations, and thoughts. Memory defects are a symptom of many diseases. Recall may fail because memories have been obliterated or suppressed psychologically, because there has been organic brain damage by drugs, disease (or age), or because of a temporary interferance with normal brain function by drugs or disease. See AIDS DEMENTIA.

memory T cell   A T cell that bears receptors for a specific foreign antigen encountered during a prior infection or vaccination. After an infection or a vaccination, some of the T cells that participated in the response remain as memory T cells, which rapidly mobilize and clone themselves should the same antigen be reencountered during a second infection at a later time. See IMMUNITY.

meninges   The three membranes that ensheathe the brain and spinal cord: the pia mater (internal), the arachnoid (middle), and the dura mater (external).

meningitis   An infection of the MENINGES, the membranes that envelope the brain and the spinal cord. The most common cause of meningitis in people with HIV infection is CRYPTOCOCCUS.

meningoencephalitis   Inflammation or infection of the brain and its meninges. The usual cause is a bacterial infection, but free-living amoebae such as the genera *Naegleria* and *Acanthamoeba* have also caused this condition.

menopause   The period during which menstruation ends permanantly; the end of a woman's period of fertility. Diagnosis of menopause is indicated by the absence of menses accompanied by symptomatology and strengthened when serum LH and FSH are found to be elevated, indicating failure of the ovaries to produce estrogen in the presence of adequate hypothalamic/pituitary stimulation. Definitive diagnosis is indicated by the completion of 12 months without menses. Women generally develop some signs of estrogen depletion prior to the cessation of periods. Until the periods have stopped for 12 months, conception is still possible and contraceptive measures should be taken. Menopause usually occurs naturally between ages 45 and 55. It may also be surgically induced, or occur prematurely. Early onset of menopause is not uncommon in HIV-positive women. Compounding a possible association with HIV are factors such as anemia, chronic illness, weight loss, tobacco use, use of street drugs (particularly heroin), and possible effects of antiretrovirals such as AZT or ddI.

Estrogen replacement therapy is generally offered to menopausal women to reduce bothersome or debilitating symptoms (hot flashes, insomnia, decreased sexual functioning, decreased appetite, night sweats, weight loss, fatigue, vaginitis, dysuria, etc.), to prevent demineralization of bones (leading to osteoporosis), and to offset changes in lipid metabolism related to heart disease. Estrogen is supplemented with progestin to offset the documented increase in endometrial cancer and potential increased risk of breast cancer in women with unopposed estrogenic stimulation. The use of exogenous hormones in HIV-positive women presents incalculable risks, including unknown drug interactions with HIV medications and uncertain effects on immune response.

menses   See MENSTRUATION.

menstrual blood   Blood that is shed from a woman's uterus during her menstrual period.

menstruation   The cyclic discharge of blood and mucosal tissues from the UTERUS through the VAGINA; also called menses. It is brought on by reduced production of ovarian HORMONES and in healthy women occurs at approximately four-week intervals, except during pregnancy, throughout the reproductive period of a woman's life (from puberty to MENOPAUSE). It is the culmination of the menstrual cycle.

Menstrual disorders often accompany chronic illness. Specific menstrual disorders encountered by HIV-positive women may be exacerbated by anemia, weight loss, medications, street drugs and psychogenic factors, particularly depression. In addition, women with HIV infection also experience the usual range of menstrual difficulties that afflict non–HIV-positive women. HIV-positive women frequently complain of changes in their menstrual cycles such as irregular periods, abnormally heavy or light periods, or an increase in premenstrual symptoms such as breast pain, cramping, fluid retention, anxiety, or depression. These changes may be due to HIV itself or to specific medications, particularly AZT. Other variables include the use of prescribed medications, the use of street drugs (particularly heroin), and weight loss. The immune system and the endocrine system interact with one another in ways that are not entirely understood. We cannot be certain of the effects of exogenous hormones in an immunocopromised individual.

Current standards of care for HIV-positive women neither approve nor forbid the use of hormone therapies or oral contraceptives for birth control or menstrual regulation. There is no present information that would alter treatment strategies for AMENORRHEA, DYSMENORRHEA, premature or natural menopause, or premenstrual syndrome in immuno-

compromised clients. Research into the etiology as well as the effect of absent menstruation on the immune and endocrine health of women is needed.

Menstrual problems can adversely affect a woman's health during HIV illness. Blood loss from heavy periods can predispose to or exacerbate anemia. Irregular or absent periods may signal significant systemic illness. Intermenstrual bleeding and amenorrhea should be investigated in all women, even if it is a long-standing complaint.

mental health   The capacity of an individual to form harmonious relationships with others; to participate in or contribute constructively to changes in one's social and physical environment; and to achieve a harmonious and balanced satisfaction of one's own potentially conflicting drives. Mental health is a highly variable concept influenced by both biological and cultural factors. It is often defined as the absence of any identifiable or significant mental disorder, or it may simply refer to mental status.

mental health professionals   Persons who work with the behavioral, social, and emotional problems of the emotionally or mentally disturbed. Mental health professionals treat symptomatic and causative elements affecting clients' ability to respond appropriately to their environment.

mental health services   Examination, treatment, and care of emotional and mental disorders and accompanying conditions.

mental status   The psychological or psychiatric state of an individual. The assessment of mental status based on a case review or examination may include consideration of behavior, appearance, responsiveness to stimuli of all kinds, speech, memory, and judgment.

meprobamate   An antianxiety drug, or tranquilizer, that acts on the CENTRAL NERVOUS SYSTEM much as BARBITURATES do. As do barbiturates, meprobamate can cause drowsiness, lethargy, and lack of coordination. Continued use for weeks or months may increase tolerance; higher doses are then required for the same effect. Continued use may also cause psychological and physical dependence. Withdrawing the drug suddenly after prolonged, regular use may cause severe reactions. Other side effects can include stomach irritation and allergic reactions. Trade names are Equanil and Miltown.

metabolic acidosis   A disturbance that results in excessive acid in body fluids due to an increase in acids other than carbonic acid. It may be caused by such conditions as severe infection, dehydration, shock, diarrhea, renal dysfunction, or hepatic dysfunction.

metabolic encephalopathy   Neuropsychiatric disturbance caused by metabolic brain disease. It may be the result of disease in other organs, such as the lungs or kidneys, or it may be caused directly by low blood sugar (hypoglycemia), low oxygenation (hypoxia), or decreased blood flow (ischemia).

metastasis   Transfer or spread of a disease, especially cancer, or its manifestations from one organ or part to another not directly connected with it; change in location of bacteria or body cells from one part of the body to another.

metastasize   To spread to other parts of the body by METASTASIS; to form new foci of disease in distant parts of the body by metastasis.

methadone hydrochloride   An opiate commonly used to control withdrawal symptoms from addictive morphinelike drugs, particularly heroin. Side effects are those shared by all morphinelike drugs that depress the CENTRAL NERVOUS SYSTEM: dizziness, mental clouding, depression, and sedation. Although used to assist addicts kick their drug dependence, methadone may itself cause physical dependence. Stopping it abruptly after prolonged and regular use can cause withdrawal symptoms. Methadone can be given orally or injected intravenously. Methadone maintenance is permitted only in programs approved by the FOOD AND DRUG ADMINISTRATION and the designated state authority. Trade names are Dolophine Hydrochloride and Methadose.

methadone maintenance clinics   Clinics which dispense methadone for treatment of drug dependence due to use of opium derivatives. These clinics may be community-based or hospital-based. Because methadone is a habit-forming agent, its use should be carefully supervised. The major goal of methadone maintenance is for the client to stop using illicit drugs, develop a productive life, and become a valued member of society. HIV/AIDS is an additional assault to these clients' self-esteem and is often a new reason to resume taking nonprescribed drugs. It is safe to say that the onset of HIV/AIDS has had an enormous impact on the clinics and staff involved in methadone maintenance as a drug treatment modality.

Most methadone maintenance clinics are managed by a medical director, and staffed by a number of mental health providers, including counselors. Often, some of these counselors are former IV drug users. Clinics function to provide access to medical care and counseling. Clinic services include seeing people every day, providing psycho-social support for them, and dispensing methadone and/or other "meds." Effective treatment is composed of first forming a working relationship with people who are or who have been at the bottom-most rungs of our society. The staff must convey understanding, respect and commitment, as well as insight in order to develop a therapeutic alliance.

Clients on methadone are different from and often more difficult to work with than other chemically dependent clients. Historically, they have had more social and health problems. They have also experienced an inordinate number of problems at work. Very often, their heroin addiction has related to a history of criminal activity and violence. For the most part, these are not people who have a history of tolerating intra-psychic distress. Their primary way of coping has been to take drugs. With the onset of HIV/AIDS, their social and health problems have increased dramatically. Very often they have been using drugs intravenously for many years before beginning to take methadone. In many cases, they continue to use illicit drugs or abuse alcohol even while on methadone. Patients on methadone frequently struggle with issues of poverty, homelessness, and crack. Many patients face all of these issues simultaneously on a daily basis. These people do not usually trust either the health care establishment or drug treatment professionals since most often they are not treated with respect, care, or gentleness.

Today, most urban methadone maintenance programs are experienced with working with clients whose lives are impacted by HIV/AIDS. These programs provide an alternative to the rejection many clients experience from their families and friends. They provide one safe place for their clients to discuss fears and concerns. The challenges the clients present to staff are enormous, but by not rejecting them the staff make a significant difference in their clients' lives. Somewhat ironically, one further problem confronts people with HIV/AIDS who want methadone or another form of treatment for their drug addiction—a current shortage of methadone maintenance clinics.

methaqualone hydrochloride   A hypnotic sedative that has become a drug of abuse. Because of the illegal abuse of this drug, it is no longer distributed in the United States.

methotrexate (MTX)   An immunosuppressive drug that like cyclophosphamide (CY), is used at high doses as a cancer chemotherapy. At lower doses, MTX suppresses inflammation in immune disorders such as Wegener's granulomatosis, rheumatoid arthritis, and psoriasis. At low doses, MTX has anti-inflammatory effects, and can reduce levels of various markers of immune activity, particularly serum antibodies and rheumatoid factor, a component of immune complexes characteristic of rheumatoid arthritis. Numerous side effects are associated with MTX treatment. BONE MARROW SUPPRESSION has been seen but is infrequent at the lower doses used for arthritis. The most common side effects of lower doses of MTX are GASTROINTESTINAL (nausea, diarrhea, anorexia, oral ulcers). Such toxicities appear to be lessened by coadministration of folic acid. Even at the low doses used in autoimmune disease, though, MTX treatment for periods of more than three months is associated with development of opportunistic infections, especially PNEUMOCYSTIS CARINII pneumonia and varicella zoster. Previously used name was amethopterin. Trade names Mexate and Folex.

methylphenidate   A stimulant used primarily to treat narcolepsy (recurrent spells of uncontrollable drowsiness and sleep) and attention-deficit disorders in children. Additional uses include the treatment of mild to moderate depression, and the management of apathetic and withdrawal states in the elderly. Nervousness and insomnia are two possible side effects. It is sold under the trade names Ritalin and Ritalin-SR.

meticorten   See PREDNISONE.

metronidazole   An antiamebic, antibacterial, and antitrichomonal drug appearing as whitish to pale yellowish crystals or crystalline powder. It is taken by people with HIV infection for common intestinal infections and common dental problems like gingivitis (inflammation of the gums) and periodontitis (infection of the structures that support the teeth). It may be administered orally or, in women, intravaginally. Side effects are unusual, primarily nausea and stomach pain. Side effects may be reduced if the drug is taken with meals or if the dose is reduced. Taking this drug for periods of months may cause pain in the feet that resembles the pain of HIV neuropathy. The pain usually goes away when the drug is stopped. The trade name is Flagyl.

MHC   See MAJOR HISTOCOMPATIBILITY COMPLEX.

microbe   A microscopic one-celled organism—bacterium fungus, protozoan, or virus—not distinguishable as vegetable or animal. Microbes cause infectious diseases and may be carried from one host to another by human and animal sources, air, contact infection, food, fomites (inanimate objects) such as linens, books, cooking utensils and clothing, insects and soil. The microbes that commonly cause the opportunistic infections associated with HIV infection are: bacteria—MYCOBACTERIUM AVIUM-INTRACELLULARE, MYCOBACTERIUM TUBERCULOSIS, SALMONELLA, NOCARDIA; fungi—CRYPTOCOCCUS, HISTOPLASMA, CANDIDA ALBICANS; parasites—TOXOPLASMA GONDII, PNEUMOCYSTIS CARINII, CRYPTOSPORIDIUM, *Isospora;* and viruses—CYTOMEGALO-VIRUS, HERPES SIMPLEX, HERPES ZOSTER, MOLLUSCUM CONTA-GIOSUM. HIV is itself a virus.

microbicide   An agent that kills MICROBEs.

microbiology   Science that deals with the study of microorganisms, including bacteria, fungi, and viruses.

microhemagglutination assay for T. pallidum (MATP)   A treponemal test for SYPHILIS based on agglutination of red cells to which ANTIGENS from the microorganism *Treponema pallidum* have been attached. The treponemal variety of syphilis tests look for *T. pallidum*, the corkscrew-shaped organisms that cause the disease.

micronutrient   An essential nutrient, as a trace mineral, that is required in minute amounts. Micronutrients are essential to the body in small amounts because they are either components of enzymes or act as coenzymes in managing chemical reactions.

microorganism   An organism of microscopic scale, not perceptible to the naked eye; a MICROBE.

Microspora   An order of parasitic protozoa; also called Enidosporidia and Microsporidia.

It is conjectured that there are many different species and classes of microspora, which can cause a variety of problems in people with HIV. However, these are very difficult to detect by the current available diagnostic tests. Although best known as a cause of diarrhea, microspora can also cause infections of the eye, kidney, liver, muscles, brain, and several other tissues. See MICROSPORIDIOSIS.

Microsporida   An order of parasitic protozoa. Also called Enidosporidia and Microsporidia. See MICROSPORIDIOSIS.

Microsporidia   An order of parasitic protozoa, also called MICROSPORA. See MICROSPORIDIOSIS.

microsporidiosis   An intestinal infection that causes diarrhea and wasting in people with AIDS. It is caused by two different species of MICROSPORA (or MICROSPORIDIA) an order of protozoal parasites. Although difficult to detect, a variety of microspora is widespread in animals and humans. The most common type is called *Enterocytozon bieneusi*, which invades the small intestine and seems to cause severe chronic diarrhea. Prior to the HIV/AIDS epidemic, only eleven cases of microsporidiosis had been reported in world medical literature.

The mode of transmission of microsporidiosis is unknown, although many patients with it have a history of extensive foreign travel or residence. Other suspected forms of transmission include unprotected sexual activity and eating food contaminated with microsporans. Symptoms such as diarrhea, abdominal cramps, fever, and weight loss do not always occur immediately after exposure.

Small obscure microsporans are thought to exist in the intestine, liver, muscles, cornea, and other tissues. They rarely show up with routine methods of detection and in fact often evoke little or no response. Examining stool with an electron microscope may be the only means to recognize or classify microspora. However, because there is not yet an accepted standard technique to detect microsporans in human stool, diagnosis of intestinal microsporidiosis must be done by small bowel BIOPSY. It is noted that there is beginning to be some success with deteching spores in stool by light microscopy.

Examining urine under an electron microscope may lead to detection of microsporidiosis of the kidney. However there seem to be no symptoms of microsporidiosis with kidney infection that would lead a doctor to make such a diagnosis. The parasite seems to shed or to be cast off through the system, so patients with diarrhea caused by microsporans may have the organism elsewhere in the body as well.

Presumptive diagnosis of microsporans in the eye can be made by examining a scraping of the cornea under an electron microscope. Diagnostic confirmation still requires biopsy.

To date, there is no known effective therapy for microsporidiosis. A variety of old and new agents are under investigation and a few scattered reports have shown partial success with albendazole, metronidazole (Flagyl), and 566c80. Antidiarrheal drugs may provide symptomatic relief.

migrating cheilosis   See PERLECHE.

milk thistle   See SILYMARIN.

milzbrand   See ANTHRAX.

mind-body therapies   Alternative and holistic therapies that focus on the mind, body, and spirit; includes meditation, image/visualization, biofeedback, hypnosis, expressive therapies (music, art, dance/movement), therapeutic healing, touch, and spiritual healing. Many believe such therapies enhance immunity in people with HIV/AIDS. A person living with HIV can learn about these approaches from a variety of practitioners and then integrate them with standard medical care in collaboration with an HIV-experienced physician. See also ALTERNATIVE MEDICINE, ALTERNATIVE TREATMENT.

mineralocorticoid   The hormones secreted by the adrenal cortex that affect fluid-ELECTROLYTE balance; aldosterone is the major hormone in this group. See CORTICOSTEROIDS.

minimal dose   The smallest dose of a medication that produces an effect.

minimum effective dose (MED-50)   The lowest dosage of a drug required to produce the desired effect in 50 percent of subjects.

miscarriage   Termination of pregnancy at any time before the fetus has attained extrauterine viability. HIV-infected women are three times more likely to experience a miscarriage than healthy women. Researchers have suggested four possible factors that alone or in combination contribute to fetal demise in HIV-infected women: direct toxic effects of HIV on the fetus; fetal thymic dysfunction; placental changes; and elevated uterine levels of the inflammatory CYTOKINES IL-4, IL-6 and TNF.

mistletoe   An extract of European mistletoe (*Viscum album*) has been used since the 1960s in Europe as an anticancer agent. It is purported to possess both antitumor and immunostimulatory properties. Mistletoe is potentially hazardous; however, it is also used safely to treat high blood pressure and cancer and has been shown to regenerate cells more quickly than normal when damaged by X-ray radiation. Lung and ovarian cancers have been treated with mistletoe. Mistletoe should be used only under the supervision of a physician. It is sold under the trade name Iscador.

mite   Any arthropod of the order Acarina except the ticks. Mites are minute arachnids related to the spiders. Some are parasitic and are causative agents of such conditions as mange or scabies. Others serve as intermediate hosts and carry causative organisms of disease from infected to noninfected individuals.

mitochondria   Slender microscopic filaments or rods, 0.5 micrometer in diameter, that can be seen in cells by using phase-contrast microscopy or electron microscopy. They are the source of energy in the cell and are involved in protein synthesis and lipid metabolism.

mitogen   A protein substance derived from plants that is used in the laboratory to stimulate cells to divide (mitosis). Frequently used IN VITRO, q.v. to study the proliferation of lymphocytes from blood drawn during a research study.

mixed lymphocyte reaction/mixed lymphocyte culture (MLR/MLC)   An assay system for T-CELL recognition of allogenic cells in which response is measured by proliferation in the presence of the stimulating cells.

mobilization   The making movable of a fixed or ankylosed part; restoration of motion to a joint; making an organ free or movable; the freeing, or making available, of substances held in reserve, such as glycogen or fat.

mode of transmission   See TRANSMISSION.

molecular biology   The field of biology in which biological systems are analyzed in terms of the physics and chemistry of their molecular components.

molecular mimicry   Immunological cross-reactivity between determinants on an environmental antigen, such as a virus and a self-antigen, a notion that has been proposed to explain autoimmunity.

molluscum   See MOLLUSCUM CONTAGIOSUM.

molluscum contagiosum   A common skin disease that is persistent and sometimes disfiguring in HIV-infected individuals and others with weakened immune systems. Molluscum contagiosum can appear on the epithelium of the genitals or other areas of the skin and is caused by a poxvirus infection. Spread by skin-to-skin contact, it is considered to be benign, but may cause itching and rapid spreading. The virus causes small dome-shaped (3 to 5 millimeters in diameter) bumps called papules. In people with healthy immune systems, the papules are usually few in number and generally resolve spontaneously within a few months. Treatment, when needed, is usually akin to that used for warts: freezing, treatment with caustic agents, removal with a sharp instrument, or electrocautery. In people with HIV infection, molluscum contagiosum is often a progressive disease resistant to treatment. In HIV-infected individuals with relatively intact immune systems, MCV papules are usually few in number, localized to the groin or face. Once an individual's CD4+ T cell count falls below 200 cells per cubic millimeter of blood, the lesions tend to proliferate and spread. At this stage of HIV disease, a person may have more than 100 papules on the face (including the eyelids), trunk, and groin. Lesions sometimes coalesce to form giant lesions that measure 1.5 centimeters in diameter. In patients with CD4+ T cell counts lower than 50/mm the lesions may extend onto mucosal surfaces of the lips or conjunctiva. MCV is one of only two poxviruses known to specifically infect people. The other human poxvirus is a distant relative: variola virus, which causes smallpox. Whereas smallpox is a sudden and severe infection that either the immune system quickly controls or death results, molluscum contagiosum is a slow disease that evokes a minimal immune response.

Moniliaceae   A family of colorless to light-colored, imperfect fungi belonging to the order Moniliases. These include the genera *Aspergillus, Blastomyces, Coccidioides, Histoplasma, Penicillum, Sporothrix, Trichoderma, Trichophyton, Trichothecium,* and *Verticillium.*

moniliasis   Infection of the skin or mucous membranes by MONILIACEAE, yeastlike fungi. Usually localized in skin, nails, mouth, vagina, bronchi, or lungs, it may invade the bloodstream. See CANDIDIASIS.

monoamine oxidase inhibitors (MAO inhibitors; MAOI)
A class of antidepressants that increase levels of neurotransmitters in the brain by interfering with an enzyme—monoamine oxidase—that breaks them down.

Depression is thought to be caused by a reduction in the level of certain chemicals, neurotransmitters, in the brain. MAO inhibitors increase the levels of these chemicals in the spaces (synapses) between nerve cells in the brain. Monoamine oxidase inhibitors differ from the other classes of antidepressants, the tricyclics and serotonin reuptake inhibitors, which prevent cells from absorbing certain neurotransmitters and thus increase their levels in the synapses.

MAO inhibitors are potentially toxic and must be used with caution because they deactivate enzymes in the body that break down chemicals found in many foods such as meat, cheese, yeast extracts, and red wine. Eating these foods while taking an MAO inhibitor can cause a dramatic rise in blood pressure (hypertension).

monoclonal   Derived from a single clone. See MONOCLONAL ANTIBODY.

monoclonal antibody   An antibody produced for a specific ANTIGEN by a hybridoma (a clone resulting from the division of a hybrid cell produced from artificial fusion of a normal antibody-producing B cell with a B cell tumor cell. Chemically and immunologically homogenous, their exceptional purity and specificity make them useful as laboratory reagents in various tests, such as the ELISA test. They are also used experimentally in cancer immunotherapy.

Monoclonal antibodies have two properties that lead scientists to believe they may be useful therapeutically. In some cases, they are directly cytotoxic; monoclonal antibodies, on their own, may destroy unwanted cells. In other cases, the monoclonal antibodies have no destructive effects themselves but can carry toxins or radioactive particles directly to target cells or tissues. Monoclonal antibody therapy has been used to treat HODGKIN'S DISEASE (HD) and NON-HODGKIN'S LYMPHOMA (NHL).

monocyte   A mononuclear phagocyte (white blood cell) derived from the MYELOID stem cells. Monocytes are formed in the BONE MARROW, and are short-lived, with a half-life of approximately one day. They circulate in the bloodstream, from which they move into tissues, where they mature into long-lived macrophages. Monocytes produce INTERLEUKIN-1, a substance that activates T LYMPHOCYTES in the presence of ANTIGEN.

Monocytes and MACROPHAGEs form one of the first lines of defense in the inflammatory process. This network of fixed and mobile phagocytes that engulf foreign antigens and cell debris is commonly called the RETICULOENDOTHELIAL SYSTEM.

monogamous   In a long-term sexual relationship with only one partner. See MONOGAMY.

monogamy   Literally, the practice of being married to one person at a time. In contemporary usage the term also refers to the practice of maintaining unmarried relationships between two people in which the partners have sexual relations only with each other. Monogamous relationships have become more widespread among single adults in the 1980s and 1990s as the AIDS epidemic has spread.

monokine   A chemical mediator released by MONOCYTEs and MACROPHAGES during the immune response. Monokines affect the growth and activity of other white blood cells. INTERLEUKIN-1 is the most important monokine.

monolaurin   A saturated fatty acid with a mode of action believed to be similar to that of lecithin extracts. It is a chemical constituent of mother's milk, known to confer immunity on nursing infants until their development of independent immunity. It is known to be safe and is licensed by the USDA as a food additive for the purpose of preventing the growth of bacteria and viruses in food products. It has demonstrated antiviral activity against lipid viruses. Many people use this substance in combination with BHT as a CMV prophylaxis.

mononeuritis multiplex (MM)   Inflammation of nerves in separate body areas. MM tends to occur during the asymptomatic early period of HIV infection, but a more severe type, attributed to CMV infection, has been observed in people with advanced AIDS.

mononuclear phagocyte system   Mononuclear cells found primarily in the reticular connective tissue of lymphoid and other organs that are prominent in chronic inflammatory states.

mononucleosis   A condition characterized by the presence of an abnormally large quantity of mononuclear LEUKOCYTEs (monocytes) in the blood. INFECTIOUS MONONUCLEOSIS is an acute infectious disease that primarily affects lymphoid tissue.

monotherapy   Medical treatment consisting of a single drug, such as AZT or ddI, administered alone (as contrasted to COMBINATION THERAPY with one or more drugs, such as AZT and DDC or AZT and ddI). Trials and studies continue to probe the clinical benefits but often quickly become irrelevant because new and more potent drugs are constantly being added to the therapeutic arsenal, and treatment options are increasing. When to employ which regimen is affected by such issues as CROSS-RESISTANCE, synergy, and TOXICITY, as well as whether trial participants had prior experience with AZT or were AZT-NAIVE. Questions abound about the optimal time to start therapy or when to switch regimens. The general feeling today is that AZT monotherapy is not the best treatment available, whether as initial therapy or in the drug-experienced. See ANTIRETROVIRAL THERAPY.

morbidity   Frequency of disease occurrence in proportion to the population. Also, the condition of being diseased.

morning-after pill   A regimen administered as a morning-after treatment to prevent AIDS infection after a possible exposure to HIV, and as of 1997, one of the latest medical advances in the battle against AIDS. Despite the lack of studies supporting the use of the morning-after pill, some doctors are using it for patients who have engaged in high-risk sex. The use of expensive AIDS drugs as a morning-after remedy raises troubling questions about who has access to such treatment. While affluent Americans may soon be able to drop by their doctors' offices to get the miracle pills, AIDS sufferers in the developing world receive woefully inadequate medical care and die much sooner than they might have had they received proper medication. Physicians and researchers are concerned that if the public perceives morning-after pills together with condoms, as part of a new, improved "safe sex" package, the result may be reinforcement of the potentially dangerous idea that any form of sex with anybody at any time is indeed safe. If people know there is a morning-after remedy, they may do things the night before that they might otherwise have avoided, and whose dire consequences the treatment may not ultimately prove capable of preventing.

mortality   The number of deaths in proportion to the population, over a specified time. Also, the state of being mortal.

mortality tables   Actuarial tables used by the insurance industry to predict the survival and death rates of large groups of people.

mother-to-child transmission   See TRANSMISSION.

mother-to-fetus transmission   See TRANSMISSION.

mother's milk   HIV has been isolated from the breast milk of infected women. A few reports demonstrate that HIV is transmissible through the milk of an infected mother to her breast-fed child. Physicians estimate the risk of transmission via breast milk at 29 percent for mothers who are postnatally infected. The risk is even higher, as high as 43 percent for women who are infected prenatally, in addition to the risk of transmission IN UTERO or during delivery.

The World Health Organization (WHO) recommends bottle feeding for HIV-infected mothers who reside in the United States or Europe. Formula feeding in many developing countries is not considered as safe; after reviewing the various risks for the two alternatives, WHO judged that breast-feeding is preferable to the risk of bottle-feeding in these areas, irrespective of the presence of HIV in the mother.

motor dysfunction   Abnormal, disturbed, or impaired functioning of a muscle, nerve, or center that effects or produces movement.

motor function impairment   See MOTOR DYSFUNCTION.

Motrin   See IBUPROFEN.

MRI   See MAGNETIC RESONANCE IMAGING.

mucocutaneous infection   The invasion by and multiplication of a pathogenic agent in a mucous membrane or the skin.

mucopurulent cervicitis   Infection of the CERVIX, often by STDS.

mucosa   A mucous membrane; the epithelial lining of a body cavity (mouth, vagina, rectum, or urethra) that opens to the environment.

mucosa-associated lymphoid tissue (MALT)   Generic term for LYMPHOID tissue associated with the GASTROINTESTINAL TRACT, bronchial tree, and other MUCOSA. This tissue produces a unique immunoglobulin (secretory IGA) and T-CELL immunity for these mucosal surfaces.

mucosal homing   The ability of immunologically competent cells that arise from mucosal follicles to traffic back to mucosal areas.

mucous membrane   The surface tissue lining various tubular structures of the body that communicate with air, such as the mouth, nose, nipples, urethra, anus, vulva, and tip of the penis. It consists of a surface layer of EPITHELIUM, a basement membrane, and an underlying layer of connective tissue. Mucous membranes are kept moist by the secretions of mucus-producing glands.

mucous membrane exposure   Exposure to infection via the mucous membranes such as the lining of the mouth, nostrils, or vagina.

mucus   The thick fluid secreted by mucous membranes or mucous glands.

multiagent therapy   Treatment with more than one drug. See also MONOTHERAPY.

Multicenter AIDS Cohort Study (MACS)   The Multicenter AIDS Cohort Study is one of the largest prospective HIV studies in the world. Begun in 1983, MACS enrolled its first participants in 1984. Of the 5,579 men who entered the study, 2,191 were infected with HIV. During the study, 488 men have become HIV infected. MACS clinical sites are located in Baltimore (Johns Hopkins), Los Angeles (UCLA), Pittsburgh (University of Pittsburgh), and Chicago (the Howard Brown Memorial Clinic/Northwestern University). The men come to the clinical sites twice a year for exams and laboratory testing as well as to answer questions about any preventive and treatment medications they take. From enrollment through March 30, 1995, 1,362 men have developed AIDS, of whom 1,158 died. Another 101 HIV-infected men died before they developed AIDS. At enrollment, MACS men were 83.1 percent white, 10.1 percent African American and 5.3 percent Hispanic, while the rest were from other or unknown racial groups. The men ranged in age from 18 to 70, and more than half had college degrees when they entered the study.

By studying the outcome of various medications in real clinical practice, MACS provides an observational database that indicates the unsuspected value of available therapies. Important MACS accomplishments and findings: the identification of more than 60 HIV-infected men who are long-term nonprogressors, many of whom have served as critical sources of information on this phenomenon in studies conducted at several United States laboratories; the discovery that prevention of PNEUMOCYSTIS CARINII PNEUMONIA can delay the first AIDS-defining illness by six to 12 months; the finding that ZIDOVUDINE (AZT) therapy given with ACY-CLOVIR may significantly increase survival of AIDS patients; the discovery that response of CD4+ T CELLS to AZT predicts AIDS-free time and survival among HIV-infected patients; the finding that risk factors for AIDS-related dementia include anemia, lower body mass, older age, and the presence of such symptoms as fever, fatigue, diarrhea, or thrush before an AIDS diagnosis; and the finding that symptoms of depression do not independently predict poorer outcomes to HIV infection. MACS collaborations with the National Cancer Institute, a component of the National Institutes of Health, and the Agency for Health Care Policy and Research (AHCPR), an agency of the United States PUBLIC HEALTH SERVICE, part of the United States DEPARTMENT OF HEALTH AND HUMAN SERVICES, have supported studies on HIV-related cancers and the impact of treatments on patients' use of health services.

multidrug-resistant tuberculosis (MDR-TB)   See MULTIPLE DRUG-RESISTANT TUBERCULOSIS.

multifocal giant-cell encephalitis   See AIDS DEMENTIA COMPLEX.

multiple allergic reactions   Increased severity of reactions (fever, rash, swelling, itching) to insect bites or common medications such as sulfa or penicillin.

multiple drug-resistant tuberculosis (MDR-TB)   A strain of TB that does not respond to two or more standard TB drugs. MDR-TB usually occurs when treatment is interrupted, thus allowing drug-resist MUTATIONs to occur in the organism.

mushrooms   Any of various fleshy fungi, including the toadstools, puffballs, coral fungi, and morels. The subject of immune potentiators and antivirals from medicinal fungi is, as one might expect, very large. Within the context of HIV/AIDS, commercial product literature, medical studies, and reports have been published that discuss both the potential of different varieties of mushrooms as immune modulation agents and their mechanisms.

Shiitake is an edible mushroom traditionally cultivated in Japan and now used as a delicacy in cooking throughout the world. Traditionally, shiitake has been used as a folk remedy in Japan. Lentinan, a substance found in shiitake, has important effects on the immune system, and is well accepted by physicians in Japan to increase T-CELLS for cancer treatment. Japanese scientists have found that the drug can be used orally and that it has very little toxicity. It has immune potentiating effects and may also be antiviral against HIV.

The problem is we don't know how much lentinan is in the mushrooms. Too much can result with the opposite of the intended effect. We do know that lentinan should not be used every day; ingesting lentinan every other day or every fourth day has worked best. Traditional cooking recipes may give the best available information about how much of the mushroom to use and how to prepare it. There has been increasing interest in the medicinal use of shiitake and lentinan as possible treatments for AIDS. More studies are needed

to determine if lentinan is an effective therapy for delaying or preventing the development of AIDS in persons at early stages of illness.

mutation   A change in the genetic material of a virus or a cell that may lead to a change in the structure or functioning of an organism; a change in the genetic material of a gene that is transmissible to offspring.

mutually monogamous sexual relationship   A relationship in which each partner agrees to be MONOGAMOUS.

myalgia   Tenderness or pain in a muscle or muscles.

Myambutol   See ETHAMBUTOL HYDROCHLORIDE.

Mycelex G   See CLOTRIMAZOLE.

Mycobacterium   A genus of acid-fast organisms that belongs to the Mycobacteriaceae family and includes the causative organisms of TUBERCULOSIS, LEPROSY, and MAC. They are slender, nonmotile Gram-positive rods and do not produce spores or capsules.

mycobacterial infection   Invasion by and multiplication of mycobacteria, members of the genus that includes the pathogenic causative organisms of TUBERCULOSIS and LEPROSY. These acid-fast organisms are slender, nonmotile Gram-positive rods that do not produce spores or capsules.

mycobacteriosis   An infection caused by any mycobacterium.

Mycobacterium avium complex (MAC)   A serious bacterial infection that causes lung and other organ system infections in individuals whose immune systems are severely damaged. Evidence of MAC has been found in approximately 50 percent of adult AIDS patients at AUTOPSY. It is caused by two similar bacteria (*Mycobacterium avium* and *Mycobacterium intercellulare* [MAI]) found in soil and dust particles. In AIDS, MAC can spread through the bloodstream to infect LYMPH NODES, BONE MARROW, liver, spleen, spinal fluid, lungs, and intestinal tract. Typical symptoms include night sweats, weight loss, fever, fatigue, diarrhea, and enlarged spleen. MAC is usually found in people with CD4 counts below 100; the risk of MAC increases when T4 CELLS are below 50. Treatment of the infection is complicated, requiring the use of four to seven drugs; prophylaxis is not yet standardized. Clarithromycin remains the most potent drug for the treatment of disseminated MAC infection (500 mg, twice daily in combination with other antibiotics, is the standard of care). Treatment often results with improvement in symptoms and clearing of bacteria from the blood. However, relapse may occur several months after treatment. While some studies have suggested that a higher dose (1000 mg) might be more effective, recent studies have ruled out high-dose clarithromycin for AIDS-related MAC. The data from these studies suggest that a higher dose is associated with higher mortality.

Initiating prophylaxis without such data is not without some risk. Many potential drug interactions and toxicities are unstudied and unknown; it is known, however, that clarithromycin alters the ability of the body to absorb and distribute AZT. The risk of developing resistance is another serious concern. Organisms often become resistant when an ANTIBIOTIC is used for a long time, and the risk is particularly acute with clarithromycin because microbacteria are known to develop resistance quickly. RIFABUTIN has been shown to delay the occurrence of MAC.

Mycobacterium avium-intracellulare (MAI)   See MYCOBACTERIUM AVIUM COMPLEX.

Mycobacterium kansasii   A slow-growing, photochromogenic organism that causes a TUBERCULOSIS-like pulmonary disease in humans.

Mycobacterium leprae   The causative agent of LEPROSY in humans. It typically occurs in rounded masses, groups of bacilli, or intracellular clumps.

Mycobacterium tuberculosis   The microorganism that causes tuberculosis in mammals.

mycoplasma   One of a group of very small organisms in which the ability to form a cell wall has been lost. There are more than 70 organisms in this group, including 12 species that infect humans.

Human mycoplasma infections are usually cervical and pelvic. It has been speculated that mycoplasma is a necessary cofactor in HIV-related disease progression, but research to date has shown that the presence of mycoplasma DNA in the blood of HIV-infected patients is transient and not prognostic.

mycosis   Any disease caused by a fungus.

Mycostatin   See NYSTATIN.

myelin sheath   Many layers of membrane of Schwann cell (in peripheral nerves) or of oligodendrocyte (central nervous system) wrapped in a tight spiral around a nerve axon forming a sheath that prevents leakage of current across all of the surrounded axon membrane except at the nodes of Ranvier.

myelitis   Inflammation of the BONE MARROW or the SPINAL CORD.

myeloma   A LYMPHOMA produced from cells of the B-CELL lineage.

myelopathy   A general term denoting any pathological condition of the spinal cord or BONE MARROW. The term is used to refer to nonspecific lesions, as opposed to inflammatory lesions, which are termed MYELITIS.

myelosuppression   The suppression of BONE MARROW activity, causing decreased production of red blood cells (anemia) or white blood cells (leukopenia). Myelosuppression is a side effect of some drugs, such as AZT.

myelosuppressive   Concerning inhibition of BONE MARROW function.

myelotoxic   Destructive to BONE MARROW.

myocardial   Concerning the heart's muscle mass.

myocardial dysfunction   Abnormal, disturbed, or impaired functioning of the muscular walls of the heart; MYOCARDIOPATHY.

myocardiopathy   See MYOCARDIAL DYSFUNCTION.

myocarditis   Inflammation of the MYOCARDIUM.

myocardium   The middle layer of the walls of the heart, composed of cardiac muscle.

myometrium   The muscular layer of the uterus.

myopathy   Inflammation of muscle tissue due to infection or adverse reaction to a medication. Myopathy may arise as a toxic reaction to AZT or as a consequence of HIV infection itself.

myositis   Inflammation of a muscle, especially a voluntary muscle.

N

N-9 A contraceptive film containing a commonly used spermicide, NONOXYNOL-9. Studies have shown that this film does not block the TRANSMISSION of HIV. Nor does it give women protection against GONORRHEA or CHLAMYDIA. Public health officials and scientists have been searching for microbicides to protect women against AIDS, preferably in a way that women could control. Condoms do not provide perfect protection, and men are not always willing to use them. Researchers had hoped that the N-9 film might increase a women's available options for HIV and STD protection. The chemical does kill the AIDS virus in the test tube, and studies are ongoing about whether it is effective against the virus in other topical forms. There is some evidence that it might irritate or disrupt cells in the genital tract, making women more vulnerable to infection. Until safe and effective vaginal microbicides are developed, the Centers for Disease Control and Prevention (CDC) recommends consistent and correct use of male latex condoms, with or without the use of a spermicide, to prevent sexual transmission of HIV and other STDs in high-risk populations. The CDC does not currently recommend the use of spermicide alone.

N-acetylcysteine (NAC) A naturally occurring substance that is metabolized into the amino acid CYSTEINE, a component of the major cellular antioxidant GLUTATHIONE, whose levels are decreased in people with HIV. Clinical studies of oral and INTRAVENOUSLY administered NAC are evaluating its usefulness in decreasing HIV activity.

naive T-cell A T cell arising from the immune system's production of fresh cells in the BONE MARROW. Naive T-cells respond to PATHOGENs containing ANTIGENs the immune system has not encountered before. The naive T-cells' activation and proliferation create an acquired immune response to the newly encountered pathogenic agent. After the disease is eradicated, a portion of the T cell population engendered by the activated naive T-cells constitutes a reservoir of memory cells, which proliferate and respond very quickly to any recurrence of the disease.

Naprosyn See NAPROXEN.

naproxen A nonsteroidal, anti-inflammatory drug used for the treatment of a number of inflammatory diseases, including osteoarthritis and rheumatoid arthritis, and for the relief of mild-to-moderate pain. Naproxen is quickly absorbed into the bloodstream. Pain relief is usually evident within an hour after the first dose, but its maximum effect on arthritis or other inflammatory disorders may not be observed for up to a month of continual dosing. Trade names are Naprosyn, Anaprox and Aleve.

narcotic Producing stupor or sleep; loosely, anything that soothes, relieves, or lulls; a drug that in moderate doses depresses the CENTRAL NERVOUS SYSTEM, thus relieving pain and producing sleep, but that in excessive doses produces unconsciousness, stupor, coma, and possibly death. Most are habit-forming. Examples include opium, morphine, codeine, papaverine, heroin, and many synthetics.

nasal ulcer An open sore or lesion of the nose, accompanied by sloughing of inflamed necrotic tissue.

nasopharyngeal carcinoma A cancer of the lining of the area of the pharynx (above the palate) that connects the mouth and nose with the esophagus. Symptoms may include pain and pressure in the cheek, toothache, persistent draining of the sinus after tooth extraction, a nasal quality to the voice, a lump in the cheek, or bloodstained discharge from the nose. Diagnostic procedures may include direct visual examination, X rays of the facial bones, nasopharyngoscopy, and BIOPSY. The National Cancer Institute has identified four stages of the disease, as well as recurrent nasopharyngeal cancer (in which the cancer returns after treatment to the original location or another part of the body). Treatment depends on the stage of the disease, the general state of health of the patient, and other factors. The most common treatment is RADIATION THERAPY. External or internal radiation therapy may be used. Surgery may be performed if the cancer does not respond to radiation therapy. CHEMOTHERAPY may also be used.

nasopharynx The part of the pharynx above the soft palate.

natural and alien An apparently fundamental conceptual opposition within AIDS discourse; like the opposition normal/abnormal, it distinguishes self from nonself. The AIDS virus is linguistically identified with that which is alien, or unnatural. See KNOWLEDGE AND IGNORANCE.

natural history studies Studies that observe the course of a disease. Concerning women and HIV, for example, much attention has been given to natural history studies designed to answer the question, Are there gender differences in HIV disease? At the VIII International Conference on AIDS (Amsterdam, July 1992), data was presented that compared men and women with HIV disease who were similar in a number of ways, including disease progression, age, and mode of transmission.

natural killer cell (NK cell) A type of large LYMPHOCYTE that performs surveillance against bacteria, viruses, and cancer cells and attacks and destroys foreign, infected, and cancerous cells. NK cells kill on contact by binding to the target cells and releasing a lethal burst of chemicals. Normal cells are not affected by NK cells. NK cells are thought to play a major role in cancer prevention by destroying abnormal cells before they have a chance to pose a real threat. NK cells are not targeted at specific ANTIGENS the way CYTOTOXIC T-CELL LYMPHOCYTES are. While they are not B or T lymphocytes, they are thought to be precursors of T-suppressor cells.

naturopathic medicine A specialty of alternative medicine; a combination of natural therapies that includes nutritional therapy, herbal medicine, HOMEOPATHY, spinal manipulation, exercise therapy, hydrotherapy, electrotherapy, stress reduction, and natural cures. Naturopathic medicine assumes that the body is always striving for good health. Disease is viewed as a result of a healing effort of nature. If an illness develops, the symptoms accompanying it are the result of the organism's intrinsic attempt to defend and heal itself. A naturopathic physician focuses on aiding the body in its effort to regain its natural health instead of initiating a treatment that might interfere with this process. Naturopathic doctors prefer nontoxic and noninvasive treatments that minimize the risks of harmful side effects. They are trained to distinguish which patients they can treat safely and which need referral to other health care practitioners. Naturopaths currently are licensed to practice in nearly all the states in the United States. Naturopathic physicians who have attended an accredited four-year program are trained in most of the same scientific disciplines taught in conventional medical schools. Consequently, most naturopaths use medical tests for diagnosis. Many naturopaths may use modern medicine for certain crisis situations. During the first visit, a naturopath uses history-taking, physical examination, laboratory tests, and other standard diagnostic procedures to learn as much as possible about the patient. Diet, environment, exercise, stress, and other aspects of lifestyle also are evaluated. Once a good understanding of the patient's health and disease is established, doctor and patient work together to establish a treatment and health-promoting program.

nausea Unpleasant sensation in the stomach, usually including the urge to vomit. It is present in seasickness, early pregnancy, diseases of the CENTRAL NERVOUS SYSTEM, neurasthenia, and hysteria. It may be provoked by the sight or odor or mental images of obnoxious matter or conditions. It may be present, without vomiting, in certain gallbladder disturbances and in carsickness and other types of motion sickness.

Although not all CHEMOTHERAPY patients experience nausea and vomiting, they are the most common side effects of chemotherapy. They may also result from other strong medications, RADIATION therapy to the gastrointestinal tract, liver, or brain, or from an illness or cancer itself. Nausea is one of the most dreaded side effects of such treatments and can have a psychological as well as physical impact on a patient. Nausea and vomiting can lead to nutrition depletion and a general deterioration of the patient's physical condition. It could also lead a patient to quit a potentially curative or useful treatment as well as to neglect self-care and reduce functional ability. Antiemetic drugs are the greatest defense against nausea and vomiting; other methods include hypnosis, acupuncture, distraction, relaxation techniques, and imagery.

NDA NEW DRUG APPLICATION. See DRUG APPROVAL PROCESS.

nebulized pentamidine See PENTAMIDINE.

nebulizer An apparatus for producing a fine spray or mist. This may be done by rapidly passing air through a liquid or by vibrating a liquid at a high frequency so that the particles produced are extremely small.

necropsy An examination of a dead body to determine cause of death or pathological condition; an AUTOPSY.

necrosis The death of areas of tissue or bone surrounded by healthy parts; the constellation of morphological changes indicative of cell death and caused by the progressive degenerative action of various enzymes. Necrosis may be caused by a variety of factors: insufficient blood supply; physical agents such as trauma and radiant energy; or chemical agents acting locally, acting internally following absorption, or placed into the wrong tissue.

needle access Increasing access to sterile injection equipment, including needles and syringes, has been the primary HARM REDUCTION strategy by governments to reduce TRANSMISSION of HIV among INJECTION DRUG USERs (IDUs).

A variety of programs has been implemented to accomplish this end, including lifting restrictions on sales; pharmacy-based interventions; vending machines; and equipment exchanges. Different types of service may be used by different subpopulations; for example, recreational or occasional drug users may prefer the "normality" of the pharmacy and gay users may prefer programs targeted to their particular group by nongovernmental organizations. The overall impact of increased access, however, has been difficult to assess. Moreover, in the United States there has been substantial public disagreement about the propriety of allowing protected access to needles and syringes, even while the possession of some such equipment remains illegal in many jurisdictions. See NEEDLE EXCHANGE PROGRAM; NEEDLE-PRESCRIPTION LAW; DRUG PARAPHERNALIA LAWS; DRUG ABUSE.

needle exchange program Any HARM REDUCTION in which INTRAVENOUS DRUG USERS may exchange used needles and syringes for sterile ones. Such programs have been created in an effort to remove contaminated works from this community and reduce the spread of HIV via this route of transmission. The concept is controversial. Those who oppose needle exchange programs believe that they encourage an illegal, destructive, and undesirable activity—drug addiction. Those who support such programs believe that AIDS prevention measures, to be effective, must deal practically with the world as it is, and that moralizing about drug abuse will only make it harder to reach the very people who are at the greatest risk and who pose the greatest danger to the larger community. The AMERICAN FOUNDATION FOR AIDS RESEARCH (AMFAR) was the first foundation willing to take a stand on this issue and fund an AIDS prevention program aimed at a group of people often considered to be expendable. Exchanges are generally conducted by outreach workers in a variety of settings—in vehicles and health care clinics, on the streets, or in visits to addicts' homes. Usually materials are provided free of charge, and each exchange involves an encounter between a drug user and a program staff member. Programs have taken various forms: Some distribute needles, others sell needles and syringes as well as exchange them, and still others conduct a strict exchange of one used for each new needle or syringe.

Exchange programs have been initiated by governmental and nongovernmental agencies. In some areas, exchange has been organized by drug users themselves. In the United States, most of the operating exchange programs began in defiance of drug paraphernalia laws, in effect as acts of civil disobedience. Some are still illegal or unsanctioned, although there are some government-sponsored programs.

Needle exchange programs have several advantages. They remove financial barriers to low-income drug users' obtaining sterile equipment. They allow exchange personnel to deliver prevention messages, incorporate high-risk users into a helping system, and reduce biowaste. Disadvantages are the high cost of materials, staff, and implementation, and that they provide less coverage of the injection drug-using population than do other NEEDLE ACCESS programs.

needle-prescription law Drug paraphernalia laws do not prohibit or regulate the sale of hypodermic needles and syringes if the seller has no reason to believe that the equipment will be used for injection of illicit drugs. Accordingly, over-the-counter sales of hypodermic syringes and needles are permitted in most states. Pharmacists are not obliged to question buyers' intentions in purchasing the equipment, and wide variations in sales practices exist. Some states, however, significantly restrict over-the-counter sales. These jurisdictions prohibit the sale, distribution, or possession of hypodermic needles or syringes without a valid medical pre-

scription. Needle-prescription laws are more onerous than drug paraphernalia laws because they do not require criminal intent. Under needle-prescription laws, physicians may write prescriptions for hypodermic needles and syringes for patients under their care only if there is a legitimate medical purpose for them to do so. A wholesale druggist or surgical supplier must keep careful records of the sale of this equipment. People charged with illegal possession have the burden of proving that they have sufficient authority or license.

Proposals for statutory reform consistent with public health objectives call for narrowing the focus of drug paraphernalia laws and repealing needle-prescription laws. It is argued that this repeal would be less controversial than needle distribution programs because the state would not be directly involved in the distribution of drug injection equipment. Repeal of these laws would have no revenue impact for state legislatures. It would simply remove the state as an affirmative obstacle to providing IV drug users with sterile equipment necessary to protect their health. Repeal of needle-prescription legislation is already supported by numerous public health and bar associations. Additionally, experience in jurisdictions that already permit over-the-counter sales of hypodermic needles and syringes shows that they are better able to control the needle-borne spread of HIV and that allowing over-the-counter sales does not result in greater drug use. See also DRUG PARAPHERNALIA LAWS.

needle sharing The act or practice of using a hypodermic syringe in common with another person or persons. Generally the term refers to the reuse of needles by drug addicts, without sterilization, after they have been used by others.

People who use needles to inject drugs can get the HIV virus by sharing works with other users who have the virus in their blood. INTRAVENOUS DRUG USERS can reduce their chances of infection if they do not share works (needles, syringes, or cookers), or rent or buy works that have been used by someone else. They can also reduce their chances of infection if they clean their works with either ethyl alcohol or household bleach before and after use.

needlestick The unintentional puncture of the skin with a hypodermic needle. See UNIVERSAL PRECAUTIONS.

nef An HIV regulatory protein whose functions are not well understood. HIV without nef appears to be less infectious.

nef-deleted vaccine A live-attenuated HIV vaccine composed of HIV with NEF, a key component of the virus, deleted to lessen its ability to replicate or reproduce.

nef gene The gene in the HUMAN IMMUNODEFICIENCY VIRUS that encodes the NEF protein and affects virus replication by decreasing production.

negligence In forensic medicine, the failure to act as a reasonably prudent person with the same knowledge, experience, and background would under similar circumstances, causing injury or damage to a person. There are four elements of negligence: duty owed, breach of duty or standard of care, proximate cause or causal connection, and damages or injuries. Nurses are legally liable for their own negligence, as well as the negligence of others of which they have knowledge but do not report. In law, the failure to exercise a reasonable degree of care, especially for the protection of other persons. Negligence may be an act of omission or commission, characterized by intention, recklessness, inadvertence, thoughtlessness, or wantoness. In health care, negligence resulting in legal liability is the failure to exercise that degree of care and skill ordinarily practiced by other professionals of similar skill and training under similar circumstances. The failure to exercise ordinary professional care must have caused an injury to the patient in order for there to have been a negligent act.

negotiated safety   A term coined by researchers in Australia to denote the practice of HIV-negative gay couples who have decided to forgo the use of condoms because they believe that if neither partner is infected, the virus cannot be transmitted between them. The question of negotiated safety forces partners to weigh their trust in each other against the consequences of betrayal, and to do so amidst homophobia, gay men's freewheeling sexual culture, and the epidemic itself. The subtext of negotiated safety is that gay couples can be strong and trustworthy, and should be. Despite considerable criticism from researchers and public health officials, Australian prevention workers have launched prevention campaigns to educate couples on how to responsibly forgo condoms. They insist that the issue is not whether people will contract HIV through negotiated safety, but rather whether fewer people will contract HIV through clarified negotiation.

Prevention researchers point out that making this strategy work requires honest communication about emotionally volatile subjects. They worry that negotiated safety could elevate unprotected intercourse to the ultimate test of true love. They offer an alternative term—"negotiated danger." Those who support teaching negotiated safety counter that current prevention campaigns already mystify sex by prescribing a simple dogmatic truth, rather than presenting a complex and honest discussion. Critics point out that even if promulgated in counseling sessions or other controlled settings, the negotiated safety regimen may be too demanding for most couples. Others note that the complex dynamics of negotiated safety may be most difficult for those most at risk. Public health officials urge counselors to emphasize the use of condoms with every partner, and remain wary of muddying the condom message.

The crucial prevention question is can HIV-negative couples abandon condoms and still be safe? Is it a "reasonable decision" for HIV-negative couples to have unprotected sex? Should AIDS workers offer such guidance?

Studies show that men in relationships in which both partners have the same HIV status are much more likely to have unprotected anal sex than men in sero-discordant couples or men who don't know whether their partner is infected. Research consistently indicates that gay men are far more likely to forgo condoms when having sex with a lover than with a casual partner. It is clear that the dynamics of a long-term relationship increase the likelihood of sexual risk-taking. The risk for HIV-positive couples is mutual reinfection, although this remains the subject of much debate. By exchanging semen, HIV-positive men might also contract other sexually transmitted diseases, thus weakening their immune systems. But clearly, the stakes are lower for these couples than for partners who are negative.

Neisseria gonorrhoea   A type of GRAM-NEGATIVE BACTERIA, belonging to the genus *Neisseria*, that causes gonorrhea.

neonate   Newly born; a newborn infant.

nelfinavir   Agouron's PROTEASE INHIBITOR. Nelfinavir presents fewer problems that RITONAVIR while still boosting SAQUINAVIR levels five times by inhibiting the liver enzymes (as does indinavir, which also does not cause diarrhea to the extent that nelfinavir and Fortovase do). Trade name is Viracept.

neoplasm   An abnormal growth of tissue in which the expansion is uncontrolled, progressive, and serves no useful function. Neoplasms may be benign (not spreading by METASTASIS or infiltration of tissue) or malignant (infiltrating tissue, metastasizing, often recurring after attempts at surgical removal). Other kinds of neoplasms include histoid (in which the structure resembles the tissues and elements that surround it); mixed (composed of tissues from two of the germinal layers); organoid (similar to some organ of the body); multicentric (arising from a number of distinct groups of cells); and unicentric (having origin in one group of cells).

neoplastic   Pertaining to, or of the nature of, a NEOPLASM (new, abnormal tissue formation).

neopterin   A molecule produced by MACROPHAGEs in response to GAMMA INTERFERON and found in serum, urine, and CEREBROSPINAL FLUID. Neopterin levels have been used to predict HIV disease progression much in the same way as beta-2 microglobulin. The neopterin level is approximately 5.4 nanomoles per liter of blood (nmol/l). Elevated neopterin levels have been reported in individuals in all phases of HIV disease. According to some studies, high neopterin levels are associated with a poor prognosis; low levels correlate with a better prognosis. Serum neopterin levels are measured in some studies as an additional SURROGATE MARKER for HIV disease.

nephropathy   Any disease of the kidney. The term covers inflammatory (nephritis), degenerative (nephrosis), and sclerotic (arteriosclerotic) lesions of the kidney.

nephrotoxicity   The quality of being toxic or destructive to kidney cells.

nerve cell   See NEURON.

nerve growth factor (NGF)   A naturally produced substance that has many roles in the maintenance of nerves and nerve cells, especially sensory ones. Synthetic, recombinant NGF is a proposed therapy for HIV- and drug-associated neuropathies.

neuroleptic malignant syndrome A rare, sometimes fatal, idiosyncratic reaction to the use of neuroleptic (antipsychotic) drugs. The principal features of the reaction are hyperthermia (temperatures of 102 to 104 degrees F), marked muscle rigidity, and coma. Other symptoms include rapid heart beat and breathing, profuse sweating, tremors, and seizures. Two-thirds of reported cases occurred in men, one-third in women. The mortality rate is 15–20 percent.

neurologic, neurological Relating to the nervous system, including the brain and spinal cord.

neurologic assessment Assessment of diseases of the nervous system.

neurologic complication A disease or abnormality of the nervous system that is superimposed upon another disease without being specifically related to it, yet affecting or modifying the prognosis of the original disease.

neurological disease Cytomegalovirus (CMV) infections of the CENTRAL NERVOUS SYSTEM (CNS). CMV can cause a number of distinct neurologic syndromes, in addition to retinal infections. These include mononeuropathy multiplex (inflammation or disease involving individual nerves in unrelated portions of the body), myelitis/polyradiculopathy (inflammation of a large number of spinal nerves accompanied by pain, muscle wasting, and paralysis), and two forms of encephalitis: diffuse micronodular encephalitis (DME) and ventriculoencephalitis (VE).

Mononeuropathy multiplex occurs when CMV infects the cranial and peripheral nerves resulting in face, wrist, and foot palsies. Mild forms that resolve spontaneously often strike patients fairly early in the course of HIV disease. Polyradiculopathy is strictly a late stage AIDS event. It starts out as weakness or pain in the legs or back, but within a couple of weeks can progress to paralysis of the lower extremities and loss of bladder control leading to an inability to urinate or loss of anal-sphincter control. Polyradiculopathy or myelopathy may accompany or lead to CMV encephalitis. The two CMV-encephalitic syndromes are distinguished by the site of infection within the CNS. For both syndromes, symptoms of dementia, delirium, confusion, apathy, and lethargy are common. Some symptoms of DME depend upon the location of the nodule lesions. Patients with VE often experience cranial nerve palsies and nystagmus (rhythmic involuntary eye movement). Both conditions are rapidly fatal.

The actual rate of CMV infection of CNS is unclear; however, recognizing the infection is a different story. In aggressive cases, the onset of symptoms is so abrupt, and the progression so rapid, that the encephalopathy may kill the patient within the time it takes clinicians to distinguish it from other AIDS-related neurologic conditions. There are some distinguishing features of CMV neurologic disease, though. For example, CMV encephalitis occurs very late in the course of HIV disease, while signs of the most common alternate diagnosis, HIV encephalopathy, appear earlier and more gradually. Other hallmarks of CMV CNS infection, such as electrolyte abnormalities, pleocytosis (an abnormally high level of white blood cells in the CSF), and contrast enhancement of the brain's ventricles on MRI brain scans, suggest CMV infection, particularly in the presence of CMV retinitis. These markers allow for a presumptive, but not a definitive, diagnosis, since they also may occur in other neurologic conditions as well.

To date, there have been no prospectively controlled studies of the treatment of CMV CNS disease, and the case reports are scant. Thus, there are no clear data on what is the best drug or dose to use or the duration of treatment. Examples of the nagging questions surrounding CMV CNS disease follow. To what extent are standard treatments for CMV retinitis (ganciclovir or foscarnet, for example) adequate as therapy for CMV infections in the brain? What effect will improvements in the treatment of CMV-retinitis have upon the development of CMV-related neurologic syndromes? How effective are quantitative CMV DNA polymerase chain reaction and CMV branched DNA as assays for disease severity, progression, and response to therapy? And what is the role of drug resistance in the evolution of CMV CNS disease and in treatment failure?

neurologic dysfunction Abnormal, disturbed, or impaired functioning of the nervous system.

neurology The branch of medical science dealing with the study of the nervous system and its disorders.

neuromuscular therapy Physical therapy that emphasizes the role of the brain, spine, and nerves in muscular pain. One goal of the therapy is to relieve tender congested spots in muscle tissue and compress nerves that may radiate pain to other areas of the body.

neuron Major cell of nervous tissue; the structural and functional unit of the nervous system, specialized for transmission of information in the form of patterns of impulses. The brain cells influence neurons by secreting neurotransmitters that alter the affected cell by physically contracting it. Alternatively, a neuron may release neurohormones into the bloodstream. The nucleus and its surrounding cytoplasm comprise the cell body, or perikaryon, which may be the site of multiple synaptic connections with other nerve fibers. In non-receptor cells, numerous projections from the cell body, or dendrites, provide a large surface area for synaptic connections with other neurons. One or more regions of the cell body (axon hillocks) extend into long thin axons and carry impulses away from the cell body to other neurons and to effectors, making contacts via synapses through the secretion of neurotransmitters. There are many different types of neurons: some distinguished by function, others by process, and still others by location.

neuronal cell death The death of a NEURON or nerve cell.

neuropathology The branch of medicine that deals with the study of diseases of the nervous system, as well as microscopic and macroscopic structural and functional changes occurring in them.

neuropathy An abnormal, degenerative, or inflammatory condition of the PERIPHERAL NERVOUS SYSTEM. Nerves are responsible for, among other things, the movement of muscles and the sensation of touch, including the sensation of pain. The symptoms of neuropathy can therefore be weakness of a muscle or pain and tingling. In people with HIV infection, the most frequent symptoms of neuropathy are painful feet and legs. Often, individuals experience numbness or tingling in the hands and feet, weakness in the legs, arms, and hands, or a burning pain in the soles of the feet and the ends of the fingers and toes. The pain can be severe and, depending on where it occurs, may interfere with walking or using the hands. Neuropathy may be a neurological complication of HIV infection itself, or it may be caused by certain drugs like alcohol, ddC, ddI, ISONIAZID, or VINCRISTINE.

Ascending neuropathy is a pathological condition of the nervous system that ascends from the lower body to the upper. Descending neuropathy, on the other hand, is a similar condition that descends from the upper part of the body to the lower. Pathological changes in a nerve due to its inflammation in a confined space is referred to as *entrapment*. Neuropathy associated with enlargement and tenderness of two or three nerves of the head and neck area is called hypertrophic mononeuropathy.

Peripheral neuropathy is damage to or disruption of the cells of the peripheral nervous system, which consists of the nerves outside the brain or spinal cord.

neuropathy drug   A drug, such as amitriptyline, nortriptyline, mexiletine, or nimodipine, that is used to treat neuropathy. Amitriphyline and nortriphyline are tricyclic antidepressants; mexiletine is an antiarrhythmic; nimodipine is a calcium channel blocker. To date, there is no effective treatment to halt or reverse the nerve damage in peripheral neuropathy. The most practical approach is to identify the cause of the disorder and, if possible, eliminate it. Treatment of neuropathy is currently aimed at reducing painful symptoms. Choice of medication is usually based on the severity of symptoms. People with mild symptoms and no functional impairment can take nonnarcotic pain relievers such as ibuprofen. Moderate symptoms with some functional limitation are often treated with tricyclic antidepressants such as amitriptyline or nortriptyline. Severe symptoms with functional limitation may be treated with narcotic pain relievers such as methadone or the fentanyl patch.

neuropsychiatric complication   A nervous or mental disease or difficulty superimposed upon another disease without being specifically related to it, yet affecting or modifying the prognosis of the original disease.

neuropsychiatry   The branch of medicine concerned with the study of nervous and mental disorders.

neuropsychological defect   An alteration in behavior that is related to a central nervous system illness and interferes with the ability to function in an age-normative fashion.

neuropsychological test   A test designed to measure certain aspects of brain function, such as memory, concentration, attention, and visual-motor skills.

neurosyphilis   A form of advanced syphilis in which the infection has spread to the central nervous system. The treatment of syphilis in HIV-infected patients is controversial. Although there is some evidence to the contrary, there has been documentation of an increased incidence of treatment failures and a more rapid progression to neurosyphilis in HIV-infected individuals with syphilis. Patients with syphilis should be tested for HIV infection, and HIV-infected individuals should receive testing for syphilis. Altered mental status, facial palsy, hemiplegia or hemiparesis, ocular symptoms, and hearing loss may occur in neurosyphilis. Neurosyphilis is confirmed with a positive cerebrospinal fluid (CSF) serology in the absence of gross blood contamination. A CSF examination is generally recommended for HIV-infected patients with syphilis for over one year or latent syphilis. The antibiotic penicillin is used to treat neurosyphilis; Ceftriaxone is used if the patient is allergic to penicillin. Patients with documented neurosyphilis should have repeat CSF examinations after six and 12 months.

neurotoxicity   Having the capability of harming nerve tissue.

neutralization   1. The opposing of one force or condition with an opposite force or condition to such a degree as to cause counteraction that permits neither to dominate. 2. In chemistry, the process of destroying the peculiar properties or effects of a substance (e.g., the neutralization of an acid with a base). 3. In medicine, the process of checking or counteracting the effects of any agent that produces a morbid effect, e.g., the process by which ANTIBODY or antibody in complement neutralizes the infectivity of MICROORGANISMs, particularly VIRUSes.

neutralizing antibody   A protein produced by B CELLS, that can directly inactivate an invading MICROORGANISM, such as a VIRUS or BACTERIUM.

neutropenia   A decrease in the number of NEUTROPHIL cells in the blood.

neutrophil   A granular LEUKOCYTE (white blood cell or corpuscle) with the properties of adherence to immune complexes, CHEMOTAXIS, and PHAGOCYTOSIS. Performing many of the same phagocytic and degradative functions as MACROPHAGEs, neutrophils play the primary role in inflammation, easily recognizing foreign ANTIGENS and destroying them through phagocytosis. An inadequate number of neutrophils (NEUTROPENIA) leaves the body at high risk for infection from many sources and requires protective precautions on the part of health care workers. Neutrophils may also overreact to stimuli and become involved in tissue destruction (e.g., neutrophil activity in rheumatoid arthritis, myocardial reperfusion injury, respiratory distress syndrome, and ulcerative colitis). The term also denotes any cell, structure, or histologic element that stains easily with neutral dye.

nevirapine   The first in a new class of antiretroviral drugs known as NONNUCLEOSIDE REVERSE TRANSCRIPTASE INHIBITORS (NNRTIs) It will be marketed under the name

Viramune. NNRTIs inactivate reverse transcriptase, the same HIV enzyme targeted by the nucleoside analog drugs AZT, ddI, ddC, d4T and 3TC. In combination with nucleoside analogs, nevirapine could be used as first-line therapy or as an alternative treatment for patients who either show no improvement with other drugs or experience adverse reactions to them. The additional COMBINATION THERAPY regimens made possible by nevirapine could help physicians devise better strategies for avoiding drug resistance. Another attractive aspect of nevirapine is its long half life; nevirapine remains active much longer than other antiretrovirals and can be administered less frequently. Nevirapine must be used in combination with other agents because HIV easily mutates to resist nevirapine's effect when it is administered alone. It does induce liver metabolism of some drugs, and early data suggests it can cause a slight reduction in levels of saquinavir.

new drug application (NDA) See DRUG APPROVAL PROCESS.

newborn screening The testing of human infants less than one month old to determine the presence of a particular disease (i.e., HIV/AIDS), or of certain risk factors known to be associated with that disease. Today, AIDS testing and screening of large groups of people remain controversial issues; whether or not HIV testing provides a net benefit both to the public health and to persons infected with HIV is still debated. One heavily debated issue concerns screening programs for all pregnant women and newborns. Advocates argue that such a program would be reasonable, given the accuracy of new confirmatory tests and the fact that perinatally acquired HIV infection is less common than congenital syphilis or phenylketonuria (both are tested for routinely). Infected women, it is further argued, could make more informed choices about family planning, and infected newborns could be treated earlier.

Opponents argue that testing newborns for the presence of HIV antibodies is medically ineffective and inconclusive. They argue that with an increase in screening, discrimination arises once a person (or an infant) is known to be infected. They characterize newborn screening as counterproductive and coercive, as it does not confront the difficult reality of treating newborns with HIV/AIDS. They argue that only when those with HIV infection are assured of receiving all the medical care they need, can we pursue the basic elements of infection control more resolutely and thus spare others the tragedy of this disease. See also TRANSMISSION.

NGO See NONGOVERNMENTAL ORGANIZATION.

NGU See URETHRITIS.

night sweats Profuse sweating during sleep at night, often an early sign of disease, especially if accompanied by intermittent fever. Night sweats are considered a symptom of HIV only when the body is drenched. Slight to moderate sweating is not a symptom. In addition to being an early sign of HIV disease, severe night sweats may also be a symptom of several HIV-related conditions, including TUBERCULOSIS.

nimodipine A calcium channel blocker used primarily to improve nerve damage caused by stroke. It works by slowing the amount of calcium that enters cells, resulting in blood vessels opening wider, allowing more blood to flow through them. (Most calcium channel blockers are used to treat heart conditions.) It is also occasionally used for the treatment of migraine headaches. In people infected with HIV, nimodipine is sometimes used as a treatment for neurological damage caused by HIV, especially PERIPHERAL NEUROPATHY.

nipple The structure on the breast through which milk is exuded (in women). In men it is vestigial. Also a source of erotic enjoyment.

nitazoxanide (NTZ) A broad-spectrum antiparasitic originally formulated for veterinary use. NTZ is currently being studied as a treatment for CRYPTOSPORIDIOSIS. In early 1996, the FOOD AND DRUG ADMINISTRATION approved a compassionate use program providing very limited access to nitazoxanide.

nizatidine Primarily an antiulcer agent; also used for the prevention of recurrent ulcers and gastroesophageal reflux disease, a condition where stomach acid backs up into the esophagus. Nizatidine inhibits the action of histamine, a substance secreted by specialized cells (mast cells). Histamine has a number of effects, including accelerating heart rate, inflammation, and increasing secretion of acid in the stomach. Nizatidine prevents the action of histamine by blocking the surface receptors that bring the compound into cells. Brand name Axid (Lilly).

nizoral See KETOCONAZOLE.

NK cells See NATURAL KILLER CELLS.

NMRI See MAGNETIC RESONANCE IMAGING.

no code An indication on a terminally ill patient's chart that he or she does not want heroic, lifesaving measures or artificial life support when death is imminent. Also called no code blue or no code blue status. See also POWER OF ATTORNEY, MEDICAL DIRECTIVE, and LIVING WILL.

no code blue See NO CODE.

no code blue status See NO CODE.

Nocardia A genus of GRAM-POSITIVE aerobic bacteria. Some species are ACID-FAST and thus when stained may be confused with the causative organism for TUBERCULOSIS. The species pathogenic for humans causes the disease NOCARDIOSIS.

nocardiosis An acute or chronic pathological condition caused by infection from any species of NOCARDIA. It may occur as a pulmonary infection but has a marked tendency to spread to any organ of the body, especially the brain. It results in abscesses in the lungs, brain, skin, or other areas.

node   A knot, knob, protuberance, or swelling; a small mass of tissue in the form of a knot or swelling.

nodular lesion   A circumscribed area of pathologically altered tissue that possesses the characteristics of a NODULE.

nodule   A small knot or protuberance that can be detected by touch.

Nolahist   See PHENINDAMINE.

non-communicable disease   A disease that cannot be directly or indirectly transmitted from host to host.

nondirective counseling   A type of counseling in which the counselor supplies information and helps the client to arrive at a decision that reflects the client's needs and wishes.

nongonococcal urethritis   See URETHRITIS.

nongovernmental organization (NGO)   Any private non-profit voluntary organization or institution that provides health; rescue; human rights; charitable, financial, economic development; or other aid and services wherever they are needed, but mainly in poorer countries. Nongovernmental organizations have been at the forefront of the response to AIDS in most countries of the world. In economic terms, NGOs focus on social needs that cannot be met otherwise, for economic or political reasons. Politically, NGOs provide public good to groups of people too small or marginalized to be served by the state. Most observers agree that NGOs working in AIDS typically offer the advantages of being cost-effective and responsive to new needs and of having access to target communities. For volunteers and activists involved in NGOs, the chief strength of the organizations would almost certainly be seen as their ability to represent effectively the needs and values of a particular constituency. Although they have recognized weaknesses, NGOs clearly serve certain functions well and can effectively complement and improve governmental response. NGOs encompass a wide variety of organizational styles and missions, and their role in response to AIDS has varied accordingly. Today, short- and long-term financial issues are a major concern of both governmental and nongovernmental AIDS programs.

non-Hodgkin's lymphoma (NHL)   A LYMPHOMA (cancer of the lymphatic system), other than Hodgkin's disease, that is prevalent among AIDS patients. As people with AIDS live longer, the chances increase for appearance among them of the less common opportunistic diseases. AIDS-related malignancies, especially non-Hodgkin's lymphoma (NHL), are becoming an epidemic within an epidemic. Lymphoma is a disease that involves the uncontrolled multiplication of dysfunctional LYMPHOCYTEs (a type of white blood cell). This process can happen either in the LYMPH NODEs or in extranodal parts of the body such as the BONE MARROW, GAS-TROINTESTINAL TRACT, or brain and SPINAL CORD. Non-

Hodgkin's lymphoma is the most common lymphoma that affects people with HIV/AIDS. It primarily involves the uncontrolled proliferation of abnormal B CELLS (lympho-cytes responsible for ANTIBODY production) and frequently appears as nodular or diffuse tumors in extranodal tissues.

Other lymphomas such as Hodgkin's disease occasionally affect people with HIV/AIDS, but unlike NHL, these do not seem to be increasing in incidence. The major difference between Hodgkin's disease and non-Hodgkin's lymphoma is that the former almost always includes a specific type of cell called the Reed-Sternberg cell (a large cell of unknown origin with an unusual bilobed nucleus). Hodgkin's disease also starts out as localized nodular tumors, which disseminate as the disease progresses.

One of the first signs of NHL is the presence of what are called "B symptoms," which include fever, night sweats, and weight loss of greater than 10 percent of body weight. Many other AIDS-related complications have similar symptoms. Other symptoms of lymphoma can be enlarged and asymmetrical lymph nodes.

Extranodal NHL is very common among people with HIV/AIDS. It has been reported that NHL can occur at practically any site on the body. The most common extranodal sites are the CENTRAL NERVOUS SYSTEM (brain and spinal cord), GASTROINTESTINAL TRACT, BONE MARROW, and LIVER. NHL also has appeared in such unusual sites as the anus, rectum, mouth, muscle, and other soft tissue.

A definitive diagnosis of lymphoma can be made only through a surgical BIOPSY of the involved tissue. If lymphoma is found, it is graded based on how rapidly the cancerous cells are growing. It is designated either high, intermediate, or low grade. The lymphoma is also staged (I through IV), based on the extent of tissue involvement. Staging requires one or more of the following procedures: X rays, whole body gallium scanning, CT or MRI scans, bone marrow biopsy, and spinal tap. Stage I indicates very limited involvement at only one site, whereas stage IV indicates very extensive involvement in multiple sites.

Lymphomas are also classified according to shape and size of the B cells that make up the tumor. Lymphoma cell types common in people with AIDS include small non-cleaved cells (lymphomas made up of cleaved cells, or cells with clefts in their nuclear membranes, are more common in non–AIDS-related NHL); large-cell immunoblasts (B-cells that have been stimulated by the presence of ANTIGEN to produce antibodies); and diffuse large cells. Several non-cleaved cell lymphomas are also referred to as BURKITT'S or Burkitt's-like lymphoma.

Whether a person can survive NHL depends on a variety of factors. Although NHL is one of the few cancers that can actually be cured, severe immune deficiency often complicates a patient's ability to tolerate and respond to treatment. Low CD4 CELL count (less than 100), central nervous system involvement, previous opportunistic infections, stage IV disease, and low ability to perform daily activities have been reported to be associated with poor survival. Patients with higher CD4 cell units (greater than 199), no extranodal disease, no previous opportunistic infections, and near normal ability to perform daily activities have a greater survival rate and potential for cure.

Exactly what causes NHL is not completely understood. Most researchers agree that it may be a combination of factors such as EPSTEIN-BARR VIRUS infection, gene mutations, and CYTOKINE dysregulation (IL-1, IL-4, IL-6, IL-10 and TNF [TUMOR NECROSIS FACTOR]), coupled with the underlying immune suppression in AIDS.

As with other cancers, NHL is treated with a combination of chemotherapies administered in cycles. There are two standard treatments for AIDS-related NHL: CHOP (cyclophosphamide, hydroxydaunomycin [doxorubicin], Oncovin [vincristine], and prednicosone) and mBACOD (methotrexate [low dose], bleomycin, Adriamycin, cyclophosphamide, Oncovin, and dexamethasone). The exact response rate to treatment is difficult to determine. Although the lymphoma may be completely cleared for a period of time, the typical person with AIDS-related NHL remains severely immunosuppressed. She or he may experience NHL relapse (recurrence either at the same or another site). Chemotherapies are immunosuppressive in their own right, and people with AIDS are often less able to tolerate them. These regimens can result in numerous adverse reactions. Side effects include nausea, vomiting, fatigue, diarrhea, swollen or sensitive gums, mouth sores, hair loss, and PERIPHERAL NEUROPATHY. Drugs such as Zofran can be prescribed to control the nausea and vomiting.

Since chemotherapy, because of its bone marrow toxicity, has a significant impact on decreasing white blood cell count, it increases the risk of bacterial infections. Administration of COLONY-STIMULATING factors such as G-CSF (Neupogen) or GM-CSF (Leukine) can increase white blood cell production and reduce the risk. Chemotherapy may also cause anemia by reducing red blood cell counts and spontaneous bleeding due to low platelet counts. Infusions of Epogen (synthetic erythropoeitin) can stimulate red blood cell production, and the cytokine IL-3 has proved of value in reversing both low white blood cell and platelet counts in AIDS patients on chemotherapy.

If primary central nervous system (CNS) lymphoma is suspected, a brain biopsy and/or spinal tap is required to provide a definitive diagnosis. CT or MRI scans usually show "single ring enhancing lesions"—lesions that appear with a ring of contrasting material around them. Symptoms of CNS lymphoma include seizures, headache, memory loss, confusion, fatigue, partial paralysis, and changes in personality. Once a diagnosis is made, treatment usually includes full brain radiation with or without systemic or intrathecal (spinal) chemotherapy.

One complication of NHL relapse is that the lymphoma may come back as secondary CNS lymphoma. For this reason, many researchers believe that intrathecal prophylaxis, consisting of ARA-C (cytosine arabinoside) or METHOTREXATE injected directly into the spinal canal, is beneficial. Some researchers argue that this treatment should be given to patients with AIDS-related NHL; others that intrathecal prophylaxis should be reserved for patients with particular types of disease, such as bone marrow, epidural (the outermost covering of the brain and spinal cord), or sinus involvement.

A number of clinical trials of new NHL treatments are currently in progress. These include CDE (cyclophospha-mide, doxorubicin, etoposide), an alternative chemotherapy that has shown improved survival and reduced toxicity administered in combination with ddI and G-CSF; anti-B4-blocked ricin, an experimental treatment being tested in combination with CHOP to improve response rates; MGBG (methylglyoxal-bisguanylhydrazone), a novel chemotherapeutic agent; and camptothecins, a new class of chemotherapeutic agents, including topotecan, CPT-11, and 9-AC, that inhibit cell division in cancer cells. Other experimental strategies target EBV antigens on the surface of tumor cells. Of course, anti-EBV therapies are unlikely to show activity in lymphomas with no evidence of EBV infection.

The most difficult part of dealing with lymphoma is that treating the lymphoma is treating only one aspect of the disease process in a person with AIDS. Research continues to make only incremental advances in the treatment of the overall condition. Until effective treatments are found against HIV, the treatment of lymphoma and other AIDS-related malignancies will continue to be a stopgap.

nonnucleoside reverse transcriptase inhibitor (NNRTI) A member of a class of compounds, including delavirdine, (brand name: Rescriptor), loviride, and nevirapine (Viramune), that acts to directly combine with and block the action of HIV's REVERSE TRANSCRIPTASE. NNRTIs appear to be very effective in treating early HIV infection when combined with other types of HIV drugs. The non-nucleoside drugs are similar to NUCLEOSIDE ANALOGS; they both change the function of reverse transcriptase (RI), an enzyme that HIV needs to replicate. However, the non-nucleoside drugs do not have to be activated by cellular enzymes. While inhibitory mechanisms of nucleoside analogs include tricking reverse transcriptase into making faulty DNA copies from strains of RNA, the non-nucleosides disarm reverse transcriptase by binding directly to it.

Their role in HIV therapy has always been uncertain because HIV rapidly develops resistance when exposed to the current members of the class, particularly when these drugs are taken alone. A better solution seems to be first-line therapy in combination with fresh nucleoside analogs. Then, the PROTEASE INHIBITORS could be saved for when HIV levels are very high or for when they stubbornly resist treatment with other drugs. The best solution, though, might be to combine maximum suppressive therapy with the less resistance-prone protease inhibitors.

NNRTIs continue to suffer from HIV's ability to rapidly mutate and become resistant to their effects. However, the quick development of resistance associated with the nonnucleosides, combined with their potency and rapid absorption, make them ideal for situations that require short-term therapy. See also DELAVIRDINE, LOVIRIDE, and NEVIRAPINE.

nonoxynol-9 A detergent chemical agent in some spermicides and lubricants that may reduce the risk of infection with HIV. In a test tube, it kills the virus that causes AIDS.

nonprogressor A person with HIV whose infection has not progressed to successive stages in the normal amount of time. Long-term nonprogressors are defined as individuals infected with HIV for seven or more years and with stable

CD4+ T CELL COUNTs of 600 or more, no HIV-related diseases, and no previous ANTIRETROVIRAL THERAPY. They may have low levels of virus in their blood and LYMPH NODES although HIV replication persists. A National Institute of Allergy and Infectious Diseases study has also found that the internal structure of these individuals' lymph nodes, unlike those of most people with HIV infection, appear essentially undamaged, and their immune function remains virtually unimpaired. Long-term nonprogressors also have higher levels of neutralizing antibodies than patients with progressive disease, and the blood of each long-term nonprogressor tested has had the ability to kill HIV-infected cells. Higher levels of neutralizing antibodies, together with consistent HIV-specific cytotoxic immune responses, indicate that both antibody and cell-mediated responses are preserved in long-term nonprogressors, suggesting that these individuals are constantly exposed to HIV antigens, yet somehow control the infection.

Researchers feel that it is likely that long-term nonprogressors are a heterogenous group: Some may be infected with a weakened virus, while others are examples of how host factors such as the immune system can, in some circumstances, contain HIV disease.

nonresponder   A mammal unable to respond to an ANTIGEN, usually because of genetic factors.

nonsteroidal anti-inflammatory drug   A type of drug that has analgesic, anti-inflammatory, and antipyretic action; similar to aspirin and aspirinlike drugs. These drugs have been used extensively in treating arthritis, dysmenorrhea, and inflammation in general. Even though effective as analgesics and in moderating inflammation, there is no evidence that they alter the pathological progression of disease. Side effects may include gastrointestinal irritation and hemorrhage of such severity as to require discontinuing the use of the drug(s). Antiulcer therapy is ineffective in preventing gastrointestinal ulcers in those who develop this condition while taking these drugs. HEPATOTOXICITY is a rare but important undesired side effect.

normal   1. In medicine normal connotes standard, natural, regular; performing proper functions. 2. In biology, it indicates unaffected by experimental treatment; occurring naturally and not because of disease or experimentation. 3. In psychology, it means free from mental disorder, or of average development or intelligence. 4. In chemistry, it is a term for a solution so made that 1 liter contains 1 gram equivalent of the solute.

Norplant   See PROGESTERONE IMPLANT.

northern blot technique   A procedure for separating and identifying RNA fragments. Fragments are separated by electrophoresis on an agarose gel, blotted onto a nitrocellulose or nylon membrane and hybridized with labeled nucleic acid probes.

nortriptyline hydrochloride   An antidepressant drug of the tricyclic class. Trade names are Aventyl Hydrochloride and Pamelor.

Norwegian scabies   A rare, severe form of scabies, characterized by an extremely heavy infestation of mites, that appears in patients with poor sensation, severe systemic disease, senility or mental retardation, and immunosuppression.

nosocormial infection   An infection acquired in a hospital or other health-care institution.

notifiable disease   A disease whose occurrence must, by law, be reported to health authorities. Among the diseases that the laws of various states require to be reported are all communicable or contagious diseases, such as scarlet fever and diphtheria; enteric fevers, such as typhoid; epidemics of acute diarrheal disease; cholera; typhus; meningococcal meningitis; AIDS; acute anterior poliomyelitis; polioencephalitis; encephalitis lethargica; tuberculosis; rubella; chicken pox; gonorrhea; and syphilis.

notification of partners   See PARTNER NOTIFICATION.

nuclear magnetic resonance imaging (NMRI)   See MAGNETIC RESONANCE IMAGING.

nucleic acid   A compound that carries genetic information, found in all viruses and living organisms. DNA and RNA are the two principal forms.

nucleoside   A building block of DNA or RNA, the genetic material found in living organisms. Before being added to a DNA or RNA sequence, nucleosides must have a phosphate group added.

nucleoside analog   A type of antiviral drug, such as AZT, ddI, ddC or D4T, whose makeup constitutes a defective version of a natural nucleoside. Nucleoside analogs may take the place of the natural nucleosides, blocking the completion of a viral DNA chain during infection of a new cell by HIV. The HIV enzyme REVERSE TRANSCRIPTASE is more likely to incorporate nucleoside analogs into the DNA it is constructing than is the DNA polymerase normally used for DNA creation in cell nuclei.

nucleoside analog therapy   Anti-HIV therapy with nucleoside analog reverse-transcriptase inhibitors.

nucleotide   A glycoside (any of a group of sugar derivatives that, when combined with water, yields a sugar and one or more other substances) formed by the combination of a sugar (pentose) and a purine or pyrimide base.

null cell   A white blood cell that is a lymphocyte but lacks the specific identifying surface markers for either T or B LYMPHOCYTEs.

Nuprin   See IBUPROFEN.

nurse   An individual who provides health care. The extent of nursing care varies from simple patient-care tasks to the most complex medical techniques necessary in acute life-threatening situations. The roles of nurses constantly change in response to the growth of biomedical knowledge, changes in patterns of demand for health services, and the evolution of professional, relationships among nurses, physicians, and other health care professionals.

Also, to nurse is to feed an infant at the breast; to perform the duties of caring for an invalid; or to care for a young child.

nursing home   An extended-care facility for persons who need medical attention and general care too taxing to be done at home but not requiring hospitalization.

nutrient   Any substance that supplies the body with elements necessary for metabolism. Carbohydrates, fats, proteins, and alcohol are nutrients that provide energy. Water, electrolytes, minerals, and vitamins are nutrients that are essential to the metabolic process. Nutrients containing carbon are organic food nutrients.

nutrient deficiency   There are many causes of nutrient deficiency in people living with HIV, including malabsorption because of damage to the intestines (by HIV or other infections); the high demand for antioxidants; the increased metabolism that begins in the earliest disease stages; and decreased intake of food because of mouth or throat problems, loss of appetite, loss of taste, fever, nausea, and vomiting. The resulting serious deficiency of nutrients critical for supporting immune function, and malnutrition, are common among people with HIV and frequently contribute to the development of opportunistic infections and general deterioration that are the immediate causes of death.

Recent research has made it clear that HIV-associated nutrient deficiencies and malnutrition are not just late-stage occurrences. Many nutrient deficiencies begin in early disease stages when patients appear to be well and free of symptoms and have CD4+ counts upwards of 400. Because nutrients seldom work alone in the body, a deficiency of one nutrient may cause other nutrients to work improperly. Research has shown that people living with HIV need to consume much more than the standard recommended daily allowances (RDA) of nutrients to maintain normal levels— diet is far more important in treating HIV disease than most people realize. But even the most nutritious diet may not be sufficient to fully meet the needs of people living with HIV disease.

nutrient supplementation   An optimal approach to managing HIV disease includes a rational nutrition program encompassing both sound dietary choices and nutrient supplementation. The goal is to provide optimal levels of nutrients in order to help prevent damage, manage symptoms related to HIV, and boost the body's capacity to heal. Multiple vitamin and mineral supplements that supply the basic level of nutrients most important to body functions are a common type of nutrient supplementation. Because of the serious deficiencies and the increased need for a number of nutrients, many nutritionists believe that it is necessary to take additional supplements such as antioxidants, essential fatty acids, carnitine, acidophilus, and digestive aids such as pancreatic enzymes or hydrochloric acid supplements, both to increase dosage levels and to include nutrients not usually found in multiple supplements. Studies have also shown that some nutritional supplements like zinc, selenium, and vitamins C, A, E, and B together with AZT may increase AZT's antiviral effect while at the same time strengthening the immune system. Additionally, there is increasing evidence for an autoimmune aspect of HIV infection that may be treated with antioxidants and other nutrients, like glutathione, coenzyme Q10, vitamins C, E, and A, selenium, and zinc, that protect cell membranes and dampen the inflammatory response of the body to the infection. Maintaining a good supplementation program helps prevent deficiencies and loss of immune function. In addition, symptoms that result from deficiencies can often be eliminated with an appropriate supplement program. Symptoms that may be related to nutrient deficiencies and may be reversible with appropriate supplementation include serious fatigue, memory loss or other cognitive dysfunction, skin problems, neuropathy, weight loss, loss of the senses of smell or taste, appetite loss, muscle pain or cramps, digestive problems, night blindness, canker sores, constipation, depression, anxiety, menstrual cramps, and menopausal problems.

nutrition   All the processes involved in the taking in and utilization of food substances by which growth, repair, and maintenance of activities in the body as a whole or in any of its parts are accomplished. Nutrition includes ingestion, digestion, absorption, and metabolism. Some nutrients are capable of being stored in the body in various forms and drawn upon when food intake is not sufficient.

Today medical practitioners are increasingly aware that good nutrition is a fundamental component of the care of people with HIV/AIDS. Specially-designed nutritional programs, including NUTRIENT SUPPLEMENTATION, have been shown to boost immune function, increase the efficacy of medical treatments, and improve energy levels and general quality of life. Conversely, malnutrition may contribute to the development of opportunistic infections and physical deterioration that may be the immediate cause of death. Registered dieticians and naturopaths may know more about general nutrition than medical doctors, since they have much more extensive training in the area. Many are also knowledgeable specifically about nutrition in people with HIV. See NUTRIENT DEFICIENCY; MALNUTRITION; PARENTERAL NUTRITION; WASTING.

nutritional deficiency   See NUTRIENT DEFICIENCY.

nutritional supplement   See NUTRIENT SUPPLEMENTATION.

Nydrazid   See ISONIAZID.

nystatin   An antibiotic appearing as a yellowish-to-tan powder. It is an antifungal used in the treatment of cutaneous, intestinal, oral, or vaginal candidal infections. Nystatin may be administered orally or topically. It works by interfering with the ability of fungi to build their cell walls. Nystatin rarely causes side effects, although nausea or irritation of the mouth or vagina are occasionally reported. Large oral doses may cause diarrhea, stomach upset, vomiting, or rashes. Also called Fungicidin. Other trade names are Mycostatin, O-V Statin, and Pedi-Dri.

OASDI See OLD AGE, SURVIVORS, AND DISABILITY INSURANCE.

obscene Defined by *Webster's* as "disgusting . . . abhorrent to morality or virtue," the term is commonly used to apply to offensive depictions of sexual activity. It is used in this sense as a legal term.

Although everyone seems to know what the word means, obscenity is notoriously difficult to identify, since what offends one person or group may not offend others. Accusations of obscenity are therefore routinely countered with accusations of censorship and defenses of freedom of speech, and no legal determination of obscenity has ever been generally accepted as proper.

obstetrics The branch of medicine concerned with the care of women during pregnancy, childbirth, and the puerperium.

occupational exposure The risk of exposure to a communicable disease through the normal procedures associated with a specific profession (e.g., a NEEDLESTICK during a surgical procedure). In June 1996, the Public Health Service published guidelines for treating occupational exposure to HIV (Centers for Disease Control and Prevention. *MMWR* 1996; 45: 486–472). According to these recommendations, doctors, nurses, and other health care workers who are accidentally exposed to HIV-tainted blood should promptly receive antiretroviral therapy. The guidelines address type of exposure (percutaneous, mucous membrane, and skin), source material (blood, fluid containing visible blood, other potentially infectious fluid), antiretroviral prophylaxis, and antiretroviral regimen. The recommendations specify two- or three-drug treatment regimens depending on the degree of risk associated with the exposure. If possible, treatment should begin within one to two hours of exposure. It is recommended that therapy be administered for four weeks, if tolerated, although optimal duration of treatment is also unknown.

octreotide An antidiarreal used for refractory secretory diarrhea. Side effects may include pain or burning at the injection site, abdominal cramps and pain, diarrhea or loose stools, nausea/vomiting, and postprandial hyperglycemia. Brand name is Sandostatin.

ocular Relating to the eye.

ocular herpes A HERPES infection of the eye, usually caused by touching an infected area of the body and then touching the eye.

odynophagia Pain upon swallowing.

off-label An "off-label" drug is one approved by the FOOD AND DRUG ADMINISTRATION for some uses, but prescribed for another use for which it has not been approved. Drug therapy administered to people with AIDS often involves off-label use of medications. Frequently, off-label use of a drug merely anticipates Food and Drug Administration approval for that use. Obtaining insurance reimbursement for off-label prescriptions may be problematic. Patients who do not have insurance or who are members of health maintenance organizations (HMOs) often have less chance of receiving off-label therapies.

ofloxacin An antibiotic used primarily to treat responsive infections in adults of the lower respiratory tract (lungs and bronchial tubes); the urinary tract (kidneys, bladder, urethra, and prostate gland); skin and related tissues; and certain sexually transmitted diseases such as gonorrheal and chlamydial infections of the urethra and cervix. By interfering with the bacterial enzyme DNA gyrase (necessary for DNA synthesis and cell reproduction), this drug in low concentrations arrests bacterial growth, and in high concentrations destroys bacteria. Ofloxacin is currently a drug of choice for starting treatment of urinary tract infections (before results of culture and sensitivity tests are known) and for treating infections due to *Pseudomonas* bacterial strains often resistant to other anti-infective drugs. Ofloxacin has a broad spectrum of antibacterial activity; is capable of establishing effective drug levels throughout the prostate gland; is an effective one-dose treatment for uncomplicated gonorrheal infection of the urethra; and has no significant effect on kidney function. There have been no reports of serious drug-induced colitis. Possible mild adverse effects include allergic reactions, headache, dizziness, weakness, drowsiness, nervousness, insomnia, visual disturbances; decreased appetite, altered taste, dry mouth, nausea, vomiting, indigestion, and diarrhea. Serious adverse effects include anaphylactoid reactions and central nervous system stimulation. Trade name is Floxin.

OI   See OPPORTUNISTIC INFECTION.

oidiomycosis   See CANDIDIASIS.

oil-based lubricant   See LUBRICANT.

Old Age, Survivors, and Disability Insurance (OASDI) Collectively, the range of worker-based income insurance programs operated by the Social Security Administration for the insured aged, disabled, and their families. The term is no longer used.

Omnipen   See AMPICILLIN.

onanism   The practice of withdrawing during coitus to ejaculate. The term is often used incorrectly to mean masturbation.

oncogene   A gene associated with cancer. Oncogenes are of either viral or mammalian origin and are found widely in the living world, including in human cells. When oncogenes are "turned off" their function is unknown. When they are "turned on" they begin to form products that may transform the host cells into cancer cells.

oncovirus   One of a subfamily of retroviruses that includes tumor-causing agents such as the Rous sarcoma virus and the BOVINE LEUKEMIA VIRUS.

oocyst   The encysted form of a fertilized gamete occurring in certain sporozoa.

"Opal" trials   Trials conducted in Australia, Austria, Belgium, Denmark, France, Finland, Germany, Iceland, Italy, Luxembourg, the Netherlands, Norway, Spain, Sweden, and the United Kingdom to determine the best time to start treatment of HIV infection based on the presence or absence of clinical symptoms. See also CONCORDE.

open-label study   See OPEN-LABEL TRIAL.

open-label trial   A study in which both researchers and participants know what drug participants are taking and at what doses.

ophthalmoscopy   Examination of the interior of the eye.

opiate   Any drug containing or derived from opium.

opium, tincture of   An antidiarrheal analgesic commonly used to treat diarrhea refractory to other agents. Side effects

may include constipation, drowsiness, hypotension, nausea/vomiting, sweating, and dizziness. Anticholinergics may add to the effects of tincture of opium. CNS depressants can have an increased effect. Tolerance to antidiarrheal effects may develop with repeated use.

opportunistic   Of a pathogen, usually able to produce disease only in an immunologically compromised host.

opportunistic infection (OI) and disease   Any of a number of rare bacterial, fungal, protozoal, and viral infections that can be caused by common microorganisms in the environment, but that do not cause disease except in persons with seriously damaged or compromised immune systems. Healthy people are able to fight off these opportunistic infections, but those with weakened immune systems can be overwhelmed by them. In conjunction with HIV, such infections become virulent and life-threatening. There are about 100 microorganisms that can cause opportunistic infections in people with HIV.

Opportunistic infections cause most of the morbidity and mortality in AIDS. The AIDS-defining opportunistic infections are convenient indicators of the severity of immunodeficiency, are easily observable, and do not require frequent laboratory monitoring, as is the case with CD4 cells. In fact, the presence of any such opportunistic infection in a person who is HIV infected is AIDS-defining and must be reported to local and national health authorities for epidemiological purposes. Although a CD4 count below 200 without symptomatic disease is also an AIDS-defining condition, physicians rely primarily on the presence of opportunistic infections to make a diagnosis.

The most common opportunistic infections in cases of HIV and AIDS affect the lungs, skin, GASTROINTESTINAL TRACT, LYMPH NODES, eyes, and brain. The lungs are most commonly affected because they are the point of entry for inhaled microorganisms. The lungs are the principal target for PNEUMOCYSTIS CARINII and are also commonly the site for CYTOMEGALOVIRUS, CRYPTOCOCCUS NEOFORMANS, and a variety of typical and atypical tuberculous bacteria. The skin is the commonest site for the cancer KAPOSI'S SARCOMA. HERPES SIMPLEX and VARICELLA-ZOSTER VIRUSES can cause painful, deep, and destructive ulcers in many different locations on the skin. MOLLUSCUM CONTAGIOSUM, a disfiguring viral disease, sometimes affects the genitals and the anal region with venereal warts. The gastrointestinal tract can be affected anywhere between the lips and the anus. Commonly found microorganisms there include the herpes simplex virus, which can cause an inflammation of the esophagus called ESOPHAGITIS and CANDIDA ALBICANS, a fungus that causes both oral thrush and esophagitis. Other microorganisms cause intestinal disturbances resulting in debilitating diarrhea and malabsorption of food. These microorganisms include CRYPTOSPORIDIUM, CYTOMEGALOVIRUS (CMV), ISOSPORA BELLI, and MYCOBACTERIUM AVIUM-INTRACELLULARE. ORAL HAIRY LEUKOPLAKIA is an important early symptom in persons with HIV infection.

The lymph nodes can undergo changes from direct infection by organisms such as cryptococcus or tuberculous bacteria, infiltration by tumor cells of Kaposi's sarcoma, or as the result of infection in parts of the body drained by those nodes. Many persons with AIDS suffer from cytomegalovirus, an inflammatory condition of the retina. Most persons with AIDS also suffer from dramatic changes in the functions of the brain sometime during the course of their disease. Opportunistic infections causing brain disease in persons with AIDS include toxoplasmosis from the protozoan TOXOPLASMA GONDII, meningitis from *Cryptococcus neoformans* and PROGRESSIVE MULTIFOCAL LEUKOENCEPHALOPATHY, a viral illness that kills selected cells in the brain.

The development of opportunistic infection prophylaxis (prevention of opportunistic infections) is desperately needed in HIV treatment. An effective prophylaxis has been documented for *Pneumocystis carinii* pneumonia (PCP), and is assumed to be popular. However, physicians tend to be less aggressive with prophylaxis for other opportunistic infections such as CMV, MYCOBACTERIUM AVIUM COMPLEX (MAC) or fungal infections, and tend to differ in their rationales for recommending prophylaxis, their choice of agents or therapies, and their choice of patient population.

Identifying patients at risk for developing OIs remains difficult. According to the *Journal of the American Medical Association*, one in four people infected with HIV is seriously immunosuppressed and at greater risk for contracting serious infections. Studies have documented a correlation of T4 counts with the occurrence of specific OIs. The OIs that can occur early in HIV disease are tuberculosis and CANDIDIASIS (thrush) in the mouth, esophagus, or vagina. These are most likely to develop when T4 counts are between 500 and 250. As T4 counts drop from 250 to below 100, the OIs more likely to develop include PCP, toxoplasmosis, cryptococcal meningitis (CM), and MAC. A high percentage of cases of CMV retinitis develop when T4 counts are below 90.

The correlation between T4 counts and OIs may help in assessing the appropriate time to initiate therapy. The key to successful prophylaxis is determining the exact point at which the benefits of preventive drug therapy outweigh the risks. Useful measurements in determining the status of the immune system and the activity of HIV include the ratio of T4 cells to all lymphocyte cells; the ratio of T4 cells to T8 cells; and the amounts of Beta 2 microglobulin and of neopterin present.

Prevention strategies for the various OIs vary. (See, for example, TUBERCULOSIS, TOXOPLASMOSIS, MAC, CRYPTO-COCCAL MENINGITIS and CMV.) Vaccines also play a crucial role in preventing common infections in people with HIV disease. Yearly immunizations for influenza and a one-time-only immunization for bacterial pneumonia are generally recommended for all HIV-positive people. One problem with these vaccines is that HIV-positive people may not achieve the high levels of protective antibodies that the vaccine is meant to trigger; however, merely increasing this protection may be beneficial. Other preventive measures currently recommended include a purified protein derivative (PPD) skin test for tuberculosis (most accurate in early HIV illness), and, if positive, treatment with ISONIAZID (INH); a syphilis test at least once, and repeatedly if other STDs are present; a toxoplasmosis blood test for antibodies

against the parasite, and, if negative, a retest once a year; not changing cat litter, or wearing a mask and gloves when doing so; avoiding undercooked meat; an eye exam for CMV, repeated every three months if T4 cells are below 100; PAP smear and pelvic exam every six months; a hepatitis B virus test, and the hepatitis B vaccine if antigen and antibody negative.

The National Institutes of Health (NIH), the CENTERS FOR DISEASE CONTROL AND PREVENTION (CDC), and the Infectious Diseases Society of America have formulated comprehensive guidelines for the prevention of opportunistic infections in HIV-infected persons. The guidelines provide up-to-date information to help medical practitioners better treat people with HIV, thus increasing the quality and duration of their lives and to reduce the overall cost of care. The guidelines discuss many new drugs and drug strategies addressed in clinical trials and stress early diagnosis of HIV infection and encourage HIV testing for all pregnant women. Also stressed is prevention of opportunistic infections as a critical part of the health care program once HIV is diagnosed. The guidelines make it possible for practitioners and patients to remain abreast of important findings. These guidelines can be found in a supplement to the August 1995 *Clinical Infectious Diseases* (Volume 21, Supplement 1, pp. S1–S141).

opsonization   A process by which PHAGOCYTOSIS is facilitated by the deposition of opsonins (e.g., ANTIBODY and C3b) on the ANTIGEN.

optimal health   The highest state of well-being attainable at a particular time of life. Although the optimal health for an HIV-infected person may be different from that of someone who is HIV-negative, optimal health, defined in terms of the individual patient, should still be the goal for care of an HIV-infected individual.

oral-anal sex   See ORAL SEX.

oral cancer   Cancer in the mouth (oral cavity), including the lips, gums, cheeks, tongue, tonsils, and floor of the mouth. The primary cause of oral cancer is tobacco use. Other risk factors include certain nutritional deficiencies and poorly fitting dentures and bridges. Oral cancer can also develop in people with precancerous conditions such as LEUKOPLAKIA and ERYTHROPLAKIA. Diagnostic procedures include a manual exam, X rays, and BIOPSY.

oral candida   See ORAL CANDIDIASIS.

oral candidiasis   Infection of the skin or mucous membranes in the mouth with any species of *Candida*. Despite the presence of oral lesions, patients are often asymptomatic during early stages of the disease. Some patients complain of oral discomfort, a burning sensation when eating, or an altered sense of taste. Diagnosis is made by scraping the lesion and examining the collected material under a microscope using KOH preparation. Mycelia will be evident. Several therapies are available for oral candidiasis: clotrimazole troches and nystatin swish and swallow are commonly recommended topical therapies. Systemic therapy with ketoconazole, fluconazole, or itraconazole is also available. Also called pseudomenbraneous candidiasis and thrush. See CANDIDIASIS.

oral coitus   See ORAL SEX.

oral contraceptive   A method of birth control (known as "the pill") in which a synthetic HORMONE pill is taken regularly by mouth to prevent conception. The pill interferes with ovulation, fertilization, and implantation of a fertilized egg in the uterus. Oral contraceptives were first made available and became popular during the early 1960s. The formulation has changed since its introduction, and newer versions provide a significantly lower dose of hormones than the original. The major advantages of oral contraceptives are their effectiveness, ease of use, ease of discontinuing use, and regulation of effects of the menstrual cycle. Many women cannot take them, however, because they have conditions that countraindicate their use, including known or suspected breast cancer or tumor; genital bleeding of unknown origin; circulatory disorders; cerebral-vascular or coronary-artery disorders; severely impaired liver function; cystic fibrosis; sickle-cell disease; or a past history of these disorders;

oral diagnosis   The compilation and study of the patient's dental history, along with a detailed clinical examination of the oral tissues and radiographs to assess the level of oral health, often with the object of developing a treatment plan to restore tooth structure, proper occlusions, and better oral health.

oral eroticism   A psychoanalytic term for pleasure derived from activities involving the mouth, including oral-genital contact, kissing, sucking, eating, biting, chewing, thumb-sucking or smoking. Some of these activities are considered unsafe sex practices with high risk of HIV transmission (oral-anal contact). Others are considered possibly unsafe practices with unclear risk of HIV transmission (fellatio, cunnilingus). Other activities, such as wet kissing, are considered low-risk practices with some risk of HIV transmission. See ORAL SEX.

oral examination   See ORAL DIAGNOSIS.

oral ganciclovir   See GANCICLOVIR.

oral-genital contact   See ORAL SEX.

oral-genital sex   See ORAL SEX.

oral hairy leukoplakia (OHL)   The symptoms of oral hairy leukoplakia are white lesions or patches on the tongue and elsewhere in the mouth; the lesion appears raised with a corrugated, or "hairy," surface. These patches produce no symptoms, but may distort taste or cause pain. They are caused by the same virus that causes INFECTIOUS MONONUCLEOSIS and EPSTEIN-BARR disease. The patches often appear similar to those of thrush. In fact, oral hairy leukoplakia is often diagnosed when people who appear to have thrush do not respond to the usual treatment. It can be diagnosed with a BIOPSY. Oral hairy leukoplakia occurs mainly in people with declining immunity; and without treatment for HIV, the first AIDS-defining illness is likely to appear within two or three years of a diagnosis. The treatment for oral hairy leukoplakia is the antiviral drug ACYCLOVIR.

oral herpes   Canker sores, fever blisters, and cold sores. See HERPES.

oral HIV test   An HIV test which uses mouth secretions. It is believed that the new test will encourage more people at risk of AIDS, particularly minorities, to get tested, because it does not involve a needle and can be given easily outside of a clinic. Patients take the oral test by placing a flat, inch-long cotton swab, attached to a stick, between their gums and their cheeks for two minutes. The swab, treated with a salt solution, draws fluid from the mucous membrane. The fluid contains HIV antibodies in people infected with the virus.

oral lesion   A circumscribed area of pathologically altered tissue or skin in the mouth.

oral sex   Sexual activity in which the genitals and anus are stimulated with the tongue and/or mouth. Contact between the mouth and the genitals is probably the most common form of oral sex (FELLATIO is the oral stimulation of the penis; CUNNILINGUS is the oral stimulation of the clitoris). Oral sexual activities may include kissing, biting, sucking, licking, exploring the partner's body including erogenous zones and genitals with the tongue and lips, and tasting and swallowing the partner's sexual secretions. Oral sex, particularly oral-anal sex, is considered high-risk—many SEXUALLY TRANSMITTED DISEASES (particularly AIDS, SYPHILIS, GONORRHEA, and HERPES) can be transmitted through it—but because individuals who engage in it rarely do so to the exclusion of other forms of sexual contact, it is difficult to attribute transmission in any particular case to oral sex rather than to other types of sexual activity. The role of oral sex as a route of transmission of HIV is, at best, poorly studied in populations other than homosexual men.

Slang terms include blow job, eating out, giving head, going down, pussy licking, and ass licking.

oral thrush   A fungal condition in the mouth caused by an overgrowth of fungus that commonly appears as creamy white or yellow patches or red splotches on the roof or corners of the mouth. The infections can sometimes extend down the throat and cause pain in swallowing and eating. When oral thrush extends down the throat, it is called ESOPHOGEAL CANDIDIASIS and is a life-threatening AIDS-defining illness. See THRUSH; CANDIDIASIS; ORAL CANDIDIASIS.

Orasone   See PREDNISONE.

organ   A body structure with specific functions; made of two or more tissues.

organ donation   The transplantation of an organ from a donor to a recipient. Organ transplants have become a routine medical practice that has dramatically improved and—sometimes—saved lives. Successful transplantation is increased by matching donors and recipients of the same racial and ethnic groups. The organ recovery process may involve several steps, including obtaining medical examiner approval, obtaining next-of-kin consent, reviewing medical and social history for organ safety, and testing blood to lower the risk of spreading infectious diseases. Once a recovery team surgically removes the organs without disfiguring the body, the organs are evaluated for transplant. People who receive organs are generally selected according to the United Network for Organ Sharing guidelines. There is no cost to the donor family for any organ presentation or donation procedures. Donor cards are legal documents under the Uniform Anatomical Gift Act. Signing a donor card signifies a donor's commitment to make a gift of any needed organs and/or tissues for the purpose of transplant, medical study, or education. The transplant takes effect after the donor's death.

organ donor   To prevent transmission of HIV, the CENTERS FOR DISEASE CONTROL AND PREVENTION (CDC) has recommended voluntary testing for exposure for anyone donating organs, tissues, sperm, or blood.

organ system   A group of related organs that work together to perform specific functions (i.e., the digestive system, the reproductive system). The immune system is the organ system that fights disease.

organic   A chemical compound that contains carbon-hydrogen covalent bonds; includes carbohydrates, lipids, proteins, and nucleic acids.

organic brain damage   Physiological harm to the brain cells, causing impairment of brain function. HIV infection of the central nervous system can cause such damage.

orgasm   A state of physical and emotional excitement, especially that which occurs at the climax of sexual intercourse. It is the third stage of the sexual response cycle, after the excitement and plateau phases. In the male, it is accompanied by the ejaculation of semen. In the female, tension is released in a series of involuntary and often pleasurable muscular contractions that expel blood from the pelvic tissue. Women may feel contractions in the vagina, uterus, and rectum. Some women describe orgasm without contractions. Orgasm can be mild, like a hiccup, a sneeze, a ripple; it can be a sensuous experience; it can be intense or ecstatic. Today, it is generally understood by sexologists and researchers that all orgasms are not physiologically the same. No one is sure as to how many types of orgasms there are and which kind is better, stronger, or more satisfying. Slang terms include the "big O."

orgy   An event consisting of uninhibited excessive group indulgence in a variety of pleasurable activities, including sex, drinking, singing, or dancing.

ornithosis   An acute generalized infectious disease of wild birds and domesticated fowl, communicable to humans.

orogenital contact   See ORAL SEX

orphan diseases   Rare, debilitating illnesses that strike small numbers of people. See ORPHAN DRUG and ORPHAN DRUG ACT.

orphan drug   Drugs that are effective for certain ORPHAN DISEASES but, for a variety of reasons, are not profitable for manufactures to produce. See ORPHAN DRUG ACT.

Orphan Drug Act   The United States FOOD AND DRUG ADMINISTRATION–sponsored Orphan Drug Act of 1983 was passed to encourage development of drugs that could not be patented and for which there would be only a limited market. Orphan status is granted before FDA approval, and afterward the manufacturer is allowed tax benefits and seven years of marketing exclusivity.

orphan drug status   See ORPHAN DRUG ACT.

orphan   See AIDS ORPHAN.

orphanage   One of today's challenges (and tomorrow's problems) is the impact of AIDS-related deaths on both the lives of community members and the individual lives of children and adolescents. To deal with this growing problem, some advocate that the institution of orphanages be revived. Today, the term conjures up images from Dickens—starving children abused by heartless masters. It is true that child care practices in some institutions in the past, especially during the nineteenth century, seem punitive and rigid by contemporary standards. But some orphanages in the United States today provide good care. An example is transition homes for HIV-infected orphaned babies. These have been successful in providing appropriate health care as well as emotional nurturing. They were created to offer an out-of-hospital environment for such babies until longer-term placement can be arranged. Those who support the return of the orphanage as an institution call for creating small-scale institutions that can offer children nurturing and care as well as shelter. They hold that congregate care is both a useful and temporary option and that orphanages are the only answer to the failure of families or foster care. On the other hand, the primacy of family life has been stressed repeatedly in the 1990s. The jury is still out with respect to institutional child care settings. A rigorous, unemotional analysis of the appropriate role of congregate care, and the services that are needed to make it work in the interests of children, is essential.

otitis   An inflammation of the ear, differentiated as externa (inflammation of the external auditory canal), media (inflammation of the middle ear), and interna (inflammation of the labyrinth of the ear).

otopharyngeal   Concerning the ear and pharynx.

otopharyngeal complication   A disease, involving the ear and pharynx, that is superimposed upon another disease without being specifically related to it, yet affecting or modifying the prognosis of the original disease.

otopharyngeal tube   The passage between the tympanic cavity and the pharynx.

ototoxic   Having a detrimental effect on the eighth nerve or the organs of hearing.

ototoxicity   The quality of being ototoxic.

outercourse   A term originating in the anti-AIDS, safe-sex movement, designating forms of sexual expression, such as massage, hugging, caressing, mutual masturbation, and rubbing bodies together that do not involve the exchange of body fluids. These forms of sexual expression are considered practices with no risk of HIV transmission.

outreach worker   A professional or paraprofessional health or social services worker who actively seeks out patients in their own environments and communities and provides education and medical services.

ovarian cancer   Cancer of the ovaries, the female reproductive organs in which the ova, or eggs, are formed and estrogen is produced.

The cause of ovarian cancer is not known, although a number of factors have been associated with its occurrence. It appears that HORMONES play a role in the development of ovarian cancer. Exposure to high levels of radiation may also cause ovarian cancer. The most common type of ovarian cancer is the EPITHELIAL carcinoma in the ovary's outer layer. Frequently there are no symptoms in the early stages of ovarian cancer, making it difficult to obtain an early diagnosis, when there is the greatest chance for effective treatment. An ovarian tumor can grow for some time before pressure or pain can be felt or other problems are noticed. When symptoms do occur, they may include abdominal swelling or bloating, discomfort in the lower part of the abdomen, a full feeling after a light meal, lack of appetite, nausea, vomiting, gas, indigestion, weight loss, constant need to urinate, diarrhea, or constipation, and nonmenstrual bleeding. Procedures used in the diagnosis and evaluation of ovarian cancer may include an internal exam of the uterus, vagina, ovaries, fallopian tubes, bladder, and rectum, a PAP SMEAR, ultrasound, blood and urine tests, and X rays. Additional procedures that may be done are a CT SCAN, lymphangiography, IVP, lower GI series, exploratory laparotomy and biopsies.

Treatment depends on the stage of the disease at the time of diagnosis, the type of cells that make up the tumor, and how fast the cancer is growing. Current medical options for treating ovarian cancer include surgery, chemotherapy and/or radiation. Biological therapies are also now available. These therapies are evolving as a result of research, which continues to offer hope for improving the outcome of treatment for women with ovarian cancer.

ovary   The major female reproductive organ that produces eggs (ova) and the female sex hormone estrogen. There are two ovaries, one on either side of the uterus.

overdose   A dose of a drug sufficient to cause an acute reaction, such as mania, hysteria, coma, or even death. While an overdose is often one that clearly exceeds the normal dosage range recommended by the manufacturer, the optimal dose of many drugs varies from person to person. What may be an average dose for most people may be an overdose for some and an underdose for others. Numerous factors such as age, body size, nutritional status, and liver and kidney function have significant influence on dosage requirements. An overdose may be accidental or deliberate and may result from accumulation of prescribed daily doses.

over-the-counter (OTC) drugs   Drug products that can be purchased without prescription. Like the more potent drug products sold only on prescription, they are chemicals that are capable of a wide variety of actions on biological systems. Within the last 30 years, many OTC drugs have assumed greater importance because of their ability to interact favorably with widely used prescription drugs. Serious problems in drug management can arise when the patient fails to tell the physician of the OTC drug(s) he or she is taking and when the physician fails to note the inclusion of OTC drugs when asking the patient about what medicines the patient currently uses. During any course of treatment, whether medical or surgical, the patient should consult with the physician regarding any OTC drug that the patient wishes to take. The major classes of OTC drugs for internal use include allergy medicines, antacids, antiworm medicines, aspirin and aspirin combinations, aspirin substitutes, asthma aids, cold medicines, diarrhea remedies, digestion aids, diuretics, iron preparations, laxatives, menstrual aids, motion sickness remedies, pain relievers, reducing aids, salt substitutes, sedatives and tranquilizers, sleeping pills, stimulants, sugar substitutes, tonics, and vitamins.

oviduct   The tube through which the egg passes from the ovary to the uterus.

ovine-caprine lentivirus   Any lentivirus associated with sheep or goats.

O-V Statin   See NYSTATIN.

ovulation   Release of the egg from the ovary, generally fourteen days after the end of a woman's last menstrual period.

oxidation   A chemical reaction resulting from exposure to oxygen or other electron-donating atom or molecule. On the cellular level, oxidative reactions are the source of energy, but free radicals and other oxidizing agents can damage cellular components such as membranes and interfere with cells' regulatory systems.

oxidative stress   A condition within cells that forces them into a highly activated state due to interference with their regulatory systems by a highly oxidized environment. Oxidative stress is thought to promote HIV replication.

oxophenarsine hydrochloride   An antitrypanosomal compound containing 30 percent arsenic. *Trypanosoma* is a genus of parasitic, flagellate protozoa found in the blood of many vertebrates, including humans. It is transmitted by insect vecters.

P

P1 lab facility   A basic laboratory such as could be found lining the hallways of university science departments, found within the CENTERS FOR DISEASE CONTROL AND PREVENTION's high-security laboratories.

P2 lab facility   A laboratory within the CENTERS FOR DISEASE CONTROL AND PREVENTION's high-security laboratories. Entry is limited to trained, authorized personnel who perform research work under hoods that suck air away from the experiment, up a ventilator duct, and past scrubbers that disinfect the air with ultraviolet light and microscopically gridded fibers.

P-3 biosafety level   Applicable to clinical, teaching, research, or production facilities in which work is done with agents that may cause serious or potentially lethal reactions as a result of exposure by inhalation. Special airflows and filters and an antechamber with a sink, must be installed. Protective garments must always be worn, and nothing may be taken out of the room without being sterilized. See P1 LAB FACILTY, P2 LAB FACILITY, P3 LAB FACILITY.

P3 lab facility   A lab within the CENTERS FOR DISEASE CONTROL AND PREVENTION's high-security laboratories in which scientist perform high-security research. Researchers are generally required to pass through a series of guarded locked doors, presenting their security pass for entry. All personnel shower before and after entry with disinfectant soap and wear head-to-toe protective clothing, a gauze face mask, double latex gloves, and a radiation badge that monitors levels of exposure to isotopes used in research. One enters the inner core of the facility after passing through two or more double air-locked doors lined with microbe-killing ultraviolet lights. Rooms in the inner core of the facility are generally kept under pressure and direct all air—and all microbes—toward special ventilators in which the microbes are destroyed by ultraviolet lights. The remaining air is filtered through several layers of sheets that strain out anything bigger than a large molecule.

p24   A protein ANTIGEN from HIV's core. The p24 level can be measured in blood and other body fluids; this level has been used to monitor viral activity. This is not considered a very accurate method, however, due to the existence of p24 ANTIBODY that binds with the antigen and makes it undetectable.

p24 antigen test   A laboratory test (also called the p24 antigen capture assay) that detects the presence of HIV in the blood. p24 is one of the several proteins that make up HIV; its presence therefore indicates the presence of HIV. This test is not especially sensitive, and most people with HIV infection test negative.

Levels of p24 are highest early and late in the disease. The number of HIV viruses is likewise highest at those times. Some physicians therefore suggest that the p24 antigen test might help track the course of the disease in people with HIV infection. It might identify people with HIV infection who are likely to develop symptoms and who are most likely to transmit the virus to others. It might also help evaluate response to antiviral drugs.

package insert   A printed information sheet from a drug manufacturer approved by the FOOD AND DRUG ADMINISTRATION for a prescription drug product, which accompanies the product in its packaging. The insert is usually not enclosed by a pharmacist with a dispensed prescription. Intended mainly for the use of prescribing professionals, principally physicians, the insert gives the recommended uses, mode of administration, dosage, and contraindications to use of the drug, with appropriate warnings.

pain   Physical suffering, typically from injury or illness. Pain is a common companion of persons living with HIV and AIDS. Pain occurs at all points on the HIV/AIDS continuum and is the most common reason for people with AIDS to be hospitalized. It appears that as people with AIDS survive longer, pain is becoming an increasingly severe complaint. Pain in HIV/AIDS can be traced to HIV infection and its complications, medical treatments, or causes independent of HIV. Pain is often complicated by multiple concurrent diagnoses as well as chemical dependency and dementia. It is crucial that medical practitioners understand the sources of pain in people with AIDS as well as the pharmacological factors affecting use of pain relievers in this population. Active pain management is fundamental to the provision of care.

pain management   Active management of pain, which seeks to ensure the greatest comfort and functioning with minimal medication-related side effects is key to relieving the effects of AIDS. Since multiple illnesses often coexist in PWAs, the importance of identifying and appropriately treating underlying causes of pain is primary. Treating the disease may eradicate the pain all by itself. While the cause of pain is being determined, pain management with appropriate analgesics should be initiated. There is much that can be done to ameliorate pain, but drug therapy is the mainstay of any treatment program.

The World Health Organization has developed a four-step ladder approach to the treatment of cancer pain, and this has been adapted for the treatment of HIV-related pain. The first step is to use acetaminophen or other nonsteroidal anti-inflammatory drugs, such as ibuprofen, sulindac, or aspirin. If these measures do not provide adequate relief, then a weak opiate, such as codeine or oxycodone, is added. If this is inadequate, a stronger opiate, such as morphine, hydromorphone, fentanyl, or levorphanol, is used. The fourth step, which can be incorporated at any point in the process, is to add adjuvants, such as hydroxyzine, that boost the effectiveness of pain medications.

Alternate routes of administration of drugs is an important element in pain management. Dehydration, malnourishment, and ELECTROLYTE imbalance due to vomiting, diarrhea, and anorexia impede the effectiveness of oral medication. In the case of vomiting, rectal or topical routes are advised. For difficulties with swallowing, liquid or rectal preparations are suggested. Few people with AIDS require injected opiates if the appropriate analgesics are prescribed in adequate doses via the most suitable route. However, skin patches releasing fentanyl, designed to last up to 72 hours, are a convenient way to administer topical pain relief.

Other interventions include general comfort measures, radiation or chemotherapy, nerve blocks, and complementary therapy believed by some to offer relief, such as aromatherapy, therapeutic touch, and relaxation and imagery techniques. Massage, acupuncture, physical therapy, heat, ice, music, and topical mentholated products may also provide additional comfort.

pain threshold   The extent of neurological or emotional stimulation required to produce the sensation of pain.

paleopathology   The study of diseases in ancient remains of bodies and fossils.

palinavir   A protease inhibitor introduced in 1995, characterized as having excellent antiviral activity, good bioavailability, and an acceptable safety profile in animals. Palinavir has some of the same problems as other PROTEASE INHIBITORS in development: It is a complex molecule and will probably be difficult to manufacture. It also binds to alpha acid glycoprotein, the naturally occurring blood protein that was found in 1994 to bind to and inactivate another protease inhibitor. Unlike that compound, however, plasma levels of the drug should still be high enough to suppress HIV—assuming that palinavir is absorbed well by the intestines. HIV does become resistant to the compound in lab cultures. One mutation occurs that makes the virus slightly less susceptible to pali-navir, but a second mutation is required to develop substantial resistance. One of these mutations is unique to palinavir while the other is also seen in lab cultures treated with the drug AG1343. The mutant virus is not cross-resistant with saquinavir, but there does appear to be some decreased susceptibility to the Merck protease inhibitor.

palliative   Offering comfort or relief of symptoms without ameliorating the underlying disease process; also a treatment or device that has such an effect.

pancreas   A compound acinotubular gland situated behind the stomach in front of the first and second lumbar vertebrae in a horizontal position, with its head attached to the duodenum and its tail reaching to the spleen. The pancreas produces both an external and an internal secretion. The external secretion, called pancreatic juice, passes through the pancreatic ducts into the duodenum, where it plays an important role in the digestion of all classes of foods. The internal secretion, elaborated by the beta cells of the islets of Langerhans, includes the HORMONES insulin and glucagon secreted by the alpha cells. These hormones, in conjunction with hormones from other endocrine glands, play a primary role in the regulation of carbohydrate metabolism.

pancreatic enzyme   One type of pancreas-produced protein that aids digestion of fats, carbohydrates, and proteins.

pancreatitis   Inflamed condition of the pancreas. An occasional side effect of ddI, pancreatitis can result in severe abdominal pain and death. Its onset can be predicted by rises in blood levels of the pancreatic enzyme AMYLASE.

pandemic   An epidemic over a wide geographic area, usually worldwide, affecting large numbers of people at the same time.

Pap smear   See PAPANICOLAOU (PAP) SMEAR.

Pap smear screening   The need for rigorous surveillance in HIV infection has given rise to the argument for routine Pap smear screening in HIV-positive women. At the time of screening, it is equally important to examine the vulva and vagina, culture the cervix for STDS (gonorrhea and chlamydia), and diagnose and treat any vaginitis present, including atrophic vaginitis. Management strategies also include liberal referrals for colposcopic evaluation, particularly for vulvar and vaginal lesions that cannot be definitively diagnosed, so that colposcopically directed biopsies can be obtained.

Most clinicians feel that Pap smear screening should be performed every six months for the majority of HIV-positive women. It is equally important to utilize a cytology laboratory that is consistently accurate and that uses the 1988 Bethesda system for reporting. Using this system, all Pap smears with recurrent atypias, CERVICAL INTRAEPITHELIAL NEOPLASIAs of all grades, and carcinoma-in-situs should be referred for colposcopic evaluation within six weeks. See also PAPANICOLAOU (PAP) SMEAR.

Pap test   See PAPANICOLAOU (PAP) SMEAR.

Papanicolaou (Pap) smear   A test for detecting cancer in women in its early stages. It is a standard component of routine gynecological examinations. It involves removal of a smear of loose cells from the surface of the cervix and examining them under a microscope. Cells are graded from class I (no abnormalities) to class V (cancer cells observed). The Pap test usually does not detect uterine lining cancer (endometrial cancer). The accuracy of Pap smears, long considered the standard method for detecting abnormalities that might develop into cervical cancer, has been called into question, particularly in the case of women with HIV. Studies have shown that Pap smear screening does not always uncover cytological abnormalities that were evident from colposcopically directed biopsies obtained at the same time. Moreover, HIV-positive women frequently have lower genital tract infections that may obscure Pap results.

HIV-positive women are found to have approximately a tenfold increase in abnormal cervical cytology. Abnormal findings include inflammatory changes, vaginal pathogens, cellular atypia, CERVICAL INTRAEPITHELIAL NEOPLASIA (CIN) of all grades, and cervical cancer. The severity of the abnormality is believed to correlate with the degree of immunosuppression. The entire lower tract may be affected and at risk of development of squamous cell cancers. In immunocompromised women, this type of disease tends to persist, recur, and extend, even with conventional treatment. It is accepted that the vast majority of squamous cell abnormalities in the genital tract are associated with HUMAN PAPILLOMA VIRUS INFECTION (HPV) and specifically with particular strains of HPV. It is also known that immunocompromise accelerates the progress from viral infection to neoplasias in both renal transplant patients (on immunosuppressive therapy) and in HIV-positive women with lowered CD4 counts.

Risa Denenberg, a family nurse practitioner in the AIDS Clinic at New York's Bronx Lebanon Hospital cautions that the accuracy of Pap smears can vary greatly from one clinical setting to another. She advises that patients and clinicians remember the following: The best smears are obtained mid-cycle; smears taken during a period or when bleeding for any other reason are unacceptable; patients should not douche, use tampons, or have sexual intercourse for 48 hours before a Pap smear; Pap smears require two tissue samples; lubricants interfere with obtaining proper tissue samples; as a preservative measure, it is necessary to apply fixative within ten seconds after spreading samples on microscope slides; proper labeling of slides is the clinician's responsibility; and patients and clinicians should only accept Pap smear results from a lab that uses the standardized Bethesda system to report results.

papillary tumor   A neoplasm composed of or resembling enlarged papillae.

papilloma   An EPITHELIAL tumor of skin or mucous membrane consisting of hypertrophied papillae covered by a layer of epithelium. Papillomas are often found in the genital area. Included in this group are warts, condylomas, and polyps. Most are caused by a strain of the HUMAN PAPILLOMA VIRUS (HPV). There are more than 40 types of HPV infections. Certain viral strains predispose women to and indeed probably cause cervical, vaginal, and vulval cancer. Women known to have HPV infections need to be monitored carefully with PAP SMEARS and at times COLPOSCOPY and BIOPSY. Cryosurgery or laser surgery may be necessary if precancerous changes occur. Male partners of women with HPV infections should be evaluated by a physician familiar with this problem, as HPV infections can be invisible to the naked eye and require special staining techniques and/or colposcopy to evaluate.

papillomavirus   A virus that causes papillomas or warts in humans and animals. Papillomaviruses belong to the papovavirus family or group.

papovavirus   One of a group of viruses important in viral carcinogenesis. Included are polyoma virus, simian virus 40, and papillomaviruses.

papule   A red elevated area on the skin, solid and circumscribed. Papules often precede vesicular or pustular formation and may appear in erythema multiforme, eczema papulosum, prurigo, syphilis, measles, and smallpox. They may develop after use of bromides, iodides, or coal tar preparation.

paracrine   Effects of a HORMONE that are only local.

parallel track   A FOOD AND DRUG ADMINISTRATION–approved program to allow patients who are not in trials, but who meet certain criteria, to take an experimental drug. In the program, doctors monitor patients' response and report data to the pharmaceutical company sponsoring the drug and the program.

paralysis   Temporary or permanent loss of function, especially loss of sensation or voluntary motion. Paralyses are divided into two groups: spastic, when due to lesion of upper motor neuron, and flaccid, when due to lesion of lower motor neuron.

Temporary paralysis can also result from a psychological disorder. Psychic inhibition of motor function occurs most characteristically in hysteria. Evidence of organic disease is always lacking in hysterical paralysis.

parasite   An organism whose survival depends on food from a host organism. A parasite does not necessarily cause disease.

parenteral   Introduced into the body by a route other than through the GASTROINTESTINAL TRACT; the term usually refers to intravenous or intramuscular administration of substances such as therapeutic drugs or nutritive solutions. See PARENTERAL NUTRITION; CATHETER.

parenteral nutrition   The INTRAVENOUS administration of liquid nutrients to patients who are unable to eat or to absorb nutrients normally. It is most often used for patients suffering moderate to severe WASTING associated with cancer or HIV/AIDS. The nutrient solution generally contains protein, carbohydrates, vitamins, minerals, and electrolytes, with the formula adjusted for individual patient's needs. An infusion pump is generally required; infusions can take from

12 to 14 hours a day. No definitive studies have been published on the side effects of parenteral nutrition.

PARTIAL PARENTERAL NUTRITION (PPN) may be used in combination with solid food to treat moderate wasting. TOTAL PARENTERAL NUTRITION (TPN) is used in cases of severe wasting, to provide patient's entire nutritional needs. In addition to the nutrient mix described above, TPN also supplies essential fats.

Studies indicate that patients receiving TPN gain significant amounts of body cell mass and weight if they are free of systemic infections. Other studies have shown that administering TPN during secondary infection can increase weight gain and improve quality of life by improving the ability to fight infection. TPN has also been shown to have favorable effects on immune cell responsiveness.

In a home care environment, TPN is expensive. It is usually used to support someone through a limited period of acute illness but may be required for more lengthy periods.

Adequate and balanced nutrition is the key to maintaining lean body mass in people with HIV. Vitamins and nutrient supplements may be appropriate at all stages of HIV disease. Opportunistic infections of the intestines should be treated aggressively to prevent malabsorption. Appetite stimulants such as megestrol or dronabinol may be appropriate to treat symptomatic loss of appetite. Wasting may also be treated with hormone therapy or cytokine manipulation, both experimental procedures.

paresthesia   Abnormal sensations such as burning or tingling. Paresthesia may constitute the first symptoms of PERIPHERAL NEUROPATHY, or it may be a limited drug side effect that does not worsen with time.

paromomycin sulfate   An antibiotic used in treating intestinal AMEBIASIS and various tapeworms, CRYPTOSPORIDIOSIS in particular. (It should be noted that there is no standard treatment for cryptosporidiosis.) It is not effective against extraintestinal infections with amoebae. Paromomycin is an antibiotic of the aminoglycoside class, similar in action to neomycin, streptomycin, erythromycin, and others. It is poorly absorbed into the bloodstream, so high concentrations stay in the gut where many parasites that cause diarrhea multiply. Paromomycin is available in tablet form. Paromomycin generally causes few side effects, but among possible side effects are nausea, abdominal cramps, and diarrhea. Trade name is Humatin. Other names are Aminosidine; AMS.

parotitis   Inflammation of the parotid gland.

paroxetine   An antidepressant of the class known as serotonin reuptake inhibitors. It is primarily used for the treatment of depression but is also used for obsessive-compulsive disorder. It has become widely used because it is effective and tends to have fewer side effects than older antidepressants. It is available in tablets. Paxil is the trade name.

paroxysm   A sudden, periodic attack or recurrence of symptoms of a disease; a sudden spasm or convulsion of any kind. It also pertains to a sudden emotional state, as fear, grief, or joy.

Part A   See MEDICARE.

Part B   See MEDICARE.

partial parenteral nutrition   See PARENTERAL NUTRITION.

partialism   Erotic responsiveness to a part of the body, for example a foot partialism.

partner negotiation   Negotiation of the terms of a sexual encounter; the primary strategy for living by safe-sex guidelines. The first step is becoming clear in one's own mind about what one is and is not willing to do, would like to do, or might be talked into doing. The second step is negotiating an agreement about it with one's partner. Negotiation involves finding out about the partner's background and other sexual relationships, past and present. It involves finding out whether he or she is easy to talk to, comfortable discussing sexual details, flexible in his or her sexual habits, caring, imaginative, and creative.

Negotiating safer sex may not be easy for many reasons. Many people don't like to change their habits. Others may assume that safer sex will be too complicated, not worth the effort, unromantic, a poor substitute for the real thing, or a compromise. Still others may be embarrassed to do some of the things that are safe. Buying condoms or spermicides may be uncomfortable for some persons. Often, individuals don't know how to bring up the subject with someone they've just met. Others may fear they will offend or lose their partners by suggesting safer sex. Some persons resent all the advance planning required by safer sex, and just want to follow their feelings. Today, books about sexual management include advice on living by the guidelines and negotiating safer sex.

partner notification   The process of informing sex or needle-sharing partners of an HIV-infected person that they have been or are at risk of contracting HIV. Notification may be done by the HIV-infected person, a HEALTH CARE PROVIDER, or a PUBLIC HEALTH worker.

Partner notification for STDS (including HIV) encompasses two distinct approaches: patient referral and provider referral. All partner notification activities within STD/HIV prevention programs are based on some combination of these. With patient referral, the HIV-infected person is encouraged to inform partners of their risk for infection, so that partners can seek appropriate medical services. Provider referral (previously called CONTACT TRACING) is a voluntary, confidential process in which health professionals obtain partner names and identifying information from an infected person, then notify the partners and help them to seek or obtain appropriate services. Partner notification has been considered an essential component of sexuallly transmitted disease control programs in North America and Europe for more than 40 years.

With no curative therapy for HIV infection, partner notification for HIV control has been controversial. Concerns about the potential for discrimination against patients and identified partners have to be weighed against the rights of exposed individuals to be informed of their risk. Although the development of antiviral treatment and prophylactic antimicrobials has provided clear benefits for the early detection and treatment of HIV infection, thereby reducing opposition to partner outreach, many countries lack the resources to provide these costly therapies and long-term care. The debate worldwide has continued to center on the role partner notification should play in HIV prevention programs relative to other preventive interventions.

The ability of any country to develop a formal HIV partner notification program is influenced by a number of factors, including the organization and strength of services for STD diagnosis and treatment, the epidemiology of HIV infection in that country, the attitude of HEALTH CARE PROFESSIONALS who must carry out partner notification in conjunction with other health care services, and the government structure for setting health policy. In many countries only a small proportion of STD cases—and presumably HIV cases—are seen in STD or other health clinics. Treatment services are often fragmented and delivered by a variety of health care providers with limited skills in provider referral. Clinicians responsible for STD treatment and partner management, in general, have had little support from organized HIV prevention programs and receive no special training for carrying out complex partner notification activities.

See PRIVACY.

passive immunity   Protection against infection achieved in a nonimmune host by introduction of preformed ANTIBODY or immune cells from another person. Passive immunity usually lasts only a short time.

passive immunotherapy (PIT)   Passive immunotherapy for HIV involves the transfer of plasma (the fluid portion of the blood without the cells) from asymptomatic HIV-infected donors with high HIV ANTIBODY levels to individuals with advanced HIV infection or AIDS and low levels of HIV antibodies. The hope is that the HIV antibodies in the transferred plasma will help preserve the recipient's health. PIT's originator and chief promoter, Abraham Karpas, Sc.D., an AIDS researcher at the University of Cambridge in England, published his first paper on PIT in 1988. Challenges facing PIT researchers have included the lack of a well-funded backer, the high cost of the technique, and the difficulty of finding enough eligible plasma donors.

Pasteurella multocida   A small nonmotile GRAM-NEGATIVE coccobacillus that can cause cellulitis, abscesses, osteomyelitis, pneumonia, peritonitis, or meningitis.

pathogen   A disease-causing MICROORGANISM. There are four types of pathogens: bacteria, fungi, protozoa, and viruses.

pathogenesis   The development of morbid conditions or disease; more specifically, the cellular events and reactions and other biological processes occurring in the development of disease.

pathogenic   Productive of disease. See PATHOGENESIS.

pathological   Diseased, or due to a disease; concerning pathology.

pathology   A condition produced by disease; also, the study of the nature and cause of disease.

pathophysiology   The study of how normal physiological processes are altered by disease.

patient   One who receives HEALTH CARE services from a health care practitioner and who gives consent for the practitioner to provide that care.

patient advocate   A person in an institutional setting responsible for meeting the personal and social needs of patients, with a special concern for high quality patient care, and for responding to patient inquiries and concerns about the care given by a practitioner or by a hospital or other health care facility. The patient advocate speaks and acts on behalf of patients, investigates the patients' problems and complaints, and mediates between the patients and the hospital or other health care facility. The patient advocate is also called a PATIENT REPRESENTATIVE or *ombudsperson*.

patient pay   See SPEND DOWN.

patient referral   See PARTNER NOTIFICATION.

patient representative   See PATIENT ADVOCATE.

Patients' Bill of Rights   A HEALTH CARE provider or facility–adopted document that defines the rights of patients or clients. The American Hospital Association House of Delegates approved a document entitled, "Statement of a Patients' Bill of Rights" in 1973. The statement has become a standard for advocacy on behalf of patients' and families' rights. Many hospitals make the Patients' Bill of Rights available to patients through a patient information booklet.

Patients have rights that all medical care organizations and HEALTH CARE providers should honor as a matter of routine. In times of critical medical emergencies, it becomes even more important to ensure patients' rights: to ask questions and to have them answered completely; to have all medical procedures explained completely; to refuse any test, procedure, or medication; to go to another health care provider or get a second opinion; and to be assured of the confidentiality of their medical records and especially their HIV test results.

PCOD   The proximate cause of death, one of two separate designations for the cause of death distinguished by AUTOPSY pathologists. See also ICOD.

PCM-4   PCM-4 is a product combining two components purported to have immunodmodulating effects. The two components are an extract (the polypeptide, or *P*) from the porcine spleen and a highly concentrated form of Siberian ginseng. The oral dosage of these two extracts was developed in 1987. The pill was developed after initial studies done with Siberian ginseng suggested that the combination might be capable of increasing T CELLS. Studies have shown that patients with cancer of the stomach who experienced immune suppression had general improvement with the use of the porcine spleen extract. To date, there are reports of some studies in HIV-infected people being conducted, but these studies are either incomplete or have not been published.

PCM-4 is available at health food stores in drops, tablets, and capsules. No toxicities from PCM-4 have been reported, but it is suggested that the compound not be used by those with high blood pressure.

PCP   See PNEUMOCYSTIS CARINII PNEUMONIA.

PCP prophylaxis   See PNEUMOCYSTIS CARINII PNEUMONIA PROPHYLAXIS.

PCR test   See POLYMERASE CHAIN REACTION TEST.

pediatric AIDS   AIDS in children. The CENTERS FOR DISEASE CONTROL AND PREVENTION (CDC) defines pediatric cases as those occurring in children under 13 years of age.

The original CDC case definition of pediatric AIDS, like the early case definition of AIDS in adults, focused exclusively on some of the most severe consequences of HIV infection. In 1987, public health officials at the CDC, acknowledging the need for a framework that included the entire spectrum of HIV-related disorders in children, published the "Classification System for Human Immunodeficiency Virus (HIV) in Children Under 13 Years of Age" (*Morbidity and Mortality Weekly Report* 36 (1987), 225–230, 235). In children, a Class P-0 includes children under 15 months of age who have antibody to HIV—indicating that their mothers are infected with the virus—but who do not meet other criteria for HIV infection.

Class P-1 consists of children who are infected with HIV but who have no symptoms. Subclass A represents children with normal immune function; Subclass B, children with abnormal immune function; and Subclass C, children with immune function not tested.

Class P-2 includes all children with clinical disorders associated with HIV infection. It encompasses both AIDS cases and cases that previously would have been grouped under the nonspecific heading "AIDS-related complex." Subclass A represents children with nonspecific findings; B, children with progressive neurologic disease; C, children with lymphoid interstitial pneumonia; D, children with secondary cancers; and F, those with other diseases possibly due to HIV infection. (For the equivalents of these classifications for adults, see GROUPS I–IV.)

peer review organization (PRO)   A nonprofit organization, usually an arm of a state medical society, which reviews appropriateness of care and length of stay under MEDICAID and MEDICARE.

peliosis hepatis   The presence of blood-filled lakes in the body of the liver. The condition may be associated with use of ORAL CONTRACEPTIVES or ANABOLIC STEROIDS. It has also been reported in patients with HUMAN IMMUNODEFICIENCY VIRUS infection.

pelvic examination   Physical examination of the VAGINA and adjacent organs by palpation. One hand is placed intravaginally and the other on the abdominal wall, and tissues between the fingers of the two hands are palpated. This is called a bimanual examination. Visual examination of the vagina and CERVIX is made with the use of a speculum inserted intravaginally.

pelvic infection   Any infection involving any of the pelvic structures (endometrium, ovaries, tubes) or extending beyond the peritoneum, as in the perihepatitis known as FITZ-HUGH–CURTIS SYNDROME. There may be an acute initial episode following infection by a sexually transmitted pathogen, most commonly GONORRHEA or CHLAMYDIA, less frequently a MYCOPLASMA. Later it may become a chronic and recurrent syndrome. When sexually transmitted PATHOGENs ascend from the vagina into the upper pelvic organs, the resulting infection is generally polymicrobial in nature. At this point, cervical and vaginal cultures are not useful in determining therapy. Often the outcome of a pelvic infection, or PELVIC INFLAMMATORY DISEASE, is recurrent infections, tubal infertility, formation of tubo-ovarian abscesses, and chronic pelvic pain syndrome.

pelvic inflammatory disease (PID)   Any serious inflammatory disorder of the upper genital tract in women. PID is difficult to diagnose and has not received much attention in the United States. PID takes different courses in different women, but can cause abscesses and constant, severe pain almost anywhere in the genital tract. PID may include endometritis, salpingitis, tubo-ovarian abscess, and pelvic peritonitis. Sexually transmitted organisms may also cause PID. Clinically, physicians report that PID seems to occur more frequently in HIV-infected women than in those who are HIV-negative, and is often more severe, requiring longer hospitalizations and more frequent surgery for treatment of abscesses.

A woman's pelvic region, including the cervix, uterus, fallopian tubes, abdominal cavity, and ovaries, may be infected by a SEXUALLY TRANSMITTED DISEASE such as GONORRHEA. The infection may spread more rapidly if an INTRAUTERINE DEVICE (IUD) is used. The condition may lead to infertility and cause such symptoms as low abdominal pain, pelvic tenderness upon palpation, cervical manipulation tenderness, adnexal tenderness or suspicion of pelvic mass, nausea, fever, and irregular menstrual cycles. These are usually accompanied by temperature above 100.5°F, elevated white blood count, elevated erythrocyte sedimentation rate, positive gram stain, wet mount loaded with white blood cells, mucopurulent cervicitis, positive culture for gonorrhea or CHLAMYDIA or pelvic mass. In persons who are immunocompromised due to HIV infection, bacterial infections are often recurrent, chronic, and extensive. In these cases PID may fail to yield the usual signs. Failure to mount an immune response may cause the inflammation and pain by which a diagnosis may be made.

PID diagnosis can most easily be made by examining the abdomen with a laparoscope. Because there exists no suitable diagnostic test and LAPAROSCOPY is not always available, a diagnosis of PID is often based on imprecise clinical findings and culture or ANTIGEN detection tests of specimens of the lower genital tract. Detection of PID in HIV-infected women may be extremely difficult. In some, particularly those infected with HIV, there may be resistance to therapy. Pelvic inflammatory disease is one of the gynecological problems Social Security Disability Determination Service specialists consider when assessing the degree to which disease affects a woman's ability to function.

Consideration is usually given to hospitalization of HIV-positive women with clinical evidence of PID. Some considerations that favor immediate hospitalization are suspicion of tubo-ovarian abscesses, suspicion of ectopic pregnancy, upper peritoneal signs, uncertain diagnosis with signs of acute abdomen, inability to tolerate or comply with outpatient regimen, and failure to improve within 48 hours on oral antibiotics and bed rest.

The outpatient regimen for oral antibiotics in PID recommended by the CENTERS FOR DISEASE CONTROL AND PREVENTION is the same as in the treatment for chlamydia. Bed rest and abstention from sexual activity are also part of the standard treatment regimen. Failure to improve in 48 to 72 hours is an indication for immediate hospitalization and for IV antibiotics. Many experts recommend that all patients with PID be treated with PARENTERAL ANTIBIOTICS.

Since most PID is caused by sexually transmitted diseases that are not detected, it is important for all women to have regular gynecological exams and PAP SMEARS. HIV-positive women should get Pap smears every six months.

pelvic mass   Routine pelvic examination will occasionally find a pelvic mass with or without significant symptomatology. Further examination is necessary to identify it; possibilities include an ovarian cyst, pelvic inflammatory disease, a tubo-ovarian abscess, fibroid tumor, normal or ECTOPIC PREGNANCY, malignant tumor, genital tuberculosis, and lymphoma.

The initial workup is intended to rule out pregnancy. A thorough history and careful pelvic exam will help to focus the remainder of the workup in the appropriate direction. It is logical to obtain a pelvic sonogram, if it can be done promptly. A diagnosis must be definitive and may require exploratory surgery.

penicillin   One of a group of antibiotics biosynthesized by several species of molds. Penicillin is antibacterial, inhibiting the growth of most GRAM-POSITIVE BACTERIA and certain GRAM-NEGATIVE forms. It is also effective against certain molds, spirochetes, and rickettsiae. It is also used to treat SYPHILIS. There are many different penicillins, including synthetic ones, and their effectiveness varies for different organisms.

Penicillin was one of the first antibiotics to be discovered and used. It interferes with a bacterium's ability to build cell walls, thus preventing it from multiplying. Penicillin is available in tablet form and solutions for oral and INTRAVENOUS administration. The most common reactions to penicillin include nausea, vomiting, stomach upset, diarrhea, and black, hairy tongue. Allergic skin reactions and anaphylactic shock occur less frequently. Trade names include Bicillin, Wycillin, Ledercillin, Pen-Vee, and Veetids.

Penicillium   A genus of molds belonging to the class Ascomycetes. These are the blue molds that grow on fruit, bread, and cheese. A number of species are sources of penicillin. Occasionally in humans they produce infections of the external ear, skin, or respiratory passageways. They are common allergens.

penis   A male's external sex organ. It contains the urethra, the tube through which urine and semen flow. Slang terms include cock, dick, joint, joy stick, prick, and rod.

peno-vaginal intercourse   Sexual activity with the penis inside the vagina; COITUS.

pension   A generic term for any public or employer retirement or disability income benefit.

pentamidine   An antiprotozoal agent; used to treat or prevent PNEUMOCYSTIS CARINII PNEUMONIA (PCP). It can be administered INTRAVENOUSLY or delivered directly into the lungs as an aerosol, using a breathing machine. Common side effects of intravenous pentamidine are low blood pressure, low blood sugar, high blood sugar, kidney failure, liver disease, low blood counts, or inflammation of the pancreas. Because it doesn't go directly into the bloodstream, aerosol, or nebulized, pentamidine rarely causes severe side effects (the most frequent are coughing and tightening of the chest that interferes with breathing). Fatigue, metallic taste in the mouth, decreased appetite, dizziness, rashes, nausea, irritation of mouth or nasal cavities, congestion, night sweats, chills, and vomiting also occur. It does not, however, affect PCP in parts of the body other than the lungs, so intravenous treatment is usually preferred for advanced PCP infections. Generally it is felt that pentamidine should be dispensed with caution if given with other drugs that can damage the kidneys. In addition, other substances that cause pancreatic damage, such as alcohol, ddI, and RIFAMPIN, may be dangerous if taken concurrently with pentamidine. Trade names include NebuPent, Pentam, and Pentacarinat.

pentoxifylline   A blood flow agent, xanthine, that reduces levels of TUMOR NECROSIS FACTOR (TNF). Pentoxifylline is a FOOD AND DRUG ADMINISTRATION–approved treatment for a circulation disorder called intermittent claudication, caused by a narrowing of the arteries. For this condition it is essentially used to thin the blood. Pentoxifylline has had variable results in AIDS patients in attempting to halt weight loss which may be caused by tumor necrosis factor. The drug once was thought to hold promise for HIV-infected people but trial data have shown otherwise. Possible side effects include nausea and other digestive upset, dizziness, and headache. Brand name is Trental.

people living with aids (PLWA)   At the October 1987 March on Washington for Lesbian and Gay Rights, persons with AIDS from all over the United States took the naming of their condition one step further, announcing that they are "people living with AIDS." As with "PEOPLE WITH AIDS," the insistence here upon naming as a key to identity, though partially aimed at the press, the public, the government, and the medical profession, is primarily an act of self-acclaim.

People With Aids   The People With AIDS movement started from support and counseling networks and has had a complex and often turbulent relationship with the mainstream AIDS organizations. In the early 1980s, new political perspectives developed; people with the AIDS virus began to acknowledge that they could use insights gained from their personal struggles with AIDS to contribute to the larger political battle against the disease. Groups exclusively containing people infected with the virus, developed in New York, San Francisco, and other cities. At the 1983 AIDS Forum in Denver, some of these groups consolidated under the name People With AIDS (a name attributed to Mark Feldman) and together claimed the right to be included in the leadership of all AIDS organizations. The following year, an attempt was made to establish a national association of people with AIDS with its own hot line and newsletter, the latter of which began appearing in June 1985.

"People" With AIDS remind us that they are more than "victims" or "patients" with AIDS. Primarily as an act of self-acclaim, the naming demonstrates how they should be viewed by others:

> We do not see ourselves as victims. We will not be victimized. We have the right to be treated with respect, dignity, compassion, and understanding. We have the right to live fulfilling, productive lives—to live and die with dignity and compassion . . . We are born of and inextricably bound to the historical struggle for rights—civil, feminist, disability, lesbian and gay, and human. We will not be denied our rights!
>
> (National Association of People with AIDS, "Statement of Purpose," September 1986)

In several cities People With AIDS has been a key organization in the AIDS movement and has been involved in supportive, educational and lobbying work. Since 1983, members of People With AIDS have been prominent figures in Gay Pride marches across the country, often including many members who march with great physical and emotional pain and difficulty. The expertise of those who have experienced the disease offers a new perspective to our understanding of AIDS not usually discussed by academic science and medicine.

Today, People With AIDS furnishes a broad variety of support services to the rising numbers of AIDS sufferers, and continues to campaign for the acceleration of availability of experimental drug therapies.

People With AIDS Coalition (PWA)   Founded in 1985, this New York City–based nonmembership organization provides local support networks for persons afflicted with AIDS. Programs include: public forums, a drop-in lounge, liaisons with social service agencies, a meal program, and an apartment referral service. PWA also operates a speakers' bureau and maintains a library.

peptide   One of a class of amino acids compounds. Because some peptides function as the active portions of many HORMONES, growth factors, and neurotransmitters, they play important roles in digestion, immunity, and emotion. These peptide components interact with key cells in the responsive organs by means of receptor molecules located on the cells' surfaces.

peptide T   A synthetic amino acid compound created in 1986 at the National Institute of Mental Health (NIMH). It was one of the first drugs to be designed specifically as an AIDS therapy. The drug's developers suggest that peptide T can slow or reverse the neurological and cognitive effects of HIV, including AIDS dementia, fatigue, and pain, although an NIMH study shows no such benefit.

Peptide T is designed to mimic the attachment sequence in GP120, the protein on the outer surface of the HIV virus, to CD4 receptor sites, taking its place and preventing HIV from interfering with brain function. However, the process leading to HIV-associated nerve tissue damage is extremely varied from one individual to another. The inflammatory process that arises in response to the presence of HIV in the brain can disrupt the operation of neurons and their support cells, which form a complex and delicate interactive network. Another important factor is the opening up of the calcium channels on neuron membranes; too much calcium can poison cells. In addition, other HIV proteins, besides gp120, seem to be toxic to cells in neural tissue. Moreover, many researchers suspect that when gp120 links up with the CD4 sites on the immune system's T-HELPER CELLS it leads to a cascade of events fatal to these cells.

Peptide T has been found to reduce levels of TUMOR NECROSIS FACTOR-alpha (TNF-alpha). Release of this CYTO-KINE has been associated with HIV disease progression. Excess TNF-alpha is widely alleged to contribute to WASTING syndrome, increased replication of HIV, immune cell dysfunction, nerve cell damage, and death. Peptide T is very similar to the active section of vasoactive intestinal peptide (VIP), a naturally occurring regulator of digestion that may have growth-promoting functions in the CENTRAL NERVOUS SYSTEM. VIP seems to interact with the CD4 immune system cells, too, leading some researchers to suggest that peptide T can supplement VIP in promoting general mental and physical health.

Despite the lack of clinical evidence for action against the neurological and cognitive damage caused by HIV/AIDS, peptide T is one of the top sellers of the AIDS underground. Its status is fueled by widespread anecdotal accounts of increases in quality-of-life variables and relief from AIDS dementia, cognitive impairment, and the pain of PERIPHERAL NEUROPATHY.

Reported side effects of peptide T have been relatively minor. Potentially troubling side effects include hormonal and emotional changes.

percutaneous   Through the skin. The term refers to the application of a medicated ointment by friction, or the removal or injection of a fluid by needle.

pericarditis   Inflammation of the pericardium.

pericardium   The double membraned fibroserous sac enclosing the heart and the origins of the great blood vessels. It is composed of an inner serous layer and an outer fibrous layer. The space between the two constitute the pericardial cavity, which is normally filled with a small amount of serous fluid.

perinatal   Near the time of birth, and specifically the period beginning after the 28th week of pregnancy through the 28 days following birth.

perinatal transmission   See TRANSMISSION.

period   See MENSTRUATION.

periodontal disease   Disease of supporting structures of the teeth, the periodontium, including the alveolar bone to which the teeth are anchored. The most common symptom is bleeding gums, but loosening of the teeth, receding gums and teeth, and necrotizing ulcerative gingivitis may be present as the process continues. Proper dental hygiene will help to prevent periodontal disease.

In the early stages of the disease, curettage of the irritating material from the crown and root surfaces of the teeth may be the only treatment required. In more advanced stages, procedures such as gingivectomy, gingivoplasty, and correction of the bony architecture of the teeth may be required. Adjustment of the occlusion of the teeth and orthodontic treatment may be used in order to prevent recurrences.

peripheral lymphoid organs   Those lymphoid organs not essential to the development of immune responses, such as the SPLEEN, LYMPH NODES, tonsils, and PEYER'S PATCHES.

peripheral nervous system   That portion of the nervous system outside the CENTRAL NERVOUS SYSTEM. Included are the 12 pairs of cranial nerves, 31 pairs of spinal nerves, and their branches to the entire body. Also included are the sensory nerves, the sympathetic and the parasympathetic nerves.

peripheral neuropathy   Any functional disturbance and/or change in the PERIPHERAL NERVOUS SYSTEM, characterized by sensory loss, pain, muscle weakness, and wasting of muscle in the hands, legs, or feet. It may start with burning or tingling sensation or numbness in the toes and fingers. In severe cases, paralysis may result. Peripheral neuropathy may arise from an HIV-related condition or as a side effect of certain drugs, some of the NUCLEOSIDE ANALOGS in particular. Two types of peripheral neuropathy are most common to HIV infection: inflammatory demyelinating polyneuropathy (IDP), which arises in the early stages of infection, and sensory axonal polyneuropathy, a late-stage complication.

IDP morbidity stems from the progressive breakdown of the fatty envelope around the neurons—the myelin sheet—which impairs conduction of signals to and from the brain. In most cases, this complication appears even before susceptibility to opportunistic PATHOGENS and is thought to be an autoimmune disease. Patients experience mild sensory problems, decreased clinical reflexes, and chronic progressive weakness, similar to Guillain-Barré syndrome in HIV-negative patients. Symptoms can be managed with CORTICOSTEROIDS.

The major symptom of sensory axonal polyneuropathy is painful tingling or burning sensations. AZT is ineffective in treating this; tricyclic antidepressants have been found useful, particularly low-dose AMITRIPTYLINE. Brief bursts of pain can be treated with the anticonvulsants phenytoin or carbamazepine. Topical capsaicin has also been tried. ACUPUNCTURE is now under evaluation, alone or in combination with amitriptyline.

peritoneal cavity   A space between layers of the parietal and visceral peritoneum, containing a small amount of fluid. The fluid minimizes friction as the viscera move against each other or the wall of the abdominal cavity.

peritoneal dialysis   Dialysis (passing solute through a membrane) in which the lining of the peritoneal cavity is used as the dialysis membrane. Dialyzing fluid introduced into the peritoneal cavity is allowed to remain there for one or two hours and is then removed. The procedure may be repeated as often as indicated. The use of strictly sterile instruments helps prevent the development of peritonitis. Three related types of dialysis are intermittent peritoneal dialysis (performed using automated equipment), continuous cyclic peritoneal (treatments are performed every night with fluid remaining in the cavity until the next night), and continuous ambulatory peritoneal dialysis (a type of maintenance dialysis that uses an implanted peritoneal catheter).

peritoneum   The thin, strong lining of the abdomen. The serous membrane reflected over the viscera and lining the abdominal cavity.

peritonitis   Inflammation of the peritoneum, the membrane lining the abdominal cavity and investing the viscera.

perleche   A disorder marked by fissures and EPITHELIAL desquamation (shedding of the epidermis) of corners of the mouth, usually seen in children. It may be due to oral CANDIDIASIS or may be a symptom of dietary deficiency, especially of riboflavin.

perphenazine   Used to treat acute and chronic psychotic disorders; may be used as a tranquilizer to help agitated and disruptive behavior in the absence of true psychosis; sometimes used to treat severe nausea and vomiting. By inhibiting dopamine, perphenazine acts to correct an imbalance of nerve impulse transmissions thought to be responsible for mental disorders. Perphenazine belongs to a class of psychoactive drugs called phenothiazines, which have potent effects on the CENTRAL NERVOUS SYSTEM and other organs. They can reduce blood pressure, stop seizures, control nausea and vomiting, and control the symptoms of psychosis. Perphenazine is available as tablets, oral concentrate, and solution for injection. It is also available in a number of combination products with the tricyclic antidepressant AMITRIPTYLINE. Drowsiness, stuffy nose, dizziness, blurred vision, tremors, and constipation are common side effects. Brand names are APO-Perphenazine, PMS-Perphenazine, Elavil Plus, Entrafon, Etrafen, Etrafon-A, Etrafon Forte, Phenazine, PMS-Levazine, PMS-Perphenazine, Triavil, and Trilafon.

Persantine   See DIPYRIDAMOLE.

persistent generalized lymphadenopathy (PGL)   A disorder of the LYMPH GLANDs. PGL is diagnosed when the lymph glands are swollen for at least a month at two different sites, not counting the groin area, and in the absence of any current illness or drug use known to cause such symptoms. PGL often occurs early in HIV infection and is generally of little consequence.

person living with AIDS (PLWA)   See PEOPLE LIVING WITH AIDS.

person with AIDS (PWA)   See PEOPLE WITH AIDS.

person with AIDS-related complex (PWARC)   An individual exhibiting signs and symptoms indicative of the AIDS-RELATED COMPLEX (e.g., fever, persistent generalized LYMPHADENOPATHY, and weight loss accompanied by the presence of HUMAN IMMUNODEFICIENCY VIRUS antibodies). It is noted that AIDS-related complex was originally used in cases of HIV-infected individuals not diagnosed with AIDS but with compromised immune systems and decreased T-CELL counts. The term is now widely considered to be obsolete. Similarly, the term *person with AIDS–related complex* is also now widely considered to be obsolete. See also AIDS-RELATED COMPLEX.

personal care service   Assistance with activities of daily living, such as dressing, walking, getting up and down, preparing food, eating, and taking medication.

personal needs allowance   The amount long-term hospital patients and nursing home and board care residents are permitted to retain for "spending money," with the balance of their incomes applied to the cost of care; the monthly and SSI benefit paid to institutionalized MEDICAID patients with no other income.

PET   See POSITRON EMISSION TOMOGRAPHY.

petting   Sexual activity including fondling, hugging, kissing, and mutual masturbation, but not COITUS.

Peyer's patches   Collections of lymphoid tissue in the submucosa (the layer of connective tissue below the mucosa) of the small intestine that contain LYMPHOCYTEs, plasma cells' germinal centers, and T-cell–dependent areas.

PGL   See PERSISTENT GENERALIZED LYMPHADENOPATHY.

pH   A formula for measuring acidity and alkalinity, expressed as a number on the pH scale. This measurement is a diagnostic tool used on vaginal discharges.

phagocyte   A cell in blood or tissue that binds to, engulfs, and destroys MICROORGANISMs, damaged cells, and foreign particles.

phagocytosis   The process by which PHAGOCYTEs engulf material and enclose it within a vacuole (phagosome) in the cytoplasm.

phallus   The PENIS.

pharmaceutical industry   The drug industry.

pharmacokinetics   The actions of drugs within the body during absorption, distribution, metabolism, and elimination; the study of such actions.

pharmacology   The branch of medical science that deals with the study of the action of drugs on living systems.

pharyngeal gonorrhea   GONORRHEA in the throat.

phase I   See CLINICAL TRIAL.

phase II   See CLINICAL TRIAL.

phase III   See CLINICAL TRIAL.

phenindamine   An antihistamine used to temporarily relieve runny nose, sneezing, itching of the nose or throat, and itchy, watery eyes due to hay fever or other upper respiratory allergies. In people with HIV, the drug is also used to reduce certain drug-induced allergic side effects, including skin rashes, swelling, hives, and breathing difficulties. Drowsiness is the most common side effect; less often, dry mouth, nervousness, insomnia, and increased irritability or excitement may occur. Available over the counter in tablets under the trade name Nolahist.

phone zap   A technique used by AIDS activists and others to bring pressure on a corporation, organization, or government agency to take a certain action. It consists of a systematic mass campaign of telephone calls to the selected target over a period of time.

phosphorylation   The addition of a phosphate group (phosphorous plus four oxygen atoms) to an organic molecule.

photopheresis   A process by which a light-sensitive drug called psoralen is used to treat various autoimmune diseases. The drug is injected into the body; after an interval blood containing psoralen is removed from the body and exposed to ultraviolet light, thus activating the drug in white blood cells. Finally, the blood is returned to the body by reinfusion. The whole procedure is usually performed on two consecutive days at monthly intervals and takes about four hours per session. Photopheresis is an approved therapy for a skin cancer called cutaneous T-CELL LYMPHOMA. In the test tube, it has been shown to work to inhibit viruses that involve RNA and DNA including HIV.

photosensitivity   Heightened skin response to sunlight or ultraviolet light (rapid burning when exposed to the sun).

PHS   See PUBLIC HEALTH SERVICE.

physical dependence   See ADDICTION.

physician-assisted suicide   The question of whether physicians should be allowed actively to assist competent, terminally ill patients who wish to end their intolerable suffering is currently the subject of widespread debate. (This is a separate question from that of merely forgoing or withholding treatment, which is legal in some circumstances.) Although the activities of Dr. Jack Kevorkian have dominated public discussion, the issue is by no means limited to his highly controversial methods. Those who favor the practice argue that the obligation to relieve suffering and to respect patients' wishes for their own treatment makes it ethical. Those who oppose it feel that it is never right for a physician to cause or bring about a death. To date, none of Dr. Kevorkian's cases has involved an AIDS patient, but several studies have shown that AIDS patients kill themselves at a much higher rate than people with other serious diseases. See also SUICIDE.

physiological leukorrhea   A normal but persistent whitish vaginal discharge that is not a symptom of infection. Usually white or yellow mucous discharge from the cervical canal or the vagina. It may constantly be present but somewhat increased preceding and following menstruation, and during sexual excitement. Leukorrhea may be abnormal if it is increased in amount, has a change of color, is malodorous, or contains blood.

PI   See PRINCIPAL INVESTIGATOR.

PICC line   See CATHETER.

PID   See PELVIC INFLAMMATORY DISEASE.

piercing   The practice of placing rings or bars through the body for adornment and/or sexual excitement. Since the needle(s) used for piercing do come into contact with blood, it is possible to become infected with HIV if the needle(s) was (were) previously used on an HIV-infected person and not properly cleaned or sterilized.

pinocytosis   The process by which cells absorb or ingest nutrients and fluid. A hollowed-out portion of the cell membrane is filled with liquid, and the area closes to form a small sac or vacuole. The nutrient, now inside, is available for use in the cell's metabolism.

piss   Slang for URINE.

Pitresin   See VASOPRESSIN.

placebo   A pharmacologically inactive substance designed to look like and taste like a new drug. It is often used in studies as a control with which to measure clinical responses to pharmacologically active substance. Also called "sugar pills."

placebo-controlled study/trial   See CLINICAL TRIAL.

placebo effect   A positive or therapeutic benefit resulting from the administration of a placebo to someone who believes the treatment is real.

placenta   The blood-filled organ that connects the fetus by the umbilical cord to the uterine wall. It is the source of

blood exchange between the mother and the developing fetus during pregnancy.

placenta barrier   A membrane that encloses the embryo. It is a composite of several structures. At the center of the concave side is attached the umbilical cord through which the umbilical vessels pass to the fetus. Maternal blood enters the intervillous spaces of the placenta through spiral arteries, branches of the uterine arteries. It bathes the chorionic villi and flows peripherally to the marginal sinus, which leads to uterine veins. Food substances, oxygen, and antibodies pass into fetal blood of the villi. Metabolic waste products pass from fetal blood into the mother's blood. In general, there is no admixture of fetal and maternal blood.

While it is known that HIV may be transmitted from mother to fetus during pregnancy or from mother to child through childbirth or breast-feeding, at present it is unclear when the TRANSMISSION of HIV to the child occurs. The virus has been isolated from the placenta, the amniotic fluid, and the fetal tissue. Infection may occur prenatally, at delivery, or through breastfeeding. Present research suggests that mother-to-fetus transmission is most likely to occur during the birth process itself, generally through exposure to infected blood and mucus in the birth canal.

plague   Severe, acute, or chronic bacterial infection caused by *Yersinia pestis*. The most common form of plague is bubonic, marked by formation of buboes (inflamed, swollen or enlarged lymph nodes that occur commonly after infective disease due to the absorphan of infective material). Plague characterized by septicemia before the formulation of buboes is known as septicemic. Pneumonic plague is a highly virulent form of plague with extensive involvement of the lungs. In ordinary usage, the term has often referred to any widespread contagious disease associated with a high death rate.

plasma   The liquid part of the lymph and of the blood. In the blood, corpuscles (blood cells) and platelets are suspended in plasma. The plasma consists of serum, protein. and chemical substances in aqueous solution. The aqueous solution also contains solids and dissolved gases, among which are electrolytes; glucose; proteins, including enzymes and hormones; fats, bile pigments, and BILIRUBIN. Plasma serves as the medium for transporting these substances to the body's structures, as well as transporting waste products from them to sites of clearance, that is, the lungs, liver, kidneys, and spleen. Different constituents of plasma have specific functions within the blood. Normal plasma is thin and colorless when free from corpuscles and has a faint yellow tinge when seen in thick layers. See also BLOOD.

plasma cell   A fully differentiated antibody-synthesizing cell that is derived from B lymphocytes.

plasma viremia   Presence of viruses in the plasma (the liquid part of the lymph and of the blood). Currently the most reliable virologic marker to monitor the effect of ANTIRETROVIRAL THERAPY, plasma viremia is a valid indicator of virus replication in the lymphoid organs. Its down regulation may reflect a systemic decrease in virus replication.

plasmacytosis An excess of plasma cells in the blood.

plasmapheresis Removing blood from the body and centrifuging it in order to separate the cellular elements from the plasma. The red cells then are suspended in a physiological solution. They may be reinjected into the donor or injected into a patient who requires red cells rather than whole blood.

Plasmodium A genus of protozoa belonging to subphylum Sporozoa, class Telosporidia. This group includes causative agents of malaria in humans and lower animals.

Plasmodium falciparum The organism that is the causative agent for malignant tertian malaria.

platelet A component of the blood that plays an important part in clotting. Platelets are also involved in immune response, especially in inflammation. Without platelets any wound could result in death by bleeding. The number of platelets is often low in people with HIV infection—sometimes so extremely low that the person is prone to bleeding. The cause of low platelets may be HIV infection itself, or the drugs used to treat it.

PLWA See PERSON LIVING WITH AIDS.

PML See PROGRESSIVE MULTIFOCAL LEUKOENCE-PHALOPATHY.

PMPA One of a class of antiviral compounds (AZT is the most familiar) known as NUCLEOSIDE ANALOGs that inhibit REVERSE TRANSCRIPTASE, an enzyme essential to HIV replication. Unlike other nucleoside analogs, however, PMPA is already activated. Thus it can enter uninfected as well as infected cells and form a reservoir of drug that prearms them against the virus. In contrast, AZT and similar drugs work only in cells that have the machinery to activate the drug. The impetus to develop PMPA came from laboratory and animal model studies showing it to be potentially better tolerated than its parent compound, PMEA.

In recent findings, PMPA was given to 25 macaque monkeys up to a day after they were exposed to SIMIAN IMMUN-ODEFICIENCY VIRUS (SIV) and safely blocked all traces of infection. Although further research is necessary to determine PMPA's potential for human use, the compound will be important for understanding AIDS PATHOGENESIS, at least in the comparative context of SIV. For example, researchers now have the means to study early stages of virus infection in "freeze frame" by stopping the virus life cycle with PMPA.

pneumocandin One of several experimental antifungal drugs currently being tested against fungal infections resistant to standard treatment, a growing problem for people with HIV.

pneumococcal vaccine A vaccine to immunize against the most common cause of bacterial pneumonia in HIV-negative people, the bacterium *Streptococcus pneumoniae* or pneumococcus. Pneumococcus is also a common cause of pneumonia in people with HIV infection. Pneumococcal vaccine is recommended for anyone who is especially prone to frequent or severe infection by pneumococcus. It is best for those with HIV to take this vaccine relatively early in the course of the disease when the immune system is strong.

pneumococcus An oval-shaped, encapsulated, non-spore-forming, GRAM-POSITIVE bacterium occurring usually in pairs having lancet-shaped ends. There are more than 80 serological types of pneumococci. In addition to causing pneumonia, pneumococci are found to cause infections such as bronchitis, conjunctivitis, keratitis, mastoiditis, meningitis, otitis media, and bloodstream infections. A pneumococcal vaccine is available. Pneumococcal infections are effectively treated with PENICILLIN or with erythromycin in a patient allergic to penicillin.

Pneumocystis carinii A protozoan (or possibly a fungus) that infects the lungs causing fever, inflammation, and impaired gas exchange in immuncompromised people.

Pneumocystis carinii pneumonia (PCP) The most common OPPORTUNISTIC INFECTION in untreated HIV-infected patients in the United States. The onset of pneumocystis pneumonia is insidious with early, nonspecific symptoms of fever, fatigue, weight loss, diarrhea, and malaise. Cough, either nonproductive or productive of scant, thin, clear mucous is variable at the onset but becomes more prominent later in disease. Shortness of breath and dyspnea on exertion are suggestive of PCP. In patients receiving pentamidine PROPHYLAXIS, the presentation is often subtle. Other organs may be involved, and disseminated pneumocystis has been seen. Tachypnea, fever, cyanosis (in severe PCP), wheezes, crackles, or rales may be present in PCP. Generally, CD4 counts are <200 in patients with PCP. While not excluding PCP, counts >200 suggest other pathogens. It is important to obtain arterial blood gases in individuals with suspected PCP because the arterial blood gas is often markedly abnormal despite a seemingly comfortable patient. Sputum induction, gallium scan, and bronchoscopy are other means of diagnosis.

Treatment for mild PCP is outpatient oral therapy with TRIMETHOPRIM-SULFAMETHOXAZOLE (TMP-SMX), dapsone, atovaquone, or CLINDAMYCIN. CLINICAL TRIALs have found atovaquone to be associated with more treatment failures and a lower survival rate than TMP-SMX. There is, however, less toxicity with atovaquone compared to TMP-SMX. For moderate to severe disease, hospitalization is recommended for supplemental oxygen, close monitoring, and IV TMP-SMX, pentamidine, or trimetrexate. Several new therapies are under investigation for PCP treatment in patients intolerant of TMP-SMX. These include clindamycin with primaquine as well as atovaquone and eflornithine. Treatment with corticosteroids have been shown to decrease mortality in moderate to severe PCP.

pneumonia An inflammation of the lungs usually associated with infection with a MICROORGANISM. The usual symptoms are cough, fever, and shortness of breath. Pneumonia can be caused by viruses, mycoplasmas, cocci, protozoa, bacilli, chlamydia, fungi, and rickettsiae, as well as by oil aspiration, radiation, chemicals, vegetable dusts, infections associated with silo-filler's disease, and chemical irritants. There are more than 50 potential causes.

pneumonitis   Inflammation of the lung.

polio vaccine   There are two types of vaccine for the prevention of poliomyelitis, live and inactivated. Both immunize against the three types of polio virus. The live vaccine contains live, attenuated polio viruses and is suitable for both children and adults. It is administered orally. The inactivated vaccine contains inactive viruses and is also suitable for children and adults, although it is preferred for adults because of the slightly high risk of vaccine-associated paralysis. It is administered parenterally.

polycillin T   See AMPILLICIN SODIUM.

polyclonal   Derived from different cells. Pertaining to cells or cell products derived from several lines of clones.

polymerase chain reaction (PCR)   A synthetic process that permits making, IN VITRO, unlimited numbers of copies of genes. This is done beginning with a single molecule of genetic material, DNA. One hundred billion similar molecules can be generated within a few hours. The practical importance of this method of investigating genetic material is enormous. The technique can be used in investigating and diagnosing bacterial diseases, viruses associated with cancer, genetic diseases such as diabetes mellitus, pemphigus vulgaris, and various diseases of the muscles and the blood, such as SICKLE-CELL ANEMIA.

polymerase chain reaction test   An extremely sensitive but still experimental test that detects the presence of HIV DNA or RNA in cells and tissue. (DNA and RNA are the gene particles that carry instructions for making more HIV.) The PCR test is able to detect the HIV virus whereas other tests may report false negatives. The test works by amplifying segments of genetic DNA or RNA of known composition with primers in sequential repeated steps. Unlike the standard blood test for HIV infection, which detects antibodies to HIV, the PCR detects HIV itself. The test is very accurate.

The great majority of people who take the standard antibody test for HIV infection need not take the PCR test, which is most useful when the results of the antibody test are ambiguous. It is also useful for early detection of perinatally infected infants and monitoring patients on clinical trials. PCR is similar to a culture for HIV but is substantially less expensive. Neither PCR nor cultures for HIV, however, are available in most laboratories.

polymerase technology   Molecular technology that permits the measurement of total body viral load, including activity in the LYMPH NODEs and MUCOSA, and that has rendered blood measurements such as P24, NEOPTERIN, and CD4 cell counts increasingly useless. See POLYMERASE CHAIN REACTION TEST.

Polymox   See AMOXICILLIN.

polyneuropathy   Any disorder or affliction of the peripheral nerves. The term is usually restricted to disorders of a noninflammatory nature.

polyomavirus   A virus of the papovavirus family that produces malignancies in some animals, but not in humans.

poppers   See ISOBUTYL NITRITE INHALERS.

pornography   Writing or pictures that explicitly depict sexual activity, with the purpose of arousing the reader or viewer sexually.

porphyria   A group of disorders that result from a disturbance in porphyrin metabolism, causing increased formation and excretion of PORPHYRIN or its precursors.

porphyrin   Any of a group of nitrogen-containing organic compounds that occur in protoplasm and form the basis of animal and plant respiratory pigments, obtained from hemoglobin and chlorophyll.

port   See CATHETER.

positive attitude   Attitudes measured or proceeding in a direction assumed as beneficial or progressive. People living with HIV disease frequently attest that the overall attitude a person with HIV takes toward his or her illness makes a difference. They challenge the notion of the person with AIDS as "helpless victim," and stress the importance of persons with AIDS being active participants in their health care.

Michael Callen's book, *Surviving AIDS* (1990), is infused with this attitude. The author presents the stories of fourteen long-term survivors illustrating some of the methods and approaches by which some people are living with and indeed surviving AIDS. "Anything is possible. Miracles happen. It's as reasonable to believe that you'll be lucky as it is to believe you are doomed. The worst thing that might happen is that you'll fail. But then again, you may live just long enough to be around for the cure that community-based research is going to find. Stick around for the celebration. It's gonna be some party." (*Surviving AIDS*, p. 201.) See also POSITIVE THINKING.

positive thinking   Negativity and fear were rampant in the beginning of the AIDS epidemic. Today, the new facts about AIDS inspire optimism, not fear, and positive thinking has, for the most, supplanted negativity and fear. A disease once viewed as an automatic death warrant is now in the process of becoming a chronic, potentially long-term treatable illness. Today we know that not everyone who is exposed to HIV becomes infected. We know too that not everyone who is infected with HIV gets AIDS. And, we know that not everyone with AIDS dies from it. Components of positive thinking include having a positive attitude about survival, and feeling one is in charge of one's medical care and the medical knowledge surrounding that health care. Similar to positive attitude, positive thinking has been shown to have a direct immunological and physical effect. Several of the common denominators of long-term survivors of AIDS are examples of positive thinking in action—they gather information about the disease, they talk to people and tell them what is going on, they make a commitment to life and to others who will have AIDS, and they want to make a difference. See POSITIVE ATTITUDE.

positron emission tomography (PET)   A noninvasive technique for scanning the brain that utilizes radiolabeled substances such as glucose to measure some body functions. More recent applications of PET include demonstrations of brain response to hearing, vision, memory applications, and psychological stimuli.

"possibly safe" sex   Once it is recognized that the AIDS virus is transmitted through bodily fluids and that any exchange of these fluids during sex is unsafe, it is possible to consider various ways of reducing the risk. Even some otherwise "unsafe" sexual practices can be made safer. Each person has to decide for him or herself if the risk is worth taking. Still, it is useful to list and think about some of the "possibly safe" sexual practices individually.

The precautions listed below should be considered very seriously and applied conscientiously in order to achieve a reduction of risk. And, of course, the fewer sexual partners one has, the smaller the overall risk. The most important elements that can make otherwise "unsafe" sex somewhat less risky are condoms and certain spermicides and lubricants. Their use does not guarantee complete safety but, in general, condoms and spermicides can and will play an important role in reducing the risk of infection with the AIDS virus. The following practices remain only "possibly safe" or "possibly unsafe."

Condom use is considered only "possibly safe" and not absolutely safe, as they are often used incorrectly. To correctly use a condom, always use new condoms. Keep a ready supply of condoms where they cannot be damaged by moisture or heat. Never test a condom by blowing it up. Put a dab of lubricant into the tip of the condom to increase sensation. Prevent any air bubbles from forming that could cause the condom to break. Put the condom on the fully erect penis and roll it down all the way to the bottom of the shaft. Generally, lubricate the vaginal entrance or the anus before entry. Use only a water-soluble lubricant. Upon withdrawal, hold tightly onto the base of the condom. After use, throw the condom away. You should use a lubricant that contains NONOXYNOL-9, a mild detergent that kills not only sperm cells but also all kinds of other organisms, such as amoebas, the HERPES VIRUS, bacteria that could cause gonorrhea and syphilis, as well as the AIDS virus.

Vaginal intercourse should be somewhat safe if the man uses a condom correctly and the woman uses a spermicide containing nonoxynol-9. This double precaution does reduce risk of infection and is strongly recommended whenever partners cannot be completely certain if either of them carries the virus.

Generally speaking, using a condom during anal intercourse does not offer the same level of protection as with vaginal intercourse. Nevertheless, a lubricant containing nonoxynol-9 should still be used as it does further reduce the risk. One should never use the same condom for both anal and vaginal intercourse.

French kissing, also called deep kissing or tongue kissing, is not considered completely safe, even though there has been no known case of HIV transmission in this way. The AIDS virus *has* been found in saliva, albeit in very low concentrations. An infection through kissing therefore is not very likely. If one of the partners carries the virus and the other suffers from bleeding gums or other injuries within the mouth, there could be danger. It seems wise, therefore, to consider long and intimate deep kisses to be somewhat risky.

Oral intercourse with precautions is also considered "possibly safe" (oral intercourse with no precautions is definitely unsafe). Sucking the penis is also considered "possibly safe." One way of reducing the risk of infection is to avoid swallowing semen. One should also avoid swallowing the clear pre-ejaculatory fluid. A better practice is to suck the penis after it has been thoroughly covered with a condom.

Licking the female sex organs is also considered "possibly safe." Using spermicides containing nonoxynol-9 in and around the vaginal opening or licking it through the covering of a dental dam are two safer options.

Playing with urine ("golden showers") is also considered "possibly safe." As long as urine comes in external contact only with unbroken skin, there should be no risk of infection. It is sometimes difficult to be certain that the skin is intact everywhere. Slight cuts, bruises, or pimples are easily overlooked. Therefore persons playing with urine, even if only externally, need to be extremely careful.

post-infection immunization   See THERAPEUTIC VACCINE.

postmortem examination   See AUTOPSY.

postnatal transmission   See TRANSMISSION.

postpartum period   The period after a woman gives birth. There have been a number of documented cases of HIV transmission through breast-feeding, but the mechanism for transmission is unclear. See TRANSMISSION.

post-sex vaginitis   Vaginitis that appears a few hours after sexual activity, with itching and other symptoms. It often disappears on its own.

postsurgical PID   A condition in which an already-present infection is aggravated and worsens to an acute PELVIC INFLAMMATORY DISEASE (PID) after a surgical procedure.

post-traumatic stress syndrome (PTSD)   A clinical psychological disorder that arises in response to a catastrophic, or traumatic, event. The best-known instances are those of men traumatized in combat, but it also afflicts those who have survived or witnessed other extremely traumatic events. PTSD responses may be acute, chronic, or delayed. Their central feature is that the survivor reexperiences elements of the trauma in dreams, uncontrollable and emotionally distressing intrusive images, and dissociated mental states. There may be a feeling of numbing, loss of normal affect and emotional responsiveness, and loss of interest and involvement in work and personal relationships. Secondary symptoms include startle response, hyperalertness or hypervigilance, memory impairment, depression, survivor's guilt, avoidance of situations associated with the trauma, emotional explosiveness, and loss of capacity for intimacy. Posttraumatic stress syndrome was first defined in the *Diagnostic and Statistical Manual* of the American Psychiatric Association in 1980. In the revised edition of 1987, it was classified as a disorder.

Therapists and health care providers who work with people with HIV and AIDS are exposed to traumatic experiences through their patients. Families and others also experience secondary, or vicarious, trauma from their day-to-day contact with men, women, and children struggling to live with AIDS. Exposed to the emotional and psychological hazards intrinsic to these relationships, these individuals often manifest symptoms of traumatic stress similar to these observed in survivors of catastrophic events.

postural hypotension   A decrease in blood pressure upon assuming an erect posture. To a degree, this is normal, but in some circumstances it may be severe enough to cause fainting, as in persons who stand up after having been lying in bed for several days.

poverty level   An amount determined by the United States DEPARTMENT OF HEALTH AND HUMAN SERVICES, based on a calculation of the minimum amount of money necessary for basic living costs. It is used as a standard for MEDICAID and other needs-based programs.

power of attorney   A legal document with which one person gives another the right to act on his or her behalf in legal or financial matters. Powers of attorney may be restricted in various ways or be virtually unqualified. They are most often given by people in poor health who want their interests protected if they become unable to act for themselves.

PPD   See PURIFIED PROTEIN DERIVATIVE.

PPD test   See PURIFIED PROTEIN DERIVATIVE TEST.

preclinical testing   The testing of experimental drugs in the test tube or in animals before CLINICAL TRIALs in humans may be carried out.

prednisone   A synthetic STEROID HORMONE, with the same effects as CORTISONE, that is used to treat a wide variety of conditions, including hormone deficiencies, arthritis, lupus and other rheumatic, autoimmune diseases, connective-tissue disease, certain blood disorders, inflammation of the brain, multiple sclerosis, and as a palliative treatment of certain cancers. Less often, it is used in combination therapy to prevent organ or tissue transplant rejection. In people with HIV, prednisone is commonly used to counteract allergic drug reactions and as part of combination chemotherapy for the treatment of AIDS-related lymphoma. In this population, prednisone is also frequently used to treat people with severe PNEUMOCYSTIS CARINII PNEUMONIA and low blood oxygen to reduce lung inflammation and improve oxygenation of the blood. It is available as tablets or as a liquid for oral administration. At low doses, prednisone rarely causes serious side effects. Large doses, taken over prolonged periods, may cause indigestion, mood changes, bone or muscle weakness, fluid retention, acne, diabetes, facial rounding, abnormal hair growth, and high blood pressure. Trade names are Deltasone, Liquid Pred, Meticorten, Orasone, and SK-Prednisone.

pre-existing condition   Under some state laws, an individual has a preexisting medical condition if, before taking out a health insurance policy, he or she had symptoms of, or sought medical treatment for, such a condition. Most health insurance policies have a preexisting condition clause which states that, for a certain period of time (commonly 12 months) any such condition will not be covered. Most policies do cover such conditions after the expiration of the specified period. In many states, if an individual had been covered by a previous policy within 60 days before the start of the new policy, the new policy must give credit for the time on the old policy. Under federal law, which applies to group self-insured plans, there is no standard definition of a preexisting condition and no limit on the amount of time an individual can be excluded from coverage for such a condition.

preferred Rx   Preferred medical product, including prescription(s); the written direction or order for dispensing and administering drugs. It is signed by a physician, dentist, or other practitioner licensed by law to prescribe such a drug. Today, many people with HIV/AIDS are taking a wide variety of therapies simultaneously—ranging from experimental and approved ANTIVIRALS and PROPHYLAXIS for OPPORTUNISTIC INFECTIONS to complementary approaches and over-the-counter medications. As more drugs have become available to treat HIV and to prevent opportunistic infections and HIV-related malignancies, the potential for drug interactions has become an increasing concern. Not only does every therapy have potential side effects, but how each therapy might augment or diminish the benefit of another must be considered when making treatment decisions. How therapies interact is not always considered and may play a major role in the success of any plan for managing HIV disease. A medication review for safety, appropriateness, compatibility, and instructions for use will help decrease the likelihood of drug interactions.

pregnancy   The impact of pregnancy on the course of HIV infection is a subject of debate. Some researchers have suggested that pregnancy alters the clinical course of HIV infection and AIDS and results in a shorter survival time. Their reports indicate that HIV increases complications during pregnancy and that pregnancy itself may accelerate progression from one stage of HIV infection to another. Pregnancy outcomes do not seem to be markedly affected by HIV infection, but women can, of course, give it to their unborn children while they're pregnant or when they give birth (or later, through breast-feeding).

Studies have found that infected women who were pregnant had very slight, if any, increases in the rate of depletion of CD4 levels and the rate of development of clinical illness. Those whose CD4 counts dropped to very low levels, however, were the most prone to development of OPPORTUNISTIC INFECTIONS during pregnancy. It is generally recommended that pregnant women who are known to be HIV infected should be closely monitored during the course of pregnancy.

In guidelines published in July 1995 the U.S. PUBLIC HEALTH SERVICE recommended that all pregnant women should be offered an HIV test and routine prenatal counseling. The Public Health Service developed the guidelines after studies showed that treatment of HIV-infected pregnant women with AZT sharply reduced transmission of the virus to their babies. The recommendations mark a shift in policy for the Public Health Service, which had previously recommended testing only for women at high risk of infection, such as INTRAVENOUS DRUG USERS and prostitutes. The guidelines also suggest that women who do not receive prenatal care should be offered HIV testing for themselves or their babies after birth. The long-term effects of AZT therapy on mothers and children are not yet known. The CDC is continuing to monitor patients for long-term side effects but stresses that a woman should make a decision about taking AZT only after she discusses the benefits and potential risks for herself and her child with her HEALTH CARE PROVIDER.

These guidelines call for women's test results to be kept confidential unless state law prohibits it. Studies have shown that most women who have received HIV counseling choose to be tested for the disease.

For several years the CDC tested a national sample of newborn infants for HIV. A positive result shows that antibodies to the virus are in a baby's blood and is evidence that the mother is infected—but not necessarily the baby. The testing was conducted solely to track the progress of the disease within the population and was performed anonymously. The program was discontinued in 1995.

pregnancy counseling   Advising a woman of childbearing age of her options regarding pregnancy. Women who are pregnant or thinking about getting pregnant are advised to consider the risks; to consider taking the AIDS antibody test; and to get help making decisions from their partner, a counselor, a health worker, or an AIDS information agency.

Decisions about pregnancy and AIDS are not easy to make. A woman may decide not to have children if she or her partner is infected. If a woman is pregnant and infected, she needs to decide whether to continue the pregnancy. If a woman wants to have a child, and is infected, it is important for her to get regular medical care from a health worker or doctor who knows about AIDS. It is also important to get emotional support from a counselor or group.

premium   Amount paid periodically by an insured person or employer to secure insurance coverage. Premiums for health insurance are paid either to MEDICARE or a private insurer or health plan.

prenatal   Existing or occurring before birth.

prenatal care   Care of a woman and her fetus during pregnancy. Routine care includes periodic examination for determination of blood pressure, weight, changes in the size of the uterus, and condition of the fetus; urinalysis; instruction in nutritional requirements, preparation for labor and delivery, and care of the newborn; and assistance and support to deal with the discomforts of pregnancy. Examinations at regular intervals offer the opportunity to detect any untoward changes in the condition of a mother or fetus so that necessary treatment can be instituted.

Medical care besides this routine testing and preparation includes screening for hepatitis; serological testing for toxoplasmosis; treating opportunistic infections per standard medical protocols; using aggressive therapy if warranted for syphilis; providing women on methadone increases in dosage if needed; and, to optimize fetal outcome, fetal surveillance through ultrasound and biophysical profiles. For women with HIV, CD4+ count is followed by testing once a trimester at a minimum. For CD4+ counts of less than 200 mm, current National Institutes of Health and CENTERS FOR DISEASE CONTROL AND PREVENTION treatment recommendations are followed; for CD4+ counts between 200 mm and 500 mm, the decision to start medication is left to the patient. See also INTRAPARTUM and POSTPARTUM PERIOD.

prenatal testing   See PRENATAL CARE.

prescription drug   A drug available to the public only upon prescription written by a physician or other practitioner licensed to do so.

preseminal fluid   The milky fluid that escapes from the penis before ejaculation. Also called pre-cum.

presumptive diagnosis   A diagnosis by a HEALTH CARE PROFESSIONAL that an infection or disease is present, based on certain signs and symptoms, rather than clinical tests. It cannot be considered definitive.

presumptive disability determination   A preliminary determination by a SOCIAL SECURITY district officer finding that a needy applicant with a specified impairment will likely be found to be disabled by legal standards. This permits SSI payments to begin immediately, meeting urgent expenses and medical care needs while a complete disability determination of the medical records is conducted. Since 1988 a diagnosis of full-blown AIDS allows for presumptive disability determination.

prevalence   The total number of cases of a disease in existence at a particular time in a specified area.

prevalence rate   The frequency of the occurrence of a disease in a population, usually expressed as the number of cases per 100,000 population.

prevention   The basic steps in the prevention of the spread of HIV and AIDS include education of the public about HIV infection; encouragement of condom use, especially among teenagers and young adults; education about the hazards of using shared and unsterile needles; education of heterosexuals, homosexuals, and bisexuals to limit their number of sex partners; screening of donated blood for HIV antibodies; and education of people with AIDS about how to avoid infecting others. Perinatal prevention efforts, or efforts to prevent transmission of HIV from mother to fetus or to infant, include routine and universal HIV counseling and voluntary testing combined with AZT therapy.

primaquine   An antiprotozoal agent used primarily as a treatment for malaria. In people living with HIV, it is sometimes used with CLINDAMYCIN to treat or prevent PNEUMOCYSTIS CARINII PNEUMONIA (PCP). Nausea, vomiting, loss of appetite, and abdominal discomfort are common side effects. Less commonly, blurred vision, allergic skin reactions, dizziness, headache, darkening of the urine, and anemia may occur.

primary brain lymphoma   A rare cancer that starts in the brain. It is an OPPORTUNISTIC DISEASE that often kills people with AIDS.

primary care   Basic health care; the point of entry into the health care system for most people. The concept encompasses continuity care, health maintenance, prevention, medical management of acute and chronic illness, immunizations, age-appropriate screening for disease, and referral and follow-up for all problems that are identified. People with HIV infection or AIDS have different primary care needs than those without, in important ways. Similarly, the primary care needs of asymptomatic HIV-positive people are different from the primary care needs of symptomatic HIV-positive people. An initial evaluation of an HIV-positive person may include lab workups, immunizations, tuberculosis testing, a complete physical examination, an ophthalmological evaluation, a dental evaluation, and a psychosocial assessment. Discussion of management strategies and therapy or treatment options for HIV infection and its complications generally follows. See ACQUIRED IMMUNODEFICIENCY SYNDROME; HUMAN IMMUNODEFICIENCY VIRUS.

primary care provider   A HEALTH CARE PROVIDER (e.g., physician, physician assistant, NURSE practitioner) who offers basic health care services and coordinates comprehensive patient care.

primary care setting   The place where basic and comprehensive care is delivered, such as a physician's office, community health clinic, or a preventive nursing service.

primary CNS lymphoma   See PRIMARY CENTRAL NERVOUS SYSTEM LYMPHOMA.

primary central nervous system lymphoma (PCNSL)   A cancer of the central nervous system occurring most often as a complication of late-stage AIDS. It takes the form of B-cell

tumor growth. B cells' normal task is to produce antibodies selectively when stimulated by CD4+ HELPER T CELLS. Factors that may contribute to their unrestrained proliferation in HIV infection include chronic stimulation, loss of T-cell control mechanisms, and infection by EPSTEIN-BARR VIRUS, which is closely associated with the development of PCNSL. Historically, this lymphoma was thought to affect only a few percent of people with AIDS, but in the MULTICENTER AIDS COHORT STUDY (MACS) survey, it was increasing at a rate faster than HIV-sensory neuropathy, TOXOPLASMOSIS, CRYPTOCOCOCCAL MENINGITIS, and PROGRESSIVE MULTIFOCAL LEUKOENCEPHALOPATHY. Symptoms include focal neurologic signs such as hemiparesis, aphasia, seizures, loss of cranial nerve function, lethargy, confusion, and memory loss. Presumptive diagnosis is established through MRI and CT SCANS, complemented with lumbar puncture and cytologic examination of spinal fluid. It has been suggested that EPSTEIN-BARR virus in spinal fluid is a marker.

Primary CNS lymphoma is unusually aggressive in people with AIDS. Survival time after the onset of PCNSL depends on CD4 count, and even with treatment, averages as little as five or six months in people with advanced symptomatic AIDS. Therapy consists of whole-brain irradiation, sometimes along with short-term administration of STEROIDS to control and shrink tissue swelling and tumors. Relapse is frequent. Use of chemotherapy for PCNSL is under investigation.

primary health care   See PRIMARY CARE.

primary HIV infection   See PRIMARY INFECTION.

primary immune response   Immune responses to the HUMAN IMMUNODEFICIENCY VIRUS during the first weeks of infection. Studies have shown that primary immune response to HIV predicts disease progression. Data suggests that the immunologic factors during this early period of infection are the critical determinants of the ultimate outcome of HIV disease. The growing understanding of the initial interaction between HIV and the immune system, and of immune responses to HIV during primary infection (both favorable and unfavorable), is important to the development of effective HIV vaccines. Once it enters the body, HIV infects a large number of CD4+ T CELLs and replicates rapidly. During this acute, or primary phase of infection, the blood contains many viral particles that spread throughout the body, seeding various organs, particularly the lymphoid organs with the virus. (Up to 70 percent of HIV-infected persons have been known to suffer flu-like symptoms.) The patient's immune system fights back with killer T cells (CD8+ T cells) and B-cell-produced antibodies. One important way in which a person's immune system responds to primary HIV infection is by mobilizing different subsets of certain white blood cells—CD8+ T cells—that can destroy cells that have been infected with HIV. Studies have shown a clear correlation between the patterns of CD8+ T cell expansion during primary infection and how well a patient clinically fared during the subsequent year and 18 months afterwards. Regardless of the amount of HIV in the blood during primary infection, patients who mobilized a broad repertoire of CD8+ T cells had slower progression of disease than individuals who showed a pronounced expansion of only a single subset of CD8+ T cells. Scientists currently do not know the reasons for the qualitative differences in the immune responses of different individuals during primary HIV infection, but they probably include factors intrinsic to the HIV-infected person, such as the genes that encode specific markers called HUMAN LEUKOCYTE ANTIGENs (HLAs) on the immune system cells.

primary infection   The acute stage of HIV disease just after transmission. Primary HIV infection usually passes unnoticed. Typical symptoms such as fevers, swollen glands, rashes, and diarrhea are frequently mistaken for the flu or the common cold. If a person undergoing primary infection does seek medical attention, HIV is rarely diagnosed unless there is good reason to suspect it, such as a known recent exposure. During primary infection, HIV replicates extensively and large quantities of HIV disseminate throughout the body, especially to the lymphoid organs. Viral load levels are extremely high, but this initial burst of viral replication is brought under control within several weeks by CYTOTOXIC T-LYMPHOCYTEs (CTLs). The CTLs can reduce virus levels by a thousand-fold or more, a greater reduction than any currently available drug can accomplish. Despite the fact that the body's immune responses following initial infection usually reduce the virus to very low levels, some HIV invariably escapes. One explanation for this escape is that the immune system's best soldiers in the fight against HIV—certain subsets of CD8+ T CELLS, multiply rapidly following initial HIV infection but then exhaust themselves and disappear, allowing HIV to escape and continue replication. In the few weeks that they are detectable, the initially expanded CD8+ T cells that effectively kill HIV-infected cells are found in the bloodstream rather than in the lymph nodes where the virus is replicating. Researchers have found that major, restricted expansion of T cells in primary HIV infection is transient, and that among these expanded cells are CTLs specific for HIV.

primary lymphoid tissue   Lymphoid organs in which LYMPHOCYTEs complete their initial maturation steps; they include the fetal liver and the adult BONE MARROW and THYMUS.

primary physician   The physician to whom a family or individual goes initially for basic medical care. See PRIMARY CARE.

primary prophylaxis   Treatment to prevent the onset of a particular disease.

primary response   The immune response (cellular or humoral) following an initial encounter with a particular ANTIGEN.

prime   To give an initial sensitization to ANTIGEN.

principal investigator (PI)   The lead researcher responsible for organizing and overseeing a CLINICAL TRIAL.

prison   The health problems that increasingly affect correctional inmate populations including HIV/AIDS, tuberculosis, and sexually transmitted diseases—pose difficult programmatic and fiscal challenges for the administrators and staff of prison and jail systems. But these problems—which are significantly associated with substance abuse, high risk sexual activity, poverty, homelessness, and poor access to preventive and primary health care in the community—also offer opportunities for correctional systems to address and help improve the health of a particularly underserved and vulnerable segment of the population. Better HIV, TB, and STD prevention programs and medical care in prisons and jails will also benefit the larger society, since the vast majority of inmates will eventually return to the community. To date, providers of correctional health care and prevention services have not taken advantage of the "public health opportunity" available to them. It remains a significant opportunity that can be addressed by carefully designed programs and a dedicated staff. Today, there is increasing recognition that addressing the challenges and opportunities of health care and disease prevention in prisons and jails requires active collaboration between correctional and public health officials. The discussion that follows begins with an overview of HIV/AIDS in correctional facilities before highlighting issues specific to persons with HIV/AIDS and STDs in correctional facilities.

The eighth national survey of HIV/AIDS in correctional facilities, sponsored jointly by the National Institute of Justice and the Centers for Disease Control, covered the prevalence and prevention of sexually transmitted diseases among inmates. According to the survey, AIDS incidence rates are substantially higher among inmates than in the total United States population. HIV SEROPREVALENCE rates are also generally higher in prison and jail populations than in the population at large. Seroprevalence rates, however, appear to be either stable or declining in most systems. Seroprevalence is also often higher among female inmates than male inmates. As in previous years, there were no documented cases of occupational HIV transmission from inmates to correctional staff. Studies have shown that inmate-to-inmate HIV transmission does occur, but at quite a low rate.

Despite continued growth of the epidemic among inmates, however, the 1994 survey indicated a continued decline in the number of correctional facilities providing face-to-face inmate HIV education. Results also suggest that there are continuing needs for improvement in HIV prevention counseling, medical care, and supportive services for inmates with HIV as well as drug treatment capacity. The survey reports that HIV knowledge among inmates is probably higher now than it was in the middle and late 1980s, but some areas of uncertainty and misinformation remain about transmission mechanisms and prevention measures. The survey reports that fewer correctional systems are offering instructor-led HIV education sessions for inmates. Moreover, only about one-third of state/federal systems offer inmate peer-based education and support programs; this number has remained flat, even though such approaches represent a promising and cost-effective way to provide services. There is a continuing need for more educational programs and materials in Spanish and more culturally appropriate materials.

Validation study results suggest that most facilities are providing the modes of education required in their systems' policies but may be expanding upon specified topics to include more controversial subjects, such as safer drug injection practices. Ongoing HIV prevention counseling (beyond pre-test and post-test counseling) does not appear to be widely offered in prisons and jails, representing a continuing weakness in the correctional response to HIV/AIDS. A sampling of issues specific to persons with HIV/AIDS and STDs in correctional facilities includes testing, counseling, confidentiality, and disclosure policies; housing and correctional management; and medical care and psychosocial services.

The 1994 survey indicates that trends in HIV antibody testing policies and notification of test results remain stable. Most systems offer HIV testing on request. About 90 percent of correctional systems conduct routine STD testing of inmates. Few correctional systems notify correctional officers of inmates' HIV status as a matter of official policy. Actual practice, however, may differ from official directives, and unauthorized disclosure to officers and others remains a problem. Staff and resource shortages have prevented many systems from providing adequate pre-test and post-test counseling.

In regards to the housing of inmates with HIV and AIDS, there has been a steady decline in segregation policies. Case-by-case decisions and presumptive general population assignments remain most common. Validation study results reveal the complexity in implementing housing policies in institutions with different security levels and different population characteristics. In most systems, inmates with HIV/AIDS are eligible for all program and work assignments. However, several systems exclude such inmates from kitchen work. This remains a controversial issue, despite strong evidence that HIV is not transmitted through food.

Medical care for inmates with HIV/AIDS continues to be uneven in quality. Although the best-known therapeutic drugs for HIV/AIDS are in widespread use, access to experimental drugs and CLINICAL TRIALS remains quite rare in correctional systems. Support groups and other supportive services are not offered as widely as they might be. Similarly, drug treatment services appear to be reaching a far smaller proportion of inmates than could probably benefit from them. In 1994, 61 percent of state/federal systems and 38 percent of city/county systems reported policies for early or compassionate release of inmates with AIDS. Discharge planning and continuity of care for inmates leaving correctional facilities remain areas in need of significant improvement.

Legal issues raised by inmates with HIV/AIDS include protection from harm by fellow inmates; challenges to mandatory testing; challenges to other testing policies; confidentiality; segregation and housing assignments; access to programs; and adequacy of medical care. Also of legal interest are patterns and trends in the criminal indictment and sentencing of persons with HIV infection. Whether and how the judicial system should consider HIV infection in its processing of persons accused and/or convicted of crimes remains a challenging question for the nation's criminal and appellate courts. Conflicting rulings appear largely related to the nature of the crime committed and to the nature of the defendant's illness. For example, while in recent years several courts have considered not prosecuting, or commuting the sentences of, defendants with HIV or AIDS who have been charged with or convicted of nonviolent crimes, defendants charged with other crimes, like having unprotected sex with teenagers, are treated quite severely. Lastly, despite evidence that HIV has never demonstrably been transmitted through saliva, over the last several years, at least two HIV-infected inmates have been prosecuted and convicted of attempted murder for biting or spitting on a correctional officer.

The American Bar Association adopted a policy on AIDS and the criminal justice system in 1989. The ABA said that appropriately funded training and education programs regarding HIV should be instituted in all correctional facilities. Further, the ABA recommended that inmates in correctional facilities should be afforded appropriate medical care for the full range of HIV-related infections and should be afforded appropriate counseling as well. The ABA policy further states that prisoners should not be segregated from the general population of the correctional facility or be placed in other special areas solely because of their known or perceived HIV status. It specifies that mass HIV-antibody testing should not be done for the purpose of segregating inmates in special cells or areas. Information about an inmate's HIV status should not be disclosed except to the warden, key supervisory staff who have a legitimate need for the information, or medical staff for care and treatment purposes. And according to the ABA, parole or temporary release should not be denied to a prisoner, nor should a prisoner be barred from participating in other community release programs, solely because of the prisoner's known or perceived HIV status.

The National Commission on AIDS has also addressed these concerns. In March 1991, it issued a report on HIV disease in correctional facilities. The report found that prisoners with HIV infection are rapidly acquiring tuberculosis and many more are at increased risk from the resurgent tuberculosis epidemic in the nation's prisons. It also found that prisoners with HIV are often subject to automatic segregation from the rest of the prison community despite the fact that there is no public health basis for this practice. Thirdly, it found that lack of education of both inmates and staff creates fear and discrimination as well as unjust policies directed toward inmates with HIV. Finally, it found that despite high rates of HIV infection and an ideal opportunity for prevention and education efforts, former prisoners are re-entering their communities with little or no added knowledge about HIV and how to prevent it. Inmates continue to be tested without their consent, to be segregated and made subject to other inmates' and staff's ridicule and animosity, and to be denied privileges available to those who are not HIV-infected.

privacy   Freedom from unwanted observation or examination, implying, in a medical context, the right of a patient to control the distribution and release of records and information concerning his or her medical history, encompassing all information the patient has provided to health care professionals and any other information contained in medical charts, records, and laboratory data. Specifically, this includes diagnoses of HIV infection, AIDS, or related disorders.

People with AIDS, their families, and others close to them often have to contend with social stigma along with their anger, guilt, grief, and denial. As a result, the right to privacy has been the subject of heated public debate. In our legal tradition, issues of HIV testing and dissemination of medical information fit into the portmanteau category of "privacy," which is protected in various ways in state and federal law and constitutions.

The U.S. Constitution and many state constitutions protect personal privacy against government and other institutional intrusion, although in all but a few state constitutions the right to privacy of medical information is not explicitly stated. Instead, it has been derived by the courts from the general tenor and purposes of these fundamental charters. Protection of privacy has been found by courts to be particularly necessary in cases of HIV-related information. Reasons for this include the moral stigma society attaches to the disease and activities associated with it (especially sexual relations and drug use), and the potential for harm in the event of a nonconsensual disclosure and the fact that the consequences of the hysteria surrounding AIDS extends beyond those who have the disease. Even in instances where courts have found release of information to be justified, they have usually been careful to make the allowable disclosure as narrow as possible. The right of privacy also encompasses the freedom to choose or refuse medical care and to decide for oneself when to release sensitive information to others.

Individual privacy is also protected by the Fourth Amendment, which establishes "the right of people to be secure in their persons, houses, papers, and effects, against unreasonable searches and seizures" by government or its agents. This means that a person has a right to expect that the privacy of his or her personal records, including medical information, will be respected and that the revelation of such information through medical testing may not be coerced. The actual degree of protection under the Fourth Amendment, however, depends on the case-by-case application of the rules by the courts. Judges assessing the reasonableness of HIV testing under the Fourth Amendment have reached varying and even contradictory decisions, and is likely that they will continue to do so for some time.

The public health consensus in support of privacy and against coercion led a majority of states to adopt measures in the late 1980s governing HIV testing and confidentiality. By the end of 1991, 36 states had enacted legislation requiring informed consent for HIV testing; virtually every state provided some degree of confidentiality. Some laws address disclosure not only of test results, but of any confidential HIV-related information developed in the course of any health or social service. A second wave of statutes that began to emerge in 1988 generally expanded the range of counseling required and information protected, but also to set forth more detailed exceptions.

Most confidentiality laws provide that information may be disclosed to health departments and hospital oversight agencies and to the subjects of tests and the physicians who order them. Most also contain exceptions based on the "need to know" (whether such needs are genuine or not has been subject to debate). In addition, many states have mandatory testing and disclosure provisions that override the general policy of voluntariness and nondisclosure. Major exceptions have been won, for example, by funeral directors, insurers, and health care providers. Some states authorize involuntary testing of, and disclosure of information about, people in prisons, mental hospitals, juvenile facilities, and residential centers for the developmentally disabled. Mandatory testing and disclosure is becoming more common in the criminal justice system. Physician warnings to third parties and testing and disclosure by court order remain two of the most debated issues in health policy.

Today it is generally recognized that the protection of privacy is important for an effective public health response to HIV in a just society. History has shown that testing and disclosure programs too often reflect a preoccupation with low but frightening risks, and a preference for identifying people whose exposure is unusual over providing services to the easy-to-identify. The claim that privacy is in conflict with public health too often reflects underlying disdain for those with, or at risk of, HIV; we have simultaneously enacted legal protections of privacy while allowing it to be needlessly compromised on too many occasions. Today those concerned with the treatment and prevention of HIV/AIDS generally agree that anyone who comes into possession of information about HIV-infected individuals or is in a position to do HIV testing must understand and respect the importance of privacy to both individuals and society. It is understood that, occasionally, this respect may bring them into conflict with legal rules and regulations.

privates   A euphemism for genitalia.

PRO 2000   A new still-experimental antiviral drug that blocks infection of CD4 cells by interfering with the binding of HIV's outer protein GP120 to cells' CD4 receptors. Though the drug seems safe thus far, there are some potential problems with long-term administration—in studies with monkeys, high doses impaired blood coagulation.

probate   The process by which an executor, if there is a will, or a court-appointed administrator, if there is not, under court supervision manage and distribute a deceased person's property.

procarbazine hydrochloride   A cytotoxic drug used in treating HODGKIN'S DISEASE and certain other neoplastic diseases. Trade name is Matulane.

Procrit   See EPOGEN.

proctitis   Infections of the ANUS and RECTUM.

proctocolitis   An inflamed condition of the COLON and RECTUM.

prodromal stages   Stages of infection that fall short of the onset of a full-blown disease. In cases of HIV infection, stages that do not meet the CDC criteria for a diagnosis of AIDS.

prodrome   A complex of physical and clinical signs and symptoms that may precede the onset of a full-blown disease.

prodrug   A compound that is converted within the body into an active form that has medical effects. Prodrugs are useful when an active drug may be too toxic to administer systemically, is absorbed poorly by the digestive tract, or broken down before it reaches its target.

progesterone   A female hormone produced by the ovaries.

progesterone implant   A surgically implanted contraceptive for women that prevents pregnancy for up to five years. It consists of six match-size flexible rubber capsules, each containing the synthetic progestin levonorgestrel, which is present in some birth control pills. This hormone is released slowly through the walls of the capsules until the capsules are removed. The capsules can be felt and sometimes can be noticed as ridges or bumps. The capsules are implanted beneath the skin of the inner arm just above the elbow. The procedure takes approximately 15 minutes and is performed in a physician's office under a local anesthetic. When the rods are removed, fertility is restored. Possible side effects include amenorrhea, menstrual irregularities, weight change, mood swings, and headache. The trade name is Norplant.

prognosis   A forecast of the probable course and/or outcome of a disease. Currently, scientists believe that all patients who are infected with HIV will progress to the AIDS stage and die. The length of time between infection and death may be brief or many years. The time from infection to clinical signs is, on the average, 10 to 11 years.

progressive multifocal leukoencephalopathy (PML)   A central nervous system disease that results in the destruction of brain tissue and the sheath that covers the nerves. PML develops in approximately 4–5 percent of HIV-infected individuals. It should be considered in cases of progressive neurologic disease in HIV-infected patients. PML results in HIV-infected persons due to infection with a virus called the Creutzfeldt-Jakob virus (JC virus). It is believed that up to 80 percent of the population contracted this asymptomatic virus of the kidney in childhood. In a person with a weak immune system, the virus is reactivated and spread to the brain by white blood cells from the bone marrow. Once in the brain, the virus infects the brain cells responsible for producing the protective sheath around the nerves. Without this protection on the nerves, nerve cells die and cause lesions in the brain. Neurologic dysfunction may follow quickly.

PML can cause a series of symptoms related to neurological impairment, including confusion, disorientation, lack of energy, loss of balance, weakness in the arms or legs, speech problems, blurred or double vision, and blindness. The onset is generally subacute with slowly progressive neurologic dysfunction. Dementia, visual defects, hemiparesis, ataxia, difficulties with speech and language, abnormal gait, sensory deficits, or other focal deficits may occur. Altered consciousness resulting from brain swelling does not occur. Physically,

focal neurologic deficits are apparent. Patients are generally afebrile. Diagnosis is by CT or MRI. These studies reveal focal or diffuse lesions in the white matter typically without mass effect or contrast enhancement. MRI is more sensitive than CT. The white matter lesions observed with PML may be mimicked by those seen with HIV encephalopathy. The definitive diagnosis rests on brain biopsy. There is no proven therapy for this disease. IV and intrathecal (spinal) infusions of cytosine arabinoside (commonly known as ara-C, trade name: Cytarabine), a drug used to treat leukemia and lymphoma, have been reported effective in some AIDS patients often weeks to months after initiation of treatment. Long term Cytarabine seems to be a good option for people with AIDS-related PML. Two other cancer drugs, topotecan and irinotecan, are also thought to be active against PML.

Although rare cases of spontaneous sustained remission have been reported, especially in those with CD4 counts >200 or those taking high dose zidovudine, the prognosis is poor with the mean length of survival <6 months after the onset of neurologic symptoms.

project inform   Founded in 1985, a San Francisco–based project that is the nation's leading and most respected community-based AIDS treatment information and advocacy organization. Services include a toll-free Treatment Information Hotline, free publications (*PI Perspective,* a quarterly HIV treatment journal, fact sheets on therapies and diseases, and position papers on complex and timely issues about HIV treatments and research), outreach ("town hall meetings"), and activism. Project Inform's Treatment Action Network (TAN) is a national grassroots network whose members respond to public issues about AIDS research and access to treatments. TAN plays an important role in protecting and increasing federal funding for AIDS research, prevention, care, and housing.

Project Inform is credited for compiling *The HIV Drug Book,* the first comprehensive, user-friendly guide to all the drugs most used by people with HIV/AIDS. Formatted for quick reference and written in nontechnical language, the handbook features an extensive master index. Drug descriptions are categorized by their specific treatments. Drug profiles include antibiotics, anticancer drugs, antidiarrheal drugs, antifungal drugs, antihistamines, antinausea/antivomiting drugs, antiprotozoal drugs, antiseizure drugs, antiulcer drugs, antiviral drugs, antiwasting treatments, corticosteroids, immune-based therapy, neuropathy drugs, pain relievers, psychoactive drugs, and vaccines.

promiscuity   Characterized by having numerous sexual partners on a casual basis. Because sexual intercourse is one of the principal routes of HIV transmission, the AIDS epidemic has fostered a new etiquette of sex. A woman or man can no longer actively or passively participate in continual one night stands or a freewheeling lifestyle and still secure a healthy future. The AIDS epidemic urges us to change the habitual sexual expectation of unprotected intercourse. Developing new habits with each of our partners is the only way to keep ourselves safe. In practical terms, this means we must scrupulously be careful to practice safer sex in all relationships except those that are long-term and monogamous—and be absolutely trustworthy. The importance of trustworthy monogamy, even among loving, lifelong partnerships, cannot be underestimated. Similarly, the risk of being promiscuous cannot be underestimated. Promiscuity does not accommodate new dating rituals, such as a period of healthy skepticism and information gathering, slower moves toward the bedroom, insistence on intimacy before intercourse, a shift toward monogamous, long-term relationships, and increased acceptance of periodic abstinence and celibacy.

prophylactic   An agent or regimen that contributes to the prevention of infection and disease. Also popular term for a condom. See PROPHYLAXIS.

prophylactic vaccine   See VACCINE.

prophylaxis   Any intervention intended to preserve health and prevent the initial occurrence (primary prophylaxis) or the recurrence (secondary prophylaxis) of a disease. The intervention may be in the form of a drug (such as a vaccine) or other treatment or the use of a device (such as a condom).

propolis   A sticky resin present in the buds and bark of certain trees and plants. It is collected by bees for the purpose of repairing combs, filling cracks, and making the entrance to the hive waterproof. There is anecdotal evidence that propolis may be of benefit in treating certain diseases. Scientific IN VITRO investigations indicate that the material inhibits the reproduction of certain viruses.

PRO   See PEER REVIEW ORGANIZATION.

Pro90   An amino acid that binds protein cyclophilin A (what HIV takes with it when it buds from a cell). The binding of cyclophilin A by Pro90 seems necessary for a viral particle to be infectious. If Pro90 is present in an abnormal form, HIV particles are not infectious, even though they appear normal. Researchers have previously hypothesized that the binding of cyclophilin A to the p24 capsid protein changes the conformation of the protein, thereby enabling the virus to release its genetic contents into a target cell. In recent experiments, Pro90 has been observed to exist in two separate conformations. It is hypothesized that one of these conformations may be necessary for the p24 capsid proteins to assemble, in order to form the viral core. The other conformation would be necessary for the core to disassemble. Pro90 may serve as a molecular switch for capsid assembly or disassembly, with cyclophilin A either flipping the switch or locking it into a particular position.

prostaglandin   A variety of naturally occurring aliphatic acid (a series of organic chemical compounds characterized by open chains of carbon atoms) with various biological activities, including increasing vascular permeability, smoothing muscle contraction, relieving bronchial constriction, and altering the pain threshold.

prostate gland   A muscular gland that surrounds the first inch of the male urethra; secretes an alkaline fluid that

becomes part of semen. Its smooth muscle contributes to ejaculation.

prostitute   Anyone who agrees to participate in sexual acts for money; a whore. Unmodified, the term generally applies to women. If male prostitutes or prostitution are discussed, they are generally so identified. Slang terms include *call girl, fille de joie, ho,* and *working girl.*

protease   A protein enzyme (of the HIV virus) that is crucial to the life cycle of HIV. Protease plays a major role in viral infectivity and replication. It is used by the virus to clip a long HIV protein molecule, known as Gag-Pol, into a number of smaller proteins. Each of these smaller units then assists in the assembly of proteins and genetic material into a mature, and infectious, viral particle. These clips can occur only because, before the process begins, protease is able to cut itself loose from the other components of the larger, inactive viral protein, a process known as autocatalysis.

HIV protease is quite small and makes an ideal target to stop HIV replication. It is a member of the aspartylprotease enzyme family that also includes the major human enzymes renin (which regulates kidney action) and pepsin (which digests protein in the stomach). See PROTEASE INHIBITOR.

protease inhibitor   Compound that blocks the protease enzyme of HIV, thereby preventing the production of infectious viral particles. Other anti-HIV drugs known as NUCLEOSIDE ANALOGS (AZT, ddI, ddC, D4T 3TC) target a different viral enzyme, REVERSE TRANSCRIPTASE.

Scientists used to think that HIV, once having infected someone went into a semidormant phase for 10 years or more before producing symptoms of illness. Now they know that for that entire period, the body and the virus are engaged in a heated battle. The virus is reproducing furiously, and the body just as furiously killing the virus. In most people, the body loses a little ground, and the virus gains a little ground each day.

As part of the process of reproducing itself in the body, the HIV virus uses an enzyme called HIV protease to wrap itself in a membrane of proteins snipped from the wall of a human cell. Protease inhibitors act at a late stage in this process, after the replicated HIV within a cell has initiated mass production of new viral components. The proteins within HIV's outer envelope first come out of the cell's protein factory in a long connected string that must be cut up. HIV protease acts like a chemical scissors. It snips out the parts of the virus core so that they reassemble in the proper configuration. This snipping process occurs as newly formed virus particles bud out of the cell. Protease inhibitors lock onto and sheathe the protease's active site (the blade of the scissors, as it were), thus disrupting the creation of mature virus particles. Studies have shown that such particles produced without protease are faulty and cannot infect other immune system cells. The aim is to tip the balance back in the body's favor, at least for a time, and to give the immune system a chance to produce more CD4 cells. The hope is that boosting the cells will ultimately slow the progression to illness and death. Unlike earlier AIDS drugs, protease inhibitors do not seem very toxic. In most who take them they seem to produce a marked reduction in virus and a concomitant boost in the immune system. While the toxicity of the new drugs has generally been low, not everyone can take them. Besides possible side effects, there's another problem: HIV quickly develops resistance to new drugs, including protease inhibitors.

It is hoped that this relatively new class of antiretrovirals will provide a more effective and less toxic alternative to NUCLEOSIDE ANALOGs. The rapid emergence of viral resistance to AZT and other reverse transcriptase inhibitors (ddI, ddC, d4T), along with their toxicities, limits their long-term usefulness in the treatment of HIV. Protease inhibitors may be less prone to this failure. It is thought that HIV is less able to alter the structure of the protease enzyme than that of reverse transcriptase. Resistance to protease inhibitors may be slower to develop and at a lower level than that for reverse transcriptase inhibitors. Nonetheless, resistance to protease inhibitors is predictable: its emergence is a consequence of the drug's effectiveness. Indeed, resistance has already been observed for some protease inhibitors. People with advanced disease commonly harbor HIV resistance to many of the new drugs, due to prior treatment with sequential monotherapies or weak combinations consisting of two nucleoside analogs. There are growing ranks of those who have become resistant to protease inhibitors after adding them to regimens of nucleoside analogs. Cross-resistance and side effects may render useless anti-HIV agents patients have not yet tried.

Combinations of different protease inhibitors or the combination of a protease inhibitor with a reverse transcriptase inhibitor may delay development of resistance. It is also hoped that the protease inhibitors will have antiviral activity against HIV strains that are resistant to AZT.

An interesting footnote to the subject of resistance is the irony that HIV makes its own protease inhibitor that is several thousand times as potent as the synthetic ones. This inhibitor, known as Vif (viral infectivity factor) could be the basis of an anti-protease drug that is virtually resistance-proof. Vif apparently binds to the same regions on the HIV polyprotein that protease breaks apart. As the HIV virion buds from cell walls, most of the Vif sticks to the lipids in the cell membrane, exposing the polyprotein to protease at the proper moment to assemble the virus core. A truncated Vif or an analog with similar structure could be created that would latch onto the polyprotein permanently and keep the protease enzyme away. Should HIV mutate its polyprotein cleavage sites to avoid the false Vif, the real Vif would not bind either, and the protease enzyme would prematurely chop up the polyprotein. There would then be no competent virus particle produced.

On December 7, 1995, the Food and Drug Administration announced approval of the first protease inhibitor. This agent, Invirase, completed an accelerated FDA approval process in the shortest time ever for any drug, three months from the filing of an application. Others have been approved since and still others are available in experimental trials. However, supplies are limited for three reasons: absorption of these oral drugs is generally poor; enzymes in the liver quickly destroy some; and they are difficult to manufacture. As a result, patients must take more of these drugs than

anticipated, and production has been slow to catch up. Pharmaceutical and biotech companies have been distributing them through large lottery programs.

In March 1996, the Food and Drug Administration approved the second and third protease inhibitors, Ritonavir and Indinavir. Ritonavir received full approval for use alone or in combination with nucleoside analog medications such as AZT in patients with advanced HIV disease. Ritonavir also received accelerated approval for patients with less advanced HIV disease. Indinavir received accelerated approval for MONOTHERAPY and COMBINATION THERAPY for the treatment of HIV infection in adults when therapy is warranted. FDA based its approval for Indinavir on data showing that the drug improves laboratory markers such as CD4+ T cell counts and VIRAL LOAD in patients at various stages of disease.

In the final analysis, all these protease inhibitors bind to the protease enzyme in similar ways and, hence, are affected by similar mutation-driven alterations in the enzyme's structure. However, several of the new protease inhibitors offer something a little different. The older protease inhibitors represented attempts to create molecules that mimic the way the natural polyprotein substrate binds to the enzyme's active site. Protease cleaves the natural polyprotein into the sturctural proteins and enzymes contained in the core of a mature virus particle. The synthetic mimics are designed to be uncleavable units that clog the protease active site. Several of the new inhibitors under development by Pharmacia & Upjohn, Bristol Myers Squibb, and Parke-Davis have novel sticky structures that bind to the active site in ways that are relatively little affected by the standard mutational alterations elicited by the older protease inhibitors.

Recent reports have confirmed that combination therapies including protease inhibitors have unprecedented effect, as indicated by dramatic drops in viral load. The reports suggest that current combinations of anti-HIV drugs will be considerably more effective than the mediocre HIV treatment options of the past.

It is doubtful that protease inhibitors will ever be a cure for AIDS all by themselves. They may be used with a wide variety of other antiviral drugs (including reverse transcriptase inhibitors) and immune modulators. Other compounds such as cytokines and antioxidant nutrients could be part of the package. To date, little is known about the long term benefits of protease inhibitors or how to optimally use them given complicating issues like toxicity and resistance. Many types of trials are required to fill in the gaps in our knowledge of optimizing protease inhibitors. Such trials include drug versus drug comparisons, screening/pilot trials to better define treatment strategies, and large-scale strategy trials.

Currently, one might characterize the response of practitioners to protease inhibitors as tempered optimism. Increased CD4 counts and decline in viral loads are viewed as encouraging, but duration of response is questioned. Drug interactions (particularly with ritonavir), side effects (particularly, gastrointestinal problems with ritonavir), and compliance requirements (particularly, coordinating three meals with thrice daily indinavir) are frequently noted as problems.

As with nucleoside analogs, there are many unknowns: To what extent do protease inhibitors work? How safe are they? When is the best time to initiate therapy—at critical CD4 level, or at a critical viral load level, always as first-line therapy, when symptoms appear, or at the patient's request? How do they compare with each other in terms of viral load response and CD4 count response? When should the combination regimen be modified? How easily can HIV evolve resistance? To what extent does reducing HIV levels translate into improvements in health?

protective equipment   CDC guidelines (*Guidelines for Prevention of Transmission of Human Immunodeficiency Virus (HIV) and Hepatitis B Virus (HBV) to Health-Care and Public-Safety Workers*) recommend that masks, eyewear, and gowns should be present on all emergency vehicles that respond to medical emergencies or victim rescues and used in accordance with the level of exposure encountered. The guidelines also recommend that masks and eyewear should be worn together, or a face shield should be used in any situation where splashing of blood or other body fluids to which universal precautions apply are likely to occur.

protein   Large molecules made up of long sequences of amino acids. Some hormones, enzymes, and cellular structures are proteins. Three-fourths of the dry weight of most cells consists of proteins.

protein S   Protein S is involved in preventing spontaneous formation of clots; a deficiency predisposes to thrombotic (clotting) episodes. It is unclear why some HIV-positive persons have protein S deficiency and are consequently at higher risk of unprovoked thrombotic episodes.

Proteus   A bacteria genus that can cause cystitis; found in feces.

protocol   The blueprint or design for an experimental drug trial that describes the trial's rationale, treatment duration, and who and how many may participate.

protozoan   A one-celled organism of the animal kingdom containing many different species. Some protozoa (plural) cause disease in humans, notably TOXOPLASMOSIS and CRYPTOSPORIDIOSIS, especially in the setting of altered immunity.

provider referral   The process by which health care providers find the sex or needle-sharing partners of people found to be infected with HIV (based on information given voluntarily by the infected people), notify them of their exposure to the virus, and refer than for examination or treatment. See PARTNER NOTIFICATION.

provirus   A copy of the genetic information of an animal virus that is integrated into the DNA of an infected cell. Copies of the provirus are passed on to each of the infected cell's daughter cells.

prozone phenomenon   A reaction that occurs in undiluted or slightly diluted serum in which ANTIBODY is present in such high concentration that it interferes with precipitation reactions with ANTIGENs. The phenomenon may distort or falsify the results of tests, especially for SYPHILIS.

prunellin   The active component of the herb prunella vulgaris (*Prunella vulgaris labiatae*), known as heal-all or self-heal, once used to treat cuts and wounds. Test tube studies have shown that prunellin can block cell-to-cell transmission of HIV. Other in vitro studies suggest that prunellin also inhibits REVERSE TRANSCRIPTASE because of its content of anionic polysaccharides, which are known to inhibit reverse transcriptase in such drugs as HEPARIN.

prurient   Having to do with, or arousing, an "unhealthy" interest in sex; from a Latin root meaning "to itch."

pruritus   Itching, as a symptom. It may be paroxysmal or constant, may be associated with skin lesions or occur independent of any skin lesion.

psittacosis   An infectious disease caused by Chlamydia *psittaci* in parrots and other birds that may be transmitted to humans. TETRACYCLINES, ERYTHROMYCIN, and PENICILLIN are effective in treatment.

psoriasis   A common chronic disease of the skin in which erythematous papules coalesce to form plaques with distinct borders. As the disease progresses, and if left untreated, a silvery yellow-white scale develops. New lesions tend to appear at sites of trauma. They may be in any location, but most frequently are located on the scalp, knees, elbows, umbilicus, and genitalia. Severity and clinical course are variable. The cause of psoriasis is unknown, but a genetic factor is present. Certain conditions, such as infection, some drugs, climate, and perhaps hormonal factors and smoking, may trigger attacks.

psychobiology   The process of interaction between body and mind in the formation and functioning of personality; also the study of such interaction.

psychological dependence   A subjective need for a specific psychoactive substance, either for its positive effects or to avoid negative effects associated with its absence. See ADDICTION.

psychological factors   The psychological or internal challenges a person with HIV/AIDS faces vary from individual to individual. Not everyone will experience all of the emotional responses or stages of the emotional responses described. Each HIV/AIDS situation is as unique as the people involved.

Due to the "terminal" prognosis associated with AIDS, diagnosis can be catastrophic to the individual, who might face catastrophic changes not only in their personal and job relationships, but in their physical bodies and in their self-images and self-esteem as well. Initially, daily routine may be interrupted; income may be disrupted or diminished. Diagnosis could lead to feeling the sense of loss of control of one's life.

Coping with an HIV or AIDS diagnosis involves confronting fear and denial while maintaining hope. After diagnosis the patients may respond with shock or disbelief. After the initial shock and disbelief may come denial, an attempt to ignore or forget the diagnosis. Hiding in denial allows a person time to regroup and become prepared to deal with the challenges ahead. After denial, a bargaining stage often occurs, hopefully followed with an ongoing commitment to work on the challenges at hand and toward recovery. Some persons with AIDS, though, give up and never allow themselves to see beyond the possibility of their own demise.

Several other possible emotional responses are noted. Coping with an HIV or AIDS diagnosis may also involve confronting or reexamining one's sexual identity and the behavioral choices one has made in support of that identity. By associating HIV/AIDS with what society has traditionally considered illicit or immoral, the person with HIV/AIDS is faced with working through his or her feelings so that his or her sexual identity may be reaffirmed in such a way as to allow him or her to feel good about himself or herself. Changing sex habits is part and parcel of living with HIV/AIDS.

In a similar vein, coping with an HIV or AIDS diagnosis may also involve confronting or reexamining one's use of drugs and/or alcohol and the behavioral choices one has made in support of that identity.

Persons with HIV/AIDS are also confronted with other people seeing them as "contagious," which may cause them to feel undesirable. This is another emotion that can cause a person with AIDS to become isolated—emotionally, geographically, or both.

One of the biggest and most destructive stressors is that of feeling isolated. This sense of isolation can stem from many factors, including the withdrawal of support by lovers, family, and friends; the isolation from friends and daily routine due to hospitalization; and the general public's ongoing failure to respond to people with HIV/AIDS as it has to others who are ill. Finally, the sexual and personal precautions persons with HIV/AIDS must take to protect themselves and others certainly underscore the feelings of being "different" and alone.

A second destructive stressor is that of feeling being dependent. In addition to having to rely more heavily on family and friends for emotional support, many people with HIV/AIDS are faced with applying for social services for the first time. The experience of applying for social services is almost always frustrating and demoralizing. Additionally, there is the conflict between continuing to work and remaining self-sufficient or forgoing work in order to be eligible for services. Applying for help is one thing; accepting and using the services is another. There is a final aspect of dependence that is potentially the most frustrating of all: the fear of a protracted illness that will drain family and friends financially as well as emotionally.

The person with HIV/AIDS will likely respond to the experience, and those described above, with a wide variety of emotions: anger, depression, fear, guilt, despair, anxiety, hurt, sadness, and, at times, joy, peace and happiness. These feelings change frequently and, if they become too intense, they can become immobilizing. Or, because it is possible to experience a combination of hopeless lows and hopeful

highs at the same time, the person with AIDS can become snared in the emotional confusion and be unable to move ahead with life.

psychological need Persons with HIV/AIDS generally experience a range of psychological needs. These needs vary with the stage in the illness plus other factors. As with psychological factors, experiences vary from individual to individual. Not everyone will experience all of the needs described below.

At diagnosis, people with HIV/AIDS may have an increased need for physical contact and emotional intimacy. These feelings may be enhanced by emotions that arise in coping with an HIV or AIDS diagnosis. But during this time, due to fear and a sense of helplessness, lovers, family, and friends may withdraw their support. When this happens, the person with AIDS may feel alone and isolated.

The need to remain independent often accompanies and increases with the progression of the illness. Accepting increasing dependency is part and parcel of living with HIV/AIDS. At various stages of the illness, people with HIV/AIDS may have an increased need for different kinds of help: help with understanding the medical aspects of their diagnosis; with coping with the diagnosis; with identifying alternative treatments; with maintaining order as concerns legal and financial matters; with their emotions; and with coping on a day-to-day basis. Asking for help is one thing; accepting and utilizing the help of friends, family members, AIDS service providers, and others is just as important.

psychological services Because HIV/AIDS effects not only the body, but also emotions and interpersonal relations, and because self-empowerment in the age of AIDS is increasingly important, the role of psychological services is often critical to the well-being of the AIDS-inflicted person. Psychological services are also designed to support AIDS caregivers and those (partners, family, friends) coping with the fear of AIDS. These services often focus on living or on dying. They may include peer counseling or counseling by social workers; support groups (either facilitated or unfacilitated); therapy groups (generally facilitated by a mental health professional); or individual therapy (provided by mental health professionals including psychologists, psychiatrists, psychiatric nurses). They may be provided independently, under the auspices of an AIDS service provider, under the auspices of AIDS-advocacy organization, or by another organization. They may be free or fee-based.

In thinking about psychological services, it is important to note that one's religion also offers human and spiritual support. Priests, rabbis, ministers, nuns, pastors of all religions give help in a similar fashion as social workers and psychologists, but they talk particularly to people strictly on a religious level. They offer advice, comfort, and company.

psychoneuroimmunology The study of the interrelationships between psychology, the nervous system, and the immune system.

psychosocial Pertaining to the effects on individuals and groups of the interaction between social conditions and psychological functioning. In a health care context, the term refers to psychological support services concerned with such effects, often needed by persons with HIV infection.

psychosis   A mental disturbance of such magnitude as to cause personality disintegration and loss of contact with reality. Such disturbances are of psychogenic origin, or without clearly defined physical cause or structural change in the brain. They usually are characterized by delusions and hallucinations, and hospitalization is generally required. Psychosis is manifest in behavior, emotional reaction and ideation. Psychotics fail to perceive ordinary reality, react inappropriately to it, and build up false concepts regarding it. Behavioral responses are inappropriate or antisocial.

psychostimulant   A drug that speeds up or increases responsiveness of the mind.

psychotic disorder   See PSYCHOSIS.

psychotropic drug   A drug that affects psychic function, behavior or experience. Many drugs are intended to be psychotropic, but others also may produce undesired psychotropic side effects.

PTSD   See POST-TRAUMATIC STRESS SYNDROME.

pubic hair   Hair growth around the genitals. Pubic hair first appears during puberty, when adult sexual characteristics develop.

pubic louse (pl. lice)   A parasitic insect that may infest the pubic area. See CRAB LOUSE.

pubis   Another term for the pubic area.

public accommodation   Since the enactment of the Civil Rights Acts of 1964, discrimination on the basis of race, color, religion, and national origin has been unlawful in places of public accommodation. The concept of public accommodation has traditionally encompassed eating establishments, hotels and motels, theaters, and other facilities open to the public. But with the onset of the AIDS epidemic, there have been calls to extend the concept to include a variety of professional services as well. Among the first such services was that provided by the funeral industry. Other professions have been affected as well. Denial of medical and dental services to those infected by HIV has been a particular problem. Institutional settings where health care is given are considered public accommodations under the law and some courts have interpreted this to include doctors' and dentists' offices as well as hospitals and clinics. Standard protective procedures adequately protect health care workers, and the medical as well as legal consensus is that people with AIDS should not be denied treatment.

public aid   A generic term for basic state social support services (welfare).

public assistance   See PUBLIC AID.

public health   The combined medical and social service discipline providing protection and promotion of community health through institutional and collective measures.

Public Health Service (PHS)   The federal agency charged by law to promote and assure the highest level of health attainable for every individual and family in the United States and to develop cooperation in health projects with other nations. The major functions of the service are to stimulate and assist states and communities with the development of local health resources and to further the development of education for the health professions; to assist with improvement of the delivery of health services to all Americans; to conduct and support research in the medical and related sciences and to disseminate scientific information; to protect the health of the nation against impure and unsafe foods, drugs, cosmetics, and other potential hazards; and to provide national leadership for the prevention and control of communicable disease and for other public health functions. The PHS has its origin in an act of July 16, 1798, authorizing marine hospitals for the care of U.S. merchant seamen. Subsequent legislation has vastly broadened the scope of its activities. The Public Health Service Act of July 1, 1944, consolidated and revised substantially all existing legislation relating to the Public Health Service. The basic PHS legal responsibilities have been broadened and expanded many times since 1944.

Public Health Service Act   Legislation signed by the president July 1, 1944, and administered by the FOOD AND DRUG ADMINISTRATION (FDA). The act gives the FDA authority to ensure safety, purity, and potency of vaccines, blood, serum, and other biological products. It also empowers the FDA to ensure the safety of pasteurized milk and shellfish, as well as the sanitation of food services and sanitary facilities for travelers on buses, trains, and planes. See also FOOD AND DRUG ACT OF 1906.

Public Health Service Act, Title VI   The section of the PUBLIC HEALTH SERVICE ACT, which, with title XVI of that act, authorizes and sets forth the requirements of the federal HILL-BURTON program.

Public Law 92–603   The 1972 federal statute that created Supplemental Security Income (SSI) and introduced a set of complex state options, some with burdensome antirecipient biases, to the system. Up until 1972, everything was relatively simple: Everyone on Aid to Families with Dependent Children (AFDC) and the old state welfare programs for the aged, blind, and disabled got automatic Medicaid cards. About half of the states also covered the "medically needy": AFDC-type families and aged, blind, and disabled people who started out "too rich" for welfare but whose medical bills "spent them down" to the Medicaid level. The changes made by P.L. 92–603, and the wide range of state options exercised under its provisions, introduced what are often described as even more Byzantine complexities into the welfare system. Highlights of 92–603 follow.

As a result of the addition of Title XVI (SSI) to the Social Security Act, states were required to allow Medicaid eligibility for SSI recipients but not necessarily automatically. Section 1634 of the amended act provided for state-SSA contracts for "automatic" Medicaid for SSI recipients, but only at state option. Section 209(B) of the law allowed states to retain some or all of the stricter Medicaid eligibility rules from their pre-SSI welfare programs. This "loophole" was added to save the poorer, less liberal states from the sudden Medicaid budget increases that would result if they had to give Medicaid to all those newly eligible under the more liberal SSI rules. However, Congress provided a "sop" to the recipients in states that take this option: If the state did not already have a "spend down" rule for those "too rich" for Medicaid, it had to allow one if it took this "209(b)" option. Finally, Section 1616 of the amended act allowed states to give higher incomes to their needy aged, blind, and disabled by having the SSA simultaneously pay out "State Supplementary Payments (SSPs)" as part of, and on top of, the SSI payment. Thus, state-financed SSPs could, in effect, "raise" the SSI (and, therefore, the Medicaid) level in those liberal states wishing to be more generous. This feature was made optional for the states.

pulmonary alveolar proteinosis   A disease of unknown cause in which EOSINOPHILIC material is deposited in the alveoli. Principal symptom is DYSPNEA. Death from pulmonary insufficiency may occur, but complete recovery has been observed. There is no specific treatment, but general supportive measures, including ANTIBIOTICS and BRONCHOALVEALOR LAVAGE have helped.

puncture wound   A wound made by piercing with a sharp instrument.

purified protein derivative   A protein-rich material derived from the MICROORGANISM M. *tuberculosis* and used as a skin-test reagent to detect current or prior infection with that organism.

purified protein derivative (PPD) test   A simple data test used to detect prior exposure to TUBERCULOSIS. PPD is injected under the skin of the forearm. After 48 to 72 hours, the injection site will exhibit a hard red bump if the subject has been infected with TB.

purine   A white, crystalline compound from which a group of compounds including uric acid, xanthine, and caffeine is derived. Also, one of several purine derivatives, especially the bases adenine and guanine, which are fundamental constituents of nucleic acids.

purpura   A skin rash of purple or brownish red spots resulting from the bleeding into the skin of subcutaneous capillaries.

PWA   The abbreviation for with AIDS. This label was devised to eliminate the moralizing character of the everyday discourse of AIDS, as in terms such as "AIDS patient," "AIDS victim," "innocent victim," "invariably fatal" and "promiscuous." PWARC and PWHIV have been used as abbreviations, respectively, for Persons with AIDS-related complex (once known as "pre-AIDS") and persons with HIV infection. See also PEOPLE WITH AIDS.

PWARC   See PWA.

pyelonephritis   Inflammation of kidney substance and pelvis, usually due to bacteria that have ascended from the bladder after entering through the urethra. Treatment generally begins with the recognition and removal of the cause substance; and includes measures to increase resistance of patient and bedrest. Alcohol and drugs irritating to the kidney should be avoided. Antipyretic drugs and an appropriate antibiotic are often administered. If there is urinary tract obstruction, surgery may be indicated. See NEPHRITIS.

pyrazinamide   An ANTIBIOTIC used in multidrug combinations to treat TUBERCULOSIS.

pyridoxine hydrochloride   One of a group of substances, including pyridoxal and pyridoxamine, that make up vitamin B_6. Trade names are Hexa-Betalin and Seesix.

pyrimethamine   An ANTIBIOTIC used to treat TOXOPLASMOSIS, usually in combination with a sulfa drug such as SULFADIAZINE or CLINDAMYCIN. The major side effect after prolonged use is ANEMIA. Other side effects include gastric intolerance, allergic reactions, and HEPATITIS, some of which are attributable to the sulfa drug that is taken with it. To avoid anemia, another drug, leucovorin, is given at the same time.

Pyrimethamine is a FOLIC-ACID antagonist that interferes with the uptake of this essential B vitamin in susceptible parasites, including those that cause malaria and toxoplasmosis, thus weakening and eventually killing these organisms. Because parasites can rapidly develop resistance to pyrimethamine, the drug is usually used in combination with a sulfa drug. The activity of the combination against parasites greatly exceeds that of either drug used alone. FOLINIC ACID is usually added to protect against BONE-MARROW toxicity. Because both drugs cross the BLOOD-BRAIN BARRIER, the combination is effective against toxoplasmosis encephalitis, a serious and potentially fatal infection of the brain. While the response to therapy is high, the relapse rate is also high when therapy is stopped, so lifelong maintenance is usually necessary. Pyrimethamine is also used alone and in combination with other drugs to prevent malaria or recurrent toxoplasmosis. Pyrimethamine is available for oral administration under the trade name Daraprim. The combination of pyrimethamine and sulfadoxine is sold under the trade name Fansidar.

pyrogen   A substance that is released either endogenously from LEUKOCYTEs or exogenously; usually from bacteria. It produces fever in susceptible hosts.

QC-PCR (quantitative competitive PCR) Method of quantitative PCR (polymerase chain reaction). In QC-PCR, a tiny amount of a control sequence, similar to the DNA sequence being tested, is added to the sample before the PCR process begins. During the successive doublings, both the target sequence (the one being looked for) and the control sequence are multiplied similarly. The quantity of the target sequence in the original sample is calculated from its ratio with the control sequence. This is more accurate than measuring the total amount of the target sequence since the inevitable errors in the doubling process equally affect the target sequence and the control sequence. Because QC-PCR is labor intensive and difficult to do, it is not available for routine medical use. It is used in CLINICAL trials, and serves as a "gold standard" by which other tests can be measured. See POLYMERASE CHAIN REACTION.

quack One who pretends to have knowledge or skill in medicine. One of the social consequences of the AIDS epidemic has been the rise in quackery in general, hardly a surprise when one considers the exploitative and sensational media coverage of the epidemic, its size and cost, the politics of medical research and funding, and the relationship between money and expertise.

quality of care In social-service terms, the impact of medical, psychological, or social support care on quality of life. Most analyses focus on medical treatment and use scales that measure changes in various indicators of health status (individual comfort, mobility, etc.). Well-known scales include the Karnofsy Index, Sickness Impact Profile, Symptom Distress Scale, Spitzer Quality of Life Index, McMaster Health Index, and Nottingham Health Profiles. Each of these has its own criteria for types of care, health status, and how different aspects of care are compared and weighed.

quality of life A subjective concept that differs for each person and may vary for the same individual as that person's situation changes. The holistic treatment of a patient requires that the health care team assess what is most important to that individual. In persons with certain diseases, it may not be possible to establish and maintain complete freedom from the signs and symptoms of the disease.

In these cases, the goal is to have quality of life be as good as possible despite the disease. In persons who have suffered disabilities, the goal is to have perceived quality of life associated with remaining capabilities rather than on what has been lost.

The Medical Outcome Study (MOS) is an example of a reliable quality of life measure for persons with HIV infection and AIDS. The basis for the MOS analysis is a questionnaire in which patients rate their perception of 20 criteria, including physical, social, and mental functioning; health perceptions; and pain. The scale is especially sensitive to symptoms associated with HIV and AIDS.

quarantine A state of physical isolation or restriction of movement imposed on carriers or potential carriers to prevent or control the spread of an infectious disease. Also, the period during which such isolation is imposed.

The possibility of quarantine has from time to time been raised by authorities, religious fundamentalists, or others as a way of restricting the spread of AIDS. Quarantine, probably the oldest public health measure, developed from concepts of spiritual uncleanliness. In the Middle Ages it was used against those suffering from either leprosy or the plague, and quarantine of lepers persisted well into the 20th century. Certain diseases are still regarded as potentially quarantinable, but it is a measure most often used to contain animal diseases. Proposals to quarantine AIDS patients or homosexual establishments such as gay bathhouses and bars have occasionally been put forward. Fear, prejudice, and ignorance about the spread of the disease are generally considered to be at their root.

Those who argue in favor of AIDS quarantine generally focus on what they call "noncompliance," the failure or refusal of those who have the virus to refrain from repeating activity that risks its further spread. The examples most often cited are the PROSTITUTE who knows that he or she is HIV-positive and who won't stop turning tricks; the promiscuous individual who knows that he or she is HIV-positive and who, out of recklessness or viciousness, refuses to stop having unprotected sex; the INTRAVENOUS drug user who continues to share needles even after being told of an HIV-positive status and of the consequences of further needle sharing.

queer Homosexual. In the early 20th century this was a derogatory term applied to male homosexuals only. In more recent usage it also applies to lesbians. Today, many gay men and lesbians, consciously refusing the implied condemnation, use the term to describe and identify themselves and their community.

The people and communities characterized as "queer" (like all other people and communities) are too diverse politically, economically, and demographically to be described adequately by a single reductive adjective. Nevertheless, in an age of identity politics, *queer* serves as an expedient term to define oneself or one's community in opposition to others, in this case the "straight" or the "mainstream".

quinone Important small hydrophobic components of the electron transport chain. Quinones carry the equivalent amount of electrons of a hydrogen atom. By alternating electron transfer between components that carry or do not carry a proton with the electron, protons can be moved across the membrane, setting up proton gradients. Most quinone molecules are not attached to proteins and diffuse rapidly in the plane of the membrane.

R

race/ethnicity   For much of the first decade of the AIDS epidemic, the source and transmission of AIDS was attributed to black people, and specifically Africans. Later people of other races and ethnicities, such as Haitians and West Indians, were added to this hypothesis. This hypothesis was a form of scapegoating and resembles an earlier hypothesis that emerged when AIDS first appeared among white American homosexuals who became the obvious scapegoat. Given the racist stereotyping of black people as dirty, disease carrying, and sexually promiscuous, it was virtually inevitable that, on the first sighting of the disease among them, they would be associated with its source. Thus the "gay plague" changed overnight to the "Haitian disease." Although the Haitian hypothesis collapsed, the idea of black people as the source of AIDS was not abandoned. Attention shifted to the African continent itself, and medical scientists and journalists escalated their search for the origin of AIDS in Africa. Today our knowledge of the disease makes it clear that preconceptions and prejudices about Africa and Africans, coupled with assumptions about Western conditions and behavior, fueled the widespread, uncritical acceptance of the AIDS-from-Africa hypothesis by the normally skeptical scientific community, the media, and the public at large.

racial differences   Today we have a relatively clear definition of the epidemiology of AIDS in most countries of the world. As the picture of AIDS becomes more clearly defined, the numbers continue to grow and change, and patterns emerge. The numbers show that there are widely variant patterns of HIV infection existing in the same population, as well as in different populations. Race may, and most likely does, influence an individual's experience of AIDS, but race in and of itself is not a risk factor for HIV infection or AIDS. On the other hand, the effects of infection on specific racial groups often varies for genetic and social reasons from the effects of infection on other groups.

radiation-resistant HIV expression in vivo (R-HEV)   A technique used in viral research since the 1960s, but until 1989 had not been previously applied to HIV. It consists of viral cultures on cells that have been treated with radiation. The goal is to measure the HIV expression levels of the patient's virus, following the theory that radiation will suppress cells carrying HIV but not express itself (radiation) in the patient.

Ordinary viral cultures are unreliable as a measure of disease progression. Part of the reason is that the latent virus, which is not causing any immediate problem, can be stimulated to become active by the culturing process itself, causing a positive result that does not reflect disease progression or poor prognosis for the patient.

In the R-HEV test, the radiation treatment causes the cells to die shortly after the time culturing begins. If the virus was latent at the time the blood was drawn from the patient, the cells containing the latent virus die without being able to infect cells in the culture medium. But if the virus was active in the patient, some of the infected cells will transmit the infection to cells in the culture medium. Eight separate wells are cultured for each test; the result reported by the R-HEV test is the percentage of wells which do grow the virus.

When it was announced, the R-HEV test promised to have great importance in speeding CLINICAL TRIALs of new AIDS drugs.

radiation therapy   Treatment of cancer with intense beams of radiation. The radiation actually kills cancer cells (and any cells it must pass through to get to cancer cells). Also, the branch of medicine that utilizes such treatment.

radiography   The making of images of the internal structures of the body through exposure to X radiation that acts on a sensitized film.

radioimmunoassay (RIA)   A very sensitive method of determining the concentration of substances, particularly the protein-bound HORMONES, in blood plasma. The procedure is based on the competitive inhibition or binding of radioactively labeled hormones to a specific ANTIBODY. It can also be used to determine the concentration of any substance that causes the production of a specific antibody or of antibodies themselves.

radioimmunoprecipitation (RIP)   Immunoprecipitation is the formation of a precipitate (a deposit separated from a suspension or solution by the reaction of a reagent that causes the deposit to fall to the bottom or float near the top) when an ANTIGEN and ANTIBODY interact.

radioimmunoprecipitation assay (RIPA) A technically demanding method of HIV ANTIBODY testing used primarily in research. The virus is detected by the phenomenon of aggregation of sensitized ANTIGEN upon addition of specific antibody to antigen in solution (immunoprecipitation). The precipitate is then washed extensively and disrupted and distributed through a polyacrylamide gel. Antibody-antigen bands are detected by autoradiography. Autoradiography is the use of radiographs formed by radioactive materials present in the tissue or individual in investigating certain diseases. These "autoradiographs" are made possible by injecting radiochemicals into the tissue and then exposing X-ray film by placing the tissue adjacent to the film.

radiotherapy See RADIATION THERAPY.

random controlled trial An experimental study for assessing the effects of a particular variable, in which subjects are assigned on a random basis to either of two groups, experimental or control. The experimental group receives the drug or procedure being tested, while the control group does not. Laboratory tests or clinical evaluations are performed on both groups (usually using the double-blind technique) to determine the results.

randomization In research, a method used to assign subjects to experimental groups. Prior to this step every attempt is made to ensure that the subjects are as equivalent as possible. Then by some random method, each individual in the study is assigned to either a treatment or nontreatment group. The purpose is to prevent inadvertent selection bias in research studies.

randomized Pertaining to a study in which participants are selected randomly to receive either the treatment being studied or a PLACEBO. See RANDOMIZATION.

randomized controlled trials See RANDOM CONTROLLED TRIAL.

randomized trial See RANDOM CONTROLLED TRIAL.

rape The coerced or forced participation in sexual acts.

rapid plasma reagin A nontreponemal serological test for detection of syphilis, the basis of which is agglutination. Unlike treponemal tests that look for *Treponema pallidum*, the corkscrew-shaped organism that causes the disease, nontreponemal tests give passive evidence of the presence of the disease.

rapid screening trial A pre-trial clinical trial. In 1989, AIDS treatment activists and government and academic statisticians joined forces in order to improve the design of CLINICAL TRIALs. They sought to develop a new kind of eight- to 15-week clinical trial to compare and prioritize new drugs that successfully complete PHASE I (early dosage and

toxicity studies). The winners from the rapid screening process would then immediately enter into larger trials designed to lead to drug approval. The impetus for the new system was that dozens of potential AIDS ANTIVIRALs were coming out of laboratories, and there was no way all could receive the full-scale clinical trials required to convince the Food and Drug Administration that the drugs were good enough for general use. Even if more money were available, it was argued that there were not enough experienced scientists, research nurses, or patients meeting entry criteria, to run so many large trials. The proposed new system was designed to speed the development of brand new therapies by quickly screening all the promising drugs, so that the more successful ones quickly could be moved into larger, definitive trials.

This drug-screening system was designed to test several different drugs at one time. Every approved volunteer randomly was offered one of the currently available drugs to take for a short period of time (about 12 weeks). Improved T-helper counts were the primary measure of efficacy. The drugs then would be compared to pick out those few that stood out from the others. They might then be made available for early access through a system like parallel track. Clinical trials experts reason that most proposed drugs do not work, so they will in effect become the placebo. The trials are kept short, probably two or three months, to avoid exposing participants to ineffective drugs for long. In some cases, a placebo or no-treatment arm might be acceptable in these trials. Since many drugs would be tested, patients would have only a small chance of receiving no treatment. Persons who were not critically ill might be willing to risk entering a no-treatment arm for two or three months.

One of the main concerns about the proposed trials is that some drugs may be valuable but not show benefits early. It is suspected that pharmaceutical companies might be afraid their products will be rejected too early. Designers argue that any drug showing potential will be followed up; the screening trials were designed to help set priorities, not to kill drugs that have other evidence in their favor.

Advantages of the concept include the fact that a screening trial would identify early activity in a high-quality study before PHASE II TRIALs begin. It would provide information to support prioritization decisions for phase II trials, give the earlier definition of a drug's efficacy, and provide much useful information to phase II trial designers. The system would also allow combination therapies to be tested as easily as single drugs. The single study would cost less than multiple small trials. The trials could easily find volunteers, both because of the short time commitment required and because it would be easier to publicize one trial than many separate ones.

Limitations and problems of the new system include the lack of long-term data, the possibility that entry and safety criteria unique to one drug might have to be applied to others to allow randomization, and the fact that the trial only identifies winners according to the criteria of early T-cell count increases, meaning that a better drug that takes longer to be effective might be missed. The question of whether drug companies would be willing to compete with other companies in terms of AIDS-related drug production and to support the program was also raised. Some scientists questioned whether or not there were enough new promising drugs that a screening system was even needed; some researchers even said that they do not know what drugs to test. It was noted that there were many scientifically promising compounds; the problem was in getting them through the pre-clinical development required for the all-important IND (Investigational New Drug approval) and then through the early phase I human test. Overall, the new proposal for screening trials did not solve this problem.

rash   A general term applied to any eruption of the skin, especially those associated with communicable diseases. Rashes are usually temporary. They are usually a shade of red, which varies with disease.

raw food   Virtually all organisms that might be present in food and that can cause infections are easily killed by even brief exposure to heat, so cooking generally eliminates any danger. Persons whose immune systems are compromised, however (especially if their CD4+ counts are below 150), are particularly advised to follow safety guidelines to avoid food-borne infections, which can cause severe diarrhea and vomiting and can be difficult to treat. Even the commonest, mildest types of "food poisoning" can be dangerous for people with HIV. Because toxic drugs are necessary to treat many infections, everything possible should be done to prevent them in the first place.

Guidelines: avoid red meat, undercooked eggs, and raw seafood, all of which can contain parasites or bacteria, as well as raw egg yolks, which can contain salmonella. Raw fruits or vegetables should be peeled or dipped in boiling water for five seconds. Cheese that has not been pasteurized (aged, ripened cheeses such as Brie, bleu, and feta) should be avoided. Uncooked root vegetables, such as radishes and carrots, that grow in the soil, as well as other salad vegetables, may be used if they are either peeled and rinsed in purified water, steamed for two minutes, or dipped in boiling water for five seconds. Vegetables with thick skins should be peeled and rinsed with purified water. Apples and pears may be eaten raw if peeled and rinsed. Bananas, oranges, and grapefruits are safe when peeled. The bottom line with raw food is: boil it, cook it, peel it, or forget it.

reagent   A substance used in a chemical reaction to detect, analyze, measure, or produce other substances. In virology, strains of HIV are reagents. The term may also be used to refer to the subject of a psychological experiment, especially one reacting to a stimulus.

rear entry   Intromission from behind. See COITUS.

reasonable charge   An allowable charge, under a health insurance policy or program, especially MEDICARE and MEDICAID.

receptive anal intercourse   Sexual intercourse in which an individual allows the insertion of a penis into his or her anus. This is a high-risk mode of transmission for the HUMAN IMMUNODEFICIENCY VIRUS. Also called *passive anal intercourse*.

receptor   In pharmacology, a cell component that combines with a drug, hormone, or chemical mediator to alter the function of the cell. In neurology, a sensory nerve ending.

recombinant   Produced by laboratory or industrial cultures of genetically engineered living cells. The cells' genes have been altered to give them the capability of producing large quantities of the desired compound for use as a medical treatment. Recombinant compounds are often versions of naturally occurring substances.

recombinant DNA   DNA prepared through laboratory manipulation in which genes from an organism of one species are transplanted or spliced to an organism of another species. When the host's genetic material is reproduced, the transplanted genetic material is also copied. This technique permits isolating and examining the properties and action of specific genes. Studies in this area must be done in a carefully controlled environment. Levels of need for containment have been defined and are designated as P-1 for the lowest level and P-4 for the highest. The P-4 level is for experiments involving animal virus DNA that contains potentially lethal genes. Experiments using DNA from pathogenic organisms, cancer-causing viruses, and viruses associated with certain toxins are prohibited in the United States.

recovery (from addiction)   The process of overcoming physical and psychological dependence on a psychoactive substance. This generally includes a period of abstinence and treatment, the return of physical and emotional health, and a commitment to sobriety. Real recovery requires such a commitment and a willingness to work at it—as the expression goes, "one day at a time."

rectal   Pertaining to the rectum.

rectal douche   A cleansing current or stream of water directed against the rectum. It may or may not be medicated.

rectal mucosa   The mucous membrane that lines the rectum.

rectum   The end of the intestines that is located between the sigmoid flexure (colon) and the anal canal. Bowel movements or stools are passed through the rectum.

red-baiting   The practice of attacking as politically radical or Communist. Such attacks are usually made against politically dissenting, nonconformist, or simply unpopular people or groups and are meant to stigmatize or demonize them or distract attention from the substance of their criticism of the social status quo.

red blood cell   See ERYTHROCYTE.

red blood corpuscle   See ERYTHROCYTE.

red tape   A popular expression for (presumably excessive or silly) bureaucratic routines that must be performed before an official action can be taken. Within the context of AIDS, such routines have been protested as endangering those who are ill by complicating or delaying urgently needed research, health care delivery, and political action.

red tape protest   See RED TAPE.

referral numbers   Telephone and/or fax numbers that direct a person to someone or for something. Within the context of AIDS, referral may be made to national, state, or local HIV/AIDS prevention, treatment, or information services. Nationwide resource groups can be useful in locating or double-checking state or local resources. Referral numbers may also lead to publications published especially for people living with HIV.

refractory   Severe and resistant to treatment.

regimen   A systematic program, or routine, as in a course of treatment or a diet.

Rehabilitation Act of 1973   More popularly referred to as Section 504, the Rehabilitation Act of 1973 requires that any program or activity that receives federal monies cannot deny access to a handicapped person. Included in its definition of handicapped are hearing, sight, and speech impairments; cancer; heart disease and diabetes; cerebral palsy; epilepsy; mental illness and retardation; muscular dystrophy; multiple sclerosis; AIDS; and drug addiction and alcoholism. Section 504 has pervasive legal ramifications because almost every aspect of daily life receives some form of federal aid.

reinfection   A possible additional "super" infection with a second strain of HIV some time after initial infection. While there is little evidence to document such a phenomenon, there is evidence that two strains of HIV can circulate simultaneously ("coinfection"). Whether there is a serious risk of reinfection for couples in which both partners are HIV positive is unknown. Aside from HIV, however, such couples have more immediately to worry about other infectious agents with the potential to affect HIV activation and replication.

Reiter's syndrome   A condition in which urethritis, arthritis, and conjunctivitis appear together, for the most part in young men. Urethritis usually appears first, but arthritis constitutes the dominant feature. The syndrome is of unknown origin and generally runs a self-limited but relapsing course.

relapse   A return to a previously worse condition of illness, after a period of recovery. In the language of addiction, relapse refers to the return to the use of alcohol or drugs after a period of abstinence or a serious attempt at recovery. A relapse can occur regardless of the length of time someone has been sober. Before returning to alcohol or drugs, the alcoholic or addict will generally exhibit an attitudinal change and emotional deterioration. Some situational changes may also signal a coming relapse. Warning signs of relapse may include: increased arguing with others for no apparent reason; decreasing or stopping 12-STEP PROGRAMS (AA, NA, etc.); returning to high-risk situations, such as socializing in a bar or returning to a drug-using environ-ment; reestablishing contacts with alcohol or drug-using friends; no longer caring about sobriety; increased negativity about life and how things are going; increased moodiness or depression; increased feelings of boredom; sudden feelings of euphoria; strong feelings of anger at oneself or another person; thinking one "deserves" alcohol or drugs after being sober for a period of time; thinking it wouldn't be harmful to substitute one drug for another; thinking that the alcohol/drug problem is "cured" due to period of sobriety.

There are a number of relapse warning signs that can help terminally ill, chemically dependent clients recognize that they are moving toward a chemical relapse and take corrective action. These include the belief that returning to the addictive use of alcohol and other drugs will make the illness more manageable or provide relief from pain; the belief that the use of previous drugs of abuse will be more effective in pain management than the use of prescription drugs; the belief that returning to alcohol or drugs will bring a quick and painless death; the belief that having a terminal illness means that there is nothing left to live for and that, therefore, alcohol and drug use is justified.

Because alcohol and drug use escalate disease progression and add pain and complications to almost any situation, staying sober is especially important to persons with HIV/AIDS. Staying sober increases the length and quality of survival time. Staying sober also gives persons with HIV/AIDS the possibility of death with dignity.

relaxation   A lessening of tension or activity; the phase or period in a single muscle-twitch following contraction, in which tension decreases, fibers lengthen, and the muscle returns to resting position. In MAGNETIC RESONANCE IMAGING (MRI), the return of an excited atom to alignment with the applied magnetic field. General relaxation refers to relaxation of the entire body and is distinct from local relaxation, which is limited to a particular muscle group or to a certain part.

remission   A period when the signs of a disease have been eliminated through treatment or the immune response. A disease may be in remission without a complete cure having been effected.

renal   Of or pertaining to the kidneys or the surrounding regions.

renal failure   Failure of the kidneys or the surrounding region. Acute renal failure may be due to trauma; any condition that impairs the flow of blood to the kidneys; certain toxic substances; bacterial toxins; glomerulonephritis; or acute obstruction of the urinary tract. Treatment includes specific therapy for the primary disease and either peritoneal dialysis or hemodialysis.

reporting requirements   See MANDATORY REPORTING; MANDATORY TESTING; PRIVACY.

reproductive counseling   The issue of reproductive choice is a most difficult and ethically charged aspect of HIV testing and counseling of women. For HIV-positive women, SERO-

STATUS is only one of many factors that influence reproductive decision-making. Others are individual, community, or religious morality or ethics regarding abortion; a desire to parent; the influence of partner, family, and friends; religious faith/optimism; risk evaluation; access to care; prior experience with HIV; maternal health concerns; cultural norms; parenting concerns; psychological adaptation to HIV; and non-HIV–related psychological issues. Counseling about reproductive options takes all these into account.

Reproductive counseling usually involves providing up-to-date information about HIV and its impact on infected women and discussing such topics as perinatal transmission, pediatric disease and assessment, and the effects of pregnancy on maternal HIV disease and on prenatal care; care of the child with HIV and plans in the event of worsening disease; and psychological support systems. Optimally, counselors should take into consideration a woman's educational level, primary language, and idiomatic or regional speech patterns. To be effective, counselors must be comfortable with the moral terrain of HIV and reproduction as well as with sexuality and drug abuse. Cultural and social or peer-group belief systems can influence the efficacy of communication.

The appropriateness of various modalities for the reproductive counseling of women also continue to be debated. For both ethical and pragmatic reasons, many care providers working with HIV-positive women espouse the generic nondirective counseling model. Here, the counselor translates medical information into personal calculations in the course of helping women to decide what is right for them and their families.

reproductive decision-making   Until fairly recently, the CENTERS FOR DISEASE CONTROL AND PREVENTION (CDC) and the American College of Obstetricians and Gynecologists (ACOG) officially recommended that HIV-positive women be discouraged from bearing children. Research has shown, however, that HIV-positive women do not differ significantly from HIV-negative women in making personal decisions regarding carrying or aborting a pregnancy. Women with HIV infection who are not overwhelmed by illness generally have the same attitudes and emotions as other women regarding childbearing.

Health care providers are generally advised to be supportive of women's rights and abilities to make informed personal decisions. An important challenge for clinicians is working with couples who wish to have a child. Couples in which only one partner is HIV-positive present an additional challenge. Support and knowledge of referrals for alternative insemination, infertility workups, and adoption agencies can assist a couple in achieving the goal of having children without practicing unsafe sex. Further, the clinician is responsible for discussing birth control choices with clients and providing the gynecological care necessary for their appropriate use.

reproductive rights   In December 1985, the CENTERS FOR DISEASE CONTROL AND PREVENTION (CDC) officially recommended that women who are HIV-positive or who have AIDS should "be advised to consider delaying pregnancy until more is known about perinatal transmission of the virus." The materials offered by the departments of health in many states go beyond that advice and recommend unequivocally that HIV-positive women should not become pregnant. Nonetheless, many infected women are having babies even when they know they are infected and have been counseled about the risks of perinatal transmission or already have a child with HIV infection or AIDS, or have lost a child to AIDS. It is generally felt that despite its gravity and consequences, HIV infection is only one of a range of conditions that can be passed from mother to fetus and should not be singled out for moral censure and coercive policies. Additionally, it is widely recognized that reproductive decisions are critical to biological and social life, and HIV-positive women must remain free to make choices that are consistent with their cultural, religious, and personal values. Given the current knowledge, there is no way to predict whether an HIV-positive woman will infect her fetus, no reliable way to determine IN UTERO or at birth whether a baby is infected (unless it is born with symptoms), and no way to foretell the likely course of the disease. This array of uncertainties is weighted very differently by public health officials and physicians and by women at risk.

reproductive system   The bodily organs and processes employed in reproduction.

research   Systematic inquiry or investigation into a subject.

research laboratories   Places where scientific research is carried on. Usually, these are affiliated with or located in government agencies, large universities, and major hospitals.

reservoir of virus   The longer-lived cells infected with HIV, such as MACROPHAGES and MONOCYTES, which continue to produce virus for weeks, functioning in effect as "reservoirs" of the virus. In contrast, an actively infected CD4 cell dies in two days. Many researchers believe that since currently available drugs do not kill infected cells, they can eliminate all of the virus from the body only if they can keep suppressing HIV replication—even in the face of mutations that confer partial resistance—for a period longer than these cells' lifetimes.

residential care facility   A live-in facility for individuals who, because of their physical, mental, or emotional condition, are not able to live independently but whose treatment does not require them to be in an in-patient facility.

residual functional capacity (RFC)   In SSA disability determinations, if a patient's medical condition does not explicitly appear in, or clearly equal, any of those in SSA's Listing of Impairments, an RFC criterion is used to assess medically his or her ability to work, taking into account the functional limitations and environmental restrictions imposed by all medically determinable impairments. The RFC method, rather than the listing, must always be used for "ARC-only" claimants. It is also sometimes relied upon for full-blown AIDS cases, as AIDS has not historically appeared in the listing.

resistance The total of all of the body's defenses against pathogens; includes non-specific barriers such as unbroken skin and specific mechanisms such as antibody production. Also, the ability of an organism to change to avoid or counteract the effects of a useful treatment. Resistance is thought to result usually from genetic mutation. In HIV, such mutations can change the structure of viral enzymes and proteins so that an antiviral drug can no longer bind well with them, thus neutralizing the effect of the drug.

Two factors are at work in allowing HIV to become resistant so quickly to many drugs. One is that when HIV inserts itself into new cells, the REVERSE TRANSCRIPTASE enzyme that makes DNA genes from the virus's RNA makes mistakes, thereby producing progeny that are slightly different from their parent cells. Many such mutations cause a new virus to be defective and others have little effect, but some allow the virus to resist the activity of therapeutic drug, since any form of the virus that survives exposure to the drug will be "selected for" and can then grow and repopulate the void left by the viruses killed by the drugs. This survival and expansion of the unaffected, or "fit," is an example of classical Darwinian evolution.

The second factor that allows HIV to produce resistant viruses quickly is the high rate at which HIV reproduces in an infected person. Over one billion virions are produced each day in an infected person. The larger the population of virus and the faster replication takes place, the faster mutant resistant virus arises and repopulates the body after the drug is applied.

At first scientists despaired over this problem, which has neutralized every effective AIDS drug over time. Now, however, it looks as though some of the drugs may serve as temporary bridges to keep people healthy until still more drugs are developed. And combinations of different drugs that attack the virus at different points in its life cycle may pack a far more potent wallop than any single drug (see PROTEASE INHIBITOR; NONNUCLEOSIDE REVERSE TRANSCRIPTASE INHIBITOR). Doctors have successfully treated tuberculosis and other diseases with such combinations for years.

Resistance detected by searching a pathogen's genetic makeup for mutations thought to confer lower susceptibility is called *genotypic resistance*. Resistance found by successfully growing laboratory cultures of the PATHOGEN in the presence of a drug is called *phenotypic resistance*. High-level resistance reduces a drug's virus-suppressing activity hundreds of times. Low-level resistance represents only a few-fold reduction in drug effectiveness. Depending on the toxicity of a drug, low-level resistance may be overcome by using higher doses.

resistant Not susceptible to the effect of a drug. See RESISTANCE.

respirator A machine that assists a patient to continue breathing by producing either intermittent or continuous positive pressure in the lungs, a process known as artificial respiration.

respiratory alkalosis A metabolic condition resulting from an excessive loss of carbon dioxide from the lungs.

respiratory burst The process by which NEUTROPHILs and MONOCYTEs kill certain microbial PATHOGENs by conversion of oxygen to toxic oxygen products.

respiratory infection An infection in the nose, pharynx, larynx, trachea, bronchi, or lungs.

respiratory syncytial virus A virus that induces formation of syncytial (of the nature of the syncytium, a multinucleated mass of protoplasm such as striated muscle fiber) masses in infected cell cultures. It is a major cause of acute respiratory disease in children.

respite care Patient care provided intermittently in an institution or at home to provide temporary relief to family members providing continuous care.

resting cell One of a large number of nondividing or "quiescent" CD4+ T CELLS, MACROPHAGEs, and other nondividing cells that harbor large quantities of HIV virus in a stable, extrachromosomal form, possibly a "primed" state ready for rapid replication upon cell activation. It is believed that these cells are probably important to the PATHOGENESIS of HIV disease.

reticulocytosis An increase in the number of reticulocytes in circulating blood. A reticulocyte is a red blood cell that contains remants of the ER, an immature stage in red blood cell formation; it indicates active erythropoiesis in red BONE MARROW and occurs after hemorrhage, during acclimatization to high altitude, and following treatment for pernicious anemia.

reticuloendothelial cell A PHAGOCYTE cell of the reticuloendothelial system. These cells are responsible for PHAGOCYTOSIS of damaged or old cells, cellular debris, foreign substances, and PATHOGENS, removing them from the circulation. Found in large concentrations in the spleen, liver, lymph nodes, and alveoli, as well as in other tissues such as the brain, blood vessels, and mucous membranes, they play a major role in the nonspecific immune response.

reticuloendothelial system Former name for the tissue macrophage system, the organs or tissues that contain MACROPHAGEs; the liver, spleen and red bone marrow.

reticulosis See RETICULOCYTOSIS.

retina The innermost layer of the eye, which receives images transmitted through the lens and is the immediate instrument of vision.

retinal detachment Separation of the inner sensory layer of the retina from the outer pigment EPITHELIUM, leading to loss of retinal function. It is usually caused by a hole or break in the inner sensory layer that permits fluid from the vitreous humor to leak under the retina and lift off the innermost layer. Blurred vision, flashes of light, vitreous floaters, and loss of visual activity are among the symptoms.

retinitis Inflammation of the retina; it is linked to CYTO-MEGALOVIRUS infection in persons with AIDS. Untreated, it can cause blindness.

retinochoroiditis An inflamed condition of the RETINA and the choroid of the eye.

retinoid Resembling a resin.

retroactive Medicaid eligibility date The date, up to three calendar months prior to the month of application, from which an applicant may be found eligible for MEDIC-AID.

Retrovir See AZIDOTHYMIDINE; ZIDOVUDINE.

retrovirus A type of virus that, when not infecting a cell, stores its genetic information on a single-stranded RNA molecule instead of the more usual double-stranded DNA. HIV is an example of a retrovirus. After a retrovirus penetrates a cell, it constructs a DNA version of its genes using a special enzyme, REVERSE TRANSCRIPTASE. This DNA then becomes part of the cell's genetic material.

There are many different kinds of retroviruses. LENTI-VIRUSES and leukoviruses, for instance, are retroviruses. HIV is the most important retrovirus to infect humans.

rev A regulatory protein produced by HIV within infected cells. Rev helps transport HIV RNA sequences from the nucleus into a cell's cytoplasm, where it directs construction of proteins for new virus particles.

rev gene The gene in the HUMAN IMMUNODEFICIENCY VIRUS that is required for viral protein RNA processing.

reverse transcriptase A viral enzyme that constructs DNA from an RNA template, an essential step in the life-cycle of a retrovirus such as HIV.

reverse transcriptase inhibitor An agent that deters or prevents RNA-directed DNA POLYMERASE. See also REVERSE TRANSCRIPTASE.

Reye's syndrome A condition first recognized in 1963, characterized by acute ENCEPHALOPATHY and fatty infiltration of the liver and possibly of the pancreas, heart, kidney, spleen, and lymph nodes. It is seen in children under 15 years of age after an acute viral infection. The mortality rate is variable, depending on severity, but may be as high as 80 percent. Symptoms include upper respiratory infection followed in about six days by pernicious nausea and vomiting and a change in mental status and HEPATOMEGALY without jaundice in 40 percent of cases.

rhesus monkey A small monkey native to India, used frequently for research purposes, especially testing the safety and efficacy of vaccines.

RIA See RADIOIMMUNOASSAY.

ribavirin A NUCLEOSIDE ANALOG approved as a treatment for RESPIRATORY SYNCYTIAL VIRUS. Ribavirin also has shown activity against hepatitis C, but its use against HIV infection is highly controversial. It is possible that it enhances the activity of ddI.

ribonucleic acid (RNA) A nucleic acid composed of ribonucleotide monomers. The base sequence of an RNA is dependent on the base sequence of a section of DNA that serves as a template for RNA synthesis (transcription). RNA controls protein synthesis in living cells and replaces DNA in certain viruses. Researchers have found that the level of HIV RNA (the genetic material of HIV) in a person's plasma is a better predictor of the risk of disease progression than the CD4+ T CELL count. Measurements of CD4+ T cells, the immune cells typically depleted during HIV infection, are routinely used as an indirect or "SURROGATE" MARKER of HIV disease progression. See also DEOXYRIBONUCLEIC ACID.

ribosome A cell organelle found in the cytoplasm; the site of protein synthesis.

ribozyme A naturally occurring RNA molecule that functions as a catalytic molecular scissors, chopping up RNA strands at selected sites. Ribozymes can be synthesized and targeted against specific RNA sequences, like antisense compounds, and have as much potential against HIV. Moreover, since ribozymes can effectively destroy many targets, according to its proponents, lower levels of drug might be needed than would be the case with antisense, and therapy could be more thorough. To date, however, chemists have not yet figured out how ribozymes can be made to reach and penetrate cells in the body.

Rickettsia A genus of MICROORGANISMs that occupies a position between viruses and bacteria. *Rickettsiae* differ from bacteria in that they are obligate parasites (they cannot survive in the free-living or parasitic mode) requiring living cells for growth, and from viruses in that they are retained by the Berkefeld filter. The Berkefeld Filter is a filter of diatomaceous earth designed to allow virus-size particles to pass through. These parasites are the causative agents of many diseases, including typhus fevers, spotted fevers, and scrub typhus, and are usually transmitted by arthropods (fleas, lice, mites, ticks), which serve as vectors.

rifabutin An oral drug approved by the FDA for preventing MYCROBACTERIUM AVIUM COMPLEX (MAC) in people with AIDS and CD4 cell counts of less than 75. Rifabutin is also used in combination with other drugs for the treatment of active MAC infection. Rifabutin seems to have fewer drug interactions than RIFAMPIN, yet like ISONIAZID (INH) can change liver enzyme production and thus alter the metabolism of Coumadin, Dilantin, Tegretol, theophylline, and the benzodiazepines (Atavin, Valium). Other possible side effects include NEUTROPENIA and eye and muscle irritation. Trade name is Mycobutin.

rifadin See RIFAMPIN.

rifampicin   See RIFAMPIN.

rifampin   An ANTIBIOTIC synthesized from RIFAMYCIN B, which is produced by fermentation of *Streptomyces mediterranei*. It is used in treating MYCOBACTERIUM TUBERCULOSIS and carriers of NEISSERIA MENINGITIS. It is administered orally. Rifampin decreases the blood levels of such common drugs as atovaquone, Coumadin, corticosteroids, cyclosporine, dapsone, digoxin, fluconazole, ketoconazole, levothyroxine, oral contraceptives, quinidine, propanolol, and theophylline. It is also called rifampicin. Trade names are Rimactane and Rifadin.

rifamycin   Any of a group of ANTIBIOTICS biosynthesized by a strain of *Streptomyces mediterranei* and effective against a broad spectrum of bacteria, including GRAM-POSITIVE cocci, MYCOBACTERIUM TUBERCULOSIS, some GRAM-NEGATIVE bacilli, and certain other mycobacteria.

right to know   One of the most controversial HIV-related legal issues is the right of medical service providers to know whether their patients or prospective patients are infected with HIV and of patients to know whether their medical service providers or prospective providers are so infected. Complicating the issue are the overlapping issues of confidentiality, testing, and the provision of professional service. Any consideration of the matter should take account of the medical/dental community's reaction to this issue, the validity of the scientific evidence of any alleged transmissions, the professional responsibility established and recommended by the professions' governing bodies, the actual risk of infection, and the role of federal and state licensing and regulatory authorities.

This issue had been simmering for some time during the first decade of the AIDS epidemic and heated up as rumors circulated that the CENTERS FOR DISEASE CONTROL AND PREVENTION (CDC) was investigating a documentable case of transmission from dentist to patient. In July 1990, the CDC confirmed that it was investigating the possibility of a transmission of HIV from a dentist with AIDS to a patient during surgery for extraction of two wisdom teeth. When speculation focused on Florida, state health officials there insisted that a confidentiality requirement prohibited them from warning the dentist's patients. Inferring that the CDC reports were of her case, the infected patient took steps to sue. Next and quite dramatically, the dentist identified himself in an emotional letter released on September 4, 1990, the day after his death. He was Dr. David J. Acer of Stuart, Florida. Less than a week later, the patient, 21-year-old Kimberly Bergalis, went public. Genetic testing later "strongly suggested" that Dr. Acer somehow infected three of his patients. Bergalis settled her claim against the dentist's insurer and against her own insurer, a dental plan that had sent her to Dr. Acer. In early June 1991, the Florida Department of Health and Rehabilitative Services announced that genetic testing by the CDC had linked two more HIV infections of Dr. Acer's patients to him.

In January 1991, the CDC was heading toward requiring mandatory testing for all health care workers. The public,

spurred by a dying Kimberly Bergalis, was feverishly pressing policymakers for harsh restrictions. Also in January 1991, the American Medical Association (AMA) and the American Dental Association (ADA) both announced new guidelines for doctors with AIDS advising HIV-infected doctors to avoid high-risk procedures without their patients' consent. In February 1991, various rights groups forced the CDC to hold a national conference to discuss the agency's policy regarding HIV-infected health care workers. A critical mass of medical workers, union leaders, public health officials, and advocates for people with AIDS opposed to mandatory testing and other restrictive policies began to form.

In April 1991, the CDC released draft guidelines recommending that doctors and dentists infected with HIV get permission from local panels of experts before continuing to perform certain operations and invasive procedures (and also that doctors and dentists should test themselves for HIV). The guidelines were less restrictive than those issued by the AMA and the ADA calling for infected health-care professionals to stop performing surgery or inform their patients.

Focusing on this issue at its annual meeting in June 1991, the American Medical Association rejected a policy endorsing mandatory HIV-antibody testing for health care workers and instead supported voluntary testing of those facing the highest risk. It also reiterated its policy that infected doctors should inform patients or refrain from doing invasive procedures. Within less than three weeks, the Academy of General Dentistry voted at its annual meeting to follow federal recommendations that dentists voluntarily take HIV-antibody tests and that those infected inform their patients. It, too, declined, however, to urge mandatory testing.

The CDC agreed. Just one day before the Academy's recommendations, the CDC released its new guidelines calling for doctors and dentists who perform procedures risking exposure to submit voluntarily to HIV-antibody tests, and that those who test positive refrain from performing such procedures until they notify prospective patients and discuss with a board of experts the conditions, if any, under which they might resume such operations. The CDC concluded that "[t]he current assumption of the risk that infected [health care workers] will transmit HIV . . . to patients during exposure-prone procedures does not support the diversion of resources" that mandatory testing would entail. The CDC then began seeking the advice of various medical groups to develop its list of "exposure-prone procedures."

In November 1991, the CDC floated a draft list containing virtually every standard surgical procedure. If adopted, this list would have effectively written into law the notion that HIV can be easily transmitted in this way—even though 10 years of the epidemic had yet to produce one case. Medical groups and AIDS advocates were invited by the CDC to Atlanta in early November to discuss its proposed list. On November 27, 1991, unable to find any support from the scientific community for its proposal, and with the threat of at least one lawsuit over its head from LAMBDA LEGAL DEFENSE AND EDUCATION FUND, the CDC jettisoned its proposal. As recommended by advocacy groups such as Lambda and public health experts around the country, it began to focus its policy efforts on proper infection control rather than mandatory testing and forced disclosure, with their potential for generating discrimination.

The case for the right of either medical/dental service providers or patients to demand testing of the other is extremely problematic. Consider, for example, the damage likely to be done to the medical/dental practices of those who adhere to the CDC recommended universal precautions, the already inadequate number of practitioners willing to treat HIV-positive patients, and the difficulty of bringing those who may have been exposed to the virus into the testing and treatment process. Many argue that strict enforcement of infection-control measures and implementation of the universal precautions recommended by the CDC would be the far better solution. See CONFIDENTIALITY; NOTIFICATION; PRIVACY.

right-wing backlash   The AIDS epidemic in the United States coincided with the politicization of religious fundamentalism that began in the late 1970s and was expressed most clearly in the growth of groups like the Moral Majority and the Christian Coalition. The spread of AIDS was linked to changes in sexual and social behavior, which in turn were part of a general shift in mores that created anxiety among those who saw their traditional values under siege and were attracted to the certainties of the religious right. It is hardly surprising that the spokespersons for the new right, already prone to cite the social acceptability of homosexuality as a sign of moral decay, were quick to seize upon AIDS as fodder for their argument. The right-wing backlash against those who suffer from AIDS and those who seek to help them has included political attacks, social stigmatization, cultural paranoia, the fear of "bad blood," documented breaches of confidentiality, calls for quarantine, discrimination and increased surveillance, and the promotion of a general attitude of moralistic hostility and punitiveness.

Rimactane   See RIFAMPIN.

ringworm   A popular term for a dermatomycosis caused by various species of fungi belonging to the genera *Microsporum* and *Trichophyton*. Red-ringed patches of vesicles, itching, pain and scaling of the skin are symptoms.

RIPA   See RADIOIMMUNOPRECIPITATION ASSAY.

ripoff   A theft, cheat, or swindle, also a person who rips off another. Responding to the surge of interest in thymic peptide drugs in the early 1990s, several groups have made various thymic products available through underground channels. Many AIDS BUYERS' CLUBS are ethical and responsible community organizations helping ailing people obtain lifesaving medication. However, there are always some blatant profiteers. Exaggerated claims of efficacy and high prices for any underground drugs are usually indicative of "thymo-ripoffs." To protect against being ripped off when buying an underground drug, find out who is selling the medication, how it has been priced, and who produced it and is ultimately responsible for it.

risk   The possibility of developing a disease or experiencing an injury. Attributable risks are those that can be attributed to known risk factors and may be estimated based on studies of factual evidence. Relative risks are those that are likely because of exposure to a PATHOGEN or injury-causing circumstances that would have been unlikely without such exposure.

risk assessment   A personal risk assessment for AIDS requires willingness to think and talk about HIV and AIDS honestly and openly. A good start would be to answer a set of questions pertaining to sex, drugs, and other common risks. If a person answers yes to any of these questions, then he or she has some risk of exposure to the HIV virus. The more yes answers, the greater the risk.

- Have you ever had unprotected sex (anal, vaginal, or oral) with anyone you know has AIDS or has tested positive for HIV?
- Have you had unprotected sex (anal, vaginal, or oral) with anyone without knowing about his or her past sexual behavior?
- Have you had unprotected sex (anal, vaginal, or oral) with anyone who has been in prison or jail?
- Have you had multiple sex partners?
- Have you had a sexual partner who has or has had other sexual partners?
- Have you ever given or received sex for money?
- Have you had one or more sexually transmitted diseases?
- Have you had sex with a partner who has had VD more than once?
- Have you ever been talked into doing sexual things you did not want to do?
- Have you had unprotected sex (anal, vaginal, or oral) with anyone who injects or has injected drugs?
- Have you or any of your sexual partners shared needles or works to shoot drugs or for any other purpose?
- Have you ever traded or given sex for drugs?
- Have you ever had sex with a new friend or stranger after doing drugs?
- Have you had sex with someone who has had sex with other people who shoot drugs with needles?
- Have you used needles or syringes that had been used by anyone before?
- Have you ever shared needles with someone who was infected?
- Have you ever had sex with someone who shared needles?
- Have you ever used alcohol or drugs to feel good in or about a social setting?
- Have you used a needle to take drugs?
- Have you used the same needle as a friend, spouse, lover or someone else to inject drugs, take vitamins or medicine, make tattoos, or do ear or body piercing?

- Have you ever shared a needle with anyone who has gotten AIDS or is HIV-positive?
- Did you or any of your sexual partners receive treatment for hemophilia between 1978 and 1985?
- Did you or any of your sexual partners have a blood transfusion or organ transplant between 1978 and 1985?

risk behaviors   Activities that may entail the risk of exposure to a PATHOGEN, or an injury. In the case of HIV/AIDs, risk behaviors are generally thought to include receipt of blood products (1978 through 1985); INTRAVENOUS DRUG use (since 1978); homosexual/bisexual activity (since 1978, predominantly males); prostitution (male and female, since 1978); and sex with a partner who participates in any of the above. In the late 1970s and early 1980s, the Centers for Disease Control and others believed that behaviors associated with "the gay lifestyle" were responsible for bringing people into contact with the virus. Among the factors considered were AMYL NITRATE "poppers," rogue genes, repeated bouts of common sexually transmitted diseases, and too much sex.

risk factor   Environmental, chemical, psychological, physiological, or genetic factors thought to create a predisposition to a particular disease or condition. The major risk factors for HIV infection are needle-sharing with INTRAVENOUS DRUG USERS and sexual contact with a person who has or may have been exposed to HIV. Another risk factor is having received blood products between 1978, when HIV infection is first known to have existed in the United States, and May 1985, when the blood supply was first screened for HIV. Other risk factors include promiscuous or casual sexual contact without precautions and being born to an HIV-infected woman. A NEEDLESTICK injury in the course of caring for people with HIV infection or AIDS is a minor risk factor. It is possible for people with HIV infection to have no clearly defined risk factor; in such cases the patients may have provided inadequate or suspect information.

risk group   An epidemiological concept referring to a group of people sharing a common behavior or characteristic placing them at greater risk for contracting a particular disease or developing a particular condition than the general population. In the case of AIDS, the syndrome was first identified in gay men, leading the Centers for Disease Control and others to speculate on the possibility that something they termed the "gay lifestyle" might itself be responsible for the condition. The discovery in late 1981 that Haitians and IV drug users were also affected by the syndrome did not support this theory, and a virus became the main suspect. The risk group concept was useful for public health, preventive purposes in the early years of the epidemic. In the media and in political debate, the epidemiological category of risk group has been used to stereotype and stigmatize people already seen as outside the moral and economic parameters of the "general population."

risk practice   This concept, that has replaced RISK GROUP for all but surveillance purposes by the National Academy of Sciences, shifts the emphasis away from characterizing and stigmatizing people as members of groups.

risk reduction   Process by which an individual changes behavior to decrease the likelihood of acquiring an infection.

Ritalin   See METHYLPHENIDATE.

ritonavir   A PROTEASE INHIBITOR that has produced drops in HIV VIRAL LOAD of greater than 99 percent in some people. Ritonavir has proved to be a relatively safe compound, but the liquid formulation has a taste that many people find intolerable, and there are frequent reports of nausea and vomiting. An encapsulated version is now available. There is a long list of drugs incompatible with ritonavir due to its impairment of liver metabolism. These include the analgesics codeine, Demerol, and Darvon; rifabutin; the antifungals ketoconazole and fluconazole; the protease inhibitor Invirase (saquinavir); the antiulcer medication Tagamet; and various psychotropic agents such as Paxil, Xanax, Valium and Halcion.

RNA   See RIBONUCLEIC ACID.

Robimycin   See ERYTHROMYCIN.

Robomox   See AMOXICILLIN.

route of administration   See ADMINISTRATION.

route of transmission   See TRANSMISSION.

routine testing   Systematic testing of everyone in a particular class (for instance, all pregnant women or all men over age 40) for a given disease or condition.

roxithromycin   A macrolide ANTIBIOTIC, like CLARITHROMYCIN and AZITHROMYCIN, being developed for use against CRYPTOSPORIDIOSIS and other bacterial infections.

rubber dam   A thin rubber tissue used by dentists to seal off a tooth from saliva during dental treatment. See DENTAL DAM.

rubber   See CONDOM.

rush   A strong contraction wave that moves down the small intestine; the first surge of pleasure produced by a drug, especially a narcotic drug. See also AMYL NITRITE inhalant and BUTYL NITRITE INHALANT.

Ryan White CARE Act   See RYAN WHITE COMPREHENSIVE AIDS RESOURCES EMERGENCY (CARE) ACT OF 1990.

Ryan White Comprehensive AIDS Resources Emergency (CARE) Act of 1990   An act that amends the Public Health Service Act, the Ryan White Comprehensive AIDS Resources Emergency Act provides emergency assistance to localities that are disproportionately affected by the Human Immunodeficiency Virus epidemic and makes financial assistance available to states and other public or private nonprofit entities to provide for the development, organization, coordination, and operation of more effective and cost-efficient systems for the delivery of essential services to individuals and families with HIV disease.

Ryan White National Fund   Founded in 1986 and named after a young victim of AIDS who died amid great public notice in 1990, this organization seeks to assist seriously ill children, particularly those with AIDS. It provides emergency financial aid, counseling, referral and placement services, promotes research, operates clinics, maintains a speakers' bureau, compiles statistics, and conducts education and awareness programs.

S & M   Also written S/M, SM, and S-M, this is a slang term for sadism and masochism, or slave/master. See SADO-MASOCHISM.

sadism   Sexual behavior in which participants obtain erotic enjoyment from inflicting physical or psychological pain on their partner or partners.

sadomasochism   Sexual behavior in which erotic enjoyment is obtained by giving or receiving physical or psychological pain. Alternate terms include S/M, S-M, S & M, B/D, D/S, and English.

sadomasochism safety   For those who practice what has been called "politically incorrect" sex—fantasy and role playing, bondage and discipline, fetishes, alternate gender identities, and especially SADOMASOCHISM (S/M)—there are now safety manuals available. These guides emphasize health and hygiene as well as emotional and psychological safety. Because many types of physical problems or injuries can arise from "doing scenes," S/M first aid has received particular attention in the age of AIDS. The consequences of anal, rectal, and vaginal problems; bleeding, abrasion, infection, or bruises; burns; fainting, dizziness, and nausea; muscle strains and nerve irritations; and broken bones and head trauma take on an entirely different dimension when one or both partners are HIV-positive or have AIDS. In addition to safety manuals, local S/M support groups also offer safe sex information. National groups, some mixed-gender, some not, can also be tapped for information or referrals to local support groups. These groups generally encourage practices that are safe, "sane," and consensual.

safe sex   Sex practices in which participants protect themselves from viral transmission. Generally, safe sex is sex in which there is no mucous membrane contact or bodily fluid (SEMEN, vaginal fluids, blood, etc.) exchange between partners. Safe sex protects from HIV as well as other sexually transmitted diseases like GONORRHEA, SYPHILIS, and CHLAMYDIA. Unfortunately, protection can never be absolute; the only absolutely safe sexual practices are celibacy and MASTURBATION. Aside from those, the best way to avoid HIV infection is to have only one sex partner who you know is not infected.

It is impossible to create an exhaustive list of sex acts and assign each a relative risk of infection with HIV. It is best to be consistent about following overall safe sex guidelines that combine precautions based on both what is known to be true and what seems reasonable based on today's state of knowledge. Some basic principles of safe sex are highlighted below.

The use of latex CONDOMS is highly recommended for protection when engaging in sexual activities that could result in the exchange of body fluids. Lambskin and other natural membrane products are not as good as latex and may allow HIV to pass through. The use of spermicidal (sperm-killing) lubricants, especially those with NONOXYNOL-9, may increase protection; but they should always be used with a condom and never instead of a condom. Many condoms are prelubricated, some with SPERMICIDES.

If neither partner has clinical or laboratory evidence of AIDS, each may safely engage in intimate sexual activities with the other, using condoms, provided that neither has outside sexual partners or other risk factors for AIDS. If both partners have evidence of infection with HIV, effective birth control measures should be employed. Any heterosexual person having casual sexual contacts should avoid anal intercourse and should use condoms. Homosexual men engaging in casual sexual activity should also avoid anal intercourse and should use condoms for all other sexual activities in which ejaculation might lead to semen's contacting the skin or mucosa of the partner.

It is also important to realize that a single negative laboratory test for AIDS may provide a false sense of security, and that the time required for AIDS to develop after infection may be years.

safe sex and bad sex   See BAD SEX.

safe sex and good sex   See BAD SEX.

safer sex   A term sometimes preferred to "safe sex," because it does not imply that sexual contact can be made 100 percent safe. The term recognizes the likelihood of human error and the inexactness of human knowledge.

Latex or plastic barriers for oral and anal-oral sex between lesbians are often recommended by safer sex educators. These educators note that lesbians are definitely at risk for HIV and other sexually transmitted diseases because exchange of blood and bodily fluids is often involved in lesbian sex. Viruses such as HERPES SIMPLEX and HUMAN PAPILLOMA VIRUS (which causes genital warts) can be transmitted by oral-genital contact, which is considered a medium-to-low risk on the spectrum of HIV transmission. Several different products can be used by lesbians as barriers. Unlubricated latex condoms can be cut into flat barriers by cutting off the tips and cutting through one edge of the condoms before unrolling them. DENTAL DAMS are larger then condoms and therefore easier to use as barriers. Plastic food wrap can also be used as a barrier. (Considerable debate has surrounded the microwavable vs. nonmicrowavable issue, but either is considered safe.)

safest sex   The safe sex practices with the least risk of infection with HIV or other sexually transmissible disease. Sexual ABSTINENCE and self-MASTURBATION are the safest sexual practices and the only ones that are 100 percent effective.

saliva   The clear waterlike fluid found in the mouth, secreted by the salivary and oral mucous glands, that begins the process of digesting food. Test-tube studies have suggested that a protein in saliva called SLPI (SECRETORY LEUKOCYTE PROTEASE INHIBITOR) inhibits HIV.

salivary gland infection   A viral infection of the oral cavity glands that secrete saliva.

Salk HIV-1 vaccine   A vaccine, also known as the Salk immunogen, made from inactivated HIV-1 (minus the gp120 envelope) with Incomplete Freund's Adjuvant (IFA), a mineral and oil emulsion used to increase the antigenicity of the vaccine. Polio vaccine discoverer, Jonas Salk, first proposed the idea of therapeutic vaccination for HIV-infected people in 1987. His concept involves inoculating with virus particles that have been both killed and stripped of their outer coat. The idea is to stimulate an immune response to HIV's inner protein appearing on the surface of HIV-infected cells. Researchers continue to harbor doubts about therapeutic vaccines, and Salk's colleagues who have continued research since his death have been unable to resolve these doubts.

Salk immunogen   See SALK HIV-1 VACCINE.

Salk polio vaccine   See SALK VACCINE.

Salk vaccine   The first successful poliomyelitis vaccine, it contains three types of formalin-inactivated poliomyelitis viruses and induces immunity against the disease. It was developed by Dr. Jonas Salk and first made available in 1954.

sallowness   Texture and temperature of skin are important signs of underlying causes. Sallowness is generally indicative of cachexia; syphilis; chronic gallbladder disease; arthritis deformans; constipation; some anemias; and gastric, pancreatic, enteric, or hepatic disorders. See also SKIN DISORDER; SKIN RASH.

Salmonella   A genus of GRAM-NEGATIVE BACTERIA belonging to the family Enterobacteriaceae. Over 1,400 species have been identified, some of which are pathogenic. The most common manifestation is food poisoning, ranging in severity from mild gastroenteritis to death.

salmonellosis   Any disease caused by infection with bacteria of the genus *Salmonella*. It can be manifested as gastroenteritis, septicemia, or typhoid fever.

salpingitis   Inflammation and infection of the fallopian tubes. Part of the PELVIC INFLAMMATORY DISEASE (PID) syndrome.

salvage therapy   The final possible treatment for people who are nonresponsive to or cannot tolerate other available treatments for a particular condition.

same-gender sexual behavior   See HOMOSEXUALITY or LESBIANISM.

sample   In the vocabulary of statistical analysis, a number of individuals selected from a population to test hypotheses about the population or to derive estimates of its characteristics.

San Joaquin Valley fever   See COCCIDIOIDOMYCOSIS.

Sandimmune   See CYCLOSPORINE A.

saquinavir   A PROTEASE INHIBITOR approved for use against HIV. Saquinavir acts on HIV, the virus that causes AIDS, by blocking an enzyme called PROTEINASE, which has a key role in the final phases of the replication cycle of HIV. As with other protease inhibitors, interference with the ability of the virus to be made results in the release of noninfectious virus. Side effects are relatively minor. Trade name is Invirase. For Invirase, resistance mutations emerged at a reduced rate compared to other protease inhibitors. Even without the advent of widespread resistance mutations, though, saquinavir trial participants' viral loads gradually rebounded on average after an initial small drop. It may be that the low saquinavir blood levels resulting from Invirase do not inhibit HIV enough to select for resistant strains. Saquinavir-resistant mutants can exist as minor, undetectable subpopulations in patients' bodies. When switching to another protease inhibitor, they continue to multiply because they are at least partially protected against the new protease inhibitor. The reduced sensitivity supports further evolution to complete resistance and drug failure.

In late 1997, Hoffman-La Roche's new version of saquinavir that comes in soft gel capsules was approved by the FOOD AND DRUG ADMINISTRATION. Packaged in a special lipid mixture and taken at twice the dose of the older Invirase formulation, Fortovase permits a total drug exposure in the body that is eight times greater than before. This is largely because the new lipids induced such a rapid absorption of saquinavir that the compound saturates the liver enzymes that can rapidly break it down. More drug therefore reaches the blood. Roche announcements have called Fortovase a"a new formulation, a new beginning" for saquinavir, whose old version, Invirase, was widely deprecated as having inferior efficacy compared to the other protease inhibitors. The daily 3.6-gram Fortovase dose requires taking 18 large oil-coated capsules a day. It represents a large additional pill burden and causes considerably more gastrointestianl problems than Invirase at the standard 1.8 gram/day dose does. Fortovase is associated with diarrhea or nausea in 10 percent to 20 percent of trial participants, but otherwise has been relatively well tolerated. One way around the onerous Fortovase dose is to combine 400 mg of Fortovase with 400 mg of RITONAVIR every 12 hours. By blocking the liver enzymes that break down saquinavir, ritonavir achieves the same effects as saturating the liver with much larger doses of Fortovase. Fortovase offers several advantages over the ritonavir/saquinavir combination. Fortovase no longer needs to be used in combination with ritonavir to increase exposure levels of saquinavir. This avoids the immediate need for refrigeration, the toxicity involved with taking two protease inhibitors, the dosing concerns with 400 mg ritonavir, and the significant drug interaction profile of ritonavir.

As of this writing, Hoffman-La Roche intends to phase out Invirase, so those who prefer the Invirase/ritonavir combination will soon have to find an alternative.

Currently available protease inhibitors include indinavir (Crixivan) and ritonavir (Norvir).

sarcoma   A malignant tumor of the skin and soft tissue.

scabies   A highly contagious skin disease caused by the itch mite. It is transmitted by close contact and is characterized by the eruption of papules, vesicles, and pustules. Eczema may result from scratching.

scapegoating   A person or group made to bear the blame for others or to suffer in their place. In the first five years of the epidemic, as AIDS virus evidence mounted, fear also erupted; exposure to Americans of the virus was much higher than had previously been suspected. As fears escalated, so did blaming so-called high risk persons or groups associated with HIV/AIDS (e.g., homosexuals, immigrants, intravenous drug users) for the continuing spread of the disease.

scat   The excrement of an animal, also slang term for sexual intercourse in feces.

scavenger cell   One of a diverse group of white blood cells with the capacity to engulf and destroy foreign material and dead tissue and cells.

Schistosoma   A genus of parasites or flukes belonging to the family Schistosomatidae, class Trematoda, that thrives on blood; the blood fluke.

schistosomiasis   A parasitic disease due to infestation with flukes of the genus *Schistosoma*. The disease is endemic throughout Asia, Africa, and tropical America. The parasite is picked up by wading or bathing in water containing cercariae (the free swimming, tailed larvae of parasitic trematodes) that have issued from snails.

SCID   See SEVERE COMBINED IMMUNODEFICIENCY.

scrapie disease   A transmissible brain disease in which the brain tissue degenerates to a spongelike condition. It is characterized by severe itching, debility, and the inability to coordinate muscle movements. Scrapie disease generally occurs in sheep and goats and is inevitably fatal.

screening   The testing, usually using one diagnostic procedure including laboratory studies, of large groups of people to determine the presence of a particular disease or of certain risk factors known to be associated with that disease. In an HIV/AIDS context screening may refer to mandatory HIV screening; screening of blood donors for HIV; screening of sperm for HIV; and/or screening through voluntary testing. Some have advocated mandatory screening for HIV infection to large portions of the population (either of the population at large or well-defined subgroups).

In psychiatry, screening refers to initial examinations to determine mental status and the appropriate initial therapy. See also MANDATORY TESTING; PRIVACY.

seborrhea   See SEBORRHEIC DERMATITIS.

seborrheic dermatitis   An acute or chronic inflammatory skin disease of unknown cause characterized by dry, moist, or greasy scaling and yellow or brown-gray crusted patches. It tends to involve the scalp but may include parts of the face, ears, genitalia, umbilicus, and supraorbital regions. Generalized seborrheic dermatitis requires careful attention, including scrupulous skin hygiene, keeping skin as dry as possible, and dusting powders. Topical and systemic cortisone preparations may be required. Also called SEBORRHEA and SEBORRHEIC ECZEMA.

seborrheic eczema   See SEBORRHEIC DERMATITIS.

secondary care setting   A place where patients are referred for special care beyond primary health care; a hospital.

secondary effect   A by-product or complication of drug use which does not occur as part of the drug's primary pharmacological activity. Secondary effects are unwanted consequences and may therefore be classified as adverse effects.

secondary infection   An infection contracted in addition to (and often due to the compromised immunity caused by) AIDS. Among the most common are MONONUCLEOSIS, TUBERCULOSIS, and PNEUMONIA.

secondary response   The immune response that follows a second or subsequent encounter with a particular ANTIGEN.

second-line therapy   A therapy used after a preferred or first-line treatment has failed. For instance, ddC may be second-line therapy for HIV after AZT therapy fails.

secretory leukocyte protease inhibitor (SLPI)   A protein in SALIVA that according to test tube studies inhibits HIV. The protein attaches to white blood cells and prevents HIV from infecting those cells. Current studies are focusing on whether SLPI has an application as an anti-HIV treatment or as a viricidal adjunct to safer sex.

Section 1619 of the Social Security Act   See SOCIAL SECURITY ACT, SECTION 1619.

sedative   Quieting, soothing, tranquilizing; an agent that has such an effect. Sedatives may be general, local, nervous, or vascular. Cardiac sedatives decrease the heart's force; nervous sedatives affect the nervous system.

segregation   In an HIV/AIDS context, the separation of people with HIV/AIDS from the general population within a large custodial institution like a prison or military organization. Segregation addresses the AIDS epidemic by imposing restrictions on individuals as a means to prevent transmission of the virus. Segregation is similar to quarantine.

Today, most knowledgable people believe that the segregation of HIV-infected people or people with AIDS is ineffective, impractical, and unsound, medically and ethically. In addition, it could convey a false sense of security, causing those who believe that the risk is reduced to take fewer precautions to avoid infection. Confining individuals who engage in behaviors that transmit HIV cannot control such a widespread epidemic. Other factors to be considered are the logistics of testing, the possibility of inaccurate test results, and the sheer challenge of finding housing for all infected personnel.

seizure   A convulsion, or episode of uncontrolled movements, of the arms and legs accompanied by unconsciousness and loss of control over urine or stool. The usual cause of seizures in people with HIV infection is an OPPORTUNISTIC INFECTION such as TOXOPLASMIC ENCEPHALITIS, CRYPTO-COCCAL MENINGITIS, or lymphoma, or an opportunistic tumor in the brain. Less commonly, seizures are caused by an imbalance of ELECTROLYTEs or by medications. Recurrent seizures can usually be controlled with such drugs are Dilantin and phenobarbital. Anyone with recurrent seizures should be careful about his or her physical circumstances: working on ladders, for instance, or driving. In many states, it is illegal for a person with seizures to drive until the seizures have been controlled for at least one year.

selenium   A chemical element resembling sulfur. It is poisonous to certain animals that feed on plants grown in soil that contains an excess of it. Selenium is one of several antioxidants that people with HIV are often advised to take because of serious deficiencies and increased need for a number of nutrients.

self-insemination   A woman's introduction of donated sperm into her own body without the help of a doctor.

To inseminate herself, a woman should have no fertility problems and her menstrual cycle should be fairly regular. Charting one's basal temperature and mucus consistency for a few months is the first step. This will indicate when one is likely to ovulate. Finding a fertile man who is willing to donate sperm is the next step. When one knows from past cycles that one is about to ovulate, the sperm donor must masturbate into a clean (preferably boiled, but cooled) jar. Within an hour after ejaculation, the woman sucks the semen into a needleless hypodermic syringe (some women use an eye dropper or a turkey baster), gently inserts the syringe into her vagina while lying flat on her back with her rear up on a pillow. She then empties the syringe into the vagina to deposit the semen as close to the CERVIX as possible. The woman should continue lying down comfortable for about 10 minutes, so that as little sperm as possible leaks out of the vagina. It is generally recommended that this procedure be repeated with fresh sperm samples in two or three days, during and after the time the woman ovulates. Most woman become pregnant after trying self-insemination during three to five cycles.

semen   A thick opalescent fluid, produced in the male reproductive organs, that is ejaculated through the PENIS during orgasm. Semen is the secretory product of various organs (the prostate, bulbourethral glands, seminal vesicles, and others) plus spermatozoa and ranges in color from milky white to yellow to grayish. Besides living sperm, semen contains water, three simple sugars (to provide nourishment for the sperm), alkalis (to buffer the acidity of the urethra and the vagina), prostaglandins (substances that cause the contractions of the uterus and fallopian tubes and are thought to aid in the sperm's passage to the womb), vitamin C, zinc, cholesterol, and a few other things. Healthy semen, in other words, does not contain anything that is bad for your health. In the age of AIDS, however, it is important to remember that, along with blood and vaginal secretions, semen is one of the primary carriers of HIV. (It can also carry the organisms that cause GONORRHEA, HEPATITIS B, and CHLAMYDIA.) Use of CONDOMS and vaginal SPERMICIDAL CREAM or jelly can reduce women's chances of acquiring the virus during sexual intercourse; use of condoms can reduce men's chances also. Treating gonorrhea, chlamydial infections, trichomonas, and other sexually transmitted diseases in HIV-infected men significantly reduces the amount of HIV in semen. Slang terms include cum, scum, spunk, and jism.

sensitivity   The degree of accuracy of a clinical test. Also, responsiveness to an ALLERGEN.

sensitization   The stimulation of allergic ANTIBODY production or DELAYED-TYPE HYPERSENSITIVITY by an initial encounter with a specific allergenic substance or hapten. Synonymous with PRIMARY RESPONSE.

sensuality   The quality of responsiveness to the senses; the capacity to experience sensual gratification. "Sensual" is sometimes used to refer to physical pleasure that is not overtly sexual, such as that derived from stroking.

sentinel animal   A susceptible animal used as an alarm for the presence of a HOT AGENT, since no instrument can detect a hot agent.

sepsis   Pathologic state, usually febrile, resulting from the presence of microorganisms or their poisonous products in the bloodstream. May be manifested as cellulitis (local dissemination of infection), lymphangitis or lymphadenitis (dispersion along lymphatic channels), or bacteremia (widespread dissemination by way of the bloodstream).

septicemia Presence of pathogenic bacteria in the blood. If allowed to progress, the organisms may multiply and cause an overwhelming infection and death. Symptoms usually include chills and fever, petechiae (small, purplish, hemorrhagic spots on the skin), purpuric pustules, and abscesses. Shock may be present.

Septra See TRIMETHOPRIM/SULFAMETHOXAZOLE.

sequential monotherapy Treatment with several drugs, one at a time. Switching from one drug to another is done either after a fixed amount of time or after a drug has failed to yield further benefit. See also MONOTHERAPY and COMBINATION THERAPY.

sero- A prefix referring to blood serum.

seroconcordance Having sex only with persons with the same HIV status.

seroconversion The process by which a person's ANTIBODY status converts from negative to positive, with the appearance of antibodies in the blood in response to infection or vaccination. The immune system usually takes several days or weeks to recognize a foreign substance like a virus and to produce antibodies to it. After transmission of the HIV virus, it may take several months or more for antibodies to develop.

serodiscordant relationships Sexual relationships in which the partners have different HIV status, or one partner doesn't know whether the other is infected.

serologic Relating to serology, the branch of medicine concerned with blood SERUM, the clear fluid portion of blood.

serologic study A study that compares the characteristics of the blood SERUM of individuals, especially those markers that indicate exposure to a particular agent of disease.

serologic test Any test performed on blood SERUM the clear, liquid portion of the blood. Often such tests are performed to determine the presence of antibodies, which would indicate the presence of an ANTIGEN such as a virus. A serologic test for SYPHILIS is required in many states for a marriage license. While technically the tests for AIDS antibodies, CHLAMYDIA antibodies, and HERPES VIRUS antibodies are all serologic tests, "serology" commonly applies to the test done for syphilis.

serologic testing See SEROLOGIC TEST.

seronegative Testing negative for antibodies to a substance or organism in the blood, such as HIV; not having such antibodies present. Synonymous with ANTIBODY nega-

tivity. In the context of HIV, the term indicates "not infected," HIV-NEGATIVE.

seropositive Testing positive for antibodies to a substance or organism in the blood, such as HIV; having such antibodies present in the blood. In the context of HIV, the term indicates HIV infection (HIV-POSITIVE).

seroprevalence The number of people with evidence of antibodies against the causative agent of a disease in a given population over a specific period or at a particular time. For HIV, the rate at which a given population tests positive on the ELISA test for HIV antibodies. The seroprevalence rate is nearly the same as the rate of HIV infection in a given population, leaving out mainly those who were recently infected.

seroreverter A person whose ANTIBODY status has changed from positive to negative. The term is used to describe perinatally exposed infants who are not truly infected and become HIV antibody negative as they lose maternal HIV antibody.

serostatus The condition of having or not having detectable antibodies to a microbe in the blood as a result of infection. One may have either a SERONEGATIVE (uninfected) or SEROPOSITIVE (infected) serostatus.

sertraline A widely used antidepressant, also used to treat obsessive-compulsive disorder. Sertraline belongs to a class known as serotonin reuptake inhibitors. It is chemically unrelated to tricyclic, tetracyclic, or other classes of antidepressants. It has become widely used because it is effective and tends to have fewer side effects than other older antidepressants. The side effects that occur most frequently are dry mouth, headache, dizziness, tremors, nausea, diarrhea, fatigue, insomnia, difficulty ejaculating, and sleepiness. Brand name is Zoloft.

serum The clear portion of any body fluid, separated from its solid elements; for instance blood serum. In medical usage the term usually refers to (human) blood serum. Also, blood serum from an animal that has been immunized against a pathogenic organism, used for passive immunization of humans. In ordinary usage "serum" is sometimes a synonym for "vaccine."

serum glutamic oxalacetic transaminase (SGOT) See ASPARTATE AMINOTRANSFERASE.

serum glutamic pyruvic transaminase (SGPT) See ASPARTATE AMINOTRANSFERASE.

serum protein Any protein in blood serum. Serum protein forms weak acids mixed with alkali salts; this increases the buffer effects of the blood but to a lesser extent than cell protein.

serum sickness An adverse immunologic response to a foreign ANTIGEN, usually a heterologous protein.

seven-year itch   See SCABIES.

severe combined immunodeficiency (SCID)   A combination of rare congenital disorders characterized by impairment of both HUMORAL and CELL-MEDIATED IMMUNITY, manifested as lack of ANTIBODY formation in response to the presence of ANTIGENS, lack of delayed hypersensitivity, and inability to reject foreign tissue transplants. Without restoration of immune function or isolation in a gnotobiotic (germ-free) environment, death usually occurs by the first birthday as a result of OPPORTUNISTIC INFECTION.

sex   The general term for erotic activity. Also, either of the biological categories *male* and *female*, with the physical and behavioral traits that distinguish them.

sex club   A private facility dedicated to the promotion and pursuit of sexual pleasure (e.g., bathhouses, orgy rooms).

sex industry   The area of commercial enterprise based on the exploitation of interest in sex—pornography, prostitution, sex clubs, sex toys, devices, and so forth. See SEX WORKERS.

sex negativism   The conviction that most sexual thoughts, beliefs, and behaviors are repugnant, immoral, and not to be trusted or tolerated. Such attitudes, grounded in religious belief, personal distaste, or psychological disturbance, have always existed, but they are particularly inappropriate and destructive as a response to the AIDS crisis, since they devalue and discourage any pragmatic approach to the problem.

sex toy   Any object used during sexual activity to enhance sensual experience. Sex toys include dildos, vibrators, specially made CONDOMS, provocative undergarments, and erotic pictures, as well as scented massage oils and feathers. Whether an object is a sex toy is largely the judgment of the user.

sex worker   A worker in the sex industry who provides sexual services for money or other considerations. Sex workers include prostitutes, exotic dancers, strippers, madams, nude models, escorts, porn actors, and workers in massage parlors. Sex work is a form of labor, and like most labor in capitalist economies, it is often alienated (that is, the worker has little or no control over working conditions and the way the work is organized). A distinction is made between voluntary and forced sex work. Forced prostitution is a form of aggravated sexual assault.

In some countries, sex workers are screened for HIV, and those found to have the virus are detained in special facilities where they are supposed to be rehabilitated or retrained. The right to protection against HIV/AIDS, the consequences of unsafe sex, and the principles and practices of safe sex are examples of training content. In other places, people with HIV are prevented from working in the sex industry by imprisonment or detention in medical or quarantine facilities. Specific legal, or quasi-legal, actions are often taken to prevent HIV-infected workers from continuing to work. These include closing commercial sex venues, taking police action again sex workers suspected of carrying HIV, and screening photos of HIV-infected sex workers on television

in the form of community service announcements. There are few protests in either industrialized or developing countries against the idea that the removal of people with HIV from the sex industry is sound policy.

The scapegoating of prostitutes for sexually transmitted diseases has a long history. Because the public has traditionally been poorly informed about the reality of sex work, it is hardly surprising that, as the AIDS epidemic grew, the scapegoating of prostitutes for AIDS became more and more commonplace. In the 1970s many organizations, were formed not only to work for women's rights but also to address the issues of sex work. Today such organizations as COYOTE (Call Off Your Old Tired Ethics) exist worldwide. Most of them are working to prevent the scapegoating of sex workers for AIDS and other sexually transmitted diseases, and to educate sex workers, their clients, and the general public about prevention of these diseases.

sexology   The scientific study of sex.

sexual abuse   The forced participation of an unwilling individual in sexual activity by use of direct or implied threats. Abuse may involve actual physical contact, acts of exhibitionism or indecent exposure, rape, sexual assault, or sexual molestation. The active person may be male, female, adult, or child, and the abused person may be of the same or opposite sex of the abuser.

sexual apartheid   The practice of selecting sex partners based on their HIV status. Prevention activists disagree on whether it is morally acceptable to select on the basis of SEROSTATUS. Others go further, saying that HIV-mixed marriages should be discouraged.

sexual assault   See RAPE.

sexual behavior   Sexual activities, ranging from touching, caressing, and looking to teasing, kissing, massaging, licking, sucking, and penetrating. What an individual does during sex, what an individual feels about her or his sexuality, how s/he wants to explore it, who s/he is with, how much love and understanding s/he feels, how comfortable all parties involved are with their bodies, how each party feels that day are matters of personal preference and ingenuity. Sexual behavior is also a reflection of sexual drives and satisfactions, both of which generally evolve throughout an individual's lifetime.

sexual double standard   The traditional view that sexual freedom is acceptable for men but not for women. In most Western countries it has become less prevalent than it was two or more decades ago.

sexual dysfunction   Any condition that prevents normal sexual functioning, up to and including sexual intercourse. Dysfunction may be temporary or persistent; it may have physiological or psychological origins. The use of some prescription drugs may cause sexual dysfunction in some people (in some cases, similar drugs without this side effect may be substituted). To some extent, sexual dysfunction is culturally defined. Recognized forms of sexual dysfunction include, for women, anorgasmia, painful intercourse, and vaginismus; for men, impotence, premature ejaculation, and retarded ejaculation.

sexual ethics   A moral code of sexual behavior; guidelines for treating partners with kindness and decency, playfulness and pleasuring. A sexual ethics might include the following: Remember the Golden Rule; take time to make yourself desirable; ask for what you want; make sure that was a yes; take no for an answer; take responsibility; respect your partner's nakedness; remember to say thank you; keep some things private. To some degree, AIDS has given rise to a new consciousness of sexual ethics and etiquette. One means of reducing the sexual transmission of HIV is to practice safe sex, and safe sex guidelines are, in many ways, a form of sexual etiquette.

sexual etiquette   Guidelines for sexual conduct. See SEXUAL ETHICS.

sexual fulfillment   A feeling of contentment after a pleasurable and satisfying sexual encounter. There is a feeling of intense fulfillment in the orgasmic and resolution phases of the sexual response cycle.

sexual health   As contrasted with sexual dysfunction, a lack of problems in sexual desire and sexual response. The World Health Organization has defined three elements of sexual health: a capacity to enjoy and control sexual behavior in accordance with a social and personal ethic; freedom from fear, shame, guilt, false beliefs, and other psychological factors inhibiting sexual relationships; and freedom from organic disorder, disease, and deficiencies that interfere with sexual and reproductive functions. Today, it is understood that sexual health is inextricably linked to total well-being—emotional and physical. The better informed we are sexually, the greater our potential health benefit. It is known that sexual problems can also be connected to depression, fatigue, headaches, diabetes, heart attacks, cholesterol, and arthritis, as well as HIV/AIDS.

A common response to the discovery of HIV infection is to shun sexual relations for some period of time. This is often a symptom of depression and may be accompanied by a poor appetite and sleep disturbances. Sexual dysfunction is also a normal, and usually temporary, initial response to learning of HIV infection. HIV+ people may need to go through the stages of grieving both in anticipation of their own death and for the loss of their identity as healthy and whole before they can actively continue healthy and safe relationships in which affection and sexuality are experienced.

sexual identity   One's sexual self-definition. An individual's sexual identity is influenced by biological and psychological components. In addition to biological gender, there are three psychological components of sexual identity: (1) gender identity (a secure sense of one's genital maleness or femaleness); (2) sexual preference; and (3) gender role identity and gender role behaviors, traits, and interests that are socially considered to be gender specific.

sexual intercourse   The physical act of sexual coupling. Sexual intercourse can be carried on between persons of the same sex or persons of the opposite sex. Genital contact between individuals is commonly involved. For heterosexuals, sexual intercourse is most commonly sexual contact that involves insertion of an erect penis into a vagina. ANAL INTERCOURSE is when a man's penis is inserted in his partner's rectum.

sexual orientation   See SEXUAL PREFERENCE.

sexual pleasure   See SEXUAL FULFILLMENT.

sexual preference   The sexual orientation one prefers in choosing his or her sex partners.

sexual risk reduction   See RISK REDUCTION.

sexual transmission   See TRANSMISSION.

sexuality   The sexual aspect of being; the capacity to respond to erotic stimuli, experience sexual feeling, and act sexually. As an aspect of being human, sexuality does not entail any specific set of behaviors or sexual preference. There are biological, cultural, psychological, and social dimensions to human sexuality, all of which help to shape an individual's attitude toward the body and his or her sense of sexual self.

Sexuality, in our culture, has perhaps been the subject of more moralizing, and the source of more conflicted emotions and psychological distress than any other human activity. This has complicated thinking about sexually charged issues and sometimes, as in the AIDS epidemic, impeded the search for a rational approach to a serious problem.

sexually transmitted disease (STD)   Any of a group of diseases, affecting both men and women, that are spread from person to person during any kind of heterosexual or homosexual activity. Some STDs can spread through skin-to-skin contact with an infected person's genital area—not just through intercourse. Sexually transmitted diseases include AIDS, CHANCROID, chlamydiosis, infestation with PUBIC LICE, GENITAL WARTs (HPV), GONORRHEA, GRANULOMA INGUINALE, HEPATITIS B (HBV), HERPES SIMPLEX, LYMPHOGRANULOMA VENEREUM, NONGONOCOCCAL URETHRITIS, PELVIC INFLAMMATORY DISEASE, SYPHILIS, and VAGINITIS (YEAST INFECTIONS, TRICHOMONIASIS). Although each STD presents unique diagnostic, therapeutic, and prevention challenges, all STDs share a common mode of transmission. Populations at risk for one STD are at risk for others, and the presence of one infection may influence the acquisition and course of another.

All STDs are preventable. Reducing the risk of contracting one requires taking certain precautions; see SAFE SEX.

At the minimum, these diseases cause discomfort. Left untreated, some STDs can cause serious long-term health problems. For example, gonorrhea and chlamydial infections can cause pelvic inflammatory disease, infertility, and ECTOPIC PREGNANCY. Several common STDs adversely affect pregnancy, resulting in spontaneous abortion, stillbirth, and premature delivery. Genital infections due to HUMAN PAPIL-LOMAVIRUS are associated with CERVICAL CANCER, one of the most common cancers in women throughout the world today. Moreover a pregnant woman can pass an infection to her baby. Infections in newborns include syphilis, herpes, gonococcal conjunctivitis (an eye disease that can lead to blindness), and chlamydial pneumonia, an infection of the lungs that can develop into a chronic respiratory disease.

Locally, STDs and genital ulcers could permit the penetration of HIV through lesions that disrupt the integrity of the genital EPITHELIUM. STDs could increase the population of HIV target cells at the site of infection by recruiting LYM-PHOCYTEs to the genital tract, increasing women's susceptibility to HIV transmission. It has been suggested that HIV might be transmitted more easily by women who have concurrent venereal infections with inflammatory secretions in the vaginal canal containing many virus-infected lymphocytes, and that the clinical status of men's penile and urethral epithelium may contribute to their susceptibility to HIV infection. There is also evidence suggesting that genital ulcer diseases (especially genital herpes, chancroid, genital warts, and syphilis; less is known about CHLAMYDIA and gonorrhea) increase the risk of HIV infection.

Effective treatments for most sexually transmitted diseases do exist and the diseases are not always fatal. AIDS is similar to these diseases in that it is passed from person to person sexually. It is different from other sexually transmitted diseases however because to date there is no effective treatment for AIDS and it is always fatal.

The term *sexually transmitted disease* is now preferred to venereal disease (VD).

sexually transmitted infection   See SEXUALLY TRANSMITTED DISEASE.

sexually transmitted vaginitis   See SEXUALLY TRANSMITTED DISEASE.

Sezary syndrome   A form of cutaneous T-CELL LYMPHOMA characterized by exfoliative dermatitis (shedding), severe itching, peripheral lymphadenopathy, and abnormal hyperchromatic mononuclear cells in the lymph nodes, skin, and peripheral blood.

SGA   See SUBSTANTIAL GAINFUL ACTIVITY.

shark cartilage   Shark cartilage—which is exactly what it sounds like—is rich in an ANGIOGENESIS-inhibiting protein called cartilage-derived inhibitor. Angiogenesis is the process whereby new blood vessels are formed to feed cancers, particularly solid tumors, such as KAPOSI'S SARCOMA. To date, studies of shark cartilage as a MONOTHERAPY for Kaposi's sarcoma in PWAs have been disappointing.

sharps container   A specialized container designed for the disposal of used needles, blades, and contaminated fluids. They are ubiquitous in doctors' offices and hospitals.

Shigella   A genus of GRAM-NEGATIVE, nonmotile rod-shaped bacteria of the family Enterobacteriaceae that fer-ment carbohydrates with acid but do not produce gas. The genus consists of several species, all of which normally inhabit the intestinal tract of humans and can cause digestive disturbances ranging from diarrhea to severe dysentery.

shigellosis   The disease produced by organisms of the genus *Shigella*.

shingles   The eruption of acute, inflammatory, herpetic vesicles along the area of an affected nerve. The blisters generally dry and scab, leaving minor scarring. In most cases the rash stays in the area of the body where it first appeared. The shingles rash seldom lasts longer than three weeks. However, the pain can continue after the rash has healed. The pain can come and go for a long time. The disease represents reactivation of VARICELLA ZOSTER VIRUS, usually acquired in childhood (when it appears as chicken pox). Shingles is not spread through person-to-person contact. It is sometimes referred to as HERPES ZOSTER and is not associated with any sexually transmitted disease. Standard treatment is with FAMCICLOVIR or ACYCLOVIR.

shiitake mushrooms   One of several immune system stimulants that serve to boost CD4+ counts. Shiitake mushrooms (*Lentinus edodes*) are a traditional Asian herbal remedy containing *Lentinan edodes* mycelia (LEM), which can be extracted as a powder. Test tube studies in Japan have shown that pretreatment of T CELL cultures with LEM protects them from both free-viral and cell-to-cell HIV infection; it has been suggested that E-P-LEM interferes in HIV interaction with the cellular CD receptor.

sho-saiko-to (SSKT)   Sho-saiko-to (SSKT) is a central formula in traditional Chinese medicine and is readily available in many countries in Asia. While SSKT is a combination of seven ingredients in precise proportion, it is speculated that the most active component is scutellariae, from which baicalein is derived. Baicalein has been synthesized in a highly purified form and is being investigated at the National Cancer Institute. Studies of the effect of SSKT on lymphocytes from HIV-infected individuals have shown a greater inhibition of HIV REVERSE TRANSCRIPTASE and reductions in P24 ANTIGEN levels in HIV-SEROPOSITIVE asymptomatic people than in people with ARC. No significant viral inhibition was found in people with AIDS. To date, however, there exist insufficient data to support use of SSKT as an anti-HIV therapy.

shoot up   In slang, to inject (illicit) drugs intravenously.

shooting gallery   A location where drug addicts meet to SHOOT UP INTRAVENOUS DRUGS, often sharing needles.

short-term memory (STM)   A memory storage capacity, also called working memory, consisting of a central "executive," visuo-spatial "sketchpad," and articulatory loop used for storing small amounts of information for periods of time ranging from a few seconds to a few minutes. It is limited to about seven or eight items of information. Information in short-term memory is rapidly forgotten unless it is refreshed by rehearsal (a method of exercising memory), following which it may eventually be transferred to long-term memory. Various memory defects occur in HIV/AIDS and the OPPORTUNISTIC INFECTIONS that often accompany HIV/AIDS.

SI See SELF-INSEMINATION.

sickle-cell anemia A hereditary chronic form of ANEMIA in which abnormal sickle or crescent-shaped ERYTHROCYTEs are present. Sickle-cell anemia is due to the presence of an abnormal type of HEMOGLOBIN, hemoglobin S, in the red blood cells. The frequency of occurence of the gene that causes this disease is high in populations of Mediterranean and African origin, particularly blacks.

sickle-cell disease See SICKLE-CELL ANEMIA.

SIDA The acronym for AIDS in French, Spanish, and other Romance languages.

side effect A normal, expected, and predictable response to a drug that accompanies the principal (intended) response sought in treatment. Side effects are part of a drug's pharmacological activity and are thus unavoidable. Most side effects are undesirable. The majority cause minor annoyance and inconvenience; some may cause serious problems in managing certain diseases; a few can be hazardous.

sigmoidoscope A flexible or rigid instrument used to examine the lower (sigmoid) COLON. See ENDOSCOPY.

sigmoidoscopy Inspection of the sigmoid colon (the S-shaped lower portion of the descending colon, located between the iliac crest and the rectum) using a SIGMOIDOSCOPE.

sign An indication of a disease or disorder. See also SYMPTOM.

significance See STATISTICAL SIGNIFICANCE.

silence = death A slogan attributed to AIDS activists, which today is part of the AIDS narrative. This slogan first appeared on Manhattan walls in 1986 in the form of a slick, stark black poster with an inverted pink triangle (a point-up version of the symbol Nazis used to designate interned homosexuals) and white lettering. The point-up version was intended to incite active fighting back, a different tactic from the silent resistance associated with the original point-down version. (The point-down pink triangle came into use as a code and symbol of resistance among the international gay movement in the mid-seventies.)

The poster was produced by the Silence = Death Collective, a group of gay men who postered New York City for several months, and then attended the founding meeting of ACT-UP, the AIDS Coalition to Unleash Power. The poster/slogan had no attribution, no author for its message. It spoke to an international, closeted language. It had a single, urgent meaning: a rallying cry to no place in particular—no march, no meeting, no group. It served as a notice to a community of camouflaged guerrillas that AIDS is not over.

The slogan has acquired many meanings over the years. Silence refers to the never spoken, the yet to set itself into language, the unique, the individual, madness, the unrepresentable, the space of that which is not to be represented, the closet. Silence also refers to the unspeakable, the perceived but best not said, the ignored, the space occupied by that which is ignored, the hidden, the safely tucked away, the camouflaged, the safety of camouflage. Silence, or rather, educators' failure to speak for fear of inciting the body to acts of pleasure that are now defined as "risks," prevents classes of people from obtaining new information—about safe sex and needle hygiene—that will save their lives: death by disinformation. Silence represents the refusal of the mainstream press to report on the epidemic in its first few years, the disadvantaged scientists seeking to unlock the "mystery" of AIDS, and the disadvantaged persons living with AIDS seeking community and affirmation.

From the mid-1980s to the present, AIDS activists have relentlessly pursued their speech, often confronting the paradox that while silence (lack of information, lack of exposure) equals death, public speech—speech seeking remedy from repression—is impossible for those most harshly affected by AIDS precisely because of the systems of information control and the politics of scientific knowledge. Activists were quick to learn that the AIDS narrative exists as a technology of social repression; it is a representation that attempts to silence not only the claims of identity politics, but the people marginalized by AIDS. AIDS activists were also quick to learn that this cannot be said; it must be performed. The insight "silence equals death" has spawned an international agitprop activism that circulates around the meanings eluded in the discourses of science, medicine, and public politics.

Silybum marianum See SILYMARIN.

silymarin The seeds of milk thistle (*Silybum marianum*) have been cultivated for centuries as a medicinal remedy, and are considered by some to have liver-protecting properties. An extract is available under the name silymarin; proponents suggest that it is useful for liver-based problems, including cirrhosis, jaundice, chronic hepatitis, and damage due to drugs, alcohol, and poisoning from chemicals and diarrhea. Some reports have suggested that silymarin may stimulate certain immune functions and may protect the liver during hepatitis. To date, no studies of silymarin in PWAs have been conducted. No toxic effects of silymarin have been reported, although it is possible that because of its purported effect on the liver and kidneys, the compound may effect the absorption of other medications. Silymarin concentrations vary in milk thistle capsules, pills, and teas, and should be taken only upon the advice of an herbalist or physician.

simian acquired immunodeficiency disease See SIMIAN IMMUNODEFICIENCY VIRUS.

simian acquired immunodeficiency virus See SIMIAN IMMUNODEFICIENCY VIRUS.

simian immunodeficiency virus (SIV)   Any of a group of viruses found in monkeys structurally similar to the HUMAN IMMUNODEFICIENCY VIRUS (HIV). Also called simian acquired immunodeficiency virus and SIMIAN T-CELL LYMPHOTROPHIC VIRUS (STLV). It has long been suspected that HIV evolved from SIV-1, a simian immunodeficiency virus, perhaps as a result of humans becoming infected with monkey viruses that mutated inside their bodies. Now, in a very suggestive finding, it is known that a chimpanzee has developed AIDS, confirming for the first time that HIV-1, the human virus responsible for most of the world's AIDS burden, can jump between species. Moreover, the human virus that infected the AIDS chimp has changed dramatically since it was experimentally injected into the animal in 1984. About 20 percent has mutated into a difference form. This finding also suggests there may be a way to test future human treatments and vaccines on chimps.

In 1993, a novel approach to creating a vaccine for preventing SIV was described. The "new" strategy described was actually a standard one for vaccines in other diseases—a live but weakened, or attenuated, SIV strain. The SIV was weakened by deleting its "NEF" gene, whose function is poorly understood. The attenuated virus produced an extremely low-level, benign, persistent infection instead of a rapidly fatal one. When the vaccine's effectiveness was tested in four monkeys more than two years after vaccination, protection was complete against two closely related SIV strains. Experiments with SIV strains that were weakened by removing three to five minor genes (including nef) have also been conducted, as has an experiment in chimpanzees using a multiply deleted version of HIV. The need for basic safety data on this vaccine in humans remains. In general, the scientific and medical communities acknowledge that there are tremendous fears about using a live, attenuated HIV vaccine on uninfected people. Professionals note that it could take 20 years to tell whether they are using a strain of HIV that produces no disease progression or only slow progression.

simian acquired immunodeficiency syndrome (SAIDS)   An AIDS-like immunodeficiency syndrome found in some macaque monkeys infected with SIV, a RETROVIRUS related to HIV.

simian retrovirus   A form of AIDS found in monkeys and apes that does not affect humans.

simian T-cell lymphotrophic virus (STLV)   See SIMIAN IMMUNODEFICIENCY VIRUS (SIV).

simian T-cell lymphotrophic virus type I   A virus very similar to HTLV-I discovered in African green monkeys and several other primate species. Researchers initially thought that the discovery of STLV-I provided a possible clue to the ancestry of the human virus. Robert Gallo speculated that HTLV-I originated in Africa, where it infected humans as well as many species of Old World primates (Robert C. Gallo, "The First Human Retrovirus," *Scientific American* 255 [1986]: 88–89).

simian T-cell lymphotropic virus type III   In late 1985 and early 1986, researchers identified a monkey virus that appeared very similar to the human AIDS virus. Evidence of the monkey virus was found in both captive macaque monkeys and wild African green monkeys. It was associated with IMMUNODEFICIENCY and LYMPHOMAS in the former species but did not appear to cause disease in the latter. Researchers named the virus STLV-III (simian T-lymphotropic virus type III).

single-agent therapy   Treatment with one drug at a time; also known as MONOTHERAPY.

sinusitis   Infection of the sinuses, the air sacs next to the nasal passages, usually as a result of a cold or allergy. Sinusitis is common, especially in people with HIV infection, although the reason for this is obscure. Symptoms are pus drainage from the nose, headache, face pain, and fever. The usual treatment is with ANTIBIOTICS taken by mouth, such as TRIMETHOPRIM-SULFAMETHOXZOLE, AMOXICILLAN, ERYTHROMYCIN, cephalexin (Keflex), CIPROFLOXACIN (Cipro), or TETRACYCLINE. Some people do not respond to these drugs, and their sinuses need to be drained.

SIV   See SIMIAN IMMUNODEFICIENCY VIRUS.

skilled nursing facility (SNF)   A facility that provides skilled nursing (such as that given by RNs) and related services requiring the most intense and professional nursing home care. Also called an extended care facility. Costs of a stay in an SNF are covered by MEDICARE, MEDICAID, and some private health insurance.

skin   The layer of tissue between the body and its environment is a major organ of the body. Skin functions include protection against injuries and parasitic invasion, regulation of body temperature, aid in elimination, and prevention of dehydration. The skin is a reservoir for food and water, a sense organ, and a source of antirachitic vitamin, which it produces when exposed to sunlight.

The term *skin* is also slang for condom.

skin disorder   The skin and mucosa are the body's first line of defense against countless microbial threats such as bacteria, fungi, protozoa, and viruses. But this defense depends on a functional immune system. When the immune system is suppressed, disorders of the skin may appear. Organ transplant and cancer patients who undergo immunosuppressive therapies can develop skin disorders such as KAPOSI'S SARCOMA or herpes outbreaks. In HIV, lesions, dry skin, and blisters are common early in the course of the infection and may recur or become chronic. Viral skin diseases in AIDS include MOLLUSCUM CONTAGIOSUM, HERPES SIMPLEX VIRUS, HERPES ZOSTER (shingles), HAIRY LEUKOPLAKIA, AND GENITAL WARTs. Viral skin disorders common in HIV-infected people are not ordinarily life-threatening, but they can cause significant pain, illness, and cosmetic frustration. In some cases, viral skin diseases can spread to infect other parts of the body, possibly resulting in life-threatening conditions such as HSV encephalitis. The early detection, prophylaxis, and treatment of skin diseases is recommended. See also SAL-LOWNESS; SKIN RASH.

skin rash Texture and temperature of skin are important signs of underlying conditions. Rashes and their causes, like scars, are diagnostic. Redness is usually seen in inflammation, skin disease, chronic alcoholism, vasomotor disturbances, and pyrexia, as well as sunburn. Local redness with pain indicates inflammation. Lesions, bumps, dry skin, or blisters are common in early HIV infection and may be caused by a number of conditions or infections, including HERPES ZOSTER, HERPES SIMPLEX, dermatitis, etc. See also SALLOWNESS; SKIN DISORDER.

skin test A test of the immune system by means of injections of certain proteins just below the surface of the skin. If the immune system is intact, a rash appears within 48 hours at the site of injection.

skip-generation parenting A situation in which children are raised by grandparents instead of parents. Although data are scarce, it appears that when parents die of AIDS, children most often go to live, at least at first, with grandmothers or aunts. The problem of skip-generation parenting is not, however, solely attributable to HIV disease. Use of drugs, especially crack cocaine, has devastated many families. Grandparents—and especially grandmothers, since women have traditionally taken on the role of family caregiving—have taken over when their own children have been unable to take on parenting responsibilities or when they have chosen to move their children to a safer environment. This problem has particularly affected African-American communities.

Two general outcomes are predictable. First, some of these grandparents, no matter how willing and devoted they are, will be unable to continue to bear the burdens of child raising—and many of these children have severe behavior or academic problems—because of illness, age, emotional exhaustion, and poverty. Second, there will be no new generation of grandparents to take the place of this generation. The mothers and fathers lost to AIDS will become a lost generation of grandparents.

slim disease See HIV WASTING DISEASE.

slow virus A virus, such as HIV, that produces disease with a greatly delayed onset and protracted course. Diseases of a chronic degenerative nature that are now suspected to be due to slow viruses include subacute sclerosing panencephalitis and progressive multifocal leukoencephalopathy.

smallpox An acute, contagious, systemic, viral disease, the constitutional symptoms of which are followed by an eruption that passes through the successive stages of macules, papules, vesicles, pustules, and crusts. Smallpox is considered to have been eradicated worldwide by vaccination programs.

smoking Tobacco smoking is harmful not only to smokers but also to those who live or work with them, regardless of HIV status. It has been associated with a higher risk of HIV infection. There are conflicting data on the effects of smoking on HIV disease progression, and the effects of pre-existing smoker's leukocytosis (see below) do not seem to be protective.

Some studies point to increased risks for certain opportunistic infections in HIV-infected smokers, especially PCP. However, the only infections in which this association has been proved are anogenital abnormalities and cancers. Other studies have shown that current smokers are more likely to develop oral CANDIDIASIS and oral HAIRY LEUKOPLAKIA, but less likely to develop cytomegalovirus disease. Heavy smokers (more than one pack a day) have been shown to be more likely to develop bacterial pneumonia compared with light smokers, non smokers, or ex-smokers. Finally, studies have shown that ex-smokers are more likely to develop PCP than nonsmokers. Despite the long time it takes many smoking-related problems to develop, smoking is by no means without health risks for the immunocompromised person.

The association between smoking and HIV infection may have a biological basis. In many, smoking degrades the lining of the oral cavity or leads to minuscule ulcerations that could facilitate HIV transmission. Smoking has a number of known negative biological effects that may affect the progression of HIV disease. These include decreased lung function, chronic inflammatory disease of the lower airways, gum and oral diseases such as periodontis, various cancers, and a lowered ability to heal wounds. Along with the chronic inflammation of the lungs, which can lead to chronic bronchitis or emphysema, smoking causes an elevation of the body's white blood cell count, a condition known as smoker's leukocytosis.

sneeze Sneezing has not been identified as a route of transmission for HIV/AIDS. To date, the virus has not been found in mucus from the nose.

sobriety A state of complete abstinence from psychoactive substances by an addicted individual, in conjunction with a satisfactory quality of life.

social disease A venereal or sexually transmitted disease.

social kiss See DRY KISS.

Social Security The United States' most extensive program to provide income for older and disabled Americans. It is paid for by a tax on workers and their employers. Qualified workers are eligible for old age and disability benefits. Benefits are also available for the spouse and dependents of a retired or disabled worker. When a worker dies, benefits can be collected by surviving family members who qualify. Over 95 percent of American workers, including household help, farm workers, self-employed persons, employees of state and local government, and (since 1984) federal workers, participate in the program. Railroad workers are covered by a separate federal program, railroad retirement, that is integrated with Social Security. The program is complicated, and the law and regulations change from time to time. Contact your local office of the Social Security Administration (SSA) for literature about Social Security benefits or to ask specific questions about your own case. They are listed in the United States Government section of your telephone directory. Or call 1-800-772-1213.

Social Security Act, Section 1619   This section allows for continued payment of SUPPLEMENTAL SECURITY INCOME (SSI) benefits to working disabled recipients, without regard to the SUBSTANTIAL GAINFUL ACTIVITY (SGA), trial work period, and extended-period-of-eligibility limitations imposed by the companion SOCIAL SECURITY DISABILITY INSURANCE (SSDI) program. Section 1619 allows disabled workers whose earnings raise them over the SSI eligibility level to continue as SSI recipients for purposes of MEDICAID coverage if Medicaid-purchased care is what is enabling them to "work their way off welfare" and if they cannot otherwise secure such medical care.

Social Security Act, Title II   The OLD AGE, SURVIVORS, AND DISABILITY INSURANCE SECTION of the Social Security Act.

Social Security Act, Title IV-A   The AID TO FAMILIES WITH DEPENDENT CHILDREN (AFDC) section of the Social Security Act.

Social Security Act, Title XIV   The AID TO THE PERMANENTLY AND TOTALLY DISABLED (APTD) section of the Social Security Act.

Social Security Act, Title XVI   The SUPPLEMENTAL SECURITY INCOME (SSI) section of the Social Security Act.

Social Security Act, Title XVIII   The MEDICARE section of the Social Security Act.

Social Security Act, Title XIX   The MEDICAID section of the Social Security Act.

Social Security Act, Title XX   Formerly, the section of the Social Security Act under which grants to states were provided for social services to the needy; since replaced by the Social Services Block Grant (SSBG) program, which is itself often referred to as "Title XX."

Social Security Administration (SSA)   See SOCIAL SECURITY.

Social Security Disability Insurance (SSDI)   A federal income insurance program operated by the Social Security Administratin for workers whom it determines are disabled. There are several means by which people become eligible for SSDI. Most qualify by working and paying Social Security taxes, which earns "credits" toward eventual benefits. Disabled widows and widowers age 50 or older, may be eligible for a disability benefit earned on the Social Security record of a deceased spouse. Disabled children age 18 or older (whose disability must have originated before age 22) may be eligible for dependents' benefits on the Social Security record of a parent who is getting retirement or disability

benefits or who has died. Children under the age of 18 qualify for dependents' benefits on the record of a parent who is getting retirement or disability benefits or on the record of a parent who has died.

social service   Activity that serves the common good of society. The term covers private and public efforts, volunteer and professional services, small enterprises, and large organized programs but is most often used to refer to large-scale welfare programs carried on under professional auspices by trained personnel, either run by a government agency or paid for by public funds.

social status   The position of an individual in relation to society. Calculations of social status, while inexact, encompass class, race, economic, and cultural factors and are largely expressions of society's biases, good and bad.

social withdrawal   A state of living or being disposed to live in isolation, rather than in companionship with others or in a community.

sodomy   Legally, a sexual act involving oral-genital, anal-oral, or anal-genital contact.

soluble CD4   A CD4 CELL that is capable of being dissolved or liquefied. CD4 has been subverted in man to serve as the receptor for HIV as it commandeers T-cells to serve as viral factories. As new viruses burst out, the T-cells rupture and die. The idea that CD4 could block the virus dates to the mid-to-late 1980s. CD4 quickly became one of the most intensively studied receptors of any enveloped virus, Research continues to date.

soluble factors   Certain proteins and other substances (e.g., IL-2, TNF, alpha interferon) found in the blood. They may have either helpful or harmful effects on disease progression.

solvent   A liquid that can dissolve other substances and hold them in solution. Ethyl alcohol and Campho-phenique are solvents used to kill organisms on the skin. The latter is used primarily for cold sores. Camphor is the primary ingredient. It can be used as a counterirritant and as a moth repellant.

somatic mutation   A process of change occurring as part of B-CELL maturation, affecting the ANTIBODY GENE regions, which permits refinement of antibody specificity.

somatostatin   A HORMONE that inhibits the release of SOMATOTROPIN. It is a hypothalamic peptide that also inhibits the secretion of insulin and gastrin. This hormone also inhibits the target tissues of the hormones it inhibits. It has been used experimentally to inhibit hormone production by tumors.

somatropin   See HUMAN GROWTH HORMONE.

somatrem   See HUMAN GROWTH HORMONE.

somewhat risky sex   ORAL-GENITAL SEX without swallowing semen or INTERCOURSE without ejaculation. See RISK; SAFE SEX; UNSAFE SEX.

sonography   See ULTRASONOGRAPHY.

sonogram   See ULTRASOUND.

sore throat   Any inflammation of the tonsils, pharynx, or larynx.

soul kiss   See WET KISS.

southern blot technique   A procedure, used to separate and identify DNA sequences, in which DNA fragments are separated by ELECTROPHORESIS onto an agarose gel, blotted onto a nylon or nitrocellulose membrane, and hybridized with labeled nucleic acid probes.

specificity   The ability of a clinical test to correctly identify a subject who is not infected.

spending down   Reducing income to the eligibility level for MEDICAID by deducting incurred medical bills.

sperm   The male germ cells, or gametes. See SPERMATOZOON.

spermatozoa   See SPERMATOZOON.

spermatozoon   A mature male sperm cell that is formed within the seminiferous tubules of the TESTES. It consists of a head with a nucleus, a neck, a middle piece, and a tail and resembles a tadpole in shape. Spermatozoa make up the element of semen that pierces the envelope of the ovum to achieve fertilization.

spermicidal   See SPERMICIDE.

spermicidal cream   Spermicidal cream or jelly are contraceptives designed primarily for use with birth control barrier methods, such as a DIAPHRAGM or CERVICAL CAP. Today many women have learned that diaphragms, correctly fitted and worn, not only prevent pregnancy, but also protect against STDs. Spermicidal cream or jelly are increasingly used for extra protection with a condom.

The cream or jelly comes in a tube with a plastic applicator. Creams are white; jellies are clear. They are available without prescription at most drugstores. When a diaphragm holding spermicidal cream or jelly is in place, up to the cervix, the sperm cannot enter the cervical canal. Sperm may move around the rim of the diaphragm and be killed by the cream or jelly. Smearing cream or jelly on the outside of the diaphragm also helps kill sperm remaining in the vagina. Repeated studies indicate that using a diaphragm with cream or jelly reduces the chance of receiving GONORRHEA or trichomoniasis infections in the vaginal canal. It also increases protection against PID and CERVICAL DYSPLASIA and may help clear up adenosis.

One possible problem to be aware of: a particular cream or jelly may irritate a woman's vagina or a man's penis. Try a different brand if this happens. A second disadvantage is leaking after intercourse. The discharge of cream or jelly can be a nuisance, although it does not stain. Using different brands, and, if necessary, using a pad or a tissue for leaking after intercourse may help. Another disadvantage is that some people find the taste of the creams and jellies unpleasant. Ways around this include washing carefully after putting in the diaphragm, and putting the diaphragm in after oral sex and before intercourse.

It is generally advised to insert the diaphragm within six hours before intercourse or vagina-to-penis contact, because the creams and jellies may start to lose their spermicidal potency in the body beyond that time. The most conservative estimates say to put it in as close to intercourse as possible. Preparation and insertion instructions usually advise putting one teaspoon to one tablespoon of cream or jelly into the shallow cup, and to spread the cream or jelly around before inserting the diaphragm. Some books say to put the cream on the rim also; others say that cream on the rim makes the diaphragm slip. An effective compromise might be to put cream or jelly around the inside of the rim and not on top of the rim. For more protection, once the diaphragm is in place, some women insert a little extra cream or jelly with an applicator.

Like the diaphragm, the cervical cap blocks sperm from entering the cervical opening. Most health workers advise using a small amount of spermicidal cream or jelly inside the cap. The cap should be filled about one-third full. If too much is used, it may break the suction. The spermicide should be spread around the inside of the cap but not on the rim. The cap may be inserted up to forty hours before intercourse or vagina-to-penis contact. For backup, some women insert cream or jelly into their vagina if they have intercourse after the cap has been in place for a few hours. Some practitioners fear this may interfere with the cap's suction. The cap must be kept in place for at least six to eight hours after intercourse.

See SPERMICIDE.

spermicidal foam   A white aerated cream that has the consistency of shaving cream and contains an effective sperm-killing chemical. It comes in a can with a plunger-type plastic applicator. Deposited just outside the entrance to the cervix at the top of the vagina, foam keeps the sperm from entering the cervix and kills them as well. Foams and suppositories used alone appear to be more effective than barrier methods used with a cream or jelly. For maximum effectiveness, it is generally recommended to use foam in combination with a condom. Problems with effectiveness arise from using too little foam, not realizing that the container is almost empty, failing to shake the container enough, not inserting the foam correctly, or inserting it after vagina-to-penis contact has begun. It is also advised to put in more foam every time intercourse or vagina-to-penis contact occurs, no matter how recent the last time was. Additionally, it is cautioned to leave the foam in for six to eight hours. Waiting before douching is essential. A minipad or tissue may be used if the foam is dripping. Foams irritate some vaginas and some penises, leading to pain, itching or the sensation of heat. Advantages include the fact that when used with a CONDOM, it is a highly effective means of birth control; it is quick; it is less drippy than cream or jelly; and it helps prevent GONORRHEA and CHLAMYDIA. Disadvantages include the fact that alone, foam is quite ineffective. Also, using it may cause a brief interruption in foreplay if it is not treated as part of sex play. Many people also think it tastes terrible. It must be inserted after oral sex play. Foam is available in most drugstores without a prescription. Trying different brands is recommended.

See SPERMICIDE.

spermicidal jelly   See SPERMICIDAL CREAM; SPERMICIDE.

spermicide   A chemical product that kills sperm or other organisms, such as viruses or bacteria, on contact. It is used to prevent pregnancy and some SEXUALLY TRANSMITTED DISEASES. CONTRACEPTIVE creams, jellies, foams, and lubricants contain spermicide, of which NONOXYNOL-9 is probably the best known. Spermicides can be used separately or, most effectively, with barrier contraceptives. Most experts recommend the use of a spermicidal jelly or cream in conjunction with CONDOM use.

In heterosexual sex, when used with a condom, the spermicide should be put directly inside the vagina. The amount of spermicide in a spermicide-lubricated condom is not enough to provide protection against HIV. Adding spermicide to the inside of a condom does not help. If the condom were to break, the semen (and any HIV) would reach the vagina before the spermicide could spread out and cover the inside of the vagina. In addition, spermicides may cause vaginal sores or irritation in some women and irritation of the penis in some men. These sores or irritations may make it easier for HIV to get into the bloodstream.

spinal fluid   See CEREBROSPINAL FLUID.

spinal tap   A procedure, also called a lumbar puncture, for obtaining CEREBROSPINAL FLUID, the fluid that surrounds the brain and the spinal cord. The procedure involves inserting a needle into the middle of the back and into the MENINGES, the membrane that contains the cerebrospinal fluid. The fluid is then analyzed for evidence of infection of the brain or spinal cord. Despite sounding unpleasant and risky, a spinal tap is a well-established medical procedure and is rarely associated with any important complications. The most common complaint is of headache following the procedure made less likely by lying flat once the spinal tap is completed.

spiramycin   An ANTIBIOTIC produced from a member of the *Streptomyces* bacteria. It is administered orally.

spirulina   See BLUE-GREEN ALGAE.

spit   See SALIVA.

spleen   A glandlike lymphoid organ with immunologic and nonimmunologic functions, not all of which are understood. It removes worn-out cells from the circulatory system and is a graveyard for red blood cells, reintroducing iron

from hemoglobin after red-cell death. Like the LYMPH NODES, the spleen produces LYMPHOCYTEs and is important early in life. Removal of the spleen has been shown to be associated with overwhelming bacterial infection in infants, children, and young adults.

splenic fever   See ANTHRAX.

splenomegaly   Enlargement of the SPLEEN.

sponge   A CONTRACEPTIVE in the form of a polyurethane disc that contains SPERMICIDE and fits over the CERVIX.

sponsor   In the context of HIV and AIDS, an organization that develops a drug and usually pays the extensive bills to do so. Almost always the sponsor is a pharmaceutical company. Occasionally, a government agency or private nonprofit organization can be a sponsor. The term also refers to a person in a 12-step program who generally has at least one year of sobriety who offers support to another member.

Sporothrix   A genus of fungi of the family Moniliaceae.

Sporothrix schenckii   Causative agent of SPOROTRICHOSIS.

sporotrichosis   A chronic granulomatous infection, caused by the fungus *Sporothrix schenckii*, characterized by abscesses, nodules, and ulcers of the skin and superficial LYMPH NODES.

sprue   A chronic disease characterized by malabsorption of essential nutritive elements, causing weakness, weight loss, anemia, and diarrhea. It occurs in both tropical and nontropical forms. The cause is unknown, but appears to be genetic and hereditary.

sputum   The mucous matter that collects in the respiratory and upper digestive passages and is expelled by coughing and/or throat clearing.

sputum analysis   A method of detecting certain infections (especially TUBERCULOSIS) by culturing of sputum and microscopic examination.

sputum examination   See SPUTUM ANALYSIS.

sputum test   See SPUTUM ANALYSIS.

SPV-30   An extract of the European boxwood tree. SPV-30 reputedly has anti-HIV properties and was initially sold in the United States by some AIDS buyers clubs and a few pharmacies. For a limited time, it was available in America through a large informal trial protocol. After controversy with the FDA over the status of the product being a dietary supplement or a drug arose, SPV-30 was taken off the shelves not to be replaced until the matter is cleared. The distributor and the FDA currently await the release of the results from an 18 month, controlled French trial. If objectively and disinterestedly analyzed, the trial's data will provide a more definitive word on SPV-30's activity.

squalamine   A compound from the immune defense system of the sand shark that, in laboratory experiments, has demonstrated activity against a broad range of bacteria and fungi. Sharks are unusual in that they appear to lack cellular immunity, do not reject grafts, and do not mount an antibody response when vaccinated; they maintain health even though they appear profoundly immunocompromised.

squamous cell   A flat, scalelike epithelial cell.

squamous-cell carcinoma   A cancer developing from squamous EPITHELIAL tissue.

squamous intraepithelial lesion   Abnormalities in cells, revealed by PAP SMEAR that may indicate cancer.

SRV   See SIMIAN RETROVIRUS.

SSA   See SOCIAL SECURITY.

SSDI   See SOCIAL SECURITY DISABILITY INSURANCE.

SSI   See SUPPLEMENTAL SECURITY INCOME.

SSI/SSP   The combined total SSI and SSP income eligibility level for poor, aged, and disabled people. The figure varies by state and with living arrangements.

SSP   See STATE SUPPLEMENTARY PAYMENT.

staging   Determining what stage in its progression a disease has reached, in order to tailor treatment accordingly.

Staphylococcus   A genus of aerobic (but under some conditions anaerobic), nonmotile, non-spore-forming bacteria containing GRAM-POSITIVE spherical cells that divide in multiple planes to form irregular clusters resembling bunches of grapes. Under anaerobic conditions, they produce lactic acid from glucose. Under aerobic conditions, they produce acetic acid and small amounts of carbon dioxide. Certain coagulase-positive strains produce toxins that are potentially pathogenic and may cause food poisoning. They are found on the skin, skin glands, mucous and nasal membranes, as well as in various food products.

Staphylococcus aureus   A species of *Staphylococcus* commonly found on the skin and mucous membranes, especially those of the mouth and nose. They are characterized by the production of golden-yellow pigment and are GRAM-POSITIVE and coagulase-positive anaerobes. They cause serious suppurative (pus-forming) conditions and systemic diseases. Various strains of the species produce toxins that cause food poisoning and toxic shock syndrome.

state supplementary payment (SSP)   A state welfare payment added to the basic federal SSI allowance, raising the minimum income for poor, aged, blind, and disabled people.

statistical significance   In terms of drug testing, the result of an analytical evaluation of the results of a comparative trial or survey. Data yielding a difference in outcome depending on treatment or environmental factors are considered statistically significant if mathematical formulae indicate that there is less than a one-in-twenty (5 percent) chance that the same results would occur through random accident.

statute of limitations   A legal time limit during which, in criminal law, charges may be brought, and in tort law, claims or lawsuits may be brought. If a claim or lawsuit is not brought during the time allowed by law, the plaintiff or injured party loses the right to do so. In medical negligence claims, the statute of limitations usually starts from the time the wrong occurred or was or should have been discovered.

Stavudine   See D4T.

STD   See SEXUALLY TRANSMITTED DISEASE.

stem cell   The cells of which all immune cells are descendants; found in the BONE MARROW in small pools, stem cells multiply and mature, when needed, into functional CD4+, T and other white and red blood CELLS. Stem cells have often been thought to be the best reservoirs for harboring anti-HIV GENES. They have been notoriously difficult to identify and purify, but a newly developed simple method for isolating and maintaining them in culture dishes has enabled new research.

Researchers are currently trying to insert disease-resistant genes into the body's blood-forming cell "factories" to help cells counter HIV infection. The goal is to be able to reconstitute the immune system of HIV-infected patients with genetically modified HIV-resistant T cells. To deliver the therapeutic genes to the stem cells, the genes are enclosed in a harmless virus, an engineered adeno-associated virus (AAV). One of the genes being used makes T cells HIV-resistant through coding for the intracellular production of antibodies against HIV. In laboratory experiments, AAV has effectively transported such ANTIBODY-coding genes into test-tube grown cells, and the antibody produced inside these cells has successfully blocked HIV growth. Researchers intend to carry out these same experiments using stem cells isolated from fragments of HIV-positive patients' bone marrow. Eventually, the HIV-resistant stem cells will be returned to the patients, where they are expected to "home" back to the bone marrow and, as needed, multiply and develop into mature immune cells that are resistant to HIV.

Researchers are also trying to combine different methods of gene therapy against HIV. One strategy is to deliver different types of anti-HIV genes at the same time, all capable of inhibiting HIV growth by blocking either the function of one HIV gene or the function of one of the virus's protein components. Each kind of anti-HIV gene targets a single but critical step in the HIV's life cycle.

Because HIV inserts its genes into its host cell's own genetic material, which other viruses such as those that cause cold, flu, and herpes do not do, it functions, in a sense, as a contagious genetic disease. This is one of the reasons why strategies such as gene therapy, which are typically applied to inherited single-gene abnormalities, are so attractive as potential anti-HIV therapeutics.

sterility   Inability of the female to become pregnant or for the male to impregnate a female; also, condition of being free from living microorganisms.

sterilization   The destruction of all MICROORGANISMs in, on, or about an object by employing various means such as chemical agents (alcohol, ethylene oxide gas, phenol), high-velocity electron bombardment, steam, or ultraviolet light radiation. Also, the act or process by which an individual is made incapable of reproduction or fertilization (e.g., castration, tubectomy, vasectomy).

steroid   A member of a large family of structurally similar lipid substances. Steroid molecules have a basic skeleton consisting of four interconnected carbon rings. Different classes of steroids have different functions. All sex HOR-MONEs are steroids. Anabolic steroids increase muscle mass. Anti-inflammatory steroids, or CORTICOSTEROIDs, can reduce swelling, pain, and other manifestations of inflammation. Side effects of steroids may include an increased appetite, mood changes, fluid retention, acne, increased blood pressure, elevated blood sugar, intestinal ulcers, and lowered resistance to infection.

Stevens-Johnson syndrome   A form of erythema multiforme (eruption of dark red papules or tubercles) that is sometimes fatal. It is characterized by systemic exfoliative mucocutaneous lesions, some of which may be severe, on or in the ears, nose, lips, eyes, anus, genitals, lungs, gastrointestinal tract, heart, and kidneys.

stigma   More than a decade into the pandemic, HIV and AIDS still carry an enormous social stigma, harming persons who are infected, persons perceived to be infected, and uninfected family members and caregivers as well. Transmission of HIV in this country has been, and still is for some, associated exclusively in the public mind with "immoral" or discreditable behavior like homosexuality and intravenous drug use. The linkage of AIDS with behaviors that society has marginalized and rejected has created a climate of fear and loathing in which it is permissible for those infected with HIV/AIDS to be despised, shunned, and even assaulted—verbally, physically, and economically. It is not surprising that some persons affected by HIV have taken the stigma and sense of shame that often accompany it as part of their own sense of identity.

To some extent, the law mitigates this situation by providing people affected with some recourse against discrimination and by giving them some control over access to medical information about themselves. Recent changes in federal laws have expanded markedly protection against HIV-related discrimination. See AMERICANS WITH DISABILITIES ACT, REHABILITATION ACT OF 1973, and FAIR HOUSING AMENDMENTS ACT of 1988.

stimulant   Any agent temporarily increasing functional activity. Stimulants may be classified according to the organ upon which they act as follows: bronchial, gastric, cerebral, intestinal, nervous, motor, vasomotor, respiratory, and secretory.

STLV   See SIMIAN IMMUNODEFICIENCY VIRUS.

stomach   A dilated, saclike distensible portion of the alimentary canal between the esophagus and the intestines, located below the diaphragm, to the right of the spleen, and partly under the liver. The stomach's basic function is as an organ of digestion.

stomatitis   Any of numerous inflammatory diseases of the mouth. Causes vary and include mechanical trauma, irritants, allergy, vitamin deficiency, and infection.

straight   Slang for a person who prefers sex with a person of the opposite sex; nonhomosexual.

streetwalker   See PROSTITUTE.

Streptococcus pneumonia   See PNEUMOCOCCUS.

streptomycin   A bacterial ANTIBIOTIC derived from the soil microbe *Streptomyces griseus*. It belongs to the AMINOGLYCO-SIDE class and is effective against most GRAM-NEGATIVE and ACID-FAST BACTERIA. It is also effective against certain GRAM-POSITIVE forms but is used mainly in the treatment of TUBER-CULOSIS.

Streptomycin was the first drug with proven effectiveness against the MYCOBACTERIA that cause tuberculosis, but because of its toxicity and the development of alternatives, it is no longer first-line therapy for tuberculosis or other bacterial infections. Streptomycin is available as a solution for intramuscular injection. Nausea, vomiting, vertigo, flushing, skin rashes, and swelling are common side effects. Less frequently, deafness, severe peeling of the skin, anaphylactic shock, muscle weakness, vision impairment, and bone-marrow toxicity occur. Rarely, kidney toxicity may occur.

stress   The result produced when a structure, system, or organism is acted upon by forces that disrupt equilibrium or produce strain. In health care, the term denotes the physical (gravity, mechanical force, pathogen, injury) and psychological (fear, anxiety, crisis, joy) forces that are experienced by individuals. It is generally believed that biological organisms require a certain amount of stress in order to maintain their well-being. When more stress occurs than the system can handle, it produces pathological changes. The amount of stress humans can withstand without having a pathological reaction to it varies from individual to individual and from situation to situation.

stressor   A factor that produces STRESS.

stroke   A suddenly occurring acute vascular lesion of the brain, such as a hemorrhage, embolism, or thrombosis, producing a condition characterized by paralysis and neurologic damage, often irreversible. Symptoms can include focal weakness, speech impediment, and impaired consciousness. Also called a CEREBROVASCULAR ACCIDENT.

stroke syndrome   The condition produced by a STROKE.

Strongyloides stercoralis A nematode, or roundworm, occurring in tropical and subtropical countries and in the southern United States that infests dogs, primates, and humans. It causes the infection STRONGYLOIDIASIS.

strongyloidiasis An infection caused by infestation with nematodes of the genus *Strongyloides*. Infestation may persist for years due to the nature of the life cycle. Infection can occur indirectly by larvae of a new generation developed in the soil. It may also occur directly by infected larvae developed without an intervening adult phase, or by autoreinfection, in which the female inhabits the intestines of the host, larvae develop within the feces of the host, penetrate the mucosa, and migrate through the venous system to the lungs, causing hemorrhage (pulmonary strongyloidiasis) and back to the intestines through blood-lung interactions.

Autoreinfection is the cause of the most serious human infections and the majority of fatalities. Their life cycle allows for massive infection sufficient to cause overwhelming systemic infection with fever, severe abdominal pain, shock, and possibly death. Severe reactions, are more likely to occur in immunosuppressed patients or patients with diseases that alter their immune status. Also called strongyloidosis. See also STRONGYLOIDES STERCORALIS.

strongyloidosis See STRONGYLOIDIASIS.

stud Slang for a virile man, or one who has sex with many partners.

subacute encephalitis See AIDS DEMENTIA COMPLEX.

subclinical infection An infection, or phase of infection, without apparent symptoms or signs of disease.

subcutaneous Under the skin, as a subcutaneous injection.

subepidemic A secondary or subordinate epidemic; within the context of HIV, a secondary epidemic existing at the same time as HIV. For example, while HIV is the most serious danger facing gay men who have unprotected sex, it is far from being the only one. Prevention experts warn that those who slip from safe sex standards run the risk of starting—or spreading—a subepidemic of other sexually transmitted diseases such as HEPATITIS A, HEPATITIS B, HEPATITIS C, CHLAMYDIA, GONORRHEA, HERPES, and SYPHILIS.

subsidized employment A job in which an employee does not fully "earn his own way," in which the paycheck is actually partial or full "disguised charity"; the term is applied by SOCIAL SECURITY to handicapped workshops and the like, where people are employed for charitable, morale, or therapeutic reasons. By extension, the term can be applied to situations in which a no-longer-productive deteriorating worker is continued on the payroll for altruistic purposes.

substance abuse See ADDICTION; DRUG ABUSE.

substantial gainful activity (SGA) A SOCIAL SECURITY term for work that brings an income of over $300 monthly, the limit of eligibility for disabled persons for SSDI.

subunit vaccine A vaccine that contains only portions of a surface molecule of a disease-producing MICROORGANISM.

sucralfate A medicine consisting of a complex formed from sucrose octasulfate and polyaluminum hydroxide. It is effective in treating peptic ulcers by forming a coating over them that stays in place for more than eight hours. Trade name is Carafate.

suicide The intentional and voluntary taking of one's own life. While many states continue to bar physicians from helping mentally competent, terminally ill adults to hasten their deaths, physician-assisted suicide still occurs in the United States. It is also a fact that while society may not approve of assisted suicide, books such as Derek Humphry's *Final Exit: The Practicalities of Self-Deliverance and Assisted Suicide for the Dying* and Sherwin B. Nuland's *How We Die: Reflections on Life's Final Chapter* continue to enjoy immense popularity. Additionally, suicide hot lines are supported in many states and counties nationwide. Psychologists and others continue to debate about whether or not assisted suicide is ever a rational choice. Some believe that suicide can be a rational act and that psychologists and other mental health professionals should be allowed to help such patients without fear of legal or professional repercussions. Others argue that suicide is a symptom of mental illness and that helping someone to commit it should continue to be banned. With regard to AIDS, many feel that suicide is a normal reaction to specific situations.

Attempts to define rational suicide outline three basic criteria. First, the patient should have a hopeless condition, which includes a low quality of life and psychological as well as physical pain. Second, the patient should be free of coercion, whether coercion consists of internal factors like ageist or able-ist beliefs or external factors like greedy relatives or cost-conscious medical professionals or institutions. Third, the patient should be engaged in sound decision making. Sound decision making, in turn, should include the following five sub-criteria: (1) the patient should be mentally competent, which eliminates patients with treatable depression and other judgment-clouding impairments; (2) the patient should nonimpulsively consider other options, such as psychotherapy, antidepressants, assisted living, or support groups; (3) the decision should be consistent with the patient's values; (4) the patient should consider the impact suicide will have on significant others; and (5), the patient should consult with others, such as religious leaders, disability advocates, physical therapists, or hospice personnel.

sulfa drug A drug of the sulfonamide group possessing bacteriostatic properties. Sulfa drugs are among the most common ANTIBIOTICs used against HIV infection. Many AIDS and HIV treatments employ antibiotic drug compounds that include sulfa, a substance to which many people with HIV disease are allergic. There are strategies that may lessen or manage this problem; desensitization, for example, is a relatively simple and safe way of overcoming sulfa allergies. See TRIMETHOPRIM-SULFAMETHOXAZOLE; SULFADIAZINE; DAPSONE; SULFASALAZINE; SULFISOXAZOLE; SULFANIMIDE.

sulfadiazine (SFDZ)   A derivative of sulfonamide that appears as a white or yellowish powder. Sulfadiazine is used to treat urinary tract infections, chancroid, and trachoma. With pyrimethamine, it is used to treat TOXOPLASMOSIS. It is also occasionally used to treat malaria resistant to chloroquine; with streptomycin, to treat meningitis; and with penicillin, ear infections. It is administered orally. The most common side effects are allergic reactions, including skin rashes, itching, anaphylactic shock, swelling, sensitivity to light, joint pain, fever, and chills. The most serious side effects are blood disorders, including reduced counts of red blood cells, white blood cells, and platelets. Other side effects include headache, peripheral neuropathy, mental depression, convulsion, weakness, hallucinations, ringing in the ears, vertigo, insomnia, and kidney toxicity. Rarely, goiter production, changes in urination, and low-blood-sugar levels have occurred in people taking the drug.

Sulfadiazine is one of a number of sulfa drugs that work by interfering with FOLIC ACID (vitamin B) metabolism in susceptible organisms, preventing them from multiplying. Because parasites can rapidly develop resistance to sulfadiazine, the drug is usually used with pyrimethamine for toxoplasmosis. The activity of the combination, called sulfadoxine, against the parasite greatly exceeds that of either drug alone. Because both drugs cross the BLOOD-BRAIN BARRIER, and the combination is effective against toxoplasmosis encephalitis, a serious and potentially fatal infection of the brain.

sulfadoxine   See SULFADIAZINE.

sulfamethoxazole   A sulfonamide appearing as a white-to-off-white crystalline powder used in the treatment of urinary tract infections. It is administered orally.

sulfasalazine (SFSZ)   A sulfa drug that is an approved treatment for a number of autoimmune diseases, including rheumatoid arthritis. In a small unblinded study in 1994, HIV-POSITIVE patients who were given sulfasalazine had substantial increases in CD4 counts.

sulfisoxazole   A sulfonamide used for treating certain bacterial infections, especially urinary tract infections. Trade names are SK-Soxazole and Gantrisin.

sulfanamide   Any of a group of compounds that consist of the amides of sulfamic acid. They are derivatives of sulfanilamide acid and are bacteriostatic. Sulfanilamide's are white, slightly bitter crystalline substances from coal tar, the parent of the azo dyes. Formerly, they were widely used in the treatment of a number of infections, but because of their toxic reactions, they have been superseded by more effective and less toxic sulfonamides. Their action on bacteria results from their ability to interfere with the functioning of the enzyme systems required for normal metabolisms, growth, and multiplication.

sunlight   Even before studies were published about the effect of sunlight on HIV, AIDS-knowledgeable physicians were cautious about the dangers of sunlight to persons with AIDS, ARC, or ASYMPTOMATIC HIV INFECTION. It had long been known that ultraviolet light can damage or suppress the Langerhans cells of the skin. These cells are an important part of the immune system, and are cells which HIV is known to infect. Strong sunlight, probably the ultraviolet rays, can impair immune response. Laying out in the sun or playing volleyball in one's swimsuit for hours at a time are examples of activities about which to be worried. T-HELPER CELL counts drop almost invariably after someone spends a long weekend at the beach. While regular exposure during daily activities is not of concern, it is noted that a number of drugs used by persons with HIV/AIDS make the skin much more sensitive to the sun than usual. Additionally, in the late 1980s, researchers at the CENTERS FOR DISEASE CONTROL AND PREVENTION found that the onset of AIDS as well as almost all opportunistic infections, peak in the summer, when ultraviolet exposure from sunlight is highest. In addition to being harmful to persons with HIV/AIDS, sunlight can provoke HERPES outbreaks.

superantigen   A foreign material produced by infectious MICROORGANISMs. Superantigens have the ability to activate many different T CELLs, resulting in large amounts of CYTOKINE production and large-scale activation of the immune system. This activation may result in shock. Many toxins that cause food poisoning in humans are superantigens. Unlike normal ANTIGENs, they are not processed and associate with MHC Class II molecules outside the peptide binding groove; recognition also is not MHC-restricted.

superinfection   A new, second infection caused by an organism different from that which caused an initial infection. The microbe responsible is usually resistant to the treatment given for the initial infection.

superoxide dismutase   One of the major cellular antioxidant enzymes. It removes surplus peroxide, an oxidizing free radical. Superoxide dismutase comes in two forms, one containing copper and zinc and the other containing manganese.

Supplemental Security Income (SSI)   A federal welfare program, operated by the SOCIAL SECURITY Administration with general revenues, that makes monthly payments to people with low incomes and limited assets who are 65 or older, blind, or disabled. As its name implies, it supplements existing, but inadequate income. The level varies from state to state and can go up every year based on cost-of-living adjustments. In addition to low income, people on SSI must have limited assets.

support group   A group whose purpose is to give emotional and psychological encouragement and confidence to its members. Support groups are often associated with psychotherapy, but many have been formed by people in similar difficulties or with similar problems, for mutual benefit. See also SUPPORT NETWORK.

support network   A therapeutic term for a group of inter-connected or cooperative individuals who give each other mutual encouragement and support. A support network tends to be an informal group linked by ties of friendship or family, rather than a purposely created formal support group.

suppository   A cylinder or cone made of a semisolid substance infused, generally, with medicine, such as soap, glycerinated gelatin, or cocoa butter, for introduction into the rectum, vagina, or urethra, where it dissolves. Suppositories are not recommended as barriers against the transmission of HIV or AIDS.

suppressor cell   See SUPPRESSOR T CELL.

suppressor T cell   Any of a subset of T LYMPHOCYTEs that suppress antibody synthesis by B CELLS or inhibit other cellular immune reactions by effector T cells. This suppressor function is presently believed to be controlled by CYTOKINEs.

suppurat   To form or emit a flow of pus.

suramin   The first compound identified, in 1984, with anti-HIV activity IN VITRO. In CLINICAL TRIALS against KAPOSI'S SARCOMA and AIDS-RELATED COMPLEX, it was found to be highly toxic, with no clinical, immunologic, or virologic benefit for HIV-infected individuals.

surgeon general   The title of the chief medical officer in the United States Army, Air Force, Navy, and PUBLIC HEALTH SERVICE.

surgical glove   A sterile, nonporous latex glove that covers the whole hand, worn by doctors and other medical personnel for surgery, examinations, and other medical procedures and in handling medical waste, blood products, and so forth. These gloves are often used for FIST- or FINGER-FUCKING and other HIGH-RISK SEX practices. Some users cut off the hand area and use the wrist/forearm area (flattened, slit lengthwise and opened) to create a DENTAL DAM/oral shield. Surgical gloves can be bought at most medical suppliers and chemists.

surrogacy   A legal arrangement under which a person or institution assumes responsibility for an adult individual judged incompetent to care for himself or to look after his affairs. There are different types of surrogacy, including attorney-in-fact, conservatorship, and guardianship. See SURROGATE.

surrogate   A person or institution appointed by a court to look after the affairs of one judged incompetent because of illness, age, or some other condition. Forms of surrogacy include attorney-in-fact, conservatorship, and guardianship. The legal process to appoint surrogates, and the legal powers granted to them vary from state to state. In California, for example, individuals demonstrating continuing grave disability as a result of mental illness may be placed under a conservatorship, subject to yearly review and renewal by the court. Anyone may file a petition for conservatorship on behalf of a gravely disabled person, and the court will inves-

tigate the need and the qualifications of the proposed conservator. If there is "clear and convincing evidence" that a gravely disabled person is so incompetent as to be unable to care for him or herself, the court may appoint a temporary conservator who will serve until the investigation is complete. A surrogate may be charged with the obligation to make health care decisions for the person judged incompetent, and be empowered to give informed consent on his or her behalf.

surrogate marker   A blood or other lab test measurement that indicates the presence and action of a virus, such as HIV, that is difficult to monitor directly.

Ever since AIDS was recognized in 1981, the medical establishment has grappled with how exactly to describe the disease and monitor its progression. A major obstacle is that measuring the amount of HIV in the human body is extremely difficult. HIV is notoriously difficult to track, since it mutates rapidly, and it is difficult to grow in the test tube. No reliable, standardized lab test that measures HIV accurately is yet available, so many health care workers have been monitoring HIV disease progression by measuring quantities, other than virus levels, that *reflect* HIV activity, such as that of T4 CELLS. These are referred to as "surrogate markers" because they provide information on HIV through its secondary effects on the immune system. This information can guide treatment decisions and monitor the efficacy of treatments.

Researchers and activists are constantly engaged in debates about which markers are the most reliable, practical, and predictive of HIV progression. As with most aspects of AIDS, the dialogue about surrogate markers resonates with political implications. For instance, the use of surrogate markers to measure an experimental drug's efficacy may significantly shorten human trials and enable the drug to be made available more expediently. Additionally, the use of surrogate markers as a way of defining AIDS will directly determine who receives a diagnosis of AIDS or ARC, who receives financial entitlements, who receives medical treatment, how research efforts are conducted, and how the scope of the epidemic is understood.

Most surrogate markers are components of the immune system. These include different types of cells, such as T4 and T8 cells. In addition, proteins secreted by immune system cells, like NEOPTERIN and BETA-2 MICROGLOBULIN, are used as surrogate markers. A current trend is to consider several markers together, as a way of accurately monitoring HIV progression. A fluctuation in a single marker may not be significant when a number of other markers remain steady. See also IMMUNOLOGIC MARKERS and VIROLOGIC MARKERS.

surveillance   In public health terms, the process of monitoring conditions such as epidemics. According to the World Health Organization (WHO), "public health surveillance is the collection of information of sufficient accuracy and completeness regarding the distribution and spread of infection to be pertinent to the design, implementation, or monitoring of prevention and control programmes and activities." Public health surveillance involves an assessment of the existing distribution and scope of infection and its likely spread in the population and is an important first step in responding to a disease. As people infected with HIV can remain asymptomatic for a very long time and because infection can be detected only with a specific test, testing has became the central issue in monitoring HIV/AIDS.

Surveillance is a term often associated with intrusions into individual privacy. For the purpose of public health surveillance it is sufficient to know how many people are infected. It is not necessary to know the identities of the infected people. See PRIVACY.

surveillance case definition   The case definition used for surveillance purposes. As AIDS cases are diagnosed among various subpopulations, epidemiologists have come to recognize a wide spectrum of clinical signs and symptoms that may be associated with the disease. This diversity has resulted with changes in the case definition used for surveillance purposes, which in turn has led to changes in the prevalence of AIDS across risk categories. The original surveillance definition for AIDS was developed primarily through studies of the natural history of the disease among homosexual and bisexual men and reflected the disease as it appeared in those individuals. It is now understood that there may be very different manifestations of the underlying immune defect across risk categories, which, including the "wasting syndrome" and AIDS-related dementia, are now included in the surveillance definition of AIDS.

In August 1987, the CENTERS FOR DISEASE CONTROL AND PREVENTION (CDC), in collaboration with public health and clinical specialists, developed a revised case definition for surveillance of acquired immunodeficiency syndrome (AIDS). This definition was intended only to provide consistent statistical data for public health purposes. (The revised definition can be found reprinted from Council of State and Territorial Epidemiologists and CDC, Center for Infectious Diseases, AIDS Program, "Revision of the CDC Surveillance Case Definition for Acquired Immunodeficiency Syndrome," *Morbidity and Mortality Weekly Report*, 36, supp. 1 [August 14, 1987], 3S-15S.) The objectives of the revision were (a) to track more effectively the severe disabling morbidity associated with infection with HUMAN IMMUNODEFICIENCY VIRUS (HIV); (b) to simplify reporting of AIDS cases; (c) to increase the sensitivity and specificity of the definition through greater diagnostic application of laboratory evidence for HIV infection; and (d) to be consistent with the then current diagnostic practices, which in some cases included presumptive (without confirmatory laboratory evidence), diagnosis of AIDS-indicative diseases (e.g. PNEUMOCYSTITS CARINII PNEUMONIA, KAPOSI'S SARCOMA).

The definition is organized into three sections that depend on the status of laboratory evidence of HIV infection (e.g., HIV antibody)—status that is unknown or inconclusive (without laboratory evidence regarding HIV infection), positive (with laboratory evidence for HIV infection), and negative (with laboratory evidence against HIV infection). The major proposed changes applied to patients with laboratory evidence for HIV infection are: (a) inclusion of HIV encephalopathy, HIV wasting syndrome, and a broader range of specific AIDS-indicative diseases; (b) inclusion of AIDS

patients whose indicator diseases are diagnosed presumptively; and (c) elimination of exclusions due to other causes of immunodeficiency. Application of the definition for children differed from that for adults. The initiation of the actual reporting of cases that met the new definition was targeted for September 1, 1987.

Clinicians were cautioned not to rely on the revised definition alone to diagnose serious disease caused by HIV infection in individual patients because there may be additional information that would lead to a more accurate diagnosis. It was emphasized that the diagnostic criteria accepted by the AIDS surveillance case definition should not be interpreted as the standard of good medical practice.

survey   A comprehensive appraisal of an area of research, particularly into a particular disease or health condition, especially its epidemiological aspects.

survival   Continued life, especially under conditions in which death would be expected to occur; a measure of drug efficacy consisting of the length of life of a person on a drug.

survival (or survivor) benefit   The amount payable to a beneficiary from an annuity or insurance policy when the policyholder dies.

survival rate   The percentage of a particular study group that survives over a given time.

susceptible host   Any organism that is easily invaded by a parasitic organism.

sweats   See NIGHT SWEATS.

swing party   A party at which participants may engage in sexual acts.

swinger   Person who engages in sex at swing parties.

swollen glands   Enlarged lymph nodes, rounded bodies consisting of accumulation of lymphatic tissue found at intervals in the course of the lymphatic vessels. In the context of HIV/AIDS, swollen glands generally refers to the condition of the lymph nodes in the region of the neck, the armpit, or the groin. Soon after AIDS was identified as a new disease, physicians noticed that a large group of previously healthy homosexual men were seeking treatment for persistent swollen glands not explained by specific illnesses or drug use. The epidemiological characteristics of this population were identical with those of the population of AIDS patients. As the epidemic progressed, similar findings were reported among intravenous drug abusers, hemophiliacs, and the heterosexual partners of some AIDS patients. When the blood test for HIV-1 antibodies became available, researchers demonstrated that LYMPHADENOPATHY (chronically swollen lymph nodes) was a frequent consequence of infection with the virus. Initially, it was believed that people who developed persistent lymphadenopathy were more likely to progress to AIDS than infected patients whose glands remained normal. Researchers in 1987 found that, in the absence of other symptoms, persistently swollen glands are not indicative of a declining immune system. (Richard A. Kaslow et al. "Infection with the Human Immunodeficiency Virus: Clinical Manifestations and Their Relationship to Immune Deficiency," *AIM* 107 [1987]: 474–480.)

symptom   Any phenomenon or circumstance accompanying something and serving as evidence of it. In medicine, a phenomenon that arises from and accompanies a particular disease or disorder and serves as an indication of it. For example, genital ulcers are one symptom of HERPES SIMPLEX, and a slowly progressive neurologic dysfunction is one symptom of PROGRESSIVE MULTIFOCAL LEUKOENCEPHALOPATHY (PML), an opportunistic infection caused by the Creutzfeld-Jacob virus.

symptomology   The complex of symptoms of a disease; also, the branch of medicine concerned with symptoms, their production, and the indications they furnish.

synapse   The point of junction between two neurons in a neural pathway, where the termination of the axon of one neuron comes into close proximity to the cell body or dendrites of another. At this point, an electrical impulse traveling in the first neuron initiates an impulse in the second neuron. The impulses travel in one direction only. Synapses are susceptible to fatigue, offer resistance to the passage of impulses, and are markedly susceptible to the effects of oxygen deficiency, anesthetics, and other agents, including therapeutic drugs and toxic chemicals.

syndrome   A group of symptoms and diseases that together are characteristic of a specific condition.

synergism   Cooperative interaction; interaction between two or more agents (e.g., drugs) that produces an effect greater than the sum of their individual effects. Also called SYNERGY.

synergy   See SYNERGISM.

synovir   See THALIDOMIDE.

synthetic baryta   See BARIUM SULFATE.

synthetic CD4   See CD4, SYNTHETIC.

syphilis   An infectious, sexually transmitted disease caused by *Treponema pallidum* that, if left untreated, can cause chronic infection of multiple organ sites, including the central nervous system. Syphilis is characterized by lesions that may involve any organ or body tissue. Syphilis usually presents initially as a single painless ulcer (which may or may not be noticed by female patients). Generally, cutaneous manifestations are exhibited, and relapses may occur frequently. Syphilis may remain asymptomatic for years. If untreated, syphilis progresses through three clinical stages: primary (ini-

tial painless ulcerative lesions at the site of inoculation); secondary (widespread mucocutaneous lesions and generalized regional lymphadenopathy); and tertiary (destructive lesions involving many organs and tissues, including the heart and central nervous system). When untreated in pregnant women, it can result in a life-threatening congenital infection in the newborn. It is usually transmitted through sexual contact (both heterosexual and homosexual), but may be acquired in utero or by direct contact with infected tissue or blood.

Diagnosis usually is based on a serologic test, run along with a confirmatory test. Treatment failures do occur and may be more common in HIV illness. Penicillin is the preferred drug for treatment. It is the only therapy that has been widely used for patients with neurosyphilis, congenital syphilis, or syphilis during pregnancy.

All sexually active patients with syphilis and their partners should be tested for HIV. Neurosyphilis should be considered in the differential diagnosis of neurologic disease in HIV-persons.

syphilitic chancre   The syphilis ulcer, the first symptom of syphilis.

syringe   Instrument for injecting fluids into cavities or vessels. A hypodermic is a syringe, fitted with a needle, used to administer drugs by injecting them into the SUBCUTANEOUS TISSUE. An oral syringe is made of plastic or glass, and is not fitted with a needle. It is graduated and is used to dispense liquid medication to children. The tip is constructed to prevent its breaking in the child's mouth.

syringe access   See NEEDLE ACCESS.

syringe exchange program   See NEEDLE EXCHANGE PROGRAM.

syringe sharing   See NEEDLE SHARING.

systemic   Relating to the entire organism, as distinguished from any of its individual parts. A systemic therapy is one that the entire body is exposed to, rather than just the tissues affected by a disease.

systemic chemotherapy   Treatment with antitumor or anticancer medication by introducing it into the veins for distribution to all tissues via general circulation.

systemic disease   Any pathologic condition involving the entire organism as distinct from an individual organ system or part.

systemic lupus erythematosus   An immune disease of unknown etiology characterized by fever, muscle pains, joint pains, skin rashes, anemia, and low white blood cell counts. It affects connective tissue as well as the kidneys, spleen, skin, heart, and the nervous system.

T

T1 cell The cytotoxic T cells involved in cell-mediated immunity.

T4 cell A LYMPHOCYTE and the most important cell in the specialized immune response, also known as a "helper" or CD4 cell. Helper T cells induce, help, and coordinate the specialized immune response, which cannot function without them. T4 cells also stimulate the production of B cells. They have an identifying surface structure called CD4 or T4.

T4-cell count A measure of the immune system; the number of T4 LYMPHOCYTEs present in a cubic millimeter of blood. A normal range is anywhere from 500 to 1,500. T4 counts are the best known and most widely used surrogate markers. Since HIV attacks T4 cells, comparing the number of existing T4 cells to the normal range (and to previous counts) is commonly used to predict progression of disease; T4 counts have been correlated with survival. T4 levels can be reported in the following ways: absolute number of T4 cells; percentage of T4 cells of all lymphocytes; and ratio of T4 to T8 cells.

To date, most research exploring T4 cells as surrogate markers for HIV disease has involved only gay and bisexual men. This information has been applied to women. Such extrapolation of research findings is common in HIV and many other areas. Research on surrogate markers in women is needed to confirm treatment recommendations such as PCP PROPHYLAXIS and anti-HIV therapies such as AZT and ddI.

T4-cell percentage What percentage of the total number of LYMPHOCYTEs is T4 cells. The normal range is between 32 and 50 percent. A change of three percentage points is considered significant, and a reduction of such size may indicate HIV progression even if absolute T4 counts remain steady.

T4-cell test T4-cell tests are significantly limited. First, T4 counts may include nonfunctioning cells, since the mechanism that counts the cells does not distinguish between healthy T4 and HIV-impaired cells. Second, it is well known that T4 counts can fluctuate dramatically even in the course of a single day, and different labs may well report different counts for the same blood sample. For individuals being tested, it is important to have blood drawn at approximately the same time of day each time, if possible, and to have samples sent to the same lab. For diagnostic purposes, the trend in T4 counts over time is more meaningful than any single T4 value.

See T4-CELL COUNT.

T4 count See T4 CELL COUNT.

T4 lymphocyte See T4 CELL.

T4:T8 ratio See T-CELL HOMEOSTASIS; T-CELL RATIO.

T8 cell Also known as a CD8 or "suppressor" cell, this LYMPHOCYTE suppresses or "turns off" the immune system when an infection has been suppressed. Without T8 cells, our immune systems would remain activated and might attack the healthy parts of our bodies. The suppressor T cell has the same identifying surface structure, called CD8 or T8, as the killer T cell. Standard lymphocyte typing does not therefore distinguish between suppressor T cells and killer T cells.

Much emphasis has been placed on the ratio of T8 cells to T4 cells. Normally, a person should have twice as many T4 CELLs as T8 cells, a ratio of 2:1. However, during HIV progression, the proportion of T4 cells decreases dramatically, and a person may have twice as many T8 cells as T4 cells. This inversion has also been interpreted as a bad sign, and some people advocate tracking the ratio of these cells. See also T-CELL HOMEOSTASIS.

Absolute T8 count, although not altogether well understood, has also been endorsed as a good surrogate marker by some AIDS clinicians.

T8 lymphocyte See T8 CELL.

T cell LYMPHOCYTE that travels from the BONE MARROW via the blood and enters the THYMUS, after which it enters the circulation again and settle in the spleen and LYMPH nodes. T cells are essential elements in cellular immunity against viruses, parasites, fungi, and malignant cells, and may be rendered ineffective by HIV. T cells also release factors that induce proliferation of T lymphocytes and B LYMPHOCYTES. T lymphocytes are found primarily in the blood, lymph, and lymphoid organs.

Immature T cells are called thymocytes. Mature T cells are "ANTIGEN-specific," meaning that each one responds only to one antigen. Unlike B cells, T cells do not recognize native antigen conformation directly, but only in association with self-antigens of the major histocompatibility complex. There are two major subsets of T cells: those expressing the accessory molecule CD4 and those expressing CD8. The former are mainly T helper cells; the latter are generally effector cells recognizing and destroying infected cells (i.e., cytotoxic cells). T helper cells recognize a specific MHC-antigen complex on the surface of a B cell and then induce its maturation and proliferation into specific antibody-screening (plasma) cells. While in the thymus, a T cell "learns" during T-cell maturation both to treat its body's Class I molecules as "self-antigens" and to recognize as foreign a specific epitope of a "non-self antigen." T cells do not produce antibody, but antibody production by B cells often requires T-cell help. T-cell receptors bind antigen on the surfaces of other cells only after it has been degraded or otherwise processed by that cell, and only after it has become physically associated with molecules of the MHC. MHC restriction refers to the process during T-cell maturation in the thymus when an individual's T cells come to recognize, and be activated by, antigen. Self-restriction occurs when T cells preferentially recognize foreign antigens encountered during their own development in the thymus. Cytotoxic T cells recognize tumor or virus-infected cells by their surface antigens in combination with their MHC markers, and will kill them. Other T cells (macrophage-activating cells) produce lymphokines, which promote macrophage activity. Suppressor T cells specifically suppress the immune response, probably through antigen-presenting cells and/or through more direct interactions with T-helper cells or B cells.

T cells are normally repopulated without regard to subset—that is, both CD4 and CD8 cells are produced to replace their loss. In people with HIV infection, CD4+ T cells are selectively infected by the virus, resulting in the preferential killing of these cells. The process of "blind T cell homeostasis" replaces lost CD4+ T cells with both CD4+ T cells and CD8+ T cells. The result is a gradual increase in the ratio of CD8+ T cells, even while the total T-cell count remains constant. Ultimately, for unknown reasons, blind T-cell homeostasis fails and CD8+ T cells, as well as CD4+ T cells, start to decrease in number.

T-cell count   The number of T lymphocytes in a cubic millimeter of blood. See also T CELLS.

T-cell homeostasis   Research indicates that the body's complex mechanisms that normally maintain levels of T cells, known as homeostasis, may contribute to the development of the abnormalities in T-cell numbers seen in HIV-infected people (i.e., falling CD4+ and rising CD8+ counts) and that the ultimate failure of T-cell homeostasis contributes to the onset of AIDS. Failure of T-cell homeostasis appears to represent a recognizable and clinically significant landmark in the natural history of HIV infection. Because of this, some researchers advocate measurements of all T-cell subsets, not just CD4+ cells. See T-CELL RATIO.

T-cell leukemia   See T-CELL LYMPHOMA.

T-cell lymphoma   An acute or subacute disease associated with a human T cell virus and characterized by LYMPHADENOPATHY, hypercalcemia, hepatosplenomegaly, skin lesions, and peripheral blood involvement. Also called T-CELL LEUKEMIA.

T-cell ratio   The relative proportions of T4 LYMPHOCYTEs (helper cells) and T8 LYMPHOCYTEs (suppressor cells) in the blood.

T-cell receptor   T CELLS need to recognize a wide variety of antigens, doing so through the cooperation of a membrane receptor (TCR) and accessory molecules. The genes encoding the receptor resemble those for antibodies and comprise variable and constant regions. As in that system, production of the TCR repertoire involves both germ-line diversity and gene rearrangements. ANTIGEN recognition by the T-cell receptors involves their binding that antigen (often a peptide fragment) when presented on another cell's surface stably bound to a protein encoded by the organism's major histocompatibility complex. Antigen-binding by the TCR activates a protein tyrosine kinase (enzymes providing a central switch mechanism in cellular signal transduction pathways, often involved in cell fate determination) and a generation of phosphatidyl-derived second messengers (a messenger produced by phospholipase, the activity as a breakdown of the major cell membrane phospholipid phosphatidy-linositol).

T-cell restriction   Alternative for MHC-RESTRICTION (major histocompatibility complex) of T CELL.

T-cell test   A test to determine T-cell count, used to monitor the immune status of someone who has HIV. See T-CELL COUNT; T4-CELL COUNT; T4-CELL TEST.

T-dependent/independent   T-dependent ANTIGENs require immune recognition by both T and B CELLS to produce an immune response. T-independent antigens can directly stimulate B cells to produce specific ANTIBODY.

T-helper cell   See T4 CELL.

T-helper cell count   See T4-CELL COUNT.

T-helper lymphocyte   See T4 CELL.

T-helper to T-suppressor ratio   See T-CELL HOMEOSTASIS; T-CELL RATIO.

T-killer cell   A type of LYMPHOCYTE, or white blood cell, that kills foreign organisms after being activated by T-HELPER CELLS.

T lymphocyte   See T CELL.

T-suppressor lymphocyte   See T8 CELL.

Tagamet   See CIMETIDINE.

tampon   A plug (made of absorbent material) inserted into the vagina to soak up menstrual blood.

tardive dyskinesia   Involuntary movements, generally of the muscles in the face or mouth. It is usually the consequence of long-term administration of certain psychoactive drugs.

tat   A gene of HIV that regulates viral activity.

tat antagonist   See TAT INHIBITOR.

tat gene   The HIV gene that enables HIV replication by encoding a transactivating genetic element of the virus that increases the production of cellular and viral proteins.

tat gene inhibitor   See TAT INHIBITOR.

tat inhibitor   One of a group of drug compounds that interfere with HIV replication by eliminating or disabling the TAT GENE. Also known as tat ANTAGONISTs or antitat compounds.

tattoo   An indelible body marking produced by injecting minute amounts of pigments into the skin. When tattooing is done commercially, sterile procedures are rarely used, and there is a serious risk that infectious hepatitis or HIV or both may be transmitted. Tattoos are usually done for decorative purposes, by those who find it attractive, but they may also be used cosmetically, to conceal a corneal leukoma, to mask pigmented areas of skin, or to color skin to look like the areola in mammoplasty.

Taxol   A chemotherapeutic drug used for the treatment of solid tumors. Taxol is an experimental treatment for KAPOSI'S SARCOMA. It works by interfering with internal cell structures, which are necessary for cell division. Consequently, it is highly toxic to rapidly dividing cells, such as those in tumors or in normal BONE MARROW. It has a long list of side effects, the most serious of which is severe and potentially fatal allergic reactions. Bone-marrow toxicity, resulting in a deficiency of white blood cells called NEUTROPENIA, is also common but is manageable and reversible. PERIPHERAL NEUROPATHY is the most common neurological side effect. Neuropathy is generally cumulative with repeated doses, and more likely to occur in people at risk for it, for instance those who have experienced neuropathy as a side effect of other therapy. Other side effects include irregular heart rhythm, hair loss, diarrhea, skin rashes, nausea, vomiting, stomach irritation, and seizures. Taxol is available as a solution for INTRAVENOUS injection. Brand name is Taxol.

TCR   See T-CELL RECEPTOR.

tears   Drops of the watery secretion of the lacrimal glands, tears are secreted continuously into the eyes. HIV has been recovered from tears but is unproved as a route of transmission of the virus. HIV is present in many body fluids, but the principal forms of transmission are limited to direct exposure to contaminated blood, sexual contact with exposure to secretions, and exchange of blood from mother to child during pregnancy or shortly thereafter.

Teldrin   See CHLORPHENIRAMINE.

Temporary Assistance for Needy Families (TANF)   A plan that replaced the AID TO FAMILIES WITH DEPENDENT CHILDREN (AFDC) program. Whereas AFDC provided direct cash assistance to families, TANF consists of block grants to the states, which were required to have their own welfare reform plans in place by July 1, 1997. New features include a requirement that most adult recipients must be working within two years of beginning welfare assistance and a lifetime limit of five cumulative years of cash assistance for each family. States can exempt up to 20 percent of their caseload from this five-year limit, but alternatively they can impose a shorter time limit on welfare recipients. States have the option of further restrictions: They can deny benefits to children born to welfare recipients, can deny benefits to unwed parents under age 18, and can maintain recipients who move in from another state at the benefit level that applied in their former state for one year. However, states must still follow the former AFDC rules with regard to eligibility for Medicaid.

temazepam   A psychoactive-sedative compound, a member of a class of psychoactive drugs called BENZODIAZEPINES. All of these drugs reduce anxiety or cause drowsiness to some degree. Compared with other benzodiazepines, temazepam is relatively long-acting and is useful for people who wake up too early. Its primary disadvantage is that it can cause a hangover the day after its use. Temazepam is available as capsules for oral administration. The most common side effects are dizziness and daytime drowsiness. Other side effects include lethargy, hangover, anxiety, diarrhea, euphoria, weakness, confusion, and vertigo. It is also sold under the name Restoril.

tenidap   A drug extensively tested for treating arthritis, tenidap is a drug under development that works to inhibit TUMOR NECROSIS FACTOR.

teratogenicity   The ability to cause malformations in a fetus. It is distinct from mutagenicity, which causes genetic mutations in sperm, eggs, or other cells. Teratogenicity is a potential side effect of many drugs, such as THALIDOMIDE.

terfenadine   A relatively new, long-lasting ANTIHISTAMINE used to treat the symptoms of seasonal allergies. In people with HIV, the drug is also used to reduce certain drug-induced allergic side effects, including skin rashes, redness, swelling, hives, and breathing difficulties. The main difference between this drug and the older antihistamines is that it causes less drowsiness and is often suitable for people who need to stay alert. Terfenadine is available as regular and extended-release tablets for oral administration. Common side effects include nausea and loss of appetite. Brand names are Contact Allergy Formula, Seldane, and Seldane-D.

terminal   Pertaining to the end phase; in medical terms, leading ultimately to death.

testes   See TESTICLES.

testicles   The male sex glands, or testes, which produce both sperm and testosterone. Located in the scrotum. Slang terms include *balls, family jewels,* nuts, and *orchids.*

testicular atrophy   A wasting away, or decrease in size and function, of the TESTICLES.

testicular cancer   Cancer of the TESTICLES.

testing   See HIV TESTING; MANDATORY TESTING; PRIVACY.

testosterone   A naturally occurring male hormone, found in both men and women. Testosterone is responsible for the masculinizing and tissue-building (anabolic) changes that occur in males during adolescence, including the growth of the reproductive tract and the development of secondary sexual characteristics. When administered as a drug it can cause gain in lean body mass, increased sex drive, and possibly aggressive behavior. Many men with HIV have low testosterone levels caused by HIV suppression of normal endocrine-gland function or by drugs (like KETONCONAZOLE) used to treat opportunistic infections. These deficiencies are associated with the loss of both energy and lean tissue mass in HIV-related weight loss. Testosterone and other ANABOLIC STEROIDS are often prescribed as part of TESTOSTERONE REPLACEMENT THERAPY.

Oral and injectable testosterone have long been available to treat testosterone deficiencies. Synthetic forms are also available. The advantages of these include lower risk of liver toxicity and fewer of the masculinizing side effects common when injectable testosterone is used. Recently, a daily-wear, no-adhesive transdermal (through the skin) testosterone patch has become available. It is applied to the scrotum and provides serum testosterone levels that mimic the normal daily pattern in healthy adults. This form of delivery also avoids the peaks and troughs in blood levels that occur with testosterone injections. For treatment of HIV-related weight loss, one manufacturer recently started a CLINICAL TRIAL of a rub-on testosterone gel. Testosterone patches are already approved for use in hypogonadal wasting. The rub-on gel must be applied to a shaved scrotum, while the patches can be placed anywhere on the body.

For treatment of HIV-related weight loss, testosterone is effective only for people with abnormally low testosterone levels. For maximum effect against wasting, both adequate nutrition and exercise should be combined with testosterone therapy. The hormone makes cells ready to build tissue but has little effect without the proper building blocks or exercise. Prolonged use of oral testosterone, however, as of other oral anabolic steroids, has been associated with severe liver toxicity and liver cancer.

Not much is known about how the use of testosterone and other anabolic steroids affects HIV replication, disease progression, or survival. Even less is known about the use of anabolic-steroid therapy in HIV-positive women.

testosterone replacement therapy   The therapeutic use of testosterone to substitute for natural testosterone that is either absent or diminished. Also used as an approach to managing weight loss.

tetracycline   Any of a group of broad-spectrum ANTIBIOTICS belonging to certain species of *Streptomyces.* They may also be produced semisynthetically. Tetracyclines are effective against a variety of organisms, including GRAM-NEGATIVE and GRAM-POSITIVE BACTERIA, CHLAMYDIAS, MYCOPLASMAS, RICKETTSIAS, and some viruses and protozoa.

Th1 cell   A subdivision of the helper T cell involved in cell-mediated immunity and characterized by its production of IFN-γ and IL-2. The cytotoxic T cells involved in this response are known as T1.

Th1 response   An acquired immune response whose most prominent feature is high cytotoxic T LYMPHOCYTE activity relative to the amount of antibody production. The Th1 response is promoted by T4 Th1 T-helper cells.

Th2 cell   A type of T-HELPER CELL that stimulates B CELLS to produce immunoglobin gamma E, immunoglobin gamma G, and proinflammatory effects in allergy and other ANTIBODY responses. They are characterized by their production of IL-4, IL-5, IL-6, and IL-10. The suppressor T cells involved in this response are known as T2 cells.

Th2 response   An acquired immune response whose most prominent feature is high ANTIBODY production relative to the amount of cytotoxic T-LYMPHOCYTE activity. The Th2 response is promoted by T2 Th2 T-HELPER CELLS.

thalidomide   A drug made infamous in the early 1960s when it caused severe birth defects in children born to women who took it during pregnancy, thalidomide has been found to effectively heal severe mouth and throat ulcers in people with HIV infection. For the many patients with HIV infection who suffer from these ulcers, eating can be excruciatingly painful, which exacerbates wasting and debilitation. Thalidomide is the first treatment shown in a scientific study to heal these ulcers. Because of its potential toxicity, treatment should be carefully monitored and limited in its duration. Possible serious side effects include irreversible, painful peripheral nerve damage, rash, and birth defects.

Thalidomide is also currently being investigated for use against primary HIV infection and AIDS-related wasting syndrome. Since the sixties, thalidomide has been found to be relatively safe in nonpregnant populations and effective in treating a number of clinical conditions, many of which are similar to each other and to symptoms observed in HIV patients. A common link may be TUMOR NECROSIS FACTOR ALPHA, a CYTOKINE, or intracellular messenger, that is possibly a key element in both wasting syndrome and HIV activation. Thalidomide has been found to selectively inhibit TNF production and release. It is a possible alternative to the immensely expensive human growth hormone, another experimental antiwasting treatment.

Trade name is Synovir.

THC   See DELTA-9 TETRAHYDROCANNABINOL; MARIJUANA; DRONABINOL.

therapeutic drug   A drug having medicinal or healing properties.

therapeutic index   The ratio obtained by dividing the lethal dose (LD-50) of a drug by its MINIMUM EFFECTIVE DOSE (MED-50). If the ratio is equal to 10 or more, it indicates that a lethal dose is at least 10 times the minimum effective dose.

therapeutic touch   Popularized by nursing professor Dolores Krieger, therapeutic touch is practiced by registered nurses and others to relieve pain and stress. The practitioner assesses where the person's energy field is weak or congested and then uses his or her hands to direct energy into the field to balance it.

therapeutic vaccine   A vaccine administered after infection with a disease-causing microorganism to modify the immune response to make it more effective. Therapeutic vaccination is a well-known medical technique first introduced a century ago for the treatment of chronic staphylococcal infections, syphilis, and tuberculosis. These early efforts with therapeutic vaccination were only marginally successful; they almost faded from use when antibiotics were introduced in the late 1940s. However, therapeutic vaccination today remains the standard of care for those believed infected with rabies and for babies born to mothers infected with hepatitis B virus. In diseases against which therapeutic vaccination does work, the vaccine retards early infection before the development of a natural immune response.

Within the context of HIV, an injected therapy consisting of synthetic HIV antigen (e.g., gp160) is administered to people who already have HIV. It is supposed to heighten and broaden the immune response to HIV, helping to halt disease progression. Since general immune stimulation via IL-2 or other agents has not offered much hope of directly restricting HIV, researchers all along have been considering ways to construct a strong specific anti-HIV immune defense. Therapeutic vaccines are the major strategy that has been proposed to preferentially increase sur–viving CD4 CELLS that could orchestrate a new defense against HIV.

After introduction of new foreign proteins (antigen) to the body, naive CD4 cells sensitive to portions of that protein eventually are activated and multiply to construct new immune defenses. The therapeutic vaccine concept is to improve on the immune defense against a particular already-existing infection by inoculating pieces of the infectious agent's protein presented in a way to trigger new naive cell activation. An immune-enhancing adjutant is frequently used to help this process along. In 1996 investigators presented evidence that therapeutic vaccines can reduce the extent and duration of genital herpes outbreaks in people with frequent eruptions and in infected guinea pigs.

Most prominent researchers have always been skeptical of the validity of the therapeutic vaccine approach for HIV.

One of the common arguments against this approach is that vaccines are not promising because the body already sees lots of HIV antigen—adding a little extra is not likely to make any difference. There is also a serious objection concerning viral diversity: Even if an induced immune response is effective, won't HIV merely mutate to rearrange the bit of viral protein that triggers the attack? Indeed, the field of therapeutic vaccines for HIV is littered with failures, despite clear demonstrations that the vaccines provoke new immune responses against HIV. To date, the most extensively tested product has been a gp160 (HIV envelope protein) inoculant made by bioengineered insect cells, developed by MicroGeneSys. Studies showed that the MicroGeneSys vaccine, though clearly "immunogenic," completely flopped in a placebo-controlled trial. After following 608 volunteers (with starting CD4 counts of at least 400) for three to five years, researchers concluded that the bimonthly injections of the vaccine were safe, but no difference existed between the placebo and vaccine groups in terms of occurrence of opportunistic infections, drop in CD4 count, rise in plasma HIV levels, or other measures of disease progression. A similar 278-person, 3-year Canadian trial had equally negative results. Findings of both trials were presented at the Eleventh International Conference on AIDS, July 7–12, 1996.

Three other, more naturally structured vaccine products (Immuno AG's gp160 produced by mammalian cell cultures, a hybrid canary pox virus with a gp160 envelope, and British Biotech's virus-like particles consisting of yeast protein particles coated with HIV p24 core protein) have also failed. Nonetheless those interested in this approach remain hopeful.

therapy   The TREATMENT of a disease or pathological condition.

THF   See THYMIC HUMORAL FACTOR.

thiazide diuretic   One of a group of related chemicals that stimulate secretion of urine, resulting in loss of water from the body; a diuretic. Thiazides are used to treat swelling due to congestive heart failure or chronic liver or kidney disease. Brand names vary as per different types—bendromethiazide, hydrochlorothiazide, hydroflumethiazide, chlorothiazide, methyclothiazide, trichlormethiazide, chlorthalidone and metalazone.

thiethylperazine   A compound belonging to a class of psychoactive drugs called phenothiazines, used as an antinausea/antivomiting agent. Although the mechanism by which these drugs work is unknown, they have potent effects on the CENTRAL NERVOUS SYSTEM and other organs and can reduce blood pressure, stop seizures, and control nausea and vomiting. Occasional cases of drowsiness, dizziness, headache, fever, and restlessness have been reported in people using thiethylperazine. Serious side effects, such as convulsions and involuntary muscle movements, are uncommon, but they have occurred. Thiethylperazine is available in tablets for oral administration and as a solution for intramuscular injection. Trade name is Torcan.

third spacing   Massive hemorrhagic bleeding under the skin.

3′-deoxy-3′ fluorothimidine (FLT)   A NUCLEOSIDE ANALOG (like AZT, ddI, and ddC) that has been under investigation for the treatment of HIV. It has been touted as the most potent nucleoside analog and is 2 to 10 times more potent than AZT. It has a long half-life and good brain penetration but causes significant toxicity to BONE MARROW, and therefore can cause severe ANEMIA (low red blood cell counts) and LEUKOPENIA (low white blood cell counts). It is hoped, research will show that toxicity may be prevented by using low doses, or managed with colony-stimulating factors.

three-drug therapy   In 1996 it was announced that a combination of one experimental and two licensed drugs appears to be the most powerful AIDS therapy ever tested on infected patients. The three-drug combination reduced the amount of HIV by 99 percent, to levels that could not be detected by standard laboratory tests in 24 of 26 patients. The two marketed drugs are AZT and 3TC, and the experimental drug is indinavir, a member of a new class of anti-AIDS drugs known as PROTEASE INHIBITORS. See also COMBINATION THERAPY; 3TC; AZT.

3TC/AZT   A combination of NUCLEOSIDE ANALOG drugs that has been approved by the FDA on an accelerated basis for use against HIV at any stage of infection.

The surrogate marker data clearly indicates that 3TC/AZT works best in people who have never taken AZT. This does not mean that 3TC/AZT is the first treatment regimen to use; a treatment that does not include AZT might be best. Also, it is unclear yet that 3TC/AZT will confer long-term benefits in people with early HIV infection, as indicated by the Concorde study, which found no advantage to early AZT monotherapy.

Resistance to 3TC/AZT is one serious concern over its use as first-line therapy. Resistance quickly develops in virtually all patients on 3TC within 12 to 16 weeks. While the mutation conferring resistance to 3TC may impair the virus's ability to replicate and postpone the development of resistance to AZT, it has been shown to decrease susceptibility to ddI and ddC by eightfold in cell culture. There are no studies showing whether this translates into a loss of response to ddI or ddC in people, and there is a chance that use of 3TC/AZT as first-line therapy may leave few options when people fail this combination. The particular mutation arising after exposure to 3TC does not seem to occur in response to ddI or ddC use in people, so it appears less likely that use of ddI or ddC before 3TC will cause a loss of susceptibility to 3TC.

thrombocytopenia   An abnormally low count (penia) of thrombocytes (or platelets), cells in the blood which facilitate clotting. The usual count of thrombocytes is 150,000 to 300,000 per milliliter of blood. Lower counts of 80,000 to 120,000 per milliliter are common in people with HIV infection. When the count is very low, from 5,000 to 25,000 per milliliter, bleeding problems may occur. People with HIV infection have thrombocytopenia because their bodies produce antibodies against their own platelets. Recent data suggest that in HIV there is diminished platelet production and decreased platelet survival, possibly resulting from direct infection of megakaryocytes (large BONE MARROW cells with large or multiple nuclei that give rise to blood platelets essential for the clotting mechanism of blood).

Presentation is generally made on laboratory testing. Bruising easily, epistaxis (hemorrhage from nose), gingival, or rectal bleeding may be present. Platelet counts as low as 10,000 are often without symptoms. Petechiae (small, purplish, hemorrhagic spots on the skin that appear in certain severe fevers and are indicative of great prostration) and ecchymoses (skin discoloration consisting of large, irregularly formed hemorrhagic areas) may be seen. Platelet counts of <100,000 define thrombocytopenia. Bone marrow biopsy often reveals decreased megakaryocytes. Some people have no symptoms but must still be careful to avoid cuts or anything that could cause bleeding.

Treatment of immune thrombocytopenia has been limited in the past by short duration of response, high cost, and sometimes serious side effects of the available therapies. There are several possible approaches to the management of thrombocytopenia in HIV: ZIDOVUDINE; PREDNISONE; intravenous GAMMA GLOBULIN; splenectomy (the surgical removal of the spleen); danazol; low-dose splenic irradiation; and no therapy. These approaches have met with some success. A conservative approach with careful observation and education for nonbleeding patients is recommended. Zidovudine, if tolerated, should be initiated because it has been found to increase platelet production in HIV-infected patients with and without thrombocytopenia. Patients with dangerously low platelet counts (<10,000) or significant bleeding should be hospitalized. In hospitalized patients, IV gamma globulin followed by platelet transfusion generally results in rapid correction. Prednisone is then begun, and the patient is discharged. Outpatient follow-up must be close, and the goal should be to taper the prednisone to the lowest possible dose that will keep the patient symptom-free and the platelet count >15,000.

thrombopenia   See THROMBOCYTOPENIA.

thrush   An infection of the mouth or pharynx caused by the fungus CANDIDA ALBICANS. See ORAL CANDIDIASIS; CANDIDIASIS.

thymic hormone   Any of the hormones produced by the THYMUS. They are believed to play a role in the maturation of T LYMPHOCYTES and overall modulation of the immune system. Versions of several are under study as anti-HIV therapies—THYMOPENTIN and thymosis-α1 in particular.

thymic humoral factor (THF)   A synthetic thymic peptide being examined as an anti-HIV treatment.

thymic humoral factor gamma 2 (THF g²)   A thymic peptide that has been developed as an immune-modulating treatment for HIV. The hope is that it will stimulate an infected person's immune system to fight HIV and diseases associated with it.

thymic peptide   Peptide produced in the THYMUS gland. Although the importance of thymic peptides remains in dispute, several investigators have reported that they can assist development of immature precursor cells into fully competent T CELLS. They also regulate the functioning of T-cells once they have matured.

Thymic peptide-based drugs have been developed as immune-modulating treatments, in the hope that they will stimulate HIV-infected persons' immune systems to fight the virus and diseases associated with it. These drugs include THYMIC HUMORAL FACTOR GAMMA 2, THYMOPENTIN, THYMOSIN ALPHA 1, THYMOMODULIN, and THYMOSTIMULIN.

thymidine   One of the basic components of DEOXYRIBONUCLEIC ACID (DNA), thymidine is the nucleoside that the NUCLEOSIDE ANALOGS AZT and D4T mimic.

thymomodulin   A THYMIC PEPTIDE, a natural extract of calf THYMUS. In Italy, where it has been approved (under the trade name Leucotrofina), it is used to treat bacterial and viral infections, food allergies in children, and immunodeficiencies in the elderly. Unlike most synthetic peptides, thymomodulin is an oral drug. It is made into syrup from the filtered freeze-dried calf thymus extract.

thymopentin   A small, synthesized thymic peptide drug, also known as TP-5 or Timunox. Thymopentin has been studied more extensively than most other thymic peptide drugs, but the results have been ambiguous due to the studies' small size and flawed design.

thymopoietin   A THYMIC PEPTIDE that stimulates differentiation of thymocytes.

thymo-ripoff   See RIPOFF.

thymosin   A THYMIC PEPTIDE that adjusts immune response when aberrations occur. Thymosin boosts the number of RECEPTORS on T CELLS, especially for ALPHA-INTERFERON and IL-2. It also increases the efficiency of T cells' response to signaling agents and causes cells to produce more of them. Intercellular signaling molecules (CYTOKINES) like alpha-interferon and IL-2 commonly have severe adverse effects. These agents are released during disease to help bolster the inflammatory response, which causes a variety of flu-like symptoms. Thymosin, in contrast, circulates in the blood at comparatively constant levels. In clinical trials to date, no serious side effects have been noted. Since thymosin promotes the action of alpha-interferon and IL-2, it is speculated that combining it with these could allow lower dosages to be used, resulting in both greater safety and greater efficacy.

The pharmaceutical development path of alpha-thymosin has been characterized by disappointments, discouragements, and contradictory data. Despite the problematic aspects of past thymosin trials, however, some believe that the drug merits further study, since it is an open question whether thymosin works or not.

thymosin alpha 1   A small synthetic peptide, first produced in the 1970s. It has been licensed in Italy for the treatment of primary immunodeficiencies and as a booster for influenza vaccine in renal dialysis patients. The drug is being tested in ongoing CLINICAL TRIALS for activity against chronic HEPATITIS B and C, HIV infection and certain forms of cancer. It is by far the most thoroughly studied of all the THYMIC PEPTIDE drugs, but published reports from ongoing trials remain inconclusive.

thymostimulin   A THYMIC PEPTIDE also known as Tp-1, thymostimulin is, like THYMOMODULIN, a natural extract from calf THYMUS.

thymus   The thymus gland has been identified as a key immune system organ. It is the central lymphoid organ in the chest (see LYMPH) and the site of LYMPHOCYTE formation and maturation as well as the secretion of THYMIC HORMONEs. The thymus seems to exert its regulatory functions through the secretion of various hormonelike products called THYMIC PEPTIDEs. An important function of the thymus is to weed out lymphocytes that react to proteins produced by the body ("self-ANTIGENS"), thus preventing AUTOIMMUNE DISEASE.

From the beginning of the AIDS epidemic, research has been done into the effect of HIV on the thymus. The research so far, however, does not offer a consistent understanding.

thymus-dependent antigen   ANTIGEN that depends on T-CELL interaction with B CELLS for antibody synthesis, (e.g., erythrocytes, SERUM proteins, and HAPTEN-carrier complexes).

thymus-independent antigen   ANTIGEN that can induce an immune response without the apparent participation of T LYMPHOCYTEs.

thyroid stimulating hormone   Hormone secreted by the anterior lobe of the pituitary that stimulates the thyroid gland. Abbreviated TSH.

thyroxine (T_4)   A hormone secreted by the thyroid gland that increases energy production and protein synthesis.

TIA   See TRANSIENT ISCHEMIC ATTACK.

Tinactin   See TOLNAFTATE.

tinea   Any fungal skin disease. Also called RINGWORM.

tinidazole   An antiprotozoal used as a first-line therapy for a variety of parasitic and amoebic infections. Trade name is Fasigyn.

Title II   See SOCIAL SECURITY ACT, TITLE II.

Title IV-A   See SOCIAL SECURITY ACT, TITLE IV-A.

Title VI   See PUBLIC HEALTH SERVICE ACT, TITLE VI.

Title XIV   See SOCIAL SECURITY ACT, TITLE XIV.

Title XVI   See PUBLIC HEALTH SERVICE ACT, TITLE VI; SOCIAL SECURITY ACT, TITLE XVI.

Title XVI state   A state that gives MEDICAID to all SSI recipients under Title XVI of the federal SOCIAL SECURITY ACT. This benefit is not automatic—it requires aged, blind, and disabled recipients to apply separately for Medicaid at a state welfare office, bringing proof of SSI eligibility.

Title XVIII   See SOCIAL SECURITY ACT, TITLE XVIII.

Title XIX   See SOCIAL SECURITY ACT, TITLE XIX.

Title XX   See SOCIAL SECURITY ACT, TITLE XX.

TJ-9   A preparation of a traditional Asian medicine known as sho-saiko-to (SSKT), or xiao chai hu tang. SSKT is a blend of seven medicinal herbs including bupleurum, *Scutelaria radix*, pinellia, fresh ginger, ginseng, jujube, and glycyrrhizin. It has been used for thousands of years to treat what the Chinese call lesser yang disorders, which include fevers, influenza, bronchitis, respiratory ailments, malaria, jaundice, and hepatitis. SSKT appears to be fairly safe, although it has been reported to induce pneumonitis in a few elderly patients. IN VITRO data suggest that the blend may have anti-HIV activity by directly inhibiting REVERSE TRANSCRIPTASE and by decreasing TNF-alpha and free-radical promotion of viral replication. The data also suggest that the herbal formula is strongly synergistic with AZT. It may also have some immune modulatory effects.

TLC G-65   Liposomal gentamicin. See GENTAMICIN.

TMP-SMX   See TRIMETHOPRIM-SULFAMETHOXAZOLE.

TNF   See TUMOR NECROSIS FACTOR.

TNF inhibitor   See TUMOR NECROSIS FACTOR (TNF) INHIBITOR.

tolerance   In cell biology, the condition in which responsive cell clones have been eliminated or inactivated by prior contact with ANTIGEN, with the result that no immune response occurs on administration of antigen. See IMMUNE TOLERANCE.

tolnaftate   A synthetic antifungal agent appearing as a white-to-creamy-white powder. It is used topically in treating various forms of TINEA. The trade name is Tinactin.

tomography   A method of producing images of the interior of the body using computer and X-ray technology. See COMPUTERIZED AXIAL TOMOGRAPHY.

toot   See COCAINE.

top   In sexual intercourse, a slang term for the partner who penetrates the body of the other.

In regard to sexually transmitted diseases, many sexually active men, both hetero- and homosexual, who prefer the top role mistakenly perceive themselves not to be at risk as tops. This is the "top mentality." It is also often assumed that it is the job of the top to be responsible for safety. See also BOTTOM.

top mentality   See TOP.

topical   Pertaining to a specific surface area.

topical microbicide   An antibacterial or antifungal compound that can be applied directly to the lining of the vagina before intercourse to thwart sexually transmitted microbes that cause diseases such as gonorrhea, syphilis, genital herpes, chlamydia, hepatitis B, and HIV infections. Today, the development of safe, effective, female-controlled topical microbicides that will block the transmission of HIV and other STD agents is a global priority and a central focus of the STD research program of the National Institute of Allergy and Infectious Diseases (NIAID). The goal is to develop safe antimicrobial products that effectively fight a combination of infectious agents, whether they are viral, bacterial, or protozoan.

The currently available mechanical and chemical products thought to prevent STD/HIV transmission have limitations. A major drawback of the male condom is that it cannot be used at the discretion of a woman without her partner's knowledge or consent, and personal, social, or cultural barriers often interfere with her ability to negotiate its use. Existing spermicides have not been clinically evaluated, and issues of safety and efficacy for STD/HIV prevention remain unresolved.

topoisomerase   An enzyme that uncoils the tightly wound DNA in cells' nuclei so that cell division and replication can take place.

topotecan   An experimental anticancer chemotherapy that inhibits TOPOISOMERASE I and blocks cell division. It is a possible therapy for HIV, having been found to inhibit HIV replication in the lab, and PROGRESSIVE MULTIFOCAL LEUKOENCEPHALOPATHY (PML), an opportunistic virus infection of the brain.

torulosis   See CRYPTOCOCCOSIS.

total parenteral nutrition   See PARENTERAL NUTRITION.

toxic   Poisonous.

toxic reaction   An unintended, sickening, sometimes severe and dangerous physiological reaction to a toxic substance in vitamin, drug, or other substance. See TOXIC SIDE EFFECT.

toxic shock syndrome   A rare disease—an extreme toxic reaction—caused by toxins that are produced by certain strains of *Staphylococcus aureus* bacteria. It is characterized by acute fever, diarrhea, vomiting, and myalgia (tenderness or pain in the muscles), followed by hypotension and possible death due to shock. Most cases have been attributed to toxins found in tampons, but cases also have been diagnosed in nonmenstruating women and in men.

toxic side effect   See SIDE EFFECT.

toxicity   Poisonousness, of a chemical, drug, or other substance.

toxin   A chemical that is poisonous to cells.

toxoid   A toxin with its toxicity destroyed but still capable of inducing the formation of antibodies on injection.

Toxoplasma gondii   The organism that causes TOXOPLASMOSIS, one of the most common causes of inflammation of the brain in people with AIDS. *Toxoplasma gondii* is an intracellular, non-host-specific, widespread sporozoan species that is parasitic in a number of vertebrates, including humans. The sexual cycle of *Toxoplasma gondii,* leading to the production of oocysts, develops exclusively in cats and other felines. An oocyte is a cell undergoing meiosis during oogenesis (the production of ova, involving usually both meiosis and maturation). It enters the body through the mouth and digestive tract from contaminated meat or contact with cat feces. It then travels through the blood to the brain, where it invades and kills neuronal cells.

toxoplasmic encephalitis   The most common form of TOXOPLASMOSIS in people with HIV infection.

toxoplasmosis   Widespread infection of an organ, usually the brain, or the whole body with the parasite TOXOPLASMA GONDII. *Toxoplasma gondii* is found in many mammals and birds, but the definitive host is cat excrement, which, with raw meat, is the most common source of infection. About 30 percent of all adults in the United States have *Toxoplasma gondii* in their bodies, but the majority are unaware of it. The parasite remains dormant and rarely causes disease unless the immune system is weakened. When symptoms do appear, they may range from a mild, self-limited disease similar to mononucleosis to a more severe, disseminated disease causing extensive damage to the brain, central nervous system, liver, and lungs. Encephalitis, hepatitis, or pneumonia are examples of such disseminating diseases. In people with HIV infection, the most common form of toxoplasmosis is an infection of the brain called TOXOPLASMIC ENCEPHALITIS.

Symptoms include fevers, headaches, confusion, lethargy, and seizures. Diagnosis is obtained by determining toxoplasma antibody levels, MAGNETIC RESONANCE IMAGING (MRI), and COMPUTERIZED TOMOGRAPHY (CT) SCANS. To date, there are no accepted prophylaxes for toxoplasmosis, although cotrimoxazole (Bactrim or Septra) and dapsone have been tried with good results. First-line therapy for active toxoplasmosis is oral pyrimethamine and sulfadiazine. Lifelong maintenance therapy to prevent recurrence is advised. Renal and dermatologic complications due to sulfadiazine occur in about 40 percent of treated patients. Alternative therapy when that occurs is a combination of pyrimethamine and clindamycin. Azithromycin is an option in patients who are intolerant to pyrimethamine, sulfadiazine, or clindamycin.

tramp   A pejorative slang term for a woman who supposedly has many sex partners.

tranquilizer   A drug that acts to reduce mental tension and anxiety without interfering with normal mental activity. The use of tranquilizers has facilitated the treatment of severely disturbed psychiatric patients. Drugs in use include chlordiazepoxide (Librium), chlorpromazine (Thorazine), diazepam (Valium), meprobamate (Miltown, Equanil), alprazolam (Xanax), and reserpine (Serpasil). Side effects, particularly from chlorpromazine and reserpine, have included jaundice, nausea, rashes, and in some instances severe mental depression.

transactivator (TAT-3) gene   See TAT GENE.

transamination   The transfer of an amino (NH$_2$) group from an amino acid to a carbon chain to form a non-essential amino acid; takes place in the liver.

transcription   The process by which a cell reproduces genetic material. Specifically, the synthesis of RNA molecules from a DNA template.

transfer factor   In immunology, a factor present in LYMPHOCYTES that have been sensitized to ANTIGENs, which can in humans be transferred to a nonsensitized recipient. Thus the recipient will react to the same antigen that was originally used to sensitize the lymphocytes of the donor. In humans, the factor can be transferred by injecting the recipient with either intact lymphocytes or extracts of disrupted cells.

transfusion, analogous   Blood TRANSFUSION in which the patient receives his or her own blood, donated several weeks before an elective surgical procedure. The blood may also be collected at the site of surgery during the procedure. Transfusion with autologous blood is the safest form of transfusion. Before 1985, autologous blood transfusions were rarely used, and many blood centers in the United States did not have procedures for handling predeposited blood. From the perspective of the HIV epidemic, the infrequent use of autologous transfusion is regrettable. Autologous blood transfusion would have been especially beneficial between 1978 and 1985 when the prevalence of HIV in the blood supply was greatest but before a specific test was available to screen donor blood. Although current testing procedures have rendered the United States blood supply extremely safe, a patient may opt for this procedure because of fear of exposure to the human immunodeficiency virus and other bloodborne infections.

transfusion, blood   The replacement in the body of blood or one of its components. The modern era of blood transfusion started during World War II, when battlefield medicine became sophisticated in the use of blood and plasma. Today, blood transfusion is a highly complex field, combining the latest knowledge of immunology and physiology with practical management of a wide range of services. The key concept in modern transfusion medicine is the provision of integrated blood transfusion services. An integrated system, a reality in industrialized countries, seeks to ensure a timely supply of adequate amounts of safe blood and blood products, where needed and at an affordable cost. The integrated system must manage donor recruitment, collection, testing and storage of blood, preparation of appropriate blood products and their appropriate use, and complex record-keeping and logistical tasks. In many developing countries, even in the major hospitals, there are no such systems. Blood is obtained from a donor, subjected (or not) to simple tests of compatibility and safety and infused into the recipient. The people of the developing world therefore rarely receive the full benefits of blood transfusion, and often suffer risks that have for the most part been eliminated in more developed countries

Effective and safe transfusion therapy requires a thorough understanding of the clinical condition being treated. In advanced countries today, there is very little chance of getting HIV from a blood transfusion. Clotting factors obtained from donated blood are equally safe. Nearly all the people infected with HIV through blood transfusions received those transfusions before 1985, the year it became possible to test donated blood for HIV. Since mid-1983, all blood donations in the United States have come from volunteers who are questioned about their risks for HIV infection. People at increased risk of infection are not allowed to donate blood. Since mid-1985, all donated blood has been tested for HIV and other viruses (seven different tests are now conducted on each blood sample). Blood that tests positive for HIV is destroyed. Donors are confidentially told that they are infected with HIV and are not allowed to donate blood again. There is no risk of getting infected by giving blood because a new, sterile needle is used for each blood donation.

transfusion-associated AIDS Acquired immunodeficiency syndrome developed as a result of a transfusion with HIV-infected blood or blood components. Widespread, accurate blood-testing procedures have greatly reduced the risk of becoming infected with HIV through a BLOOD TRANSFUSION.

transient HIV infection HIV infection that becomes undetectable in infants. Clearance of HIV infection in an infant born in 1991 was reported by National Institutes of Health–supported investigators in 1995. The boy was born to an HIV-infected mother; no HIV could be found in his blood when he was born, but viral culture tests at day 19 and day 51 did reveal the virus. Later attempts to find HIV using HIV-culture techniques, polymerase chain reaction, and antigen searches did not reveal any virus. Today he is healthy and has no evidence of HIV infection. Researchers noted the similarity of the child's experience to the likely outcome of HIV exposure after immunization—transient infection with no later evidence of virus or disease. How HIV is cleared in such cases is not known. The data do not suggest that infection in infants will automatically disappear but do raise numerous questions about the frequency and mechanism of transient HIV infections, the implications for pregnant women and their children, the HIV disease process and the body's immune response.

Three possible explanations may suggest how the transient HIV infection may have occurred. One is that the boy's immune response to HIV either eliminated or is totally suppressing the virus. A second is that the immune response could come from maternal antibodies passed during pregnancy and/or from his immune system. A third theory is that he may have been infected with a defective form of HIV that

could not adequately replicate. Each theory requires more evidence and testing.

transient ischemic attack (TIA) Temporary interruption of blood supply to the brain. The symptoms and signs of neurologic deficit may last from a few minutes to hours but are not persistent. There is no evidence of residual brain damage or neurologic damage after an attack.

translation In cell biology, the process of formation of a peptide chain from individual amino acids to form a protein molecule.

transmissible Capable of passing from one person to another through means other than casual contact.

transmissibility The property of a disease-causing organism that enables it to spread from person to person.

transmission HIV is transmitted through four principal routes, or modes, of transmission: exposure through sexual activity, contact with contaminated blood, exposure through blood and needles, and from mother to child through pregnancy and birth.

Transmission through sexual activity. This can occur via intercourse and other direct contact with infectious areas (blisters, open sores, rashes, mucous patches) or warts; contact with infected mucous membranes in the urethra, cervix, anus, throat, or eyes; and contact with clothes or bedding contaminated with infected body fluids.

Bidirectional transmission. "Bidirectional" is an adjective meaning capable of reacting or functioning in two, usually opposite, directions. In the context of HIV/AIDS, bidirectional transmission refers to the fact that the virus can be passed or spread from one individual to another bidirectionally—it travels as easily between men and women as it does between women and men, men and men, and between women and women. HIV/AIDS is a disease that does not have sexual preferences, as is evident in the course of the disease in Africa (where the rate of infection is equal between the two sexes), in the course of the disease in the United States (where statistics have changed dramatically since the first decade of the epidemic, and where the "myth" of heterosexual transmission is no longer a myth), and the continued evolution of the disease in the rest of the industrialized world (where the incidence of AIDS cases associated with heterosexual transmission has been on the rise since 1991). That HIV/AIDS is a gender-neutral disease is also evident in statistics presently available to public health officials worldwide. While the statistics on who is HIV+ or who has AIDS and how they got it vary by continent, country, city, and the particular study at hand, the statistics show that the assumption that female to male transmission is less likely than male to female transmission, although still widely believed, is unfounded. Similarly, while evidence continues to surface on whether or not it is easier for men to give HIV/AIDS to women than for women to give HIV/AIDS to men, or for men to give HIV/AIDS to men than for women to give HIV/AIDS to women, or for women to give HIV/AIDS to their fetus than for them to pass it to their infants in childbirth, today we know that the risk of infection is dependent on behavior and specifically on such factors as who your partner(s) is/are, what you do with him or her, and how often you do it.

Sexual transmission from men to women. This process is fairly well understood. Semen from an infected man contains HIV that is mostly associated with infected LYMPHOCYTEs also present. HIV introduced into the VAGINA must make its way into the bloodstream to initiate viral reproduction. Small breaks in the lining of the vagina are the presumed main route of entry into the bloodstream.

Studies indicate that sexual transmission from men to women may be substantially more effective than transmission from women to men, particularly in the strains of HIV that are widespread in the developed nations. It has been estimated that there is anywhere from a 3- to 19-fold excess risk for male-to-female over female-to-male sexual transmission among HIV-discordant couples. This difference has not been documented in Africa, where over 50 percent of those with both HIV and AIDS are women, and where heterosexual intercourse is overwhelmingly the most common means of transmission of HIV for both sexes. Other studies indicate that women may be more susceptible to infection than men after a single exposure, a difference that may be attributable to the greater number of potential entry sites in the vagina than on the surface of the penis and to the fact that the vagina is exposed to a greater volume of infectious material during intercourse than the penis is.

Sexual transmission from women to men. Although this is known to occur, the means are less clear. Women can and do transmit other SEXUALLY TRANSMITTED DISEASES (STDS) to men as well as to other women, and there are documented cases of woman-to-man transmission of HIV. HIV, like CHLAMYDIA, GONORRHEA, HERPES, SYPHILIS, and other STDs, can thrive in the vaginal juices, mucous tissues in the vagina, blood (including menstrual blood), and breast milk, as well as in urine and feces. STDs are easily passed between partners of either sex through open sores. Studies have also demonstrated a clear relationship between HIV infection in men and the presence of genital ulcers. Researchers hypothesize that genital ulcers in men serve the same function as breaks in the lining of the vagina by providing the virus a portal into the bloodstream.

Other factors undoubtedly influence transmission during heterosexual genital intercourse. The presence of menstrual fluids, simultaneous infection with other organisms, cutaneous conditions, prior exposure to chemical irritants that disrupt the skin, and other conditions may all play a part.

Heterosexual transmission is the most common route of HIV infection for women worldwide and is rapidly becoming the most common in the United States as well. HIV transmission from men to women and from women to men has occurred mainly through vaginal intercourse.

Homosexual/bisexual transmission. As of December 1989, the CENTERS FOR DISEASE CONTROL AND PREVENTION (CDC) had 117,781 cases of AIDS in the United States. Of the adult and adolescent cases, a significant majority (70,093) were attributed to male homosexual and bisexual contact. For the first decade of the epidemic, these groups, as well as IV drug users, were considered at high risk for HIV infec-

tion. Indeed, the development of the epidemic was often linked to these so-called high-risk groups, including, in addition to homosexuals and bisexuals, blood donors, hemophiliacs, Haitian immigrants, low-income women, prostitutes, and partners of individuals in high-risk groups. In the United States, the incidence rates among gay and bisexual men have stabilized, indicating changes in the epidemiology of AIDS in the United States. In the second decade of the epidemic, the focus has shifted from high-risk groups to high-risk behavior, and, while homosexuals and bisexuals pose a continuing challenge, as do IV drug users, concerns about heterosexual transmission, perinatal transmission, AIDS and adolescents, and AIDS in children equal if not outweigh concerns about homosexual and bisexual transmission.

Sexual transmission from women to women. As noted above, women can and do transmit STDs to other women during sexual activity. Cases of woman-to-woman transmission of HIV have been reported, and it is now believed that the virus can indeed be transmitted in this way, although even less is known about the process than about woman-to-man transmission. Researchers agree that while cervical secretions can carry HIV, menstrual blood does not carry it in the same potency as circulatory blood, which has a higher living cell density than other body fluids. The issue is complicated, of course, by the near-impossibility of knowing how a lesbian (or anyone else) identified as HIV-positive contracted the virus. The CDC has so far not identified any high-risk sexual behavior between women and finds no reason to believe that lesbians are a risk group.

Transmission via contaminated blood. Although safety has been a concern since the beginning of the era of transfusion medicine and although it is not unique to the AIDS epidemic, the advent of AIDS and HIV infection raised new concerns about the safety of the blood supply in the United States. Early in the epidemic, suspicions arose that AIDS could be transmitted by transfusion. In the spring of 1983, cases of AIDS diagnosed among hemophiliacs were thought to be related to clotting factor concentrates made from contaminated blood. Although the etiologic or causative agent of AIDS had not been identified in the early 1980s and no specific diagnostic tests were available, reports of cases among transfusion recipients and hemophiliacs prompted blood banks to institute a variety of procedures to reduce the risk of AIDS associated with blood transfusions. Such procedures included efforts to exclude donors who were members of groups at high risk for the disease, studies of the use of tests that measured factors considered to be surrogate markers of AIDS (e.g., antibody to HEPATITIS B core ANTIGEN, T lymphocyte ratios), the increased use of autologous donation (providing one's own blood for personal use), and the reduction of unnecessary transfusions of blood and blood components.

After the etiologic agent, HIV, was identified and blood tests for the antibody to the virus became available in March 1985, blood collection organizations added this serologic test to their screening procedures. Despite the high sensitivity of HIV antibody tests, they do not detect all infected donors. A variable length of time elapses between acquisition of the virus and development of a detectable antibody response. Generally, this period is no more than a few months, but in one study, the virus was isolated from blood samples of 27 men who did not yet exhibit antibodies for periods of as long as three years after the initial positive virus culture. During this so-called window period, the blood collected from an infected donor may test negative and thus go undetected by the serologic screening mechanisms employed in most blood banks. As of this writing, the current incidence of HIV infection from antibody-negative blood in the United States is not known.

Although HIV antibody tests cannot eliminate the possibility of transfusion-associated HIV infection, they have vastly improved the safety of the blood supply. Additional methods to detect infected units are being explored to increase the sensitivity of serologic testing. These include those based on recombinant DNA technology, synthetic peptides, and gene-amplification techniques. Other safeguards include improved donor screening and recruitment.

Transmission through blood and needles. Substance abusers compose a population severely affected by AIDS. The spread of AIDS in the substance-abusing population occurs via two primary vectors. Substance abusers transmit the HIV virus to other abusers through the use of unclean intravenous needles or other blood-contaminated drug apparatus. In addition, as with other populations at risk for AIDS, substance abusers spread HIV to other drug users and nonusers alike through unsafe sexual practices. The use of IV drugs without cleaning needles between uses and users is the prominent risk in the former category. Needle hygiene behaviors among intravenous drug users are not as frequent as they might be and not frequent enough to significantly alter the spread of AIDS through blood and needles. The AIDS risk-reduction message has, to date, not reached drug users with the same impact as it has reached gay and bisexual men. Many counselors and epidemiologists consider substance users to be the "second wave" of the AIDS epidemic.

Transmission from mother to child during pregnancy, birth, and postpartum period. In the mid-1980s, the idea that AIDS would become an epidemic of women and children would have been met with considerable skepticism. But increasingly women and children are becoming infected. Women are more vulnerable to HIV infection than men, in part because the direction of sexual spread favors male-to-female transmission. About one of every four babies born to infected women will have HIV infection. The time from birth to the development of AIDS varies from weeks to years.

The vast majority of AIDS cases in children are a result of perinatal transmission—transmission from mother to child during pregnancy, birth, or the postpartum period, the interval after birth, possibly through breast-feeding. Clinical studies have found HIV in fetuses well before delivery, in umbilical cord blood obtained from the placenta, and in maternal blood lost during delivery. Exposure to any of these sources of virus is a potential means of infection.

Transmission from mother to child during pregnancy. It is possible to transmit the virus to the fetus in the uterus, before birth, but at present it is unclear when the transmission of HIV actually occurs. The virus has been isolated from the placenta, the amniotic fluid, and the fetal tissue. Infection may occur prenatally, at delivery, or through breast-feeding. The risk in each pregnancy may depend on such factors

as how advanced the disease is, the woman's immunological state, or the gestational age of the infant at birth. The rate of transmission ranges widely. Studies have shown that women with HIV base their reproductive choices on the same criteria used by noninfected women of similar socioeconomic and psychosocial status. When providers are able to identify which fetus is infected or will be infected, women can incorporate that knowledge into their decision making. Amniocentesis, cordocentesis, and chorionic virus sampling have all been explored as prenatal HIV diagnostic techniques, but because of the blood-borne nature of the virus they themselves involve risk of transmission.

The question of whether infected mothers will give birth to infected infants has attracted enormous emotional attention in the HIV/AIDS pandemic. As early as 1982, only a few months after AIDS had been described as a new disease in adults by the United States Centers for Disease Control, children with AIDS were reported in North America and Europe. Even though the virus responsible for the disease had not yet been identified, the pediatricians involved were certain that the children had been infected either by their mothers during pregnancy or through blood transfusions. Even though the description differed from that of genetic immune deficiencies, these reports were initially received with skepticism by the medical community, in part because these cases had been identified almost simultaneously in different geographical areas under widely differing circumstances. Today we know that factors associated with perinatal transmission include the characteristics of the mother's infection (her clinical status during pregnancy, and her immune response to the virus), the integrity of the placental barrier, the virus itself, and the child's clinical status during exposure to HIV.

We now know that fetuses can be infected with HIV as early as eight weeks after conception. By then, they already have the receptors that enable HIV to penetrate their T cells. However, HIV transmission also seems to occur at a later stage in pregnancy, as indicated by both the absence of clinical signs of infection in the newborn and the low number of viruses in the blood, which therefore creates difficulties in detection by polymerase chain reaction or viral culture. Some children not infected during pregnancy probably become infected during birth.

One of the central difficulties confronting researchers seeking to uncover how HIV passes from mother to child is the determination of whether or not HIV has passed or not. Babies do not come into this world complete with their own ready-made immune systems. They inherit some antibodies from their mothers. Others they develop themselves. It takes more than a year for a child's immune system to mature, and this process is by no means uniform. Some maternal antibodies disappear more quickly than others. Some of the child's own antibodies take longer to develop than others. Although a reliable indicator of HIV infection in an adult, the presence of HIV antibodies provides no reliable indication about an infant's HIV status. And because newborns lack fully developed immune systems, they naturally remain at high risk of contracting some of the opportunistic infections normally associated with HIV during the first 15 months of life.

Some of the other questions that remain follow. What precisely is the risk of perinatal HIV transmission? What are the exact factors influencing this transmission? Does pregnancy affect the course of HIV infection, and, conversely, does HIV influence the evolution and outcome of pregnancy? What strategies could prevent or control the perinatal transmission of HIV? Issues related to transmission of HIV infection from pregnant women to their infants continue to be studied to generate interest and discussion. One of the lasting controversies emanating from the Third Conference on Retroviruses and Opportunistic Infections was the relationship between a pregnant woman's plasma HIV levels and transmission of the virus to her baby. Four studies on vertical HIV transmission were presented at the conference. These studies looked at whether higher HIV levels in blood plasma correlated with greater mother-to-child transmission. They sought to ascertain whether a threshold viral load existed below which HIV transmission did not occur. A related question was also under examination: whether an AZT-induced reduction in a woman's viral load leads to a reduced risk of her baby contracting HIV before and during birth. Only one of the presentations was sanguine about viral load's predictive power. Today it is thought that transmission at delivery is not necessarily tied to high maternal viral load during delivery and that events during delivery that expose the baby to maternal blood or cervico-vaginal secretions might promote transmission.

Transmission from mother to child during birth.   While we know that it is possible for HIV to pass from a pregnant woman to her fetus, we do not know for sure how HIV passes from a woman to her fetus during pregnancy and/or during delivery. We do know that a woman is most likely to transmit the HIV virus to the fetus either immediately after she is infected or during childbirth. A low CD4 cell count (below 300), anemia, inflammation of the placenta, the presence of other infections, and advanced AIDS in a woman may each increase the risk of transmission to the fetus and affect a woman's health and the progress of her pregnancy.

Every infant born to an HIV+ woman will have its mother's antibodies in its blood and may test positive for HIV for a period of time even if it is not infected. Because the current standard antibody test cannot distinguish between the mother's and the infant's antibodies, it has been necessary to wait a few months to determine whether the infant is infected. New tests have been developed that can determine HIV infection in infants as young as three to six months, and researchers are seeking tests that can reliably detect infection in a fetus. Testing, however, is a complex issue. Some policy makers advocate routine testing of all newborns for HIV as a means of assessing the percentage of reproductive-age women who are infected with HIV. Those concerned with women's rights strenuously oppose any testing that is done without the informed consent of the mother. They argue persuasively that the time and money involved in widespread testing could better be spent on prevention, education, and treatment of HIV disease.

A study reported in the *New England Journal of Medicine* reported that the amount of HIV in the blood of perinatally infected infants peaks at 1 to 2 months of age and then declines slowly to level off at 24 months at relatively high concentrations compared to those for an adult. Peak VIRAL LOADs at one month of age suggest that the majority of the infected infants were exposed around the time of delivery. The same study also reported that a small number of infected infants had high blood levels of HIV at birth, indicating that some may have become infected in utero. Researchers note that the dynamics of viral replication in HIV-infected infants are distinctly different from those observed in infected adults. Following a dramatic rise in viremia during their first month of life, the viral burden remains very high in infants in contrast to the sharp decline usually seen in adults. It is hypothesized that this persistently high viremia may partially explain the more rapid progression of AIDS observed in infants compared to adults and further underscore the need for early antiretroviral therapy.

Transmission from mother to child during birth   A research report published in the July 26, 1997 issue of the *British Medical Journal* notes that cleansing the birth canal with an inexpensive antiseptic solution dramatically reduced post-birth infections, hospitalizations, and deaths. The investigators report that washing the birth canal with a very safe solution—0.25 percent chlorhexidine in sterile water—at each vaginal examination before delivery, and then wiping the babies with the solution after delivery, significantly reduced postpartum infectious problems in both mothers and babies. Perhaps most significant was their finding that infant deaths related to sepsis, or bacteria in the bloodstream, were reduced threefold among babies in the intervention phase of the trial. Chlorhexidine has a long track record of safety, and the investigators noted no adverse reactions to the solution among mothers or babies. The low cost, simplicity, and safety of this approach suggests that it may have a role in reducing illness and death associated with perinatal bacterial infections, which exact a considerable toll among women and neonates, especially in the developing world. Specifically, the cost of the antiseptic solution used in the study, and the cotton to apply it, was less than 10 cents per patient, making this a feasible approach for the most resource-poor settings.

Transmission from mother to child during breast-feeding. In the developed world, breast-feeding has been advocated over formula for some time: It promotes mother-child bonding and may promote parenting skills. Today, there are a number of documented cases of HIV transmission through breast-feeding, but the mechanism for transmission is unclear. Although the virus has been isolated from breast milk, many women also have cracks and abrasions on the nipple and surrounding areas. For this reason, breast-feeding is not recommended for HIV-infected women in developed countries.

The World Health Organization (WHO), however, feels that the morbidity and mortality associated with the use of formula in developing countries outweighs the risk of transmission through breast-feeding. For two decades, doctors and public health agencies had offered uniform advice to new mothers in developing countries: Breast-feed your babies to protect their health. But now, the AIDS pandemic is upsetting that simple equation. Studies have shown that mothers infected with the AIDS virus can transmit it through breast milk at significant rates. Based on such findings, the United Nations recently estimated that one-third of all infants with HIV got the virus through their mother's milk. To a growing number of researchers and advocates of breast-feeding, the implications of such studies are as compelling as they were once unthinkable—infant formula, a product whose misuse in developing countries with poor sanitation was once blamed by opponents for killing 1 million babies a year—may now be a powerful weapon to reduce childhood deaths from AIDS. Doctors in industrialized nations have long recommended that HIV-infected mothers use formula. But as women in developing countries become aware of the risks of breast-feeding, they face excruciating choices and confront societal taboos. Physicians in the developing world are also torn. In many instances, advising new mothers to use formula would be impractical: Many lack the means to sterilize bottles or the money to afford formula. Additionally, the majority of pregnant women in developing countries are not tested for HIV and thus are unaware of the risks they and their newborns face.

Although the data are incomplete, some experts say, in the vast majority of the developing world, more infants will be imperiled by renewed promotion of bottle-feeding, with its accompanying risks of diarrhea and dehydration, than by the danger of HIV transmission through breast-feeding. These experts contend that in 90 percent of the developing world, the protection afforded by breast-feeding against the diseases of the developing world is higher than the rate of HIV transmission. Some advocates of breast-feeding are prepared to work with formula makers, their sworn enemies for decades, on combating the growing threat. Meanwhile, the United Nations has come under criticism from scientists who say that the group, in its zeal to promote breast-feeding, has not confronted the HIV issue. Others say that it is imperative to find alternatives to breast-feeding, including ways to make safe, affordable formula widely available.

Transmission from mother to child during the postpartum period. A baby born to an HIV-infected woman will test positive for HIV at birth whether or not the infant is actually infected because the positive antibodies are transferred from the mother. Since it takes more than a year for a child's immune system to develop, these antibodies may last in the child's bloodstream well into the second year of life. During that time the baby naturally remains at high risk of contracting, and dying from, the opportunistic infections normally associated with HIV.

Most babies born to HIV-infected mothers will not be infected, but they will probably become orphans because their mothers, and often their fathers, are infected and will die before they are grown.

Secondary routes of transmission. The biggest myth about AIDS is that it is easy to get. Unlike other viruses, HIV cannot live in air, food, or water. It cannot be contracted from shaking someone's hand. Aside from the three primary routes of transmission, it may be transmitted through nonsexual contact with body fluids and secretions other than blood, including CEREBROSPINAL FLUID, feces, donated sperm, transplanted organs, and vaginal/cervical secretions. Other body fluids such as tears and urine are as yet unproved as routes of transmission. Transmission via saliva may be possible through deep, or "French," kissing,

although this, too, is unproved. A few people are known to have been infected while getting medical or dental treatment, and there are apparently two cases on record of HIV being transmitted through a human bite.

See also BLOOD; DRUG ABUSE; DRUG ADDICTION; INTERCOURSE; NEEDLE SHARING; RISK; SAFE SEX; SPERM; STIGMA; TRANSFUSION, AUTOLOGOUS; TRANSFUSION, BLOOD; TRANSIENT HIV INFECTION; TRANSPLANT; UNSAFE SEX; UNIVERSAL PRECAUTIONS.

transplant Organ and tissue transplants have become a routine medical practice that can dramatically improve—and sometimes save—lives. Because HIV is present at many sites in many body fluids, products, and tissues, transplanted organs and tissue, like transfused blood, are potential sources of infection. However, all donors and potential donors are tested, and all organs and tissues are evaluated before transplant. Today, the chances of getting HIV from a transplant are minimal.

transplant-associated AIDS AIDS acquired via an organ TRANSPLANT. See TRANSMISSION.

transsexual An individual who is biologically of one sex but identifies with the other. (This identification may have more to do with socially constructed gender roles than biological sex differences). Male-to-female transsexuals may have had surgery for breast implants, removal of the testes and penis, and construction of a synthetic vagina. Even without surgical intervention, these individuals often take estrogen and/or progesterone to support desired secondary sexual characteristics, such as absence of facial hair, enlarged breasts, and change in voice quality. Female-to-male transsexuals support desired secondary sexual qualities by taking androgens.

Hormone use in male-to-female transsexuals, beside having its pros and cons in itself, may complicate the treatment of HIV and AIDS. Addressing the use of hormones enables the clinician to correctly calculate the dosing schedule of drugs, to monitor complications accurately, and to achieve desired therapeutic effects while reducing unwanted complications. The clinician must also be on the lookout for drug interactions and the risk of breast and possibly other cancers, all of which may be affected by hormones, and must monitor the unknown effect of estrogens and progestins themselves on immune response.

transvestite A man who obtains erotic enjoyment from dressing in women's clothes.

trauma Any damage or injury to the body caused by something outside the body; also, and by extension, any psychological injury caused by an extremely stressful or upsetting event or experience. See POST-TRAUMATIC STRESS SYNDROME; TRAUMATIC EVENT.

traumatic event An event or experience that causes psychological TRAUMA.

Traumatic events or experiences have come to mean those that are outside the usual range of human experience, those that would be markedly distressing to almost anyone. These events or experiences are so overwhelming that emotional reactions and affects may be extraordinarily deep and long lasting, evoking stressful feelings and other responses, and perhaps affecting patterns of behavior, long after the traumatic event has occurred. See also POST-TRAUMATIC-STRESS SYNDROME; TRAUMATIC EVENT.

traumatic lesion   A scratch, scrape, or chafing on the body. See LESION; TRAUMA.

travel restrictions   The exclusion from the United States of aliens infected with the human immunodeficiency virus (HIV). Few issues in immigration law have caused as much controversy in recent years as the issue of travel restrictions. Seemingly a straightforward question, the issue is actually quite complex and has a long and volatile history. Should persons with HIV/AIDS be allowed to travel without restriction to the United States to professional, business, or scientific conferences? Is this a question of the public interest? Or a question of the rights of persons with HIV/AIDS? Should nonimmigrants be allowed in the United States without restriction for the purpose of receiving medical treatment? What is the role or purpose of special visas, waivers, and quotas? Are these initiatives based on the best medical thinking, on sound public policy, or on prejudice? These are some of the questions that have been debated by the United States government, public health and medical authorities, the news media and AIDS activists, as well as persons with HIV/AIDS during the first and second decades of the epidemic.

The regulation of IMMIGRATION on the basis of contagious diseases dates to the adoption and ultimate codification in 1952, as part of the Immigration and Nationality Act (INA), of specific exclusions for aliens suffering from such contagious diseases as leprosy and tuberculosis. The provision was revised in 1961 to reflect changes in medical language and to incorporate more precise language. The language of the provision is that "aliens who are afflicted with any dangerous contagious disease" shall be excluded from the United States. Determination and designation of which diseases are "dangerous contagious diseases" are left to the United States Public Health Service. In mid-1987, the Public Health Service added AIDS to the list. Soon thereafter, despite considerable opposition from AIDS and immigration advocates, doctors and public interest organizations, the Public Health Service replaced AIDS on the list with Human Immunodeficiency Virus (HIV) infection, further expanding the definition of persons considered to be afflicted with a contagious disease. On July 8, 1987, the Immigration and Naturalization Service and the State Department began testing aliens seeking admission to the United States for HIV. This set the stage for what was to become a hotly contested congressional battle following the enactment of the 1990 Immigration Act to statutorily exclude HIV-infected aliens.

The Immigration Act of 1990 completely revised the grounds of exclusion and provided for the exclusion of aliens on health-related grounds who, according to Public Health Service regulations, have been determined to have a "communicable disease of public health significance." The act also permitted, for the first time, a waiver of health-related exclusion grounds for permanent resident and immigrant visa applicants. In January 1991, the Public Health Service announced its intention to remove HIV from its list of communicable diseases because it had determined that HIV is not spread by casual contact. After critical public response, the Public Health Service decided to postpone finalizing its rule.

In 1993, the Public Health Service drafted new regulations that would have removed HIV from the list of contagious diseases and, as a result, two congressional bills were introduced containing language that would deem HIV a communicable disease of public health significance for purposes of exclusion. The ensuing congressional debate led to the enactment of the National Institutes of Health Revitalization Act of 1993, which specifically codified HIV-infection as a ground of exclusion.

Current law now provides for the statutory exclusion of HIV-infected immigrants and nonimmigrants. Any person who is determined to have a communicable disease of public health significance that includes infection with the etiological agent (HIV) for acquired immune deficiency syndrome (AIDS) is excludable. Certain classes of aliens are eligible for waivers that permit nonimmigrants entry to the United States on a temporary basis and that permit immigrants the right to be admitted and remain permanently. In this context, nonimmigrants are those persons, non-citizens and non-residents seeking to enter the United States on a temporary basis for a variety of reasons, including business, pleasure, and schooling. Immigrants, on the other hand, are those persons wishing to enter the United States with the intent to remain permanently. "Excludability" and "inadmissibility" are terms used interchangeably. Although a medical examination is required for all applicants applying for immigrant visas, a medical examination is not mandatory for nonimmigrant visa applicants. However, if a consular officer suspects that an applicant is HIV-infected, a medical examination to determine whether or not the applicant is eligible for a visa may be requested. Although the grant of a waiver to nonimmigrants is discretionary in nature, there are standard factors considered by consular officers in reaching their determination. These factors include whether the person, (1) is currently afflicted with symptoms of the disease; (2) is coming to the United States for a short visit; (3) has insurance or assets that will enable the person to pay medical expenses should he or she become ill; and (4) whether there is a reason to believe that the person poses a danger to the public health in the United States.

See also IMMIGRATION.

treatment   Medical, surgical, dental, or psychiatric management of a patient. Today, "treatment" is often broadly interpreted to encompass the nutritional, psychological, psychosocial, and spiritual management of a patient. Treatment also refers to any specific procedure or substance, or course of such procedures or substances, used for the cure or the amelioration of a disease or pathological condition. An overview of primary HIV/AIDS care follows, with a focus on the medical management of persons with HIV/AIDS.

Five key components of HIV care include: (1) the prevention of TRANSMISSION; (2) the preservation of the immune function; (3) PROPHYLAXIS AGAINST OPPORTUNISTIC INFECTION; (4) early diagnosis and treatment of opportunistic infection; and (5) optimizing the quality of life. Medical management of HIV infection consists of monitoring CD4 count; offering antiretroviral therapy when CD4 count falls below 500; initiating prophylaxis against PCP at a CD4 count of 200 or less; and initiating prophylaxis against MAC at a CD4 count of 50 or less. Additionally, the HIV-infected individual must be monitored closely for the development of opportunistic processes.

Treatment generally begins with an initial patient visit in which a general history of the patient is examined. Specific questions are indicated regarding mode of infection and possible dates of infection. Occurrence of any HIV-related problems or AIDS-defining illness must be documented. Current medication should be noted, including vitamins or other substances taken for nutritional or medicinal purposes. Special attention should be paid to sexually transmitted diseases and fungal, parasitic, and mycobacterial infections. Dates and treatment should be noted. A review of systems is conducted, and the patient is asked about his or her experience of fatigue; weight loss, anorexia; anxiety, depression; fever, chills, night sweats; adenopathy; skin rash; bruises or other skin lesions; headache, sinusitis; blurring of vision or other visual changes; oral sores; dysphagia or odynophagia; shortness of breath or dyspnea on exertion; cough; abdominal pain; nausea, vomiting, diarrhea, constipation; rectal sores, genital sores; arthritis, muscle weakness; forgetfulness; and lack of coordination. A psychosocial history is also taken, and patients should be asked about familiarity and experiences with others having HIV infection. A dialogue regarding individual expectations of immediate and long-term prospects should be initiated and continued throughout treatment. Patients may have strong feelings regarding the level of intervention they desire, particularly in regard to life-prolonging measures. A complete physical examination and laboratory tests are also commonly part of the initial patient visit.

Follow up-visits are generally scheduled as soon as possible after lab results have become available. Particular emphasis should be given to the psychosocial dimensions of the patient's response to HIV infection. A review of systems should be performed at each visit, and a physical examination is also indicated at each visit. Laboratory results are reviewed and interpreted at the follow-up examination.

Prevention is a key concept in the care of HIV-infected individuals—the prevention of viral transmission, prevention of illness by immunizing patients, and prevention of opportunistic infections. Prophylactic regimens vary from opportunistic infection to opportunistic infection. Common opportunistic infections include PNEUMOCYSTIS CARINII PNEUMONIA, MYCOBACTERIUM AVIUM COMPLEX, and TOXOPLASMOSIS ENCEPHALITIS PROPHYLAXIS, fungal infections, and herpes simplex.

Antiretroviral therapy involves the use of one or more of the four antiretroviral medications currently available to physicians—zidovudine, didanosine, zalcitabine, and stavudine. All are REVERSE TRANSCRIPTASE inhibitors. There are three major considerations in the evaluation of antiretroviral therapy: the TOXICITY of the medications; the duration of effectiveness of the currently available drugs, especially in advanced disease; and the fact that reverse transcriptase inhibitors do not completely suppress viral replication. Questions about the optimal usage of antiretroviral agents remain.

Treatment for common HIV-associated infections and conditions is also a part of the management of HIV/AIDS. Candidiasis, coccidioidomycosis, *Cryptococcus neoformans*, *Cryptosporidium*, *Isospora belli*, and *Microsporidia*, cytomegalovirus, herpes simplex, histoplasmosis, Kaposi's sarcoma, HIV-related lymphoma, *Mycobacterium avium* complex, *Mycobacterium tuberculosis*, *Pneumocystis carinii*, PROGRESSIVE MULTIFOCAL LEUKOENCEPHALOPATHY, THROMBOCYTOPENIA, *Toxoplasma gondii*, and VARICELLA ZOSTER are common HIV-associated infections. Common complaints of HIV-infected individuals include dermatologic complaints; diarrhea; fatigue; fever; hepatomegaly/elevated liver enzymes; headaches, seizures and focal neurologic findings; odynophagiz/dysphagia; peripheral neuropathy; and respiratory complaints. Issues specific to the treatment of women with HIV/AIDS include gynecologic concerns; gynecologic infections; menstrual disorders; cervical dysplasia and neoplasia; pregnancy; prenatal care; opportunistic infection prophylaxis in pregnancy; intrapartum considerations; and postpartum considerations.

Issues specific to the treatment of infants and children with HIV/AIDS include when to consider testing and the challenge of providing comprehensive and anticipatory health maintenance, including prophylaxis and treatment of common pediatric HIV-associated infections and conditions.

Increasingly, the medical management for persons with HIV/AIDS involves experimental and nontraditional treatments for HIV/AIDS. In the 1980s, science could offer nothing to people with the AIDS virus. Soon, the problem may be the opposite. There will be anywhere from eight to as many as 10 or 11 partially effective drugs and treatments on the market and many possible regiments for using them. So far, scientists have produced little research to answer what is becoming the central strategic question: How should the treatments be used, in what order and in what combinations, at what stages of the illness?

AIDS researchers are the first to admit that the latest treatments could ultimately prove disappointing. First, the virus can evolve rapidly in the body to become resistant to drugs, limiting how long even the best ones will work. Second, most AIDS treatments, including the new ones, seem to work best in people who are not too sick to begin with. For the many thousands who have already progressed to severe illness, science does not hold out as much hope. Finally, tapping into the latest developments is complicated and expensive. Those with access to experimental treatments and nutritional counseling have largely been middle-class white men, while the virus is afflicting more and more poor women and minorities. This "knowledge gap" is emerging as an enormous problem. Many people with the virus don't know they have it, much less what kinds of treatment are available.

treatment access   Despite the fact that there have been vast improvements in treatment access since the first decade of the epidemic, access to treatment remains one of the more controversial areas in HIV-related research today. In the early 1980s, the medical and scientific communities were not prepared to tackle the unexpected AIDS epidemic. The slow, methodical path that experimental therapies went through from initial conception to final approval was clearly inadequate. Efforts of community groups and AIDS service organizations, among others, led to significant changes in the way clinical research is performed. Still, as the second decade of the epidemic nears its end, many aspects of CLINICAL TRIALs, drug testing, and development remain a source of confusion, frustration, and at times, anger among people living with HIV.

Of particular concern is the exclusionary nature of many clinical trials. In the past, this has been a source of frustration for women who have been discriminated against in clinical research, mainly because of pregnancy-related concerns. This has been done to protect the fetus from potentially harmful new drugs. Also in the past, children were discriminated against in clinical research—the focus was always on men first. Because children are very different from adults, most children's therapies need to be tested separately. The exclusionary nature of many clinical trials has also been the source of tremendous frustration for many people who have been willing to enter trials, only to be rejected because their CD4+ count is too high or too low, or because they have taken AZT or some other drug in the past. Although trials will always involve specific exclusion and inclusion criteria, researchers and persons with HIV/AIDS hope that they will become more open in the near future, thereby increasing access to treatment for men, women, and children.

The red-tape of the United States drug testing and development bureaucracy has historically thwarted access to promising new drugs for persons with HIV/AIDS. Today, the Food and Drug Administration has approved several mechanisms for distributing experimental drugs before those drugs are approved for general sale, including compassionate use, parallel track, and treatment IND. Also today, persons with HIV/AIDS can make use of the growing network of community-based research groups in the United States whose top priority is the prevention of OPPORTUNISTIC INFECTIONS. Supporters of the CRI movement insist that it is doing an end run around federal incompetence and indifference. They insist that through community-based research, persons with HIV/AIDS can save their own lives, and encourage persons who want to survive AIDS to make contact with the community-based research group in his or her area.

treatment (IND) (Investigational New Drug)   See INVESTIGATIONAL NEW DRUG.

treatment IND status   See INVESTIGATIONAL NEW DRUG.

treatment plan   A projected series and sequence of treatment procedures for an individual patient, based on an evaluation of what is needed to restore or improve his or her health and functioning.

treatment use regulations   FOOD AND DRUG ADMINISTRATION rules under which drug manufacturers apply to distribute drugs for the treatment of the desperately ill when the drugs have been approved only for CLINICAL TRIALs. In some cases, these rules also cover drugs that have been approved for use but not for the disease for whose treatment it is being proposed. A change in the rules in June 1987 allowed for the early release of anti-AIDS drugs.

Treponema pallidum   The microorganism that causes SYPHILIS; sometimes referred to as a spirochete because of its shape.

tretinoin   A derivative of VITAMIN A being tested as a topical and oral treatment for KAPOSI'S SARCOMA. Although the oral form appears to have an effect on the disease, it also has serious side effects, including severe nausea and vomiting, intolerable headaches, malaise, altered blood calcium levels, and inflammation of the pancreas.

triage   The classifying of sick, injured, or wounded persons according to the severity (and survivability) of their conditions and the urgency of their medical needs; the assignment of priority for treatment. Triage promotes the most efficient use of health care resources when time, personnel, facilities, and equipment are limited.

trial   The experimental testing of a drug under controlled conditions. See DRUG TRIAL; MANAGEMENT TRIALS.

trial accrual   The number of persons enrolled in a CLINICAL TRIAL at a given time.

tribadism   A sexual act between two women involving rubbing their bodies together.

Trichomonas   A genus of parasitic protozoa, most commonly sexually transmitted, that cause an infection of the urogenital tract, mainly in women, in whom it causes a copious yellow or green vaginal discharge with a fishy odor and extreme itching. Occasionally it is present and asymptomatic. Diagnosis is by examination of vaginal secretions and findings of motile trichomonads. It may coexist with other vaginal PATHOGENs. It may be a marker for the presence of additional sexually transmitted infections, particularly GONORRHEA and CHLAMYDIA. Treatment is with metronidazole. For women who can not tolerate metronidazole, garlic suppositories are a home remedy that is reported to work well.

Trichomonas vaginalis   A species of parasitic protozoan flagellates, belonging to the genus *Trichomonas*, commonly found in the urethra and vagina of women and in the urethra and prostate gland of men. It is the causative agent of TRICHOMONIASIS VAGINITIS.

trichomoniasis   A form of vaginitis caused by the protozoan TRICHOMONAS VAGINALIS.

trichomoniasis vaginitis   Acute or subacute urethritis or vaginitis due to infection with TRICHOMONAS VAGINALIS that does not invade the tissue or mucosa but causes an inflammatory reaction. Infection is venereal or by other forms of contact. It is usually asymptomatic but may produce vaginitis, with vulvar and vaginal pruritus, vaginal discharge of white or yellowish viscid fluid containing mucus and pus, and rarely purulent urethritis in males.

trichosanthin   An experimental anti-HIV drug made from the roots of the Chinese cucumber, also known as GLQ-223. GLQ-223 is a highly purified form of compound Q. In the test tube it has been found to have potent anti-HIV activity, but in clinical studies sudden and severe life-threatening allergic reactions have been observed.

trifluorothymidine   See TRIFLURIDINE.

trifluridine   An antiviral used for topical treatment of infections caused by HERPES SIMPLEX VIRUS. In people infected with HIV, it has been used topically to treat skin, genital, and perianal HSV infections resistant to acyclovir. Trifluridine works by interfering with DNA synthesis in infected cells. It has been shown to be effective for treatment, but not prevention, of herpes virus infections. It is not effective against bacterial, fungal, or chlamydial infections. Available as a sterile solution for administration into the eyes. The most common effect of the optical solution is mild, transient burning when dropping it into the eye. Also called TRIFLUOROTHYMIDINE. The trade name is Viroptic.

triglyceride   A combination of glycerol with three of five different fatty acids. These substances, triacylglycerols, are also called neutral fats. A large portion of the fatty substance in the blood is composed of triglycerides. Because these lipids are not soluble in water, they are transported in combination with proteins. About one or two grams of triglycerides per kilogram of body weight are ingested daily in the usual diet in the United States. In addition, they are produced in the liver from carbohydrates.

trimethoprim   An antimicrobial agent that enhances the effect of sulfonamides and sulfones.

trimethoprim-sulfamethoxazole (TMP-SMX)   A first-line combination drug for *Pneumocystis carinii* pneumonia prophylaxis and treatment. Possible side effects include skin rash, pruritus, cytopenia, liver abnormalities, and gastrointestinal upset. This commonly used combination antibiotic has a variety of interactions and toxicities that need to be monitored. The most common side effect associated with the sulfa component is a skin rash, usually allergic in nature, which on rare occasions spreads to other body surfaces and becomes the life-threatening Stevens-Johnson syndrome. It is also known that the drug can greaten the skin's sensitivity to ultraviolet light, so excessive exposure to the sun should be avoided while taking it. Common drugs that have been reported to interact with TMP-SMX's liver effects include Coumadin (an anticoagulant) and Dilantin (an anticonvulsant). Elevated potassium levels sometimes also occur when on TMP-SMX. High potassium may lead to abnormal heart rhythms and contractions. In the presence of kidney disease, TMP-SMX can accumulate and cause greater toxicity. Kidney-toxic drugs (e.g., amphotericin, foscarnet) and AMINOGLYCO-SIDE ANTIBIOTICS (amikacin, gentamicin, paromomycin, streptomycin) pose a special problem for people taking TMP-

SMX, as does potassium supplementation. Finally, TMP-SMX increases the effect of the anticonvulsant Dilantin by inhibiting the liver's ability to break down the drug.

Trade names are Bactrim, Septra, and Cotrimoxale.

trimetrexate glucuronate   An antineoplastic agent and antiprotozoal "orphan" drug used in the treatment of moderate-to-severe PNEUMOCYSTIS CARINII PNEUMONIA. Often used as "salvage therapy" for people with PCP who do not respond to or who are intolerant of standard treatments. Trimetrexate causes severe bone marrow, liver, kidney, and gastrointestinal toxicities. It must be administered along with LEUCOVORIN (folinic acid) to ameliorate these adverse effects. Trade name is Neutrexin.

Trimox   See AMOXICILLIN.

trip   A vernacular term used to denote a drug-induced period of hallucination or euphoria.

triple helix   A genetically engineered modification to DNA, now in development. Naturally-occurring DNA consists of two interlocking strands (the famous double-helix structure). Scientists have now developed the means to attach a third strand, effectively blocking transcription—in other words, preventing the organism from reproducing. They are now working to synthesize small strands of modified DNA targeting specific sequences of the HIV genome.

In the same way that RNA-targeted therapeutics are more efficient than drugs that bind with proteins, synthesized triple helix promises to be more efficient than the controversial antisense. The compound would bind to the DNA itself, rather than to the thousands of RNA transcripts. Thus less drug would be needed and greater efficacy achieved—transcription of the unwanted gene would cease completely. This technology is at an early stage of development and many biochemical obstacles remain.

triple therapy   A three-drug combination of antiviral medications, one of them usually from the potent PROTEASE INHIBITOR family of compounds, recommended for all people with AIDS. The rationale behind this approach is that triple therapy with three antiviral drugs greatly decreases a person's risk of getting sicker or dying of AIDS. In June 1997, the federal government launched a high-profile campaign urging aggressive treatment to fight AIDS. A detailed document prepared under the auspices of the Department of Health and Human Services tells doctors what good and what substandard care is for patients with HIV infection. Guidelines on treatment for HIV/AIDS recommend that all people with AIDS be treated with a three-drug combination of antiviral medications and that most people in the early, symptom-free stage of HIV infection get the same aggressive treatment. The recommendations represent a highly unusual effort by the government to redirect treatment of a specific disease. They are meant to let physicians and health insurers know that, for hundreds of thousands of HIV-infected Americans, there's little question about what constitutes good medical practice. The goal is to give the clinician information to move through relatively complex decisions. The guidelines released recommend that all people meeting the definition of AIDS, or with symptoms such as unexplained fever or minor mouth infections, should get triple therapy. People without symptoms and with CD4 cell counts below 500 cells per cubic millimeter of blood, or with viral load measurements of greater than 20,000 viruses as measured by the REVERSE TRANSCRIPTASE-PCR method, should be treated. Other patients should consider treatment. It is acceptable for a person to be monitored closely and not treated.

Triple therapy, along with necessary lab tests, is expensive. An estimated 750,000 Americans are infected with HIV. Of them, about 500,000 have been diagnosed and know they are infected. Of them, between 150,000 and 180,000 are taking triple therapy. There are many reasons HIV patients are not on triple therapy. Some do not want or cannot physically tolerate the treatment which often involves taking 20 pills a day. A major reason, however, is the reluctance of many physicians to recommend the expensive and occasionally toxic treatment to patients who appear healthy and have no symptoms. That attitude derives, in part, from the disappointing experience with AZT, the first antiviral AIDS drug, which had no effect on mortality when taken alone. Physicians and researchers familiar with liberal use of triple therapy, however, have doubts about its dramatic effects.

The guidelines, and a second document outlining the broad principles of HIV care, are available from the National AIDS Clearinghouse (1–800–458–5231) and on its web site (http://www. cdcnac.org) and from the HIV/AIDS treatment Information Service (1–800–448–0440) and on its web site (http://www.hivatis.org).

TSS   See TOXIC SHOCK SYNDROME.

tubal pregnancy   Pregnancy in which the egg is fertilized and remains in the fallopian tube, which later ruptures. See ECTOPIC PREGNANCY.

tubal surgery   Surgery on the fallopian tubes, generally performed to reverse the effects of PELVIC INFLAMMATORY DISEASE (scarring and infertility).

tubercle   A granulomatous lesion caused by infection with *Mycobacterium tuberculosis*. Tubercles vary in size and in histologic component proportions but tend to be circumscribed, firm, spheroidal lesions that generally consist of three zones: an inner focus of necrosis; a middle zone consisting of an accumulation of large mononuclear phagocytes, or macrophages; and an outer zone consisting of mostly LYMPHOCYTEs with a few MONOCYTES and plasma cells. Where healing has begun, fibrous tissue forming at the periphery may form a fourth zone. "Tubercle" is also used nonspecifically to refer to any granuloma.

tuberculin unit   The unit of measurement for doses of tuberculin purified protein derivative (PPD), used to test for TUBERCULOSIS.

tuberculosis (TB)   A bacterial infection, usually in the lungs (where it is infectious), caused by *Mycobacterium,* most commonly *Mycobacterium tuberculosis*. It may also occur outside the lungs. Tuberculosis is far more frequent in people with HIV infection than in the general population. It is transmitted when a person with active TB coughs or sneezes, releasing microscopic particles in the air. These, also called droplet nuclei, contain live tubercle bacteria and may cause infection when inhaled by another person. Once infected by TB, most people remain healthy and develop only latent infection. In this state they are neither sick nor infectious, but they do have the potential to become sick and infectious with active TB. Many researchers compare HIV disease to tuberculosis as both HIV and the tuberculosis bacterium tend to become resistant to drugs.

The immunological factors that allow latent TB infection to develop into active disease are unknown. It is known that HIV-positive people have a higher risk of developing active TB disease. It is also believed that some people with active HIV will develop active disease from a newly acquired infection due to their inability to mount a sufficient immune response.

Although TB is spread through the air, infection usually occurs only after prolonged exposure to someone with active TB. Documented TB outbreaks have been primarily associated with hospitals, clinics, nursing homes, prisons, shelters for the homeless, and other places where persons who may have TB congregate.

The most common site of active TB is the lungs. This is called pulmonary TB. However, TB may affect any part of the body (extrapulmonary TB), including the skin, bone marrow, liver, spleen, kidney, bones, and even the breast and may occur simultaneously as pulmonary and extra-pulmonary disease. General symptoms of disease include fever, NIGHT SWEATS, dramatic weight loss, and a feeling of malaise. Symptoms of TB in the lungs include these, an otherwise unexplained cough lasting longer than three weeks, and bloody sputum. Since the symptoms of TB can mirror the symptoms of a number of other infections, it is important that TB be considered along with PNEUMOCYSTIS CARINII PNEUMONIA and other mycobacterial infections such as *Mycobacterium avium intracellulare.*

Clinical manifestations of active TB in persons with HIV infection can vary considerably depending on the stage of disease. TB can occur early in HIV disease, when CD4 cell counts average 300 to 400. At this stage of HIV disease, TB is usually localized in the lungs and the sputum specimen is smear positive (infected matter is visible over solid culture media). As the CD4 count declines, the presentation of TB may change, with more extrapulmonary disease, miliary lung involvement, negative sputum smears, and atypical chest X-ray patterns.

In HIV-infected people who develop active TB, levels of HIV in the bloodstream increase five- to 160-fold, findings which help explain why HIV-infected people with active TB have a poorer prognosis than HIV-infected people without TB. Research has shown that high levels of HIV in the blood correlate with an increased risk than an HIV-infected person will develop AIDS or die. The fact that active TB disease boosts HIV levels in the blood underscores the importance of diagnosing and effectively treating tuberculosis in HIV-infected people. These facts also highlight the importance of preventive TB therapy in HIV-infected people. Such therapy may not only help to control the spread of TB, but also prevent the increased replication of HIV associated with active TB.

The PPD (Purified Protein Derivative) skin test is the first step in diagnosing TB. PPD is injected under the skin of the forearm. After 48 to 72 hours, the injection site will be indurated (i.e., have developed a red hard bump) if there is TB infection. This induration is caused by an immune response, immunosuppressed persons may have little or no reaction to the test, even if they have been exposed to TB. According to the CENTERS FOR DISEASE CONTROL AND PREVENTION (CDC), an HIV-infected individual with an induration of greater than or equal to 5 mm is considered to be infected with TB. Some researchers believe that even the 5 mm cutoff may underestimate the rate of true TB infection and suggest that a 2 mm induration be considered a positive skin test in HIV-infected patients. A positive PPD skin test does not mean that the person has active TB, only that the individual has been infected with the bacteria that causes TB. Lack of response to PPD skin test is more frequent when CD4 cells drop below 200.

Along with a PPD test, an HIV-positive individual should receive an anergy test (skin reaction) to verify immune competence. An anergy test consists of two or three common ANTIGENS, usually candida, mumps, or tetanus toxoid, which are injected under the skin. If there is a reaction to the antigens, the person is considered nonanergic, and the TB skin test results are considered reliable. If there is no reaction to either the antigens or the PPD, the person is considered anergic. A negative PPD reaction should never be used to exclude the diagnosis of TB infection in persons who are anergic.

A person who has a positive skin test or who has symptoms of active TB should have a chest X ray and sputum sample analysis. The sputum will be examined microscopically for the presence of ACID FAST bacilli (AFB) and cultured for TB.

TB is treated with a combination of several ANTIBIOTICs. Combination antibiotic therapy given intermittently (less than daily) has recently been shown to be an effective initial treatment for persons with HIV-related TB. Prior to this finding, the standard of care was to prescribe multidrug therapy for several months before switching to intermittent therapy for the remainder of a typical nine-month course of treatment. When effective therapy is given, symptoms typically improve within four weeks and sputum cultures become negative within three months. The standard treatment of drug-sensitive TB in HIV-positive people generally includes isoniazid, rifampin, pyrazinamide, and ethambutol. TB treatment regimens that contain rifampin are far superior to those that do not contain rifampin. Rifampin-containing regimens are usually much shorter (six to nine versus 18 to 24 months) and have faster clearance of the tubercule bacterium from the sputum, higher cure rates, and fewer relapses.

Rifamycins, the class of drugs that includes rifampin and rifabutin pose a significant problem for TB patients who are also HIV-positive. Rifampin and rifabutin heighten the activity of the liver's drug-metabolizing cytochrome P450 enzyme system, leading to subtherapeutic blood levels of the anti-HIV protease inhibitors (saquinavir, indinavir and ritonavir).

At the same time, the protease inhibitors inhibit the P450 enzymes, causing higher levels of rifampin and rifabutin with an accompanying increased risk of serious side effects (including bone marrow suppression and inflammation of various tissues and organs). In late 1996, the CDC issued guidelines for HIV-positive patients with tuberculosis who also require treatment with protease inhibitors.

The CDC recommends completion of a six-month TB regimen containing rifampin for all HIV-positive patients with active TB regardless of CD4 cell count. For TB patients already on protease inhibitor therapy, the CDC believes one option is discontinuing therapy with protease inhibitors and completing a six-month course with a rifampin-containing TB regimen. A second option is to switch from rifampin to rifabutin (150 mg per day) and to indinavir from other protease inhibitors, and suggests treating patients with a four-drug rifabutin-containing TB regimen for nine months. The CDC also recommends measuring rifabutin plasma concentrations. A third option is a four-drug rifampin-containing regimen for two months or until the sputum culture has converted to negative, followed by 16 months of continued TB treatment with isoniazid at 15 mg/kg of body weight and ethambutol at 50 mg/kg, given twice weekly. Some experts also recommend adding a third drug such as streptomycin for the continuation phase. This regimen allows for reintroduction of protease inhibitor therapy after the second month of TB therapy. This third option is not recommended for patients with INH-resistant TB.

The agency's advice is based on the best guesses of experts in the fields of HIV, TB, and drug metabolism. The regimens have not been formally tested since most trials of protease inhibitors excluded patients requiring rifamputin or rifabutin. The recommendations serve as a good starting point that will encourage practitioners who care for people with TB not to withhold potent antiretroviral therapy from patients who also have HIV. As TB is known to accelerate the rate of HIV disease, intervention with protease inhibitor therapy in this patient population is considered crucial.

TB is considered multidrug resistant (MDR-TB) if it does not respond to two or more standard anti-TB drugs. MDR-TB usually occurs when treatment is interrupted thus allowing mutations to occur which confer drug resistance. Resistance may also be the consequence of inadequate care and follow-up that resulted in undermedication of TB. However, primary infection with MDR-TB can occur as well. MDR-TB strains are difficult to treat with the existing range of medicines. In most cases, MDR-TB has led to death in people with AIDS. MDR-TB has serious public health implications due to the rapid progression to life threatening disease, the efficient transmission to others, and delays in diagnosis.

PROPHYLAXIS with anti-TB drugs can prevent the development of active TB. Therefore, TB screening should be a routine part of HIV clinical management. Persons with HIV are more likely to suffer adverse reactions to anti-TB drugs and therefore require careful monitoring. The BACILLE CALMETTE-GUÉRIN (BCG) vaccine is the only TB vaccine currently available. BCG is widely used in parts of Africa and Asia where TB is endemic. BCG is not recommended for anyone who is immunocompromised, due to reported incidents of disseminated infection with the Calmette-Guérin bacillus.

BCG vaccination should only be given to immune competent children who are at unavoidable risk of exposure to TB and for whom other methods of prevention and control have failed or are not feasible.

tubuloplasty   A surgical operation to reconstruct the fallopian tubes and restore fertility.

tumescence   A swollen and enlarged condition. The penis is tumescent when sexually aroused

tumor   Any abnormal growth, whether or not cancerous or a threat to health.

tumor necrosis factor (TNF)   A CYTOKINE produced in response to infection by circulating white blood cells called MONOCYTES. TNF helps activate T CELLS; it may also stimulate HIV activity. TNF levels are very high in people with HIV and the molecule is suspected of playing a part in HIV-related WASTING, NEUROPATHY, and DEMENTIA.

TNF is one of a wide variety of cytokines produced by the immune system, each with differing effects on immune function. These cytokines also have effects on body metabolism that parallel their role in immune response. The observed metabolic effects of chronic exposure to TNF include fever, anorexia, hypermetabolism and, finally, wasting. TNF can furthermore trigger the release of other factors implicated in wasting and other symptoms, among them such cytokines as INTERLEUKIN-1, endocrine hormones, PROSTAGLANDIN E2 and the LEUKOTRIENES. It has also been shown to activate latent HIV infection within cells.

The list of therapies promoted as TNF reducers or inhibitors is quite long, and includes thalidomide, pentoxifylline (Trental), ketotifen, tenidap (an anti-arthritis medication), vesnarinone, OPC-8212 (an oral agent used in Japan as a treatment for congestive heart failure), cyclosporine, peptide T, sulfasalazine, thorazine, many antioxidants, corticosteroids, anti-TNF monoclonal antibodies, recombinant TNF soluble receptors, marijuana, glycyrrhizin, sho-saiko-to (SSKT, a Chinese herbal formulation), L-carnitine, hyperthermia, and hyperbaric oxygen therapy. Most of these therapies have been reported to reduce TNF in the test tube. Whether any achieves this in the body is hard to tell—there are conflicting reports about several of the therapies mentioned above. Even when there is a broad consensus that a given disease elevates TNF, there is always a study or two that contradicts that conclusion.

These discrepancies could be due to a number of factors. First, TNF has a very short half-life, and if blood samples aren't tested right away, assays will probably not detect it. Sec-

ond, TNF quickly binds to soluble and cellular receptors (which makes it undetectable in many tests), but this doesn't mean that it still can't do damage. There are several laboratory tests that measure TNF, both free and bound, but researchers do not agree on which to use.

tumor necrosis factor (TNF) inhibitor   Drugs that work to inhibit TUMOR NECROSIS FACTOR.

tumor-specific antigen   A cell surface ANTIGEN that is expressed on malignant but not normal cells.

turmeric   See CURCUMIN.

turned on   A slang term for sexually excited.

12-step program   A self-help program to achieve a goal, usually sobriety, organized in a set number of stages (often but not always 12). These programs are carried out by members of such groups as Alcoholics Anonymous (AA; the original 12-step program), Narcotics Anonymous (NA), Overeaters Anonymous (OA), and so forth. In most, the focus is on a mind-body-spirit approach to a behavioral problem.

typhoid fever   An acute infectious disease acquired by ingesting food or water contaminated by human waste matter. It is characterized by sustained bacteremia and infestation of the PATHOGEN within the mononuclear phagocytic cells of the liver, LYMPH NODES, SPLEEN, and PEYER'S PATCHES of the ileum, accompanied by fever, rash, headache, malaise, and abdominal pain. Diagnosis is made by isolation of the bacteria from the blood.

typhus   Any of a group of infectious diseases caused by RICKETTSIAe. Typhus is characterized by great prostration, severe headache, generalized maculopapular rash, sustained high fever, and usually progressive neurologic involvement, ending in a crisis in 10 to 14 days. Three diseases are included in this group: epidemic (louse-borne) typhus, caused by *Rickettsia prowazekii*; Brill-Zinsser disease (recrudescent typhus), caused by *Rickettsia prowazekii*; and murine (flea-borne) typhus, caused by *Rickettsia typhi*. Although clinically and pathologically similar, they differ in intensity of symptoms severity and mortality rate. Broad spectrum antibiotics, such as tetracyclines and chloramphenical, give excellent results. Prognosis is variable. Mortality may be quite high in epidemic typhus and almost nonexistent in murine typhus.

U

ubiquinone A lipid-soluble QUINONE (important small hydrophobic component of the electron transport chain) also known as COENZYME Q10, present in virtually all cells. It is a collector of reducing equivalents during intracellular respiration. It is converted to its reduced form, ubiquinol, while involved in this process.

ulcer An open sore or lesion of the skin or mucous membrane, accompanied by the sloughing of inflammatory necrotic tissue. It may discharge pus if it becomes infected. Trauma, caustics, intense heat or cold, and arterial or venous stasis are some causes of simple ulcers (local ulcers with no severe inflammation or pain). Ulcers may also occur as a complication of varicose veins, in which stasis of blood leads to inflammation, necrosis, and sloughing of tissue, or they may be caused by a specific disease such as SYPHILIS or lupus. Ulcers of the stomach or duodenum are caused by the effect of gastric acid and pepsin. The secretion from these sores contains the causative agent *Treponema pallidum*.

ulceration The development or formation of an ulcer; an ulcer.

ultrasonic cardiography See ECHOCARDIOGRAPHY.

ultrasonography The use of ultrasonic waves to make an image of an organ or tissue by recording the echoes or pulses of the waves as they are reflected by the tissues.

ultraviolet Beyond the visible spectrum at its violet end; said of radiation whose wavelength is between that of violet light and roentgen rays (X RAYS).

ultraviolet light The HIV community has long been aware of the danger in exposure to sunlight and artificial tanning lights, and that its potential for immune suppression and viral activation may play a key role in accelerating the decline and death of people living with HIV. It is a generally held belief that ultraviolet (UV) radiation harms the immune system. Nonetheless, some physicians have recommended controlled exposure to ultraviolet light, stressing that patients should tan only without exposing themselves to enough UV light to burn. A significant number of HIV-infected individuals have dermatological conditions that may be candidates for PUVA (psoralen ultraviolet-A light) therapy, which has been claimed to activate latent HIV in the Langerhans cells of the skin. Many researchers believe that a side effect of the DNA damage caused by UVA radiation is the activation of HIV expression. Others note that in situations in which quality of life is so severely impaired by problems related to AIDS psoriasis, and other treatments are not options (due to the even more immunosuppressive side effects of other conventional therapies), moderate exposure to sunlight, which contains both UVA and UVB radiation may be advisable to obtain some degree of symptom relief. Experts do not agree about the length of exposure to UVA radiation needed to activate dormant HIV.

Tanning beds as well as sunlight give exposure to UV radiation. While specialized equipment which emits only type A radiation does exist, both UVA and UVB radiation are employed in the tanning beds that are the most commonly used in the industry.

Other treatments for HIV psoriasis include high dosages of AZT and topical steroid drugs, both of which have their own immunosuppressive side effects.

umbilicus The umbilical cord, the structure that connects the fetus to the placenta.

"undetermined" An epidemiological category that also serves a social and political function. Like "risk group," "undetermined" isolates identifiable social characteristics predictive of where a disease or condition is likely to appear, for public health purposes. This has also led, unfortunately, to stereotyping and condemnation.

unemployed parent In the AFDC (AID TO FAMILIES WITH DEPENDENT CHILDREN) program, the highest-earning parent unemployed over 30 days, whose unemployment qualifies even a two-parent family for AFDC and MEDICAID, if they are also poor.

universal precautions In 1985, the CENTERS FOR DISEASE CONTROL AND PREVENTION (CDC) developed the strategy of "universal blood and body fluid precautions" to address concerns regarding transmission of HIV in the HEALTH CARE setting. Now referred to simply as "universal precautions," the concept stresses that all patients should be assumed to be infectious for HIV, HBV, and other blood-borne PATHOGENS. In hospitals and other health care settings, universal precautions should be followed when workers are exposed to blood, certain other body fluids (amniotic fluid, pericardial fluid, peritoneal fluid, pleural fluid, synovial fluid, cerebrospinal fluid, semen, and vaginal secretions), or any body fluid visibly contaminated with blood. Since HIV and HBV transmission has not been documented from exposure to feces, nasal secretions, sputum, sweat, tears, urine, and vomitus, universal precautions do not apply to these fluids, or to saliva, except in the dental setting, where it is likely to be contaminated with blood. The precautions recommend that because the unpredictable nature of exposures encountered by emergency and public safety workers may make differentiation between hazardous and nonhazardous body fluids difficult or impossible, these workers should treat all body fluids as potentially hazardous when they encounter them. Part I of the CDC's published "Guidelines for Prevention of Transmission of Human Immunodeficiency Virus (HIV) and Hepatitis B Virus (HBV) to Health-Care and Public-Safety Workers" addresses disinfection (of equipment and surfaces), decontamination (of hands, soiled linen, protective clothing), and disposal (of needles and sharps, infective waste). Fire and emergency medical procedures and equipment are also addressed (gloves, masks, eyewear, gowns, resuscitation equipment), as are other considerations, such as handling bodies, autopsies, and forensic requirements. Part II, "Recommendations for Preventing Transmission of Human Immunodeficiency Virus (HIV) and Hepatitis B Virus (HBV) During Exposure-Prone Invasive Procedures," discusses infection control during surgery and other invasive procedures, including oral, cardiothoracic, colorectal, and obstetric/gynecologic procedures, as well as digital palpation of needle tips in body cavities or any procedure involving simultaneous presence of a health care worker's fingers and a needle or other sharp instrument in a poorly visualized or highly confined anatomic site.

The most commonly referenced principles of universal precautions include appropriate handwashing, protective barriers, and care in the use and disposal of needles and other sharp instruments. These should be maintained rigorously in all health care settings. Proper application of universal precautions is designed to minimize the risk of transmission from patient to health care worker, health care worker to patient, and patient to patient. Recommendations for Preventing Transmission of Human Immunodeficiency Virus and Hepatitis B Virus to Patients During Exposure-Prone Invasive Procedures" were published in the *Morbidity and Mortality Weekly Report (MMWR)* 40 (no. RR-8), 1991.

The CDC's "Guidelines for Prevention of Transmission of Human Immunodeficiency Virus and Hepatitis B Virus to Health-Care and Public-Safety Workers" was published in *MMWR* 38 (No. S-6), 1989.

unlabeled uses   Generally accepted uses of a drug that are not currently included in FOOD AND DRUG ADMINISTRATION approved labeling.

unprotected sex   Sexual intercourse without the use of a condom or other prophylactic or contraceptive device.

unsafe sex   Dangerous or risky sex. Unsafe sex is essentially UNPROTECTED SEX.

While the concept of "SAFE SEX" has been around since the early 1980s and the basic priorities of prevention have changed little since then, there is currently disagreement about how "safe" and "unsafe" should be defined. The biggest arguments involve oral sex, the condom-every-time message, and the pros and cons of negotiation between partners. Ultimately the arguments are over a question on which no one is an expert: How much risk is acceptable? For years the major prevention organizations and government agencies said none. By most accounts, a significant number of men, both gay and straight, have simply ignored the advice or have set a goal of safer rather than absolutely safe sex. It is difficult to draw conclusions, however, since for many reasons government agencies remain reluctant to fund research into infection trends, risk, and prevention, so most information remains anecdotal.

uremia   A toxic condition caused by chronic or acute renal failure, resulting in an excessive amount of nitrogenous substances in the blood that are normally excreted by the kidneys; the constellation of symptoms associated with this condition, including anorexia, nausea and vomiting.

ureter   The long tube that carries urine from the kidney to the bladder.

urethra   The tube that carries urine from the bladder out of the body. In the female it ends at the urethral opening in the vestibule between the vagina and clitoris. In the male it goes through the penis, where it also serves as the passage for semen.

urethritis   Infection of the urethra.

urinalysis   A laboratory test performed on urine to detect disease.

urinary tract   The four-part system, including two kidneys, two ureters, the bladder, and the urethra, that creates, processes, and removes urine from the body.

urinary tract infection (UTI)   Infections of the urinary tract usually caused by bacteria, such as *Escherichia coli*, which travel from the colon to the urethra and bladder (and occasionally to the kidneys). TRICHOMONIASIS and CHLAMYDIA can also cause UTIs; low resistance, poor diet, stress and damage to the urethra from childbirth, surgery, catheterization and so on can predispose individuals to get them. Often a sudden increase in sexual activity triggers symptoms. UTIs recur frequently in females. Pregnant women are especially susceptible (pressure of the growing fetus keeps some urine in the bladder and ureters, allowing bacteria to grow), as are postmenopausal women (because of hormonal changes). Very occasionally UTI is caused by an anatomical abnormality or a prolapsed (fallen) urethra or bladder, most common in older women or women who have had many children.

Cystitis (inflammation or infection of the bladder) is by far the most common UTI in women. While the symptoms can be frightening, cystitis in itself is not usually serious. Symptoms include urinary frequency, burning on urination, hematuria (blood in the urine), pyuria (pus in the urine), pain just above the public bone (for women), and a peculiar, heavy urine odor when one first urinates in the morning.

In HIV-positive women, particularly those with depressed immune function or AIDS, a simple UTI is generally treated with 10-day regimens of oral antibiotics, guided by the results of urine sensitivity tests. TRIMETHOPRIM-SULFAMETHSOXAZOLE (TMP-SMX) is widely used. However, in HIV-positive women who are already taking this medication as prophylaxis against PNEUMOCYSTIS CARINII PNEUMONIA (PCP), an alternative has to be chosen, unless sensitivity to TMP-SMX or its components has been established. Other antibiotics commonly used include ampicillin, nitrofurantoin, tetracycline, or sulfonamides (e.g., Gantrisin). Antibiotics often cause diarrhea and vaginal yeast infections. Eating plain yogurt or taking *acidophilus* bacteria in capsule, liquid or granule form helps to prevent this diarrhea by replacing the normal bacteria in the intestines killed by the drugs.

If cystitis persists more than 48 hours, recurs frequently, or is ever accompanied by chills, fever, vomiting or pain in the kidneys, pyelonephritis (kidney infection) may be present. Researchers estimate that 30 to 50 percent of women with cystitis symptoms also have silent kidney infections. An immunocompromised patient with a likely kidney infection should be hospitalized for treatment. Finally, women placed on oral antibiotics should receive a prophylactic treatment to prevent vaginal thrush during the course of oral antibiotics.

urine   A yellow fluid, produced in the kidneys and passed through the urinary tract, in which waste is excreted from the body. In healthy persons, urine is amber color with a slightly acid reaction, has a particular odor with a bitter saline taste, and frequently deposits a precipitate of phosphates when fresh, but especially on standing. Urine is sterile and nontoxic, except in one who is suffering from an infection. Changes in the quantity, color, transparency, odor, proteinuria (the amount of protein found in urine), specific gravity, or acidity of urine are often significant as indicators of the presence of certain substances or of certain conditions or diseases.

urine culture   A laboratory test that shows what bacteria are present in a sample of urine by creating ideal conditions for their growth.

urophilia   The erotic attraction to urine; the desire to urinated upon or to urinate upon a sex partner.

us and them   The "us" / "them" dichotomy is part of the familiar system of social classification—the way "difference" or "differentness" is conceived and made sense of—to which the discourse of AIDS, like other social discourse, is assimilated. Other such oppositions are "self and other," "heterosexual and homosexual," "homosexual and general population," "active and passive," and so forth. The effect of such reflexive opposition is to isolate the self ("general population") from the other ("AIDS victims"), justifying indifference to or unequal treatment of the other. See STIGMA.

uterus   The major female reproductive organ that nurtures the fetus during pregnancy. The lining of the uterus is excreted during the menstrual period. This is a possible site of infection.

UTI   See URINARY TRACT INFECTION.

VA   See DEPARTMENT OF VETERANS AFFAIRS

vaccination   Immunization with a VACCINE for the prevention of a specific infection or disease.

vaccine   A suspension of infectious agents, or some part of them, given for the purpose of establishing resistance to an infectious disease. Vaccines stimulate an immune response in the body by creating antibodies or activated T lymphocytes (see T CELL) capable of controlling the organism. The result is more or less permanent protection against a disease. There are four general classes of vaccines: those containing living attenuated infectious organisms; those containing infectious agents killed by physical or chemical means; those containing living fully virulent organisms; or those containing soluble parts of microorganisms. Vaccines are given by mouth or by injection. BCG (bacillus of Calmette and Guérin), cholera, DPT (diphtheria, pertussis, tetanus), hemophilus influenza B, hepatitis B, influenza, measles, mumps, plague, pneumococcal vaccine, polio, rabies, Rh immune globulin rubella (German measles), smallpox, typhoid, and yellow fever are examples of vaccines. The age administered and booster schedule vary for each vaccine.

Dr. Jonas Salk, the famous polio researcher, was the first to suggest vaccination of HIV-infected people with HIV vaccine products. As of mid-1996, at least three dozen preventive HIV vaccines were being tested in small-scale clinical trials around the world, and the quest for a vaccine continues to gain momentum. The National Institute of Allergy and Infectious Disease Control (NIAID) remains poised to move into large-scale efficacy trials as soon as a suitable product is identified. NIAID is addressing the problem in a number of ways, first and foremost through its investment in research. In March 1997, NIAID instituted a new grant program designed to speed the pace of AIDS vaccine discovery and development—the INNOVATION Grant Program for Approaches in HIV Vaccine Research. The first phase of this pilot grant program encourages three areas of research: understanding the structure and function of the HIV envelope protein; improved animal models for vaccine and pathogenesis studies; and understanding the mechanism of directing antigen processing in vivo to maximize the immune response.

NIAID also established the Reference and Reagent Repository and the research of the HIVNET program, which is carrying out epidemiologic, virologic, and behavioral research required to ensure the success of the efficacy trials in communities and individuals at risk of infection. Through HIVNET and other programs, NIAID is working to build community linkages. In addition the Institute has also provided leadership in Phase I and II clinical trials through the AIDS Vaccine Evaluation Group, and in developing better clinical methodology. Finally, since 1988, NIAID has sponsored yearly conferences on advances in AIDS vaccine development. This event brings together investigators from NIAID's HIV vaccine testing centers, these centers' community advisory boards, independent researchers, and pharmaceutical companies.

Since 1988 and through mid-1996, more than 1,900 healthy, non-HIV-infected adults have voluntarily enrolled in 25 Phase I and II experimental AIDS vaccine trials conducted in the United States by the NIAID-sponsored AIDS Vaccine Evaluation Group (AVEG). AVEG consists of six university-based clinical testing sites, two central immunology labs, and a data coordinating and analysis center. Through mid-1996, the AVEG trials have involved 16 experimental AIDS vaccines, 10 adjuvants (a substance that enhances the immune responses stimulated by a vaccine), and a variety of delivery vehicles and routes, dosages, and schedules of immunization.

Initially, AVEG trials focused on testing injections of first-generation subunit vaccines. These are genetically engineered copies of single HIV-1 proteins, generally the surface proteins gp160 or gp120. The AVEG program has since evolved to include the testing of synthesized peptides (small compounds formed by linking two or more protein building blocks) and live vaccine vectors; novel delivery vehicles and adjuvants; and vaccines made from combinations of the highly mutable surface protein and the more conserved internal HIV proteins. Inducing cell-mediated and mucosal immune responses in addition to antibody-mediated immune responses have become goals in the design and evaluation of newer trials. One of the most promising vaccines strategies tested by AVEG so far is the prime-boost approach, the sequential administration of a live vector vaccine and a purified subunit vaccine. The objective of this strategy is to combine the strengths of each type of vaccine. Vector-based vaccines—which use an attenuated virus or bacterium to carry genetic copies of pieces of HIV into the body for presentation to the immune system—primarily stimulate cell-mediated immune responses. Subunit vaccines primarily induce antibodies. Research through mid-1996 indicates that the prime-boost regimen has been much better than other HIV vaccine strategies at consistently inducing both HIV-1 neutralizing antibody and cytotoxic T lymphocyte (CTL) responses.

To date, some of the most central issues remain unsolved. Researchers have yet to agree on the so-called correlates of protection, what sort of measurable immune response—blood-borne versus mucosal, antibody versus cellular—a vaccine should trigger to confer protective immunity to HIV. Vaccines against other diseases have been developed without settling the "correlates" question, but human testing of HIV vaccines is bogged down by this controversy. Additionally, scientists have not created a generally accepted animal model for more direct testing of vaccine-generated protection.

There are numerous problems in developing an AIDS vaccine. The first problem is a risk inherent to all killed-virus vaccines. Suppose by accident some virus escapes being killed? The 1950s witnessed such a catastrophe when a manufacturing error loosed into the population a number of doses of Salk vaccine that contained live virus; they caused a rash of vaccine-induced polio that almost derailed the fight against the disease. With AIDS, the consequences of such a mistake could even be more devastating. All viruses subvert cells by ordering them to make new viral offspring instead of new cells. But the AIDS virus takes subdivision one step further: It not only invades the cell, it splices the genes into those on the cell and then hides there indefinitely, invisible to the immune system. All it might take to cause disease, then, is a single escapee, just one live virus.

A second problem is that the AIDS virus is not a single, well-identified target: It is highly variable, and existing strains are continuing to change, mutating more quickly than any other virus known. A vaccine that works against one strain of HIV might prove worthless against another. A practical vaccine will have to deal with this knotty problem of variability.

A third problem is that the most common means of human infection is sex. During sex the virus directly infects cells in the mucous membranes of the sexual organs. It is likely that cytotoxic lymphocytes (CTLs) in the bloodstream are not enough to achieve full protection from sexual exposure of HIV. The activation of specific mucosal responses will be required too. Stopping this route of infection—ensuring mucosal protection whether through vaccines or topical anti-HIV microbicides—calls for cellular immunity, a quite distinct arm of the immune system that employs antibodies in the fluid surrounding mucous membranes as well as marauding white blood cells called killer T cells. (Virus that is transmitted directly into the bloodstream as a free-floating particle is easier to stop: An effective vaccine must produce the kind of antibodies that circulate in the blood, ready to neutralize the invader before it infects cells.)

A fourth problem is that no one knows what natural immunity would consist of. Infected people don't end up safe from future infection. They end up dead, as the virus destroys the system producing the antibodies. It is possible that one or more of those antibodies would prevent infection in healthy people, but there is no guarantee.

Participants in the AIDS vaccine wars have included researchers who focus on primates as well as those who focus on people already infected with the virus. In 1986, Daniel Zagury of Pierre and Marie Curie University in Paris and Robert Gallo of the National Cancer Institute, began a series of experiments to try to immunize humans against HIV. Their experiments involved injecting people who already had symptoms with a genetically engineered vaccine containing an HIV envelope protein. The vaccine incorporated the HIV protein into the harmless vaccinia virus, originally used in smallpox inoculations, which has become an all-purpose carrier for engineered vaccines. Soon afterward, Zagury expanded the study to include uninfected volunteers. One year later, albeit with the help of an impractical regimen of booster shots, it was clear that the vaccine could indeed beef up immune defenses against HIV. Zagury himself served as one of the volunteers in the experiment.

Jonas Salk, who died in 1995, took a rather similar tack, arguing that since AIDS symptoms typically don't develop until years after the initial infection, there may be a way to augment the body's immune defenses before it's too late. He called this approach immunotherapy, to distinguish it from what people conventionally think of as a vaccine. Salk began with the premise that once in the body, HIV's main mode of spread is not through the bloodstream but from cell to cell. Infected cells often fuse with healthy ones to form unwieldy clumps filled with virus. By destroying diseased cells much of the resident virus may also be destroyed. Salk's team, who continue his research, thus hopes to prevent disease in people already infected by shoring up their immune system's ability to destroy infected cells—so-called cellular immunity. The researchers are relying on the proven techniques that served Salk so well with his polio vaccine. In contrast to Zagury and others who are using genetically engineered vaccines containing pieces of HIV, Salk's preparation contains the actual killed virus. In a further departure from the approach favored by others, Salk's killed virus contains no envelope proteins. Salk's team is after the destruction of infected cells rather than free-floating virus, so the loss of the outer proteins may not be crucial.

vaccine development No effective vaccine against HIV/AIDS has yet been developed. Developing one is a particularly difficult challenge because the virus is constantly mutating. To be effective, a vaccine would have to protect against a variety of types. One obstacle to developing a vaccine is the lack of a laboratory animal that develops AIDS after infection with HIV. Such an animal would make it much easier to test potential vaccines. Since that animal has not been found yet, scientists have to rely on human volunteers. Moreover, the biggest scientific obstacle faced in developing an HIV vaccine is that the correlates of immunity—the specific immune responses that might protect an individual from HIV—have thus far proven elusive. Tough questions such as What if a flawed vaccine caused a volunteer to develop AIDS? and How do you determine whether a vaccine works? raise serious barriers to research, and many fear that there may never be an effective vaccine against HIV. At the very least, it will take years to develop.

Developing a vaccine against the AIDS virus has been the chief goal of AIDS vaccine science. The traditional view of an HIV/AIDS vaccine required that it provided "sterilizing immunity," which means that it would prevent an individual from becoming infected with the virus. Vaccines for other viral diseases only prevent the development of acute illness, not infection itself, but this approach has been perceived as extremely risky in the case of HIV. One of the new goals of HIV/AIDS vaccine development is to prevent "disease," not infection. Another goal of vaccine research today is the development of vaccine-like agents designed to boost the defenses of people who are already infected.

Investigators have observed that a high HIV setpoint (the HIV level attained after primary infection) is associated with rapid disease progression, while a low setpoint is associated with slow progression. If a drug or vaccine is developed that can push down this initial steady state, disease progression might be slowed to a very low rate, even though an individual would remain chronically infected. Since viral load also is associated with infectiousness, a vaccine that merely limited the HIV setpoint would have substantial epidemiological impact by reducing the rate of HIV transmission. The most immediate implication for HIV vaccine research is the possibility of using plasma viral load as an endpoint measurement for vaccine evaluation studies in primates.

In another retreat from the absolutism of sterilizing immunity, the National Institute of Allergy and Infectious Diseases (NIAID) is now talking of "preventive trials" as opposed to "vaccine trials." Purportedly, this new emphasis is a recognition that behavioral modification and physical and chemical barriers are also keys to preventing HIV infection.

In an interview published in the September 1995 issue of *AIDS Agenda*, Dr. Jack Killen, director of NIAID's division of AIDS, reported that many remain optimistic that an effective vaccine against HIV can be developed. Killian outlined the criteria of an "ideal" HIV vaccine. An ideal HIV vaccine would be safe and produce few side effects; produce strong immune responses against all subtypes of HIV to which an individual is likely to be exposed; provide long-lasting protection against all potential routes of infection, especially infection at the vaginal and rectal mucosa; be inexpensive to manufacture; and be easily stored and administered anywhere in the world.

Dr. Killen felt that progress toward such a vaccine would be made in incremental steps, through fundamental research and clinical trials of multiple vaccine approaches. He claimed that the biggest scientific obstacle faced in developing an HIV vaccine was the fact that the correlates of immunity—the specific immune responses that might protect an individual from HIV—have thus far proved elusive. Continuing advances in our understanding of the basic biology of HIV disease would facilitate the design of a safe and effective vaccine.

Candidate vaccines have been, and continue to be, studied in clinical trails worldwide to determine their safety and ability to stimulate immune responses. Most of these experimental HIV vaccines have consisted of recombinant viral proteins and are based on the envelope glycoprotein precur-

sor gp160 or on the glycoprotein gp120. All the vaccine candidates tested so far have been well tolerated, producing only mild side effects. A few of them have, fairly consistently, stimulated the production of antibodies that block HIV from infecting cells in laboratory assays that use strains of the virus that are closely related to the strain from which the vaccine is derived. Although antibody levels decrease within months, HIV-specific immunologic memory cells have remained for a year or longer. None of the vaccines tested to date has stimulated antibodies that neutralize so-called field isolates, obtained directly from infected individuals.

In June 1994, following a recommendation of a special advisory panel, NIAID decided not to proceed with large-scale human testing of two vaccine products, both of which were genetically engineered versions of the HIV envelope protein gp120. Among the panel's most important arguments was the finding that the antibodies generated by these products were unable to neutralize "primary isolates" of HIV, that is, virus obtained from infected people (not laboratory strains). At the time, questions were raised about the validity of the test used to measure viral neutralization. Specifically, this assay could not detect neutralizing antibodies in the blood of several vaccinated chimpanzees that were shown to be protected from HIV infection when injected with the virus.

At the 1996 Conference on Advances in AIDS Vaccine Development in Bethesda, Maryland, results of two blind studies involving a new, more sensitive test were reported. Both the new and the conventional neutralization assay work by mixing the virus with antibodies and putting them in cell cultures to determine if, and to what degree, the presence of antibodies prevents the infection of cells. The conventional assay adds PHA to the cultures, which powerfully stimulates cell proliferation and makes the cells much more prone to infection with HIV. The new assay, known as the "resting cell assay," uses no such stimulant.

Data demonstrated that with the new assay, antibodies present in the blood of three vaccinated and protected chimpanzees did indeed neutralize HIV and that these antibodies persisted for more than a year. Furthermore, the data showed that there is an "absolute" correlation in the chimpanzees studied between protection from HIV and the presence of such neutralizing antibodies. It is now clear that the gp120 vaccines can induce neutralizing antibodies. Whether the neutralizing antibodies protect against infection may depend on whether CD4 cells are in an activated or resting state when exposed to HIV. However, the conventional assay may not accurately reflect the immune system even when activated, so it may be too high a standard for any vaccine.

Nonetheless, the possibility of reconsidering the negative decision made two years ago remains slim, mainly because the gp120 products alone do not elicit significant cellular responses, as some of the new vaccine candidates do.

The vaccine research community is enthusiastic about a number of "second generation" approaches to HIV vaccines that are already in early clinical investigation. Most of these so-called second generation approaches fall into three major classes: recombinant vector vaccines; peptide vaccines; and virus-like particle vaccines. Recombinant vector vaccines use live viruses that undergo limited replication in human cells and are genetically engineered to express one or more HIV proteins. Peptide vaccines are chemically synthesized portions of various HIV proteins designed to elicit focused immune responses aimed at important specific viral targets. Virus-like particle vaccines utilize small particles of varying complexity containing viral antigens. These particles are produced in genetically engineered expression systems.

Many researchers now believe that a successful HIV vaccine must be able to stimulate at least two different kinds of immune responses: a humoral response, essentially the production of antibodies; and a cellular response, mainly the production of cytotoxic lymphocytes (CTLs). Antibody production helps the body rid itself of free virus, while CTLs destroy infected cells. As of April 1996, the vaccine products furthest ahead in clinical studies (Genentech's and Chiron/Biocine's versions of gp120), stimulated strong antibody responses, but they did not elicit the production of CTLs. A vaccine product named the ALVAC vaccine seems to be able to elicit both a cellular and a humoral response. This vaccine consists of Pasteur-Merieux-Connaught's live canary virus (harmless to humans) carrying portions of several HIV genes (for eliciting the cellular response) plus a "booster" of Chiron/Biocine's gp120 (to trigger the humoral response). By the time of the 1996 winter Conference on Advances in AIDS Vaccine Development, data from early safety and immunogenicity studies demonstrated that close to 50 percent of trial participants in one of the studies had new cellular responses to HIV. If this pattern is sustained it is likely that a larger Phase II study will be initiated in the United States in early 1997, with even larger Phase III studies in 1998.

In 1997 the NIAID announced the INNOVATION Grant Program for Approaches in HIV Vaccine Research, designed to speed the pace of discovery and development in vaccines to prevent HIV disease. In the same year, President Clinton challenged the nation to develop a vaccine against AIDS in the next 10 years. Health and Human Services Secretary Donna E. Shalala notes that "These grants will help to foster the kind of fresh, innovative thinking we need to achieve that goal." NIAID awarded 49 grants, totaling more than $11.8 million, after an exhaustive evaluation of more than 100 applications. The AIDS Vaccine Research Committee (AVRC) endorsed the concept of the INNOVATION program.

The grant recipients will be conducting research within the following areas: understanding the structure and function of the HIV envelope protein; improving animal models for vaccines and studies on the causes and progression of disease; understanding the mechanisms of antigen processing in living organisms to maximize the immune response. NIAID created the program to encourage novel ideas and approaches while stimulating interest from a new group of scientists, including those who had not been involved in HIV research. Today it is generally acknowledged that while traditional killed vaccine or live attenuated vaccine development methods are being pursued, they may not be the most successful for HIV. Many people in the scientific community believe that to discover the best way to tame HIV infection we need to focus on the newer biomedical technologies and approaches that depart from the conventional. Because of the importance and urgency that NIAID and AVRC place on AIDS vaccine development, NIAID piloted a new streamlined grant award process with this program announcement.

Based on the encouraging response from the scientific community, a second program announcement is planned.

vaccinology   A science encompassing all aspects of vaccine from its conception in the laboratory to its production by companies and its application and distribution in the field.

vacuolar myelopathy   A pathologic condition involving vacuolization (the formation of VACUOLEs) and sometimes degeneration of the SPINAL cord.

vacuole   A clear place in the substance of a cell. Sometimes it is degenerative in character; sometimes it surrounds a foreign body and serves as a temporary stomach for digestion of that foreign matter. Also, minute space found in any tissue.

vagina   The organ in women leading from the vulva to the uterus. The vagina serves as the passage for the intromission of the penis, for the reception of semen and for the discharge of the menstrual flow, as well as the passageway through which the fetus is delivered. Slang terms include box, cunt, manhole, pussy, quiff, and quim.

vaginal candidiasis   See CANDIDIASIS.

vaginal discharge   Abnormal vaginal secretions. Healthy vaginal secretions are made up of aging cells cast off from the vaginal walls, secretions from the cervix that help protect the uterus from infection and aid in fertility, and chemicals produced by vaginal bacteria and fungi. Normal vaginal secretion is clear white. White clumps generally indicate CANDIDA; a gray thin discharge, BACTERIAL VAGINOSIS; green profuse discharge, TRICHOMONAS; clear, bloody, watery discharge, atrophic vaginitis; and yellow discharge, MUCOPURULENT CERVICITIS (MPC). Abnormal discharge is often due to infection and is frequently associated with pain, burning, itching, and painful urination. Inflammation of the vagina is the most common reason for discharges and is usually caused by infection. PELVIC INFLAMMATORY DISEASE (PID), HERPES GENITALIS, infection of the inside of the uterus, a hole in the vagina, and inflammation of the vagina due to lack of estrogen are other possible causes of vaginal discharge.

vaginal douche   A liquid pumped into the vagina for deodorant, antiseptic, stimulating, or hemostatic purposes. The vagina has the ability to cleanse itself, so there is very little reason for a healthy woman to use a vaginal douche. Douching can upset the balance of the vaginal flora and change vaginal pH, thus predisposing the woman to VAGINITIS. There is no evidence that a postcoital vaginal douche is effective as a contraceptive. It has been shown that vaginal douching is a risk factor for PELVIC INFLAMMATORY DISEASE.

vaginal fluid   All women secrete moisture and mucus from membranes that line the vagina. Vaginal fluids provide lubrication, help keep the vagina clean, and maintain the acidity of the vagina to prevent infections. The walls of the vagina may be almost dry to very wet. The vagina tends to be dry before puberty, during lactation, and after menopause, as well as during the part of the cycle right after the flow. It tends to be wet around ovulation time, during pregnancy, and when sexually aroused. When a woman is under stress, secretion also increases. The discharge is clear or slightly milky and may be somewhat slippery or clumpy. When dry, it may be yellowish. Vaginal fluids normally cause no irritation or inflammation of the vagina or vulva.

Many bacteria grow in the vagina of a normal, healthy woman. Some of them help to keep the vagina somewhat acidic in order to keep yeast, fungi, and other harmful organisms from multiplying out of proportion. These harmful organisms may secrete wastes that, in large amounts, irritate the vaginal walls and cause infections. At such times, there may be an abnormal discharge, mild or severe itching and burning of the vulva, chafing of the thighs, and, occasionally, frequent irritation.

HIV was first detected in the cervical secretions of HIV-infected women in 1986. Scientists reported that the virus could be cultured from secretions throughout the menstrual cycle, an indication that the presence of the virus was not merely the result of contamination with menstrual blood. The probable source of HIV in cervical secretions is infected cervical tissue. In male-to-female transmission of HIV, contact with infected semen could lead to local infection of susceptible cervical cells; replication of the virus in those cells might precede systemic infection with HIV. Female-to-male transmission probably results from the sloughing of infected cervical cells into cervical and vaginal fluids. As concerns prevention, while condoms reduce the risk of infection with HIV and other venereal diseases, they do not eliminate it. The only way to eliminate risk is to avoid all exposure to infectious semen, blood, and vaginal fluids. See also VAGINAL SECRETIONs.

vaginal intercourse   In heterosexual sexual intercourse, the insertion of the penis into a woman's vagina.

vaginal-manual intercourse   A sexual practice involving placing a portion of or the entire hand in a partner's vagina.

vaginal opening   The opening to the vagina, closely protected by the labia minora.

vaginal secretion   Body fluid produced by glands in the vagina. The walls of the vagina may be almost dry to very wet. Dryer times usually occur before puberty, often during lactation, and after menopause, as well as during that part of the menstrual cycle right after the flow. Wetter times are around ovulation, during pregnancy, and when sexually aroused. These continuous secretions provide lubrication, help keep the vagina clean, and maintain the acidity of the vagina to prevent infections.

vaginal thrush   See CANDIDIASIS.

vaginitis   A common inflammation or infection of the vagina. Vaginitis occurs when the normal environment of the vulva and vagina is disturbed, usually by common bacteria. Although the vagina resists disease as well as the rest of the body, vaginal imbalance and lowered resistance to infection can be caused by poor diet, lack of sleep or exercise, and stress. Causes of vaginitis include viruses, irritation from use of strong chemicals in douching, fungal infection, protozoal infection, neoplasms of cervix or vagina, irritation from foreign bodies or tampon, vitamin deficiency, and conditions such as uncleanliness or intestinal parasites. In addition, pantyhose, nylon panties, tight jeans, and wet swimwear can also lead to EPITHELIAL injury resulting in vaginitis. The presence of vaginal pathogens may predispose women to increased frequency of herpes outbreaks or recurrences of GENITAL WARTS.

vaginitis, Gardnerella vaginalis   Vaginitis due to the bacterium *Gardnerella vaginalis*. The bacilli are usually GRAM-NEGATIVE but may be gram-variable in old cultures. The disease is most probably sexually transmitted. Symptoms include a malodorous discharge, elevated vaginal ph, and wet preparation of vaginal epithelial cells that are heavily supplied with bacteria called "clue cells." Metronidazole (Flagyl) is used to treat infections due to *Gardnerella vaginalis*.

valley fever   See COCCIDIOIDOMYCOSIS.

variable   In research studies, an element or condition that changes or may change in a measurable way in relation to other elements, providing a means to value and compare results. An *independent variable* is controlled by the investigator directly to allow examination of its effects; *a dependent variable* is one which is influenced by the independent variable. See DRUG TRIAL.

varicella zoster virus   The virus that causes chicken pox in children; its reactivation in adults causes SHINGLES.

vas deferens   The tube that transfers sperm from the testicles to the seminal vesicles.

vasectomy   The surgical severing of the vas deferens, usually as a means to prevent conception. Vasectomy leaves the man's genital system basically unchanged. His sexual hormones remain operative, and there is no noticeable difference in his ejaculate because sperm makes up only a small part of the semen. A vasectomy does not offer protection from HIV transmission during a sexual encounter. The semen of an HIV-positive man can transmit HIV regardless of whether or not a man has had a vasectomy.

vasopressin   A HORMONE formed by the neuronal cells of the hypothalamic nuclei and transported to the posterior lobe of the hypophysis (pituitary gland), where it is stored through the hypothalamohypophyseal tract. It stimulates the contraction of the muscular tissue of the capillaries and arterioles, elevating blood pressure. A pharmaceutical preparation of similar nature, extracted from the posterior pituitary of domestic animals or produced synthetically, is used as an antidiuretic in the treatment of acute or chronic DIABETES INSIPIDUS. Also called ANTIDIURETIC HORMONE. The trade name is Pitressin.

VD See SEXUALLY TRANSMITTED DISEASE.

VDRL See VENEREAL DISEASE RESEARCH LABORATORIES TEST.

vector vaccine A vaccine using a non-disease–causing virus or bacterium to transport HIV or other foreign genes into the body. The GENOMES of these "vector" viruses, including HIV DNA, integrate into the host cell's genetic machinery.

Venereal Disease Research Laboratories (VDRL) test A laboratory test, named after the Venereal Disease Research Laboratory of the U.S. PUBLIC HEALTH SERVICE, where it was developed, for the presence of antibodies in the blood to *Treponema pallidum*, the MICROORGANISM that causes SYPHILIS.

venereal wart A moist reddish elevation on genitals and anus. See CONDYLOMA ACUMINATUM.

verification The process by which a benefits program or agency checks an applicant's claim of eligibility (establishes citizenship, residency, age, disability, income, and so forth).

vertical transmission See TRANSMISSION.

Veterans Administration See DEPARTMENT OF VETERANS AFFAIRS.

victim A person who suffers from a destructive or injurious action or agency. Since the beginning of the AIDS epidemic, much energy has been expended in preventing people from referring to people living with AIDS, ARC, or HIV as "victims" or "sufferers." The emphasis today is on the empowerment of persons who are HIV+ or have AIDS: people with HIV/AIDS are able to speak for or about themselves, and are able to determine policy despite their biased status. The term has also been condemned by AIDS activists, medical workers, and service providers because it elicits an improper emotional attitude in both volunteers and the so-called experts.

A second concern about the term "victim" is its relationship to violence. In this society, violence against persons who are HIV+ or have AIDS has occurred throughout the epidemic in varying degrees. "Blaming the victim" is a means by which society tells persons with HIV/AIDS that they caused it or brought it on themselves in some way. It is a myth that supports violence against persons with HIV/AIDS, violence which has been perpetrated by individuals and institutions. AIDS activists have, in many ways, successfully challenged victim-blaming views. People with HIV/AIDS have emerged; hiding is no longer an acceptable means for people with HIV/AIDS to protect themselves and their fellow PWAs (Persons With AIDS) from violence. Awareness of the "blame the victim" mentality is the first step towards prevention of AIDS-related violence.

victimization To apply "victim" status to another person or to a group of people; as regards the AIDS epidemic, the victimization of persons who are HIV+ or have AIDS. See also VICTIM.

vidarabine An antiviral agent that inhibits DNA synthesis and is effective in the treatment of HERPES SIMPLEX and HERPES VARICELLA ZOSTER VIRUS. It has also been shown to be effective against HERPES SIMPLEX ENCEPHALITIS. Also called ADENINE ARABINOSIDE and ARA-A. The trade name is Vira-A.

Videx See DIDEOXYINOSINE.

vif gene The gene in the HUMAN IMMUNODEFICIENCY VIRUS that encodes proteins of 23,000 molecular weight and effects virus replication by increasing virus production.

villoma See PAPILLOMA.

villous papilloma See PAPILLOMA.

villous tumor See PAPILLOMA.

vinblastine An anticancer agent used for the treatment of Hodgkin's disease, lymphoma, testicular cancer, and breast cancer. In people with HIV, it is used for the treatment of KAPOSI'S SARCOMA. Vinblastine belongs to a class of cancer drugs called vinca alkyloids, which are naturally occurring chemicals isolated from the periwinkle plant. Vinca alkyloids stop the growth of tumors by preventing cells from dividing. Although vinblastine can be used by itself to treat cancers, it is used more frequently in combination with other chemotherapy drugs. Vinblastine is available as a solution for intravenous injection. The most common side effect is reduction in the number of white blood cells, which occurs, to some extent, in virtually everyone using the drug. Hair loss occurs commonly. Constipation, loss of appetite, nausea, vomiting, abdominal pain, sore mouth, jaw pain, diarrhea, stomach bleeding, and rectal bleeding may occur. In general, side effects occur most frequently when large doses of the drug are used.

vincristine An anticancer agent used for the treatment of a wide variety of cancers including LEUKEMIA and HODGKIN'S DISEASE. In people with HIV, it is used primarily as part of combination therapy for NON-HODGKIN'S LYMPHOMA and KAPOSI'S SARCOMA. Vincristine belongs to a class of cancer drugs called vinca alkyloids, which are naturally occurring chemicals isolated from the periwinkle plant. Vinca alkyloids stop the growth of tumors by preventing cells from dividing. Vincristine has a relatively low toxicity to normal cells in the BONE MARROW when compared to VINBLASTINE and is often the drug of choice in people with impaired bone-marrow function.

Although vincristine can be used by itself to treat cancers, it is used more frequently in combination with other chemotherapy drugs, frequently with bleomycin. It is also used in a two-drug combination with vinblastine and a three-drug combination with bleomycin and doxorubicin. For the treatment of AIDS-related lymphoma, vincristine is used in two different combinations. The first, called m-BACOD, consists of methotrexate, bleomycin, doxorubicin, cyclophosphamide, vincristine, dexamethasone, and leucovorin. m-BACOD is toxic to bone marrow, and many HIV-positive individuals cannot tolerate it. A more tolerable lower-dose version is available. The second combination is called CHOP, consisting of cyclophosphamide, doxorubicin, vincristine, and prednisone.

The response rates for CHOP and m-BACOD are similar. People with less disease, no prior AIDS-defining illness, and no bone marrow or central nervous system involvement are more likely to respond to treatment. The most important predictor of success is not the drugs used, but the CD4+ count at the time the cancer is diagnosed. Vincristine is available for intravenous injection only. When injected weekly, reduced white blood cell counts, pain, and constipation occur but usually last less than a week. Reducing the dose will often moderate or eliminate these symptoms. The most serious side effects of vincristine are hair loss and neurological impairment, which is often progressive. Peripheral neuropathy, a condition characterized by tingling numbness or pain in the extremities, is the most common. With continued treatment, pain, loss of coordination, loss of reflexes, and eventual paralysis may occur. Convulsions, accompanied frequently with hypertension, have occurred in a number of people taking the drug. Rarely, short-term blindness may occur. See also vinblastine.

vincristine sulfate   A drug that prevents the development, growth, or proliferation of malignant cells, obtained from the periwinkle plant *Vinca rosea*. It has similar activity to VINBLASTINE but is more useful in the treatment of acute leukemia and lymphocytic lymphosarcoma. See VINCRISTINE.

Vira-a   See VIDARABINE.

Viracept (AG1343)   A PROTEASE INHIBITOR. CLINICAL TRIALS have shown substantial reductions in viral load and increases in CD4 cell counts. Mild diarrhea is a common side effect.

viral assay   A test which measures the amount of virus in the blood. Over the course of the epidemic, we have heard that these tests are useful markers which can be used by clinicians from time to time. Generally, it is felt that disease progression and/or death are the only surrogate markers that one would use to stop a study. See VIRAL TEST.

viral culture   A laboratory test that enables medical workers to grow a virus from the cells or body fluids of an infected person. Viral cultures are one of several means to estimate how much virus is present. The test consists of diluting the sample until no virus is found. Other viral tests include PCR (polymerase chain reaction), QC-PCR (quantitative competitive PCR), bDNA (BRANCHED DNA ASSAY), and the P24 antigen test. See PCR, QC-PCR, and P24 ANTIGEN TEST.

viral DNA   See DEOXYRIBONUCLEIC ACID.

viral dynamics   The rate of viral particle production and clearance within the body. It has been found that production of HIV virions and CD4 cells both can exceed a billion per day. These findings indicate the difficulties involved in relying on antiviral drugs to eliminate HIV, especially given the number of mutant, drug-resistant variants that viral production of this magnitude makes possible, and suggest the importance of starting aggressive treatment with more than one drug as early as possible. Keeping HIV levels and replication to a minimum may delay the emergence of resistance to particular therapies.

viral encephalitis   ENCEPHALITIS caused by a VIRUS.

viral epidemic   HIV is one of a long series of viruses that have recently surfaced, and it will be followed by more. The history of viral discovery over the past decades shows clearly our unpreparedness for the emergence of such viruses and our vulnerability to a new epidemic. Much needs to be done if we are to avoid being caught off-guard again.

In the last 40 or more years, numerous infectious viruses have been discovered. These "emerging viruses" are not really new but rather represent existing agents that have acquired new significance and new hosts. Most have undoubtedly existed for centuries, escaping detection because they coexisted successfully with hosts, producing symptoms that were not previously recognized as being caused by infectious agents. Improvements in viral detection technology have opened up new frontiers in human biology, showing links between previously unnoticed slow viral infections and diseases whose cause had been unknown. Viral agents recognized in the 1990s include Borna virus, hepatitis E, HHV-7, and Crimean-Congo hemorrhagic fever.

Of equal or even greater concern is the movement of viruses across biological niches or vast geographic regions. Old viruses found in new locales or using a new mode of transmission include dengue fever, Kyasanur forest disease, Argentine hemorrhagic fever, Oropuche fever, Bolivian hemorrhagic fever, Lassa fever, California Bunyamwera, and morbillivirus.

viral infections   Micro-organisms such as viruses, bacteria, parasites, and fungi all cause OPPORTUNISTIC INFECTIONs, or SECONDARY INFECTIOUS DISEASES, in persons with AIDS. Examples of infections caused by viruses include CYTOMEGALOVIRUS, HERPES SIMPLEX VIRUS, VARICELLA-ZOSTER, EPSTEIN-BARR VIRUS, and ADENOVIRUSES.

viral interference   The inhibition of the multiplication of one type of VIRUS by the presence of another virus in the same cell.

viral hepatitis   Hepatitis caused by one of several types of VIRUSes.

viral load   The quantity of free virus in plasma as measured by the concentrations of HIV RNA. Treatment-associated reductions in viral load have been shown to correlate with protection from AIDS and AIDS-related death. Today, HIV viral load is increasingly employed as a surrogate marker for disease progression. It is important as a direct measure of how many cells are being infected and killed by HIV each day. CD4 count can be imagined as a measure of the current distance from progression to AIDS and viral load as a measure of how fast the patient is getting there. It is measured by

PCR and BRANCHED DNA ASSAY tests and is expressed in number of HIV copies or equivalents per milliliter.

Diagnostic techniques that measure the amount of HIV in the blood provide a quick assessment of the effectiveness of antiviral therapies without having to wait for clinical endpoints (the onset of opportunistic infections or death). For individual patients and their physicians, these tests may ultimately provide a way to track disease progression more clearly. An increase in someone's HIV population might indicate that their current treatment had lost its effectiveness and thus point to the need to alter antiviral therapy.

Viral load is commonly checked before initiating therapy, four to eight weeks after initiating therapy, and then afterwards for every three or four months. After a patient starts a new antiviral, a consistent decrease in viral load should be seen. If viral load creeps up or increases dramatically, and assuming the patient is properly taking the antiviral, the antiviral is seen to have failed. Physicians could then think about adding or switching therapies.

Recent findings have shown that while viral load is the most powerful single predictor of outcome in HIV-infected individuals, combining it with CD4+ T cell counts allows a more precise estimation of prognosis. Studies have also found that prediction of disease progression can be optimized by measuring viral load and CD4+ T cells before, and viral load shortly after, treatment begins. Findings indicate that individuals with high viral loads and low CD4+ T cell counts are more likely to develop AIDS than were those with high viral loads and relatively higher CD4+ T cell counts.

The extent to which viral load is a stable marker in the majority of patients continues to be studied. While research has shown that HIV can be suppressed, it has not shown for how long and in whom. It is clear that present antiviral therapy needs further refinement, and that better understanding of the variation in viral load and its causes is needed.

viral load assay Viral load assays, known as POLYMERASE CHAIN REACTION (PCR) and BRANCHED-DNA ASSAY (BDNA) tests, are used to measure changes in the level of free HIV in blood plasma. They have been used to measure drug effectiveness when making treatment decisions for individual patients. Counting VIRIONs has been widely proposed as a way to radically shorten trials. Convinced that viral load reflects the balance between the immune system and the virus and is therefore the most important determinant of outcome, many researchers believe only that plasma viral load is an earlier and more accurate predictor than CD4 count. The problem has been that no one has established how predictive viral load measurements are of long-term disease course. Even more in question has been the significance of short-term reductions in circulating HIV induced by specific treatments.

See SURROGATE MARKER.

viral replication For the first decade plus, one of the widely-held myths about AIDS in conventional medicine was that HIV remains dormant for up to ten years before initiating immune damage. Today, we know that there is more viral replication occurring in the lymphoid organs, even during the asymptomatic phase, than people had suspected. During this period virtually all patients experience a gradual deterioration of the immune system, manifested particularly through the depletion of CD4 T CELLS. In certain pathologic processes involving lymphoid cells, the peripheral blood may not accurately reflect the status of disease. Furthermore, specific immune responses are generated predominantly in the lymphoid organs rather than in the peripheral blood. Because the lymphoid organs are the major reservoirs of virus and sites of viral replication, peripheral blood measurements do not accurately reflect the total body burden of HIV infection. See also CLINICAL, LATENCY.

viral test Generally, a blood test for HIV activity, and for other markers of disease severity or progression. These tests are critically important for developing new drugs and for patient care. Reliable tests might shorten the time required to show which drugs are good candidates from years to months, allowing many more potential treatments to be tested. Better viral tests could also improve medical care with the drugs we already have by showing when a course of treatment is working for an individual and when it is not, so that the physician will have rational guidance on when to add or switch therapies. Examples of viral tests include PCR (POLYMERASE CHAIN REACTION), quantitative PCR, QC-PCR (quantitative competitive PCR), BRANCHED DNA ASSAY (bDNA), P24 ANTIGEN TEST and VIRAL CULTURES. See VIRAL ASSAY.

viremia The presence of a VIRUS in blood or blood plasma. Plasma viremia is a quantitative measurement of HIV levels similar to viral load but is accomplished by seeing how much of a patient's plasma is required to start an HIV infection in a laboratory cell culture. It has been found that the presence of viremia in the blood identifies a risk for development of active disease in multiple organs.

virion A complete viral particle existing outside a cell.

virologic markers Direct measurements of the amount of VIRUS are called "virologic markers." Some virologic tests are not sensitive enough and others are too labor-intensive to be practical for everyday use. A few of the tests that have moved forward, and are being used to measure the anti-HIV effects of experimental drugs directly on HIV quantity include P24 ANTIGEN and POLYMERASE CHAIN REACTION (PCR).

See BRANCHED DNA ASSAY; POLYMERASE CHAIN REACTION TEST; SURROGATE MARKER; VIRAL LOAD; VIRAL LOAD ASSAY.

virology Study of VIRUSes and viral diseases.

virucide An agent that destroys or inactivates a VIRUS.

virus Any of a large group of submicroscopic agents, or MICROBES, capable of infecting plants, animals, and bacteria, characterized by a total dependence on living cells for reproduction and a lack of independent metabolism. Unlike bacteria, viruses can neither survive nor reproduce unless they live in a cell. Viruses consist of a core of genetic material, either RNA or DNA, surrounded by a protein coat. HIV is a virus that lives in CD4 LYMPHOCYTEs in humans. Viruses may be named and classified according to the host they dominate, or according to their origin, mode of transmission, manifestations, and geographic location where they were first isolated.

virus-hunting   Nearly discredited by the failed war on cancer, virus-hunting is the attempt to link viruses and illness. In large part due to AIDS, virus-hunting has enjoyed a spectacular revival in the 1980s and 1990s. Within the context of AIDS, virus-hunting has become a public scientific controversy. On one side stand microbiologist Peter Duesberg and a circle of defenders who believe that the HUMAN IMMUNODEFICIENCY VIRUS (HIV) has not been proved to cause AIDS. These "dissidents" argue that HIV is an innocent bystander in the AIDS epidemic, and assert that millions of dollars have been poured into research to find vaccines and therapies, and thousands of people are poisoning themselves with toxic medications, all in the goal of obstructing a virus that doesn't make anyone sick. On the other side are mainstream AIDS researchers who insist that HIV is the primary cause of AIDS.

visceral leishmaniasis   Leishmaniasis caused by *L. donovani*.

visna   A viral disease that affects sheep. The primary target is the CENTRAL NERVOUS SYSTEM. It is characterized by asymptomatic onset and partial paralysis of the hindlimbs, progressing to total paralysis and death.

visualization   The act of viewing or sensing a picture of an object.

One of many different methods used to reach a state of relaxation. With eyes closed, one becomes completely relaxed either by another method or, for example, by visualising walking down a shaded stairway, becoming more and more relaxed as one descend into comforting darkness.

Once relaxed, an image is brought to mind that may represent the desired change in any number of ways. Some people see themselves as being completely healthy. Others imagine the healing white blood cells as white knights charging forth, conquering the invading infections and visualising the "bad guys" in full retreat. For those who may have trouble focusing clearly on an image, the suggestion is made to draw the desired image on paper to give it more substance and reality. The practice of visualization or imagery is recognized as one of the most powerful healing techniques available today.

vitamin   Any of a group of organic substances other than proteins, carbohydrates, fats, minerals, and organic salts that are essential for normal metabolism, growth, and development of the body. Vitamins are not sources of energy, nor do they contribute significantly to the substance of the body, but they are indispensable for the maintenance of health. Effective in minute quantities, they act principally as regulators of metabolic processes and play a role in energy transformation, usually acting as coenzymes in enzymatic systems. Vitamins may be fat-soluble or water-soluble.

vitamin A   Discovered more than 50 years ago, retinol, known as vitamin A, was originally classified as an anti-infective agent. It plays an important role in rapid renewal of tissues associated with growth, reproduction, and bone formation. It is a fat-soluble vitamin and can be toxic at high doses. Vitamin A deficiency is often associated with protein-energy malnutrition; deficiency also adversely affects the lymphoid system.

Vitamin A was first seen as an IMMUNOMODULATOR as a result of the observation that susceptibility to infection and the development of tumors in vitamin A–deficient human subjects was easily and quickly reversed by replenishment of the vitamin. It is believed that vitamin A can, at nontoxic doses, act as an adjuvant, or enhancing agent, of the immune response. Vitamin A deficiency is also associated with the suppression of both the innate and acquired branches of the immune system. While the function of vitamin A in immunology is not clearly understood, it is known that loss of cellular integrity caused by inadequate vitamin A results in adverse consequences to individual immunity.

All impairments caused by deficiency of vitamin A can be reversed by adequate supplementation. But vitamin A in its most commonly used form is toxic at high doses and should not be consumed in daily doses exceeding 10 mg. Deficiencies can occur even in cases of adequate dietary intake, particularly in the presence of abnormalities of fat ingestion and absorption, such as those caused by intestinal infections, which are extremely common among people with AIDS. The vitamin tends to accumulate in the liver and requires zinc to release it into the bloodstream. Beta-carotene is a nontoxic substance that can be stored in the body and converted into vitamin A by the liver as needed.

vitamin B complex   A group of water-soluble vitamins isolated from liver, yeast, and other sources. Among the B vitamins are thiamine, riboflavin, niacin, pyridoxine, biotin, FOLIC ACID, and cyanocoalamin. The vitamin B complex affects growth, appetite, lactation, and the gastrointestinal, nervous, and endocrine systems; aids in marasmus; stimulates appetite; aids metabolism of carbohydrates; and stimulates biliary action. B vitamins are also used as adjuncts to some antituberculosis drugs. Deficiency disorders include beriberi, pellagra, digestive disturbances, enlargement of the liver, disturbance of the thyroid, degeneration of sex glands, and neurological disturbances. Vitamin B deficiencies induce edema, affect the heart, liver, spleen, and kidneys, enlarge the adrenals, and cause dysfunction of the pituitary and salivary glands.

vitamin B₁₂   A red crystalline substance, a cobamide, extracted from liver, that is essential for the formation of red blood cells. Its deficiency results in pernicious anemia. It is used for prophylaxis and treatment of diseases in which there is defective red cell formation.

vitamin C   A vitamin necessary for formation of intercellular substance of connective tissue and essential in maintenance of the integrity of intercellular cement in many tissues, especially capillary walls. Also known as ascorbic acid. Deficiency leads to scurvy.

Few nutrients are as active in human metabolism as ascorbic acid. It is known to be the most important water-soluble antioxidant and cofactor in cellular metabolism. Researchers have clearly demonstrated that the immune system is sensitive to intake levels of vitamin C, and that numerous immunological functions are dependent on it for their mediation. Vitamin C is possibly the most often used dietary supplement, particularly in immune-suppressed individuals and those suffering from other degenerative illnesses. It is virtually universal in the health regimens of long-term

AIDS survivors. Vitamin C can be purchased in tablet, capsule, or powdered form. If vitamin C powder is taken dissolved in water or juice, it should be drunk with a straw—ascorbic acid can, over time, erode tooth enamel.

vitamin D   One of several vitamins having antirachitic activity, vitamin D is essential in calcium and phosphorus metabolism. It is required for normal development of bones and teeth. Deficiency disorders include imperfect skeletal formation, bone diseases, rickets, and caries.

vitamin E   A fat-soluble vitamin, composed of a group of compounds called tocopherols. Seven forms of tocopherol exist in nature: alpha, beta, delta, epsilon, eta, gamma and zeta. Of these, alpha-tocopherol is the most potent form and has the greatest nutritional and biological value. Tocopherols occur in highest concentrations in cold-pressed vegetable oils, seeds and nuts, and soybeans. Wheat germ oil is the source from which vitamin E was first obtained. The vitamin is necessary for all forms of oxygen-consuming life forms. Vitamin E is an ANTIOXIDANT, which means it opposes oxidation of substances in the body. Oxidation involves a compound called an oxidizer which attacks another compound, removing an electron from it. Vitamin E protects other substances by being oxidized itself, taking the brunt of any attack on lipids or other components of the membranes.

Vitamin E prevents saturated fatty acids and VITAMIN A from breaking down and combining with other substances that may become harmful to the body. Fat oxidation results in the formation of FREE RADICALs. Free radicals are highly destructive molecules that can alter DNA and cause extensive damage to the body, from blood clots to cancer. The VITAMIN B COMPLEX and ascorbic acid are also protected against oxidation when vitamin E is present in the digestive tract. Fats and oils containing vitamin E are less susceptible to rancidity than those devoid of vitamin E. It has the ability to unite with oxygen and prevent it from being converted into toxic peroxides; this leaves the red blood cells more fully supplied with the pure oxygen that the blood carries to the heart and other organs.

Vitamin E is also of great importance in energy production. It plays an essential role in the cellular respiration of all muscles, especially cardiac and skeletal. The vitamin makes it possible for these muscles and their nerves to function with less oxygen, thereby increasing their endurance and stamina. It also causes dilation of the blood vessels, permitting a fuller flow of blood to the heart. Vitamin E is a highly effective antithrombin in the bloodstream, inhibiting coagulation of blood by preventing clots from forming. It also aids in bringing nourishment to the cells, strengthening the capillary walls, and protecting the red blood cells from destruction by poisons in the blood.

Vitamin E prevents both the pituitary and adrenal hormones from being oxidized and promotes proper functioning of linoleic acid, and unsaturated fatty acid. Since aging in the cells is due primarily to oxidation, vitamin E may be useful in retarding that process.

Vitamin E is also necessary for the proper focusing of the eyes in middle-aged people. The vitamin stimulates urine excretion, which helps heart patients whose body tissues contain an excessive amount of tissue fluid. It protects

against the damaging effects of many environmental poisons in the air, water, and food. Finally, vitamin E may possibly be involved in calcium metabolism, correcting deposition in the body of either too little or too much calcium.

Vitamin E, along with VITAMIN C, selenium and beta carotene, is an antioxidant that has been shown to have a beneficial effect on the functioning of the immune system. Studies at Tulane University suggest that vitamin E increases AZT's ability to fight symptoms caused by HIV. Vitamin E may also reduce the bone marrow toxicity caused by AZT.

vitreous humor   The gellike substance that fills the eyeball between the lens and the retina.

Vocational Rehabilitation Act of 1973   One of two federal statues that address the issue of employment of people with disabilities (the other is the AMERICANS WITH DISABILITIES ACT). Congress passed the Rehabilitation Act to promote the hiring of the disabled and to prohibit employers who receive funds under the act from discriminating against disabled workers who are otherwise able to perform their duties. Following a case brought by an employee with tuberculosis against a Florida school board [*Arline v. School Bd. Of Nassau County*, 480 U.S. 273 (1987)], the act was amended to state that while a person with a contagious disease such as AIDS does qualify as disabled, the act does not apply to individuals who pose a health or safety threat to others or who are unable to perform their duties due to illness. Both statutes require "reasonable accommodation" of the employee's disability.

volunteer organizations   The "AIDS service industry," which emerged in the 1980s, spawned a vast array of volunteer organizations, and which differ in mission, purpose, target audience, structure, staff, and funding. National, regional, and local in scope, volunteer organizations include the broad array of AIDS Service Organizations (ASOs), many of which are educational and support agencies for people with HIV/AIDS, as well as AIDS advocacy and/or activist groups (i.e. groups which promote the urgent need for biomedical research on AIDS and groups which provide updated information on experimental drug treatments for persons with HIV or AIDS), and specialized groups, such as organizations comprised of people who have been diagnosed as having AIDS, AIDS-related complex, or HIV, or others which provide education and support to women with AIDS. See also VOLUNTEERS.

volunteers   The backbone of AIDS SERVICE ORGANIZATIONS (ASOs), volunteers have been, and continue to be, the primary workforce in the AIDS service industry. This work has been characterized as a cultural response to both disease and shifting mores. Volunteers typically provide their services and/or time willingly and without pay. They care for people with HIV-related illnesses and provide a broad range of other client services, including meeting food and medical needs, daily living, prevention education, legal, and social needs of persons with HIV/AIDS. Other volunteers provide specialized services to people of color and drug users. Other volunteers may be involved with advocacy; fund raising; counseling; community, professional or general public education; policy-making; or public relations. Volunteers pursue their work in the AIDS service industry for a variety of reasons, ranging from the altruistic to the political to the self-interested. Feeling more personally engaged and less hopeless are just two possible positive outcomes of pursuing this kind of work.

vomiting   Ejection through the mouth of the gastric contents, and, in cases of bowel obstruction, intestinal contents. It may result from toxins from ptomaines, drugs, uremia, and specific fevers; cerebral tumors and meningitis; diseases of the stomach; reflex from pregnancy, uterine, or ovarian disease; irritation of the fauces (the passage from the mouth to the pharynx), worms, biliary colic; intestinal obstruction; motion sickness; or nervous affections.

von Willebrand's disease   A congenital bleeding disorder, von Willebrand's disease usually manifests at an early age, with the symptoms decreasing with age or during pregnancy.

It is characterized by prolonged periods of bleeding and a deficiency of coagulation factor VIII in the blood. It is associated with increased bleeding during surgery or trauma and excessive loss of blood during menstruation.

voyeur   One who obtains erotic enjoyment from watching others naked or engaging in sexual acts.

vpr gene   A gene in the HUMAN IMMUNODEFICIENCY VIRUS whose function is currently unknown.

vulva   The external female sex organs, including the outer and inner lips of the vagina and the clitoris.

vulvovaginal candidiasis   See CANDIDIASIS.

vulvovaginal condition   The state of health of the vulva and vagina.

waiver The procedure by which rules of regulatory and benefits programs can be set aside in extraordinary circumstances, usually for experimental, research, demonstration, or compassionate purposes.

Walter Reed Classification System A standard scale of measurement of the progression and severity of HIV disease. It distinguishes six stages following exposure. Stage 1: infection; flulike syndrome characterized by fever, myalgia, malaise, and lymphadenopathy; SEROCONVERSION. Stage 2: chronic LYMPHADENOPATHY. Stage 3: T4 count below 400. Stage 4: reduced delayed hypersensitivity response to common allergens. Stage 5: complete anergy and appearance of chronic viral or fungal infections of mucous membranes. Stage 6: AIDS as defined by CENTERS FOR DISEASE CONTROL AND PREVENTION standards; the presence of opportunistic infections in sites other than the skin or mucous membranes. The length of time a patient stays in each stage is still relatively unclear.

See AIDS CASE DEFINITION; AIDS-DEFINING ILLNESS.

wart A circumscribed elevation of the skin resulting from an increase in size or bulk of the epidermis and protuberances in the layer just under the epidermis. Warts are caused by a PAPILLOMAVIRUS. Genital, plantar, seborrheic, and venereal are four common types of warts.

Wasserman Test One of several nontreponemal variety of serological (blood) tests for SYPHILIS which give passive evidence of the disease if antibodies are present. In contrast, tests of the treponemal variety look for *Treponema pallidum*, the corkscrew-shaped organisms that cause the disease.

waste See MEDICAL WASTE.

wasting An involuntary loss of 10 percent or more of usual body weight, including lean tissue. It can be caused by a variety of conditions associated with disease and drug therapy. Wasting and weight loss accompany most major infections. In HIV/AIDS, weight loss in the absence of an identifiable cause may result directly from HIV, which can infect intestinal cells, causing inflammation and diarrhea. Wasting was added to the CENTERS FOR DISEASE CONTROL AND PREVEN-TION definition of AIDS in 1987 after an evaluation of diseases found often in INTRAVENOUS DRUG USERS.

wasting syndrome HIV- or AIDS-associated WASTING, known as wasting syndrome, is a major cause of illness and death in patients with late-stage HIV infection. It can be divided into two categories: acute WEIGHT LOSS, which often rebounds after an opportunistic infection is brought under control, and chronic weight loss, which is more difficult to reverse. Either decreased nutrient intake or alterations in metabolism can lead to weight loss. These factors may arise directly from HIV infection as well as from opportunistic infections, cancers, or preexisting gastrointestinal disease.

It is important to differentiate between mere loss in weight and the loss of protein stores (in lean tissue) that occurs during HIV infection. When acute weight loss is halted by treating an opportunistic infection, weight may be regained by adding fat rather than rebuilding lean tissue. Simply taking in more nutrients does not automatically produce recovery from wasting. An added complication of malnutrition and wasting in women is demographics. HIV-positive women are likely to be minority, poor, and drug users or partners of drug users.

AIDS-related wasting differs qualitatively from starvation. In starvation, the body's protein stores and muscle mass are conserved while basic metabolic rates slow and fat deposits are broken down for energy. During AIDS, the reverse happens. Studies have shown that death from wasting is related to the loss of lean body mass rather than just the amount of weight loss.

Primary infection with HIV or secondary opportunistic infections changes the body's metabolic pathways. Abnormal patterns of protein and lipid metabolism result, with nutrients transferred from lean to adipose (fat) tissue. Some inflammatory CYTOKINES (intercellular immune regulators), such as TUMOR NECROSIS FACTOR (TNF) and INTERLEUKIN-1, have been associated with metabolic dysregulation and wasting. Their chronic release during HIV infection seems to play a major role in HIV-related wasting.

Endocrine abnormalities, including changes in gonadal, adrenal, and thyroid function, have been noted in HIV-infected individuals and are another cause of weight loss and wasting. Finally, progressive muscle weakness (myopathy), is an ill-defined condition that may be caused by HIV itself or by extended use of AZT. It is reversible in the latter case.

Because sex hormones are important in determining the fat-to-lean tissue ratio, it is possible that HIV wasting syndrome has major gender differences. However, studies comparing patterns of body mass depletion in men and women continue to report conflicting results.

Weight gain strategies include appetite stimulants such as megestrol acetate (Megace), a synthetic progesterone that seems to promote weight gain in patients with AIDS who do not have significant diarrhea; marijuana therapy (Marinol); or appropriate treatment for underlying causes. Other strategies include parenteral nutrition (TPN), which means nutritional liquids are administered through the vein.

water-based lubricant   See LUBRICANT.

water sports   A twentieth-century slang term for sexual activities that involve URINE; also known as golden showers. While HIV TRANSMISSION has not been documented from exposure to it and UNIVERSAL PRECAUTIONS do not apply to it, the AIDS virus has been found in urine. Drinking urine is therefore considered to be very unsafe, as is any oral contact with excretions. See TRANSMISSION.

weakness   A subjective symptomatic condition; a feeling of lack of strength compared to normal. The cause may be organic or a combination of an organic and a mental state. If it is unremitting, it requires careful investigation with special attention given to potentially lethal causes that may be curable, such as anemia, cancer, neurologic conditions, or certain parasitic or infectious diseases.

weight loss   Weight loss (as distinct from wasting syndrome) is common in people with HIV/AIDS. Weight loss can be intentional or unintentional. People with HIV infection lose weight for different reasons: difficulty eating (perhaps because an infection in the mouth, such as thrush, makes eating difficult), lack of appetite, apathy and depression, prolonged diarrhea, nausea and vomiting, HIV itself, opportunistic infections that affect various organs of the body, and fever. Treatments vary, depending on the cause, and include diet adjustments, appetite stimulants, small but frequent meals, high-calorie and protein foods, nutritional supplements, or intravenous feeding (a procedure called parenteral hyperalimentation or total PARENTERAL NUTRITION). An adequate exercise program is also especially important for people with HIV infection and AIDS. Diarrhea, nausea, and vomiting, can be treated with drugs. If fever is a factor in weight loss, treatment will try to reduce fever with aspirin, acetaminophen, or ibuprofen and will try to eliminate the cause of the fever.

well-being   *Well-being* is a relative term. HIV affects not only the body but the emotions and has obvious consequences for personal relationships. In the context of HIV/AIDS well-being depends not only on fighting the disease, but on preserving mental health, keeping from giving in to hopelessness and depression. See also WELLNESS.

wellness   A condition reflecting the overall quality of life, rather than merely the absence of a (medically treatable) disorder of an individual. Maintaining optimal physical health through adequate nutrition and exercise and good mental health all contribute to wellness. Today, HIV and AIDS have added yet another dimension to the concept of wellness. See WELL-BEING.

Western blot   See WESTERN BLOT TEST.

Western blot test   A blood test that involves the identification of antibodies against specific protein molecules. ANTIGENs are separated by changing the electrical potential (electrophoresis) and are then transferred to a solid substance by blotting. (A technique for analyzing a tiny portion of the primary structure of genomic material.) The substance or membrane is incubated with antibodies. Enzymatic or radioactive techniques are then used to detect the bound antibodies.

The Western blot test displays antibodies to specific HIV viral proteins in a separate, well-defined band. A positive test result shows stripes at the locations for two or more viral proteins. A negative result is blank at these locations. This test is more specific and reliable than the ELISA test in detecting antibodies to HIV, but requires more sophisticated lab techniques and is more expensive. It is commonly used to double-check positive ELISA test results. The Western blot is also applied to diagnosing other conditions such as brain tissue degenerative diseases. See also BLOTTING METHODS.

wet mount   The most important diagnostic procedure to detect the cause of VAGINITIS or VAGINAL DISCHARGE. Often called the saline wet mount test, because it uses a saline (salt) solution. A cotton-tipped stick is dipped in saline and then mixed with a bit of vaginal discharge. It is examined immediately under the microscope for one of three common causes of vaginitis: TRICHOMONIASIS; CANDIDIASIS; or hemophilus vaginals. In some cases a woman's sex partner's urine is also examined to make certain that she is not being constantly reinfected as a consequence of sexual activity.

wet kiss   A kiss in which each partner sticks his or her tongue in the other's mouth, making exchange of saliva likely. Also called a FRENCH KISS.

wet sex   Any kind of sexual activity in which bodily fluids are exchanged.

whey   Recent experiments have suggested that whey, a protein that can be extracted cheaply from the waste product from cheese making, could provide a weapon in the battle against AIDS. Researchers have found that whey seems to block the HIV virus from entering CD4 cells, the white blood cells that are the main target when the virus infects the body. So far the milk substance has been tested only on cells in a test tube, not on animals or humans. Researchers think it might eventually be prepared as an ointment, for use along with condoms, to block transfer of the virus during sexual intercourse. Other virologists think that whey might also be used as a wash for newborns to keep them from being infected with HIV after passing through the birth canal. They speculate that it might be able to prevent mother-to-baby transmission of the virus that way. The milk protein will have to be tested to see how it affects normal tissues and if it is toxic. It is also not clear that blocking the receptors in CD4 cells will be enough to avoid infection completely because the virus can invade a few other kinds of cells.

Whipple's disease A malabsorption syndrome characterized by abnormal skin pigmentation, diarrhea, weight loss, weakness, arthritis, lymphadenopathy, and lesions of the central nervous system.

white blood cell A blood cell whose primary function is to fight infections. See LYMPHOCYTE.

whole-killed virus vaccine A vaccine composed of an intact, but killed, virus.

will 1) A legally enforceable declaration of what people want done with their property and their instructions concerning other matters when they die. Wills can be changed or revoked before the author dies. 2) The mental capacity used in choosing or deciding upon an act or thought. 3) The power of controlling one's own actions or emotions.

Having a will is important for a variety of reasons. When a person dies without having formally signed or "executed" a will, state law determines how the property is distributed. In some cases, distribution is in accord with what the deceased person would have wanted; in other cases, not. State laws vary, but all of them mandate distributions to lawful relations by marriage or blood only, with nothing going to friends or lovers, no matter what their relationships with the deceased.

Other important reasons for having a will relate to the disposition of remains and conduct of memorial services. Local medical examiners' offices, hospitals, and funeral homes look almost exclusively to family members for direction on such issues as funeral plans, burial vs. cremation, post-funeral possession of the ashes of a cremated deceased, and all of the small decisions involved in each of these issues. Unless there is clear agreement between family members and surviving friends or lovers, the latter are likely to be excluded from decision making when the deceased might have preferred either that they share responsibility or that the decisions be left in their hands entirely. This is true even if the deceased has made his or her wishes known explicitly, but not in a will, which is legally enforceable.

It is important that a will and related documents (LIVING WILL, POWER OF ATTORNEY, etc.) be made at a time and under circumstances that do not invite an inference of undue influence by a potential beneficiary. It is on this issue that most AIDS-related challenges have arisen.

window period The time in which a person is infected with HIV but has not produced enough antibodies to be found in tests of blood, body fluids, or tissues. The window period is usually from several weeks to six months.

woman-to-man transmission See TRANSMISSION.

woman-to-woman transmission See TRANSMISSION.

womb See UTERUS.

women Initially, AIDS was thought of as a disease primarily affecting gay men and INJECTION DRUG USERS (IDUs). In the early years of the first decade of the epidemic, reports of HIV/AIDS incidence or studies of HIV/AIDS therapies virtually ignored women as either a demographic or a transmission group. Little was known about the public health impact of HIV in women. Even less was known about the epidemiology, clinical manifestations (AIDS-defining illnesses, gynecologic disease, cervical neoplasia, gynecologic infections), and natural history (survival with AIDS, gynecologic care, etc.) of HIV/AIDS in women. However, as the pattern of the AIDS epidemic shifted to include more cases of heterosexual transmission, it became increasingly apparent that women had been undercounted and underdiagnosed.

This phenomenon occurred for a number of reasons. Sexism, poverty, and racism all impact forcefully on women with HIV illness. Further, women bear tremendous responsibility within the family system for the care of children, spouses, lovers, and elderly family members and often delay seeking health care for themselves because of these kinds of burdens. Equally important is the fact that many early symptoms of HIV illness in women are problems of the reproductive tract, problems that have been inadequately studied in the epidemic. Additionally, women were often underdiagnosed for HIV/AIDS because of a failure both to consider HIV as a possible cause of medical complaints and to recognize the early manifestations of immunocompromise in the genital tracts of women.

Today it is recognized that survival of women with AIDS depends upon a clear clinical understanding that AIDS is different in women inasmuch as women are different from men. Women get virtually all the HIV-related infections that men get, and some conditions diagnostic for AIDS occur more frequently in women than in men.

On January 1, 1993, a newly revised Centers for Disease Control AIDS CASE DEFINITION was implemented in the United States. This definition includes as an AIDS-defining illness invasive cervical carcinoma in HIV-infected women. Although this is a rare manifestation of both HIV and HPV disease in the United States because it is a preventable condition, its inclusion in the case definition indicated significant progress in our understanding of HIV/AIDS and women. Today, our current knowledge about gender differences in the spectrum of HIV disease and AIDS is supplemented by a research agenda, protocols, primary and gynecological care models for HIV-positive women, gynecological care manuals, and safer sex guideliness for HIV-positive women. The epidemiology of AIDS in women in the United States is carefully studied and documented, and our understanding of the modes of acquisition of HIV in women is considered as important as our understanding of them in men. See TRANSMISSION.

work incentives SOCIAL SECURITY has designed a number of special rules, called "work incentives," that provide cash benefits and continued MEDICARE or MEDICAID coverage while a recipient works. (The rules are different for Social Security and SUPPLEMENTARY SECURITY INCOME (SSI) beneficiaries.) Work incentives are particularly important to people with HIV disease who, because of the recurrent nature of HIV-related illnesses, may be able to return to work following periods of disability.

workers' compensation   A no-fault system of injury compensation for the protection of employees while engaged in the employer's business. It requires only that an injured party show that the accident occurred in the workplace. Once the causation threshold is met, administrative compensation is available in an expedited fashion for economic costs. In the United States, insurance and, when necessary, tort litigation are two means by which the cost of accidents is shifted from injured individuals to a broader pool of others.

If one contracts HIV at the workplace, the injured health care provider may choose to bring a lawsuit against a hospital, or to sue manufacturers of needles or other equipment. Lawsuits against hospitals are not easy. First, it will be somewhat difficult to define the standard of care that was violated, and, if the duty of care is not easily defined, it will likely be difficult to prove negligence. Even more important, infected health care workers must prove that their infection occurred at the workplace. While most providers should recall and report needle-stick injuries that occur, these accidents rarely are witnessed. Since transmission of HIV occurs much more commonly through sexual or parenteral transmission outside the workplace, infected health care workers will face the prospect of proving that this more common form of transmission is not the cause of their HIV infection. Hospitals will resist establishment of a legal presumption that infected health care workers contracted the virus at work, and may, in fact, investigate the private lives of litigants. Thus, the causation question represents a significant threshold to successful suits.

In light of this, some health care workers may choose to sue manufactures of needles or other equipment. These suits would be based on a claim that the equipment was designed in a substandard fashion, increasing the risk of injury.

Presumably, however, tort litigation will not play an important role in compensation of injured health care workers. Indeed, many health care workers may be unable to sue employers because of the availability of workers' compensation benefits and the attendant exclusivity doctrine that prohibits suits against employers who provide such benefits. Many health care workers, and especially support staff, nurses, and physicians employed by hospitals are eligible for workers' compensation benefits. In the past, workers' compensation boards have provided benefits for workers' infected with HEPATITIS B, and indeed have developed presumptions regarding infectious causation. This relaxation of causation standards makes workers' compensation a much more attractive alternative for shifting the costs of accidents.

This is not to say that workers' compensation is a panacea for the costs associated with occupational infection with HIV. First, workers' compensation has generally performed poorly in compensating for occupational disease. Second, benefits will be small in general, especially for nurses and physicians in training who will have their com-

pensation pegged to the salary they are earning at the hospital and not to the much larger salary they expect once their training is completed. Third, self-employed physicians and nurses will not be as eligible for benefits and will likely have to seek other alternatives.

The foregoing assumes that the health care worker has information regarding the HIV status of a patient. This is not the case in many needle-stick or other types of accidents that occur. In these situations, health care workers will want to know the HIV status of the patient. Such testing is generally prohibited without the patient's consent. A constitutional analysis also favors nontesting because it would be easier to perform serial antibody testing on the potentially infected health care worker. These arguments are complicated somewhat by the fact that some individuals do not immediately develop antibodies. Some state legislatures have balanced trade-offs and require testing of patients who may have exposed an emergency, or "first response," to health care workers. Moreover, some courts have characterized exposed parties' interests as superior to privacy rights in cases of rape and other exposures of body fluids. The law in this matter is unsettled.

works   Slang term for apparatus (needle, syringe, other equipment) used to prepare and inject INTRAVENOUS drugs.

Sharing works exposes users to HIV. Needle sharing and having unprotected sex with someone who shares drug paraphernalia are the most common ways that HIV infection is spread among women. Needles and other works, to be cleaned, must be soaked in rubbing alcohol or household bleach for at least ten minutes. The alcohol or bleach should not be injected. Works should be washed thoroughly in running water. Bleach and water must not be reused. Cookers must be cleaned with bleach-soaked cotton, then rinsed with water. The cotton must be discarded after use.

World AIDS Day   A day when the world is encouraged to focus its attention on the global plague of HIV/AIDS, the tragic human losses it has caused, and the memory of those who have died. Generally, it is held on December 1.

worried well   Persons who are healthy but who live in fear of AIDS. Because of their anxiety or imagined illness, they may frequent medical care facilities seeking reassurance. Signs of this fear include a decision that the only way to be safe from AIDS is to abstain from sex completely; loss of interest in sex; diminution of sex drive; impotence or lack of orgasm; unsociability and loneliness; curtailment of friendship with gay or bisexual persons or activity in the gay or bisexual community; sadness, anxiety, or depression for no apparent reason; sleeplessness, nightmares, or loss of appetite without an apparent cause; constant anxiety about health despite physicians' assurances that medical conditions, if any, are not AIDS-related; refusal to believe negative results of HIV antibody tests; feelings of self-rejection because of homosexuality or bisexuality; self-blame for having had lovers who were gay or bisexual intravenous drug users; guilt about one's history of intravenous drug use; psychosomatic symptoms that are known to be signs of AIDS, such as night sweats or seemingly inexplicable weight loss; strong feelings of regret or guilt over past sexual behavior. See FEAR OF AIDS.

Xanax See ALPRAZOLAM.

X ray A high-energy electromagnetic wave varying in length from 0.05 to 100 angstrom units. X rays are produced by bombarding a target in a vacuum tube with high-velocity electrons. Because of their ability to penetrate most solid matter to some extent and to act on photographic film, X rays are used to produce images of the interior of the body to enable medical diagnosis and therapy.

xenogeneic Pertaining to the relationship that exists between members of genetically different species.

xerosis Dryness of the skin, mouth, or eyes; abnormal except in the aged, in whom it is the result of normal sclerosis of tissues.

yeast Any of several unicellular fungi of the genus *Saccharomyces*, which reproduce by budding. Yeasts, especially *Candida albicans*, may cause systemic infections as well as vaginitis. Yeast infections are frequently present in patients with malignant lymphomas, severe diabetic mellitus, AIDS, and other immunocompromised individuals.

yeast infection Invasion and multiplication of body-tissue yeasts that may produce injurious effects. In women, yeast infection can cause a thick white vaginal discharge. It causes itching and may have an unpleasant odor. Millions of women get yeast infections, overgrowths of natural fungi in the body, but infections that won't go away after treatment may also be an early sign of HIV. Some common HIV medications can cause an overgrowth of vaginal yeast and trigger these infections frequently. See also CANDIDIASIS.

yellow nail syndrome A syndrome associated with an excessive amount of fluid in the body tissues due to obstruction of the lymphatics, especially of the legs. The nails become yellowish to greenish in color and may be smooth, thickened, excessively curved, or slow in growth, causing them to shed.

Yersinia enterocolitica A type of bacteria that can escape detection despite rigorous screening of the blood supply. It has killed at least 12 people due to tainted transfusions since 1985. The bacterium thrives when stored in lab refrigerators. *Yersinia* is found in unpasteurized cheese or undercooked meat. People who receive transfusions tainted with it can suffer fever, chills, and breathing trouble, and eventually die.

Yodoxin See IODOQUINOL.

yogurt Milk that has been fermented by a mixture of bacteria and yeasts forms a custard-like product. The milk is defatted and soured with *Lactobacillus acidophilus* and other bacteria that are necessary for the health of the intestine. Yogurt aids digestion and controls the action of the intestine in favorably stimulating the kidneys. It contains the B-complex vitamins and has a higher percentage of VITAMINS A and D than does the milk it was made from; it is also high in protein. Its calcium benefits women. The beneficial bacteria in yogurt make it a natural antibiotic and anticancer agent. A cup or two a day will boost the immune system. Yogurt has been found to be beneficial in treating colds and upper respiratory infections, high cholesterol levels, arthritis, constipation, diarrhea, gallstones, halitosis, hepatitis, VAGINITIS, osteoporosis, kidney disorders, cancer-causing bacteria in the colon, and skin diseases.

Z

Zalcitabine   See DIDEOXYCYTIDINE.

zap   In the vocabulary of protest, agitation, and other forms of public activities, a small strike against a selected target. The major victories of AIDS activists in transforming clinical research policy were won by a combination of tactics that included zaps in the form of telephone campaigns, street protests, and so forth. See also ACT-UP.

zidovudine (ZDV or AZT)   A synthetic thymidine (one of the basic components of DNA) that inhibits the growth and development of HIV, the virus that causes AIDS. Originally named azidothymidine (AZT) or azido-deoxythymidine, it is properly called zidovudine, but is almost universally referred to as AZT (a practice followed in this dictionary). It was the first antiretroviral therapy and the first anti-AIDS drug approved by the FOOD AND DRUG ADMINISTRATION. It is marketed under the trade name Retrovir. For a complete discussion of zidovudine, see AZT.

zinc   An essential trace mineral occurring in the body in larger amounts than any other trace element except iron. It is present in all tissues. Zinc is known for its ability to fight disease and to protect the immune system. It is involved in the Krebs cycle and energy production. Recently, blindness in the elderly has been found to be arrested by zinc. It is also credited with increasing male sex drive and potency because of its ability to regulate testosterone in the prostate. Sources of zinc include pumpkin seeds, squash seeds, sunflower seeds, seafood, oysters, crabmeat, herring, organ meats, mushrooms, Brewer's yeast, soybeans, eggs, wheat germ, meats, liver, and turkey.

Zinc has a variety of functions. It is related to the normal absorption and action of vitamins, especially the B complex. It is a constituent of more than 2,000 enzymes involved in digestion and metabolism, including carbonic anhydrase, which is necessary for tissue reproduction. Some of the enzymes are involved in alcohol detoxification, bone metabolism, protein digestion and RNA synthesis, electron transport, and aerobic and anerobic energy production. Zinc is also a component of insulin and is part of the enzyme that is needed to break down alcohol. It also plays a part in carbohydrate digestion and phosphorus metabolism. In addition, it is essential in the synthesis of DNA, the master substance of life that carries all inherited traits and directs the activity of each cell. Finally, it is essential for the taste buds and the skin's oil gland function, and is important in the healing of wounds and burns. The most common cause of zinc deficiency is an unbalanced or poor diet (high in grains and cereals and low in animal protein), although other factors may also be responsible. Zinc deficiency is clearly recognized in medicine as a critical factor in chronic disease. AIDS patients have been found to have low blood levels of zinc.

Some effects of zinc deficiency on immune competence include T-LYMPHOCYTE dysfunction and atrophy of the THYMUS gland, where T cells are produced. CELL-MEDIATED immunity is also impeded by zinc deficiency, resulting in anergic DELAYED-TYPE HYPERSENSITIVITY. Lack of zinc can result in diminished T-cell-dependent antibodies, decreased populations of cells in the monocyte/macrophage system, and lower levels of interleukin-2, a cytokine that signals the growth and differentiation of T lymphocytes. NATURAL KILLER CELL activity appears to be inhibited by zinc insufficiency, and individuals with inadequate zinc supply are more susceptible to infectious diseases and suffer more severely from them. Zinc's function of facilitating the transport of vitamin A from the liver to other parts of the body is critical. Without zinc, vitamin A deficiency can occur even in the presence of an adequate dietary supply of the vitamin.

Zinc deficiency is also a factor in stress, fatigue, susceptibility to infection, injury, and decreased alertness. Energy production, protein synthesis, collagen formation, and alcohol tolerance are all interfered with in its deficiency. Zinc levels are low during chronic infections, renal disease, cardiovascular disease, some malignancies, protein malnutrition, and I-V feeding.

Zinc has a beneficial effect on many ailments. T-helper lymphocytes, which fight infection, are increased with zinc and are of particular interest to those with AIDS.

Zinc sulfate supplementation has been used to prevent some opportunistic infections, including cryptococcus, PNEUMOCYSTIS CARINII PNEUMONIA, salmonella, toxoplasmosis and tuberculosis. No effects have been seen for CMV, and esophageal candidiasis.

Ingesting high doses of zinc can be harmful because it interferes with the absorption of copper, another essential micronutrient.

zinc finger   Chains of AMINO ACIDs found in cellular proteins that bind to DNA or messenger RNA, and play important roles in a cell's life cycle. They also appear to play a role during the earlier stages of cell infection. They are called zinc fingers because they capture and help package HIV genetic material into newly budding virions. Zinc fingers can have a number of structures. In HIV's zinc finger, four amino acids are responsible for capturing the zinc ion. The sequence is unique, found elsewhere only in other lentiviruses, the family of retroviruses that includes HIV-1 and 2, cancer-causing HTLV, feline immunodeficiency virus, and murine leukemia virus, to name a few.

Data presented by researchers from the National Cancer Institute at the Thirty-Fifth Annual Interscience Conference on Antimicrobial Agents and Chemotherapy held in September 1995 indicate that HIV's zinc fingers may be the next antiviral target. The two zinc fingers in HIV's nucleocapsid (NC), a core viral protein, are involved in binding and packaging viral RNA into new virions budding from an infected cell. To date, experiments in which the zinc fingers have been deleted have shown that new budding virions do not incorporate RNA, which instead spills out of the infected cell. The NC protein and zinc fingers also play some role in the process of reverse transcription, although its exact nature is unclear. Some speculate that it may anchor the RNA molecule while the REVERSE TRANSCRIPTASE enzyme builds HIV DNA from the RNA template. HIV that lacks zinc fingers is unable to infect new cells. The zinc fingers are therefore essential for two phases of the viral life cycle. As of early fall 1996, two zinc finger inhibitors were in clinical studies.

Research findings indicate that HIV may not be able to mutate and escape the effects of drugs targeting its zinc fingers. Moreover, since HIV's zinc fingers are identical, one antiviral compound could inhibit both. Research is under way to find such a compound.

zinc finger inhibitor   A drug that inhibits zinc finger activity, preventing HIV genetic material to be captured and packaged into newly budding virions.

zip code genocide   An expression sometimes used by dismayed AIDS activists in the first decade of the epidemic, to refer to proposed public health policies that would explicitly have confined money spent on fighting the disease to certain geographical areas in which it was, at that time, concentrated. It was feared that such policies would create virtual AIDS ghettos, with disastrous social and economic effects on those within, while trivializing the seriousness of the problem by implying that the danger was confined to a few marginal neighborhoods and groups of people, while the rest of the population shared little risk.

In the first decade of the AIDS epidemic it was often observed that AIDS was settling into certain narrow geographic and cultural parameters (minority populations in specific urban areas), and that many other areas and demo-graphic groups were virtually untouched. Sequestering the disease epidemiologically and putting money where the problems were—in specific neighborhoods in Houston, New York, Miami, San Francisco, and other cities—was often proposed as a preventative measure. It was pointed out, however, that identifying certain groups, whether infected or not, through such demographic means as zip code distribution was likely to lead to serious consequences—decreased property values, rejection of insurance coverage, higher rates of unemployment, and other forms of social and economic ostracism. Indeed it was predicted that in cities less tolerant than San Francisco, targeted groups might find their neighborhoods increasingly "ghettoized" and isolated from the larger community. Today, such segregationism is generally viewed as a dangerous idea that has racist and homophobic undertones. Also, much progress has been made in AIDS education, helping to lessen discrimination against groups severely affected by the epidemic. This was accomplished largely by shifting the focus from HIGH-RISK GROUPS to HIGH-RISK BEHAVIORS.

Zithromax   See AZITHROMYCIN.

zoning districts   See ZONING RESTRICTIONS.

zoning ordinances   See ZONING RESTRICTIONS.

zoning restrictions   Zoning or land use ordinances generally divide a community into districts and designate uses appropriate to each. There are always districts limited to residential uses, and frequently single-family and multifamily residences are assigned to separate districts. Ordinances may define the type of family permitted in residential districts and may limit the number of unrelated people who may live together. Thus they may effectively prohibit informal group living arrangements for people with HIV who wish to live together, as families in family residences, in hospices, or in group homes or similar facilities.

Zoning ordinances may provide specifically for group homes by allowing them as "special-use" or "special exception" dwellings in residential districts, if they are considered compatible with the neighborhood. A special-use designation is allowed in a zoning district only after it has been approved by the local zoning agency or municipal governing body. Although special-use provisions do not on the surface present a serious obstacle to group homes for people with HIV, opponents of such homes may use these provisions to block their establishment in locations where they are needed. Some areas specifically allow group homes as permitted uses in residential districts but limit the number of such homes or the extent to which they can be concentrated. State legislation that prohibits the exclusion of group homes from residential districts may contain similar restrictions.

Zoning restrictions on group homes and unrelated families may not serve a constitutionally acceptable purpose. They may also deny equal protection of the laws guaranteed by the Fourteenth Amendment, although the courts have been divided on the Fourteenth Amendment's application to zoning. Given the uncertainty of constitutional protection, advocates are relying on the FAIR HOUSING ACT to oppose discriminatory zoning practices. Although the act does not expressly prohibit zoning discrimination, it does prohibit acts that "otherwise make unavailable or deny" housing because of a handicap, such as HIV or AIDS. The courts have held that this language applies to discrimination that occurs through zoning ordinances.

Zovirax   See ACYCLOVIR.

APPENDIX I

Frequently Used Abbreviations

ACOG	American College of Obstetricians & Gynecologists
ACT-UP	AIDS Coalition to Unleash Power
ACTG	AIDS clinical trial group
AFB	acid-fast bacillus
AHCPR	Agency for Health Care Policy and Research
AIDS	acquired immunodeficiency syndrome
AmFAR	American Foundation for AIDS Research
AMA	American Medical Association
ARC	AIDS-related complex
ARV	AIDS-associated retrovirus
AZT	azidothymidine
BCG	bacille Calmette-Guérin
BV	bacterial vaginosis
CAIDS	community-acquired immunodeficiency syndrome
CAT	computerized axial tomography; computer-assisted tomography (see CT)
CBC	complete blood count
CDC	[U.S.] Centers for Disease Control and Prevention
CFS	chronic fatigue syndrome
CID	Center for Infectious Diseases (of CDC)
CIN	cervical intraepithelial neoplasia
CIS	carcinoma *in situ*
CMV	cytomegalovirus
CNS	central nervous system
CPCRA	Community Programs for Clinical Research on AIDS
CSF	cerebral spinal fluid
CT	computerized tomography (formerly CAT [see CAT])
ddC	2′, 3′-dideoxycytidine (Zalcitabine)
ddI	2′, 3′-dideoxyinosine (Didanosine)
DFA-TP	direct fluorescent antibody staining for *Treponema pallidum*
DNA	deoxyribonucleic acid
DOT	directly observed therapy
DUB	dysfunctional uterine bleeding
ELISA	enzyme-linked immunosorbent assay
ESR	erythrocyte sedimentation rate
FDA	[U.S.] Food and Drug Administration

FSH	follicle-stimulating hormone
FTA-ABS	fluorescent treponemal antibody absorption
G6PD	glucose-6 phosphate dehydrogenase
GLS	generalized lymphadenopathy syndrome
GMHC	Gay Men's Health Crisis
GRID	gay-related immunodeficiency disease
GUD	genital ulcer disease
HCTZ	hydrochlorothiazide
HIV	human immunodeficiency virus
HPV	human papilloma virus
HRT	hormone replacement therapy
HSV	herpes simplex virus
HTLV I, II, III	human T-cell lymphotropic virus, types I, II, or III
IDU	injection drug user
IFA	immunofluorescence antibody
IgG	immunoglobulin G
IM	intramuscular
IND	Investigational New Drug
INH	isoniazid
IRB	Investigational Review Board
IV	intravenous
KS	Kaposi's sarcoma
LAV	lymphadenopathy-associated virus
LGV	lymphogranuloma venereum
LH	luteinizing hormone
LIP	lymphocytic interstitial pneumonia
LP	lumbar puncture
MAC	mycobacterium avium complex
MACS	multicenter AIDS cohort study
MDR-TB	multidrug-resistant tuberculosis
MHA-TP	microhemagglutination assay for *Treponema pallidum*
MHC	major histocompatability complex
MPC	mucopurulent cervicitis
MRI	magnetic resonance imaging
MTB	mycobacterium tuberculosis
NHL	non-Hodgkins lymphoma
NIAID	National Institute of Allergy and Infectious Diseases (of NIH)
NICHD	National Institute of Child Health and Human Development (of NIH)
NIH	[U.S.] National Institute of Health

NLM	National Library of Medicine (of NIH)	RPR	rapid plasma reagin
OB/GYN	obstetrics/gynecology; obstetrician/ gynecologist	SIDS; SAID	simian acquired immunodeficiency syndrome
OI	opportunistic infection	SIL	squamous intraepithelial lesion
PAP	Papanicolaou (Pap test, Pap smear)	STD	sexually transmitted disease
PCP	*Pneumocystis carinii* pneumonia	TAT 3	transactivator gene
PCR	polymerase chain reaction	TB	tuberculosis
PGL	persistent generalized lymphadenopathy	TMP-SMX	trimethoprim-sulfamethoxazole
PHS	[U.S.] Public Health Service	TSH	thyroid stimulating hormone
PPD	purified protein derivative	TU	tuberculin unit
PGL	persistent generalized lymphadenopathy	UTI	urinary tract infection
PID	pelvic inflammatory disease	VAIN	vaginal intraepithelial neoplasia
PML	progressive multifocal leukoencephalopathy	VDRL	venereal disease research laboratories
PMS	premenstrual syndrome	VIN	vulvar intraepithelial neoplasia
PWA	Person With AIDS; persons living with AIDS	WHO	[U.N.] World Health Organization
		ZDV	zidovudine (AZT)
RNA	ribonucleic acid		

APPENDIX II

The Global Epidemic at a Glance

Snapshots of the Global Epidemic, 1996 (estimates in millions)[1]

New HIV infections:	Adults	2.7[2]
	Children	.4
	Total	**3.1**
People living with HIV/AIDS:	Adults	21.8
	Male	12.6
	Female	9.2
	Children	.83[3]
	Total	**22.6**
HIV/AIDS-associated deaths:	Adults	1.1
	Male	.65
	Female	.47
	Children	.35
	Total	**1.5**
Cumulative HIV infections:	Adults	26.8
	Male	15.5
	Female	11.3
	Children	2.6
	Total	**29.4**
Cumulative AIDS cases:	Adults	6.7
	Male	3.9
	Female	2.8
	Children	1.7
	Total	**8.4**
Cumulative HIV/AIDS deaths:	Adults	5.0
	Male	2.0
	Female	2.1
	Children	1.4
	Total	**6.4**

[1]Because of rounding, figures may not tally.
[2]Nearly half of new HIV infections occured in women.
[3]Many children with AIDS die from other causes; the estimated number of children living with HIV/AIDS (830,000) is therefore less than the difference between cumulative infections (2,600,000) and cumulative deaths (1,400,000) in children.
Source: UNAIDS and WHO

Countries with 1,000 or More AIDS Cases Reported as of 6/30/97

Country	cases (% males)	Country	cases (% males)
Africa	**576,972**	**Americas**	**797,227**
Angola	1,296 (48)	Argentina	10,461 (80)
Benin	1,529 (65	Bahamas	2,475 (64)
Botswana	5,337 (51)	Brazil	103,262 (75)
Burkina Faso	7,957 (57)	Canada	14,836 (91)
Burundi	8,378 (NR)	Chile	1,863 (90)
Cameroon	8,141 (50)	Colombia	7,546 (90)
Central African Republic	5,111 (47)	Costa Rica	1,133 (88)
Chad	3,457 (54)	Dominican Republic	3,717 (64)
Congo	10,223 (NR)	El Salvador	1,875 (74)
Democratic Republic of the Congo (former Zaire)	29,434 (NR)	Guatemala	1,787 (71)
Djiboutic	1,238 (48)	Haiti	4,967 (NR)
Eritrea	2,650 (67)	Honduras	6,057 (66)
Ethiopia	19,443 (NR)	Jamaica	2,060 (59)
Gabon	1,376 (NR)	Mexico	29,962 (87)
Ghana	18,730 (67)	Panama	1,327 (77)
Guinea	3,080 (NR)	Peru	5,958 (80)
Ivory Coast	31,963 (62)	Trinidad and Tobago	2,394 (66)
Kenya	69,005 (54)	United States	581,429 (82)
Lesotho	1,288 (44)	Venezuela	6,768 (89)
Malawi	46,022 (50)		
Mali	4,028 (NR)	**Europe**	**191,005**
Mozambique	4,905 (52)		
Namibia	6,784 (NR)	Austria	1,678 (78)
Niger	3,002 (NR)	Belgium	2,275 (71)
Nigeria	5,509 (NR)	Denmark	2,024 (84)
Rwanda	10,706 (NR)	France	45,395 (80)
Senegal	1,982 (NR)	Germany	16,138 (86)
South Africa	12,825 (48)	Greece	1,604 (86)
Sudan	1,595 (78)	Italy	38,418 (76)
Tanzania	82,174 (NR)	Netherlands	4,369 (84)
Togo	7,993 (57)	Portugal	4,066 (83)
Uganda	51,779 (NR)	Romania	4,599 (56)
Zambia	42,447 (48)	Spain	45,132 (80)
Zimbabwe	61,037 (56)	Sweden	1,498 (81)
		Switzerland	5,707 (94)
Asia	**70,949**	United Kingdom	14,082 (85)
India	2,996 (NR)	**Australia**	**7,033 (96)**
Japan	1,447 (92)		
Myanmar (Burma)	1,822 (81)		
Thailand	59,782 (81)	**World Total**	**1,644,183**

Source: World Health Organization (WHO), Weekly Epidemiological Record, 7/4/97.
Note: These figures reflect reported cases only. Based on available data, the WHO
has estimated that by the end of 1996, 8.4 million AIDS cases in adults and children had occurred worldwide.

Estimated Incidence of Infection—United States

Estimated incidence[1] of AIDS-related opportunistic infections (AIDS-OIs) and estimated number of deaths among persons aged ≥13 years reported with AIDS, by sex, race/ethnicity[2], exposure category, and percentage change in AIDS-OIs and deaths from 1995 to 1996—United States

	AIDS-OIs			Deaths		
	1995 No.	1996 No.	% Change from 1995 to 1996	1995 No.	1996 No.	% Change from 1995 to 1996
Characteristic						
Sex						
Men	49,360	45,240	−8	42,000	31,440	−25
Women	11,260	11,490	2	8,140	7,340	−10
Race/Ethnicity						
White, non-Hispanic	24,370	21,130	−13	21,700	14,670	−32
Black, non-Hispanic	24,090	24,030	0	18,840	16,460	−13
Hispanic	11,410	10,800	−5	9,010	7,220	−20
Exposure Category						
MSM[3]	28,640	25,530	−11	24,880	17,310	−30
MSM-IDU[4]	3,580	3,030	−15	3,310	2,490	−25
Male-IDU	12,880	12,140	−6	10,790	8,970	−17
Female-IDU	4,950	4,750	−4	3,830	3,440	−10
Heterosexual contact						
Male	3,420	3,790	11	2,300	2,120	−8
Female	5,900	6,320	7	3,980	3,640	−8
Total[5]	60,620	56,730	−6	50,140	38,780	−23

[1]Estimates are presented rounded to the nearest 10 because they do not represent exact counts of persons with AIDS-OIs but are estimates that are approximately ±3% of the true value.

[2]Numbers for races other than black and white were too small for meaningful analysis. Persons of Hispanic origin may be of any race.

[3]Men who have sex with men.

[4]Injecting-drug user.

[5]Includes persons aged ≥13 years with hemophilia/coagulation disorders, transfusion recipients, or with other or no risks reported.

Appendix III

Selected Resources for Practitioners, Researchers, and Persons with HIV/AIDS

(Note: these listings represent a selection of the resources available and are by no means complete. Inclusion in these listings does not imply endorsement by the authors or publisher.)

1. TELEPHONE LISTINGS

Associations and Organizations

ACT-UP	212/966-4873
AIDS National Interfaith Network	202/842-0010
AIDS Resource Foundation for Children (ARFC)	201/483-4250
American Cancer Society	800/227-2345
American Civil Liberties Union (ACLU)	212/549-2500
American College of Obstetricians and Gynecologists (ACOG)	202/638-5577
American Foundation for AIDS Research (AmFar)	212/682-7440
American Holistic Medical Association (AHMA)	919-787-5146
American Holistic Nurses Association	919/787-5181
American Hospital Association (AHA)	800/424-4301
American Institute for Teen AIDS Prevention	817/237-0230
American Medical Association (AMA)	312/464-5000
American Public Health Association (APHA)	202/789-5600
American Red Cross	800/842-2200
American Society of Alternative Therapists	508-281-4400
Americans for a Sound AIDS Policy (ASAP)	703/471-7350
American with Disabilities Act (ADA)	305/271-0012
Center for Infectious Diseases (CID) See CENTERS FOR DISEASE CONTROL AND PREVENTION (CDC)	
Center for Substance Abuse Prevention See NATIONAL INSTITUTES OF HEALTH (NIH)	
Centers for Disease Control and Prevention (CDC)	
24-hour hot line	800/342-2437
Public inquiries	800/311-3435

In Spanish	800/344-7432 (Mon–Fri 8–2 Eastern)
For the hearing-impaired	800/243-7889 (Mon–Fri 10–10 Eastern)
Center for Infectious Diseases (CID)	800/311-3435
National AIDS Information Clearinghouse	800/458-5231
National Center for Health Statistics (NCHS)	301/436-8500
Department of Agriculture (DA)	703/305-2039
Food Nutrition Information Center	301/504-5719
Department of Health and Human Services (HHS)	202/619-0257
Department of Housing and Urban Development (HUD)	800/569-4287
Department of Veterans Affairs (VA)	800/827-1000
Food and Drug Administration (FDA)	800/532-4440
Gay and Lesbian Medical Association	415/255-4547
Gay Men's Health Crisis (GMHC)	212/807-6664
Lambda Legal Defense and Education Fund	212/809-8585
Mobilization Against AIDS	415/863-4676
Mothers of Children with AIDS (MOCA)	718/426-8585
Names Project Foundation (NPF)	415/882-5500
National AIDS Information Clearinghouse See CENTERS FOR DISEASE CONTROL AND PREVENTION (CDC)	
National Association of People With AIDS (NAPWA)	202/898-0414
National Association of Public Hospitals (NAPH)	202/408-0223
National Cancer Institute (NCI) See NATIONAL INSTITUTES OF HEALTH (NIH)	
National Center for Health Statistics (NCHS) See CENTERS FOR DISEASE CONTROL AND PREVENTION (CDC)	

National Center for Lesbian Rights (NCLR) — 415/392-6257
National Gay and Lesbian Task Force (NGLTF) — 202/332-6483
National Hemophilia Foundation AIDS Center — 800/424-2634
National Hospice Organization — 703/243-5900
National Institute of Justice (NIJ) — 800/851-3420
National Institutes of Health (NIH) — 301/496-4000
Center for Substance Abuse Prevention, workplace hotline — 800/WORK-PLACE
National Cancer Institute (NCI) — 800/4-CANCER
National Institute of Child Health and Human Development (NICHD) — 301/496-5133
National Institute of Mental Health (NIMH) — 301/443-6100
National Institute of Drug Abuse (NIDA) — 800/843-4971
National Library of Medicine (NLM) — 888/346-3656
National Pediatric HIV Resource Center — 800/362-0071
National Resource Center on Women and AIDS — 202/872-1770
National Minority AIDS Council (NMAC) — 202/483-6622
National Native American AIDS Prevention Center — 800/283-2437
National Task Force on AIDS Prevention — 415/356-8100
National Women's Health Network — 202/347-1140
Pediatric AIDS Foundation — 310/395-9051
People With AIDS Coalition (PWA) — 212/647-1415
People With AIDS Health Group — 212/255-0520
Physicians for Human Rights (PHR) — 617/695-0041
Project Inform — 800/822-7422
Public Health Service (PHS) — 301/443-2403
Red Cross
See AMERICAN RED CROSS
Ryan White National Teen Education Program — 800/933-KIDS
Social Security Administration (SSA) — 800/772-1213
Teens Teaching AIDS Prevention Program — 800/234-8336
Women Organized to Respond to Life-Threatening Diseases (WORLD) — 510/658-6930

Education for Physicians/Practitioners

HIV Telephone Consultation Service for Health Care Providers — 800/933-3413 (Mon.–Fri., 7:30–5 Pacific)

AIDS Education and Training Centers

Arkansas, Louisiana, Mississippi — 504/568-3855
California (southern) — 213/342-1846
Connecticut, Maine, Massachusetts, New Hampshire, Rhode Island, Vermont — 508/856-3255
Nevada, Arizona, Hawaii, California (northern) — 415/502-8196
New Jersey — 201/972-3690
New York, Virgin Islands — 212/305-3616
Ohio, Michigan, Kentucky, Tennessee — 614/292-1400
Pennsylvania — 412/624-1895

Puerto Rico — 787/759-6528
Alabama (southern), Georgia, North Carolina, South Carolina — 404/727-2929
Washington, Alaska, Montana, Idaho, Oregon — 206/720-4250

Clinical Trials

AIDS Clinical Trials Information Service — 800/TRIALS-A (Mon.–Fri. 9–7 Eastern)
Community Research Initiative on AIDS — 212/924-3934
National Institutes of Health (NIH) AIDS Trials — 800/243-7644

Pharmaceutical Information

Selected Buyer's Clubs for AIDS drugs
Carl Vogel Foundation — 202/638-0750
Healing Alternatives Foundation — 415/626-2316
PWA Health Group — 212/255-0520

Payment Assistance Programs and Expanded Access Programs (by manufacturer)

Abbott (Clarithromycin) — 800/688-9118
Amgen (Filgrastim) — 800/272-9376
Astra (Foscarnet) — 800/488-3247
Burroughs-Wellcome (Acyclovir, Atovaquone, Primethamine, Zidovudine, TMP/SMX) — 800/772-9294
Fujisawa (Pentamidine) — 800/366-6323
Janssen (Itraconazole) — 800/544-2987
Miles (Ciprofloxacin) — 800/998-9180
Ortho Biotech (Erythropoetin) — 800/553-3851
Pfizer (Azithromycin, Fluconazole, Streptomycin) — 800/254-4445
Roxane (Dronabinol) — 800/274-8651
Sandoz (Octreotide acetate) — 800/447-6673
Schering-Plough (Alfa-Interferon-2b) — 800/521-7157
Syntex (Ganciclovir) — 800/444-4200
US Bioscience (Trimetrexate) — 800/8US-BIOS

Payment Assistance Programs and Expanded Access Programs (by drug)

Acyclovir (Burroughs-Wellcome) — 800/772-9294
Alfa-Interferon-2b (Schering-Plough) — 800/521-7157
Atovaquone (Burroughs-Wellcome) — 800/772-9294
Azithromycin (Pfizer) — 800/254-4445
Ciprofloxacin (Miles) — 800/998-9180
Clarithromycin (Abbott) — 800/688-9118
Dronabinol (Roxane) — 800/274-8651
Erythropoetin (Ortho Biotech) — 800/553-3851
Filgrastim (Amgen) — 800/272-9376
Fluconazole (Pfizer) — 800/254-4445
Foscarnet (Astra) — 800/488-3247
Ganciclovir (Syntex) — 800/444-4200
Itraconazole (Janssen) — 800/544-2987
Octreotide acetate (Sandoz) — 800/447-6673
Pentamidine (Fujisawa) — 800/366-6323
Primethamine (Burroughs-Wellcome) — 800/772-9294
Streptomycin (Pfizer) — 800/254-4445

TMP/SMX (Burroughs-Wellcome)	800/772-9294
Trimetrexate (US Bioscience)	800/8US-
	BIOS
Zidovudine (Burroughs-Wellcome)	800/772-9294

Journals and Newsletters

AIDS Clinical Care	800/843-6356
AIDS Treatment News	800/873-2812
BETA: Bulletin of Experimental Treatments for	
AIDS	800/327-9893
PWA Newsline	800/828-3280
Treatment Issues	212/337-3613

State HIV/AIDS Hot lines

Centers for Disease Control and Prevention	
(CDC)	800/342-2437
For a printed list:	800/458-5231
Local numbers	
Local phone directory (see *Health*	
Care [under *State Government* in Blue	
Pages])	

2. WEB SITES

General guides

AIDS Education Global Information System
   http://www.aegis.com/
AIDS Patents Project
   http://app.cnidr.org/
AIDS Resource Sampler
   http://www.nnlm.nlm.nih.gov/pnr/etc/AIDSpath.html
The Body: A Multimedia AIDS and HIV Resource
   http://www.thebody.com/cgi-bin/body.cgi
GALEN II (Digital Library, University of California,
   San Francisco [UCSF]):
   Knowledge Resources—AIDS/HIV
   http://galen.library.ucsf.edu/kr/subs/hiv/index.html
Journal of the American Medical Association(JAMA),
   HIV/AIDS site
   http://www.ama-assn.org/special/hiv/hivhome.htm
Lycos: A2Z: Health & Medicine: Illnesses & Disorders:
   AIDS/HIV
   http://a2z.lycos.com/Health_and_Medicine/Illnesses_and_
   Disorders/AIDS_slash_HIV/
NLM's ATIS-supported HIV/AIDS articles
   http://text.nlm.nih.gov/atis/list.html
Yahoo!: Health: Diseases and Conditions: AIDS/HIV
   http://www.yahoo.com/Health/Diseases_and_Conditions/
   AIDS_HIV/

HIV/AIDS agencies and organizations

AIDS Research Information Center (ARIC)
   http://www.critpath.org/aric
American Cancer Society
   http://www.cancer.org

American College of Obstetricians and Gynecologists (ACOG)
   http://www.acog.org
American Foundation for AIDS Research (AmFar)
   http://www.amfar.org
American Holistic Nurses Association
   http://www.ahna.org
American Medical Association (AMA)
   http://www.ama-assn.org
American Public Health Association (APHA)
   http://www.apha.org
American Red Cross
   http://www.redcross.org
American Soceity of Alternative Therapies
   http://www.asat.org
Assocation of Nurses in AIDS Care
   http://www.mc.vanderbilt.edu/adl/pathfinders/missions/an
   ac.html
Center for Infectious Diseases (CID)
   See CENTERS FOR DISEASE CONTROL AND PREVENTION (CDC)
Centers for Disease Control and Prevention (CDC)
   http://www.cdc.gov
Center for Infectious Diseases (CID)
   http://www.cdc.gov/ncidod/ncid.htm
Division of HIV/AIDS Prevention (DHAP)
   http://www.cdc.gov/nchstp/hiv_AIDS/dhap.htm
National AIDS Clearinghouse
   http://www.cdcnac.org
   gopher://cdcnac.aspensys.com:72/11/
National Center for Health Statistics
   http://www.cdc.gov/nchswww/nchshome.ht
WONDER on the Web
   http://wonder.cdc.gov/
Department of Agriculture (DA)
   Food and Consumer Service
   http://www.usda.gov/fcs/fcs.htm
Food Nutrition Information Center
   http://www.nal.usda.gov/fnic
Department of Health and Human Services (HHS)
   http://www.os.dhhs.gov
Department of Housing and Urban Development (HUD)
   http://www.hud.gov
Department of Veterans Affairs (VA)
   http://www.va.gov
Food and Consumer Service
   See DEPARTMENT OF AGRICULTURE
Food and Drug Administration (FDA)
   http://www.fda.gov
Food Nutrition Information Center
   See DEPARTMENT OF AGRICULTURE
Gay and Lesbian Medical Association
   http://www.glma.org/
Harvard AIDS Institute
   http://www.hsph.harvard.edu/Organizations/hai/home_pg.
   html
Jewish AIDS Network, Chicago
   http://www.shalom.com/janc.htm
Joint United Nations Programme on HIV/AIDS (UNAIDS)
   http://gpawww.who.ch/index.html
National Association of Public Hospitals and Health Systems
   http://www.naph.org

National Cancer Institute (NCI)
 http://www.nci.nih.gov
National Gay and Lesbian Task Force (NGLTF)
 http://www.ngltf.org
National Hemophilia Foundation
 http://www.infonhf.org
National Hospice Organization
 http://www.nho.org
National Institute of Justice (NIJ)
 http://www.ncjrs.org/nijhome.htm
National Institutes of Health (NIH)
 http://www.nih.gov
National Institute of Allergy and Infectious Diseases (NIAID)
 http://www.niaid.nih.gov
 Division of AIDS (DAIDS)
 http://www.niaid.nih.gov/research/divisions.htm
National Institute of Child Health and Human Development
 (NICHD)
 http://www.nih.gov/nichd
National Institute on Drug Abuse (NIDA)
 http://www.nida.nih.gov
National Institute of Mental Health (NIMH)
 http://www.nimh.nih.gov
National Library of Medicine (NLM)
 http://www.nlm.nih.gov
Pediatric AIDS Foundation
 http://www.pedAIDS.org
Physicians for Human Rights
 gopher://gopher.humanrights.org:5000/11/int/phr
Public Health Service
 http://phs.os.dhhs.gov/phs/phs.html
 Public Health Service Agencies
 http://phs.os.dhhs.gov/progorg/progorg.html
 Program Offices
 http://phs.os.dhhs.gov/progorg/ophs/
 Support Activities
 http://phs.os.dhhs.gov/psc/
Ryan White National Fund
 http://www.netwalk.com/~catf
Social Security Administration (SSA)
 http://www.ssa.gov
UNAIDS
 See JOINT UNITED NATIONS PROGRAMME ON HIV/AIDS
United States Public Health Service
 See PUBLIC HEALTH SERVICE
World Federation of Hemophilia
 http://www.wfh.org/
World Health Organization(WHO)
 http://www.who.ch/welcome.html

Publications

*Abstracts from the Fourth Conference on Retroviruses and
 Opportunistic Infections*
 http://207.78.88.28/retrovirus97/frameset5.htm
AEGIS HIV Publications Library, Table of Contents
 http://www.aegis.com/areas.htm
AIDS Book Review Journal
 http://www.library.ucsb.edu/journals/AIDS
AIDS Daily Journal (CDC)

 gopher://cdcnac.aspensys.com:72/
*MMWR Reports on HIV/AIDS: Morbidity and Mortality
 Weekly Report*
 (CDC, Division of HIV/AIDS [DHAP])
 http://www.cdc.gov/epo/mmwr/mmwr.html
Poz Magazine
 http://www.poz.com
XI International Conference on AIDS
 (Vancouver, July 7–12, 1996)
 http://www.interchg.ubc.ca/AIDS11/AIDS96.html
XI International Conference on AIDS: *Program Abstracts*
 http://sis.nlm.nih.gov/AIDSabs.htm
12th World AIDS Conference (Geneva, June 28–July 3, 1998)
 http://www.AIDS98.ch/

AIDS Consumer and Patient Organizations

Critical Path AIDS Project in Philadelphia
 http://www.critpath.org/
National Association of People with AIDS (NAPWA)
 http://www.thecure.org
National Foundation for Children with AIDS
 http://www.childrenwithAIDS.org
People With AIDS Coalition of America, Inc.
 http://jaxadnet.com/pwaca
People With AIDS Coalition of New York
 http://www.AIDSnyc.org/pwac
People With AIDS Coalition of Philadelphia
 http://www.critpath.org/wtp/
People with AIDS Coalition of Vermont
 http://www.sover.net/~vtpwac/
Project Inform
 http://www.projinf.org/

Clinical trials

Adult AIDS Clinical Trials Group
 http://aactg.s-3.com/
AIDS Clinical Trials Information Service
 http://www.actis.org/
AIDS Treatment Data Network
 http://www.AIDSnyc.org/network
Community Programs for Clinical Research on AIDS (CPCRA)
 http://www.cpcra.org
HIV/AIDS Treatment Information Service (ATIS)
 http://www.hivatis.org
National AIDS Treatment Advocacy Project (NATAP)
 http://www.AIDSnyc.org/natap/

Databases

AIDSLINE (fee charged)
 http://www.silverplatter.com/physicians
 http://www.paperchase.com
HIV Molecular Immunology Database
 http://hiv-web.lanl.gov/immuno
HIV Sequence Database
 http://hiv-web.lanl.gov/
NLM's Internet Grateful Med
 http://igm.nlm.nih.gov:80/

Newsgroups

AIDS mailing list/sci.med.AIDS newsgroup gateway
http://ds.internic.net/cgi-bin/enthtml/health/AIDS.b
AIDS.NET
http://nursing.adm.binghamton.edu/AIDSnet.html
Newsgroup:alt.sex.safe
news:alt.sex.safe
Newsgroup:misc.health.AIDS
news:misc.health.AIDS
Newsgroup:sci.med.AIDS
news:sci.med.AIDS

Terminology

AIDS Treatment Data Network Glossary: Conditions
& Symptoms
http://www.AIDSnyc.org/network/oisgloss.html
National AIDS Treatment Activist Forum. AIDS Glossary of
Medical and Statistical Terms
http://www.teleport.com/~celinec/glossary.htm
National Institutes of Health Searchable AIDS Dictionary
gopher://gopher.niaid.nih.gov:70/77/AIDS/.AIDSdict/index

Safer Sex

Boy2Boy Network
http://www.tde.com/~boy2boy/
Lesbian Safer Sex Page
http://safersex.org/women/lesbianss.html
Safer Sex Page
http://www.safersex.org/
Sexual Health Advocate Peer Education (Shape)
http://www.missouri.edu/~shape/

Community and Regional Aids Organizations and Services

ACT-UP
http://www.actupny.org

AIDS Project Los Angeles
http://www.apla.org/apla/
Community Health Project
http://www.chp-health.org
Consumer News
http://www.AIDSnyc.org/cnews
Gay Men's Health Crisis (GMHC)
http://www.gmhc.org/GMHC
STOP AIDS Project, San Francisco
http://www.stopAIDS.org/
Treatment Action Group
http://www.thebody.com/tag/tagpage.html

Law and Legislation

American Civil Liberties Union (ACLU)
http://www.aclu.org
Americans with Disabilities Act (ADA)
http://www.usdoj.gov/crt/ada/adahom1.htm
Lambda Legal Defense and Education Fund
http://www.gaysource.com/gs/ht/oct95/lambda.html

Miscellaneous

Names Project Foundation (NPF)
http://www.aidsquilt.org
Pasteur Institute, Paris
http://www.pasteur.fr/
World AIDS Day
http://www.oneworld.org/avert/worldaid.htm
http://www.wad.hea.org.uk
http://www.cyberzine.org/html/WAD/

BIBLIOGRAPHY

BIBLIOGRAPHY

The Act-Up/New York Women & AIDS Book Group. *Women, AIDS & Activism*. Boston: South End, 1990.

Altman, Dennis. *AIDS in the Mind of America: The Social, Political, and Psychological Impact of a New Epidemic*. Garden City, N.Y.: Anchor/Doubleday, 1986.

Altman, Roberta and Michael J. Sarg. *The Cancer Dictionary*. New York: Facts On File, 1992.

Alyson, Sasha, ed. *You Can Do Something About AIDS*. Boston: The Stop AIDS Project, Inc., 1988.

Ammer, Christine. *The New A-to-Z of Women's Health: A Concise Encyclopedia*. Rev. and expanded ed. New York: Facts On File, 1989.

Arno, Peter S. and Karyn L. Feiden. *Against the Odds: The Story of AIDS Drug Development, Politics and Profits*. New York: HarperCollins, 1992.

Bartlett, John G. and Ann K. Finkbeiner. *The Guide to Living with HIV Infection*. Baltimore: Johns Hopkins University Press, 1991.

Bechtel, Stefan and the Editors of *Prevention* and *Men's Health* magazines. *The Sex Encyclopedia: An A-to-Z Guide to the Latest Information on Sexual Health, Safety, and Technique from the Nation's Top Sex Experts*. New York: Simon & Schuster, 1993.

The Boston Women's Health Book Collective. *The New Our Bodies, Ourselves: Updated and Expanded for the '90s*. New York: Simon & Schuster, 1992.

Breitman, Patti, Kim Knutson and Paul Reed. *How to Persuade Your Lover to Use a Condom . . . and Why You Should*. Rocklin, Ca.: Prima, 1987.

Burris, Scott, Harlon L. Dalton, Judith Leonie Millera and the Yale AIDS Law Project, eds. *AIDS Law Today: A New Guide for the Public*. New Haven: Yale University Press, 1993.

Butler, Sandra and Barbara Rosenblum. *Cancer in Two Voices*. San Francisco: Spinsters, 1991.

Califia, Pat. *The Advocate Adviser*. Boston: Alyson, 1991.

Califia, Pat, ed. *The Lesbian S/M Safety Manual: Basic Health and Safety for Woman-to-Woman S/M*. Denver: Lace, 1988.

Callen, Michael. *Surviving AIDS*. New York: HarperCollins, 1990.

Carmichael, Cynthia G., J. Kevin Carmichael and Margaret A. Fischl. *HIV/AIDS Primary Care Handbook*. Norwalk, Conn.: Appleton & Lange, 1995.

Carrera, Michael A. *The Language of Sex: An A to Z Guide*. New York: Facts On File, 1992.

Caulfield, Charles R. with Billi Goldberg. *The Anarchist AIDS Medical Formulary: A Guide to Guerrilla Immunology*. Berkeley: North Atlantic, 1993.

Centers for Disease Control and Prevention, "Update on Acquired Immune Deficiency Syndrome (AIDS)—United States," *Morbidity and Mortality Weekly Report* 31 (1982): 507–514.

———,"The Case Definition of AIDS Used by CDC for National Reporting (CDC reportable AIDS)," Document no. 0312S, August 1, 1985.

Corea, Gena. *The Invisible Epidemic: The Story of Women and AIDS*. New York: Harper Perennial, 1992.

Crimp, Douglas. *AIDS Demo Graphics*. Seattle: Bay Press, 1990.

Crimp, Douglas, ed. *AIDS: Cultural Analysis Cultural Activism*. Cambridge: MIT Press, 1988.

DeCotiis, Sue. *A Woman's Guide to Sexual Health*. New York: Pocket Books, 1989.

Delacoste, Frederique and Priscilla Alexander, eds. *Sex Work: Writings by Women in the Sex Industry*. San Francisco: Cleis, 1987.

Denenberg, Risa. *Gynecological Care Manual for HIV Positive Women*. Durant, Okla.: Essential Medical Information Systems, 1993.

Dietz, Steven D. and M. Jane Parker Hicks. *Take Those Broken Wings and Learn to Fly: The AIDS Support Book for Patients, Family and Friends*. Tucson: Harbinger House, 1989.

Douglas, Paul Harding and Laura Pinsky. *The Essential AIDS Fact Book*. New York: Pocket Books, 1989.

Edison, Ted, ed. *The AIDS Caregiver's Handbook*. New York: St. Martin's, 1988.

Fettner, Ann Giudici. *The Science of Viruses: What They Are, Why They Make Us Sick, How They Will Change the Future*. New York: William Morrow, 1990.

Flanders, Stephen A. and Carl N. Flanders. *AIDS*. New York: Facts On File, 1991.

Ford, Michael Thomas. *100 Questions & Answers about AIDS: What You Need to Know Now*. New York: Beech Tree, 1992.

Formichella, Annamaria, Susan McIntyre and Marjorie Brant Osterhout. *Tell It Like It Is: Straight Talk About Sex*. New York: Avon, 1991.

Froman, Paul Kent. *Pathways to Wellness: Strategies for Self-Empowerment in the Age of AIDS.* New York: Penguin, 1990.

Frumkin, Lyn and John Leonard. *Questions & Answers on AIDS.* 2nd ed. Los Angeles: PMIC, 1994.

Gay Men's Health Crisis. *GMHC Treatment Issues: The Gay Men's Health Crisis Newsletter of Experimental AIDS Therapies.* New York: GMHC, Treatment Education, vol. 1, no. 1, November 1987–to date.

Geballe, Shelley, Janice Gruendel and Warren Andiman. *Forgotten Children of the AIDS Epidemic.* New Haven: Yale University Press, 1995.

Hay, Louise L. *The AIDS Book: Creating a Positive Approach.* Santa Monica: Hay House, 1988.

Heimel, Cynthia. *Sex Tips for Girls.* New York: Simon & Schuster, 1993.

Huber, Jeffrey T., ed. *How to Find Information about AIDS.* 2nd ed. New York: Harrington Park, 1992.

Humphry, Derek. *Final Exit: The Practicalities of Self-Deliverance and Assisted Suicide for the Dying.* New York: Dell, 1991.

Hwang, T. L., et al. *Journal of Neuro-Oncology* 3(4), April 1986, 335–9.

Institute for the Advanced Study of Human Sexuality. *The Complete Guide to Safe Sex.* Published for the PreVenT Group of Beverly Hills, California, by Specific Press, 1987.

——. *Safe Sex in the Age of AIDS.* Secaucus, N.J.: Citadel, 1986.

James, John S., ed. *AIDS Treatment News.* Vol. 1. Berkeley: Celestial Arts, 1989.

——. *AIDS Treatment News.* Vol. 2. Berkeley: Celestial Arts, 1991.

——. *AIDS Treatment News.* Vol. 3. Boston: Alyson, 1994.

Johnson, Elizabeth A. *As Someone Dies; A Handbook for the Living.* Santa Monica: Hay House, 1987.

Johnston, William I. *HIV-Negative: How the Uninfected Are Affected by AIDS.* New York: Plenum, 1995.

Kahn, Ada P. and Linda Hughey Holt. *The A–Z of Women's Sexuality.* New York: Facts On File, 1990.

Kain, Craig, ed. *No Longer Immune: A Counselor's Guide to AIDS.* Alexandria, Va.: American Association for Counseling and Development, 1989.

Kaplan, Helen Singer. *The Real Truth About Women and AIDS: How to Eliminate the Risks without Giving Up Love and Sex.* New York: Simon & Schuster, 1987.

Kinsella, James. *Covering the Plague: AIDS and the American Media.* New Brunswick, N.J.: Rutgers University Press, 1989.

Kirp, David L. *Learning by Heart: AIDS and Schoolchildren in America's Communities.* New Brunswick, N.J.: Rutgers University Press, 1989.

Kirschmann, Gayla J. and John D. Kirschmann. *Nutrition Almanac.* 4th ed. New York: McGraw-Hill, 1966.

Kramer, Larry. *Reports from the Holocaust: The Making of an AIDS Activist.* New York: St. Martin's, 1989.

Kübler-Ross, Elisabeth. *AIDS: The Ultimate Challenge.* New York: Macmillan, 1987.

——. *Death: The Final Stage of Growth.* New York: Simon & Schuster, 1975.

——. *On Death and Dying.* New York: Macmillan, 1969.

——. *On Life After Death.* Berkeley.: Celestial Arts, 1991.

——. *Questions and Answers on Death and Dying.* New York: Macmillan, 1974.

——. *To Live Until We Say Goodbye.* Englewood Cliffs, N.J.: Prentice-Hall, 1976.

Kurth, Ann, ed. *Until the Cure: Caring for Women with HIV.* New Haven: Yale University Press, 1993.

Kyle, Garland Richard. *Whatever Happened to Passion: Writings from the Epidemic Years.* San Francisco: Modern Words, 1992.

Lester, Bonnie. *Women and AIDS: A Practical Guide for Those Who Help Others.* New York: Continuum, 1989.

Lingle, Virginia A. and M. Sandra Wood. *How to Find Information about AIDS.* New York: Harrington Park, 1988.

Lu, Henry C. *Chinese System of Food Cures: Prevention & Remedies.* New York: Sterling, 1986.

Macklin, Eleanor D. *AIDS and Families: Report of the AIDS Task Force Groves Conference on Marriage and the Family.* Binghamton, N.Y.: Harrington Park, 1989.

Malinowsky, H. Robert and Gerald J. Perry. *AIDS Information Sourcebook.* Phoenix: Oryx, 1988.

——. *AIDS Information Sourcebook.* 2nd ed. Phoenix: Oryx, 1989.

Mann, Jonathan, Daniel J. M. Tarantola, and Thomas W. Netter, eds. *AIDS in the World.* Cambridge: Harvard University Press, 1992.

Martelli, Leonard J. with Fran D. Peltz and William Messina. *When Someone You Know Has AIDS: A Practical Guide.* New York: Crown, 1987.

Marti, James E. *The Alternative Health Medicine Encyclopedia: The Authoritative Guide to Holistic & Nontraditional Health Practices.* Washington, D.C.: Visible Ink, 1995.

McCormack, Thomas P. *The AIDS Benefits Handbook.* New Haven: Yale University Press, 1990.

Mikluscak-Cooper, Cindy and Emmett E. Miller. *Living in Hope: A 12-Step Approach for Persons at Risk or Infected with HIV.* Berkeley: Celestial Arts, 1991.

Miller, Heather G., Charles F. Turner and Lincoln E. Moses, eds. *AIDS: The Second Decade.* Washington, D.C.: National Academy Press, 1990.

Miller, Norman and Richard C. Rockwell, eds. *AIDS in Africa: The Social and Policy Impact.* Lewiston, N.Y.: The Edwin Mellen Press, 1988.

Moffatt, Betty Clare. *When Someone You Love Has AIDS: A Book of Hope for Family and Friends.* New York: NAL Penguin, 1986.

National Cancer Institute. *Advanced Cancer: Living Each Day.* National Institutes of Health, Public Health Service, U.S. Department of Health and Human Services, Revised February 1994. NIH Publication No. 94–856.

——. *Taking Time: Support for People with Cancer and the People Who Care About Them.* National Institutes of Health, Public Health Service, U.S. Department of Health and Human Services, 1990. NIH Publication No. 94–2059.

Nevid, Jeffrey S. *201 Things You Should Know about AIDS and other Sexually Transmitted Diseases.* Boston: Allyn & Bacon, 1993.

Nichols, Eve K. *Mobilizing Against AIDS.* Cambridge: Harvard University Press, 1989.

Norwood, Chris. *Advice for Life: A Woman's Guide to AIDS Risks and Prevention.* New York: Pantheon, 1987.

Nuland, Sherwin B. *How We Die: Reflections on Life's Final Chapter.* New York: Alfred A. Knopf, 1993.

Nungesser, Lon G. *Epidemic of Courage: Facing AIDS in America.* New York: St. Martin's, 1986.

O'Sullivan, Sue and Pratibha Parmar. *Lesbians Talks (Safer Sex).* London: Scarlet Press, 1992.

Patton, Cindy. *Fatal Advice: How Safe-Sex Education Went Wrong.* Durham, N.C.: Duke University Press, 1996.

———. *Inventing AIDS.* New York: Routledge, 1990.

Patton, Cindy. *Sex and Germs: The Politics of AIDS.* Boston: South End Press, 1985.

Patton, Cindy and Janis Kelly. *Making It: A Woman's Guide to Sex in the Age of AIDS.* Ithaca, N.Y.: Firebrand, 1987.

The PDR Family Guide to Women's Health and Prescription Drugs. Montvale, N.J.: Medical Economics, 1994.

Perrow, Charles and Mauro F. Guillen. *The AIDS Disaster: The Failure of Organizations in New York and the Nation.* New Haven: Yale University Press, 1990.

Pinckney, Cathey and Edward R. Pinckney. *Do-It-Yourself Medical Testing.* 3rd ed. New York: Facts On File, 1989.

———. *The Parent's Guide to Medical Tests.* 3rd ed. New York: Facts On File, 1986.

Preston, Richard. *The Hot Zone.* New York: Random House, 1994.

Project Inform. *The HIV Drug Book.* New York: Pocket Books, 1995.

Reinisch, June M. *The Kinsey Institute New Report on Sex: What You Must Know to Be Sexually Literate.* New York: St. Martin's, 1991.

Rhea, Joseph C., J. Steven Ott and Jay M. Shafritz. *The Facts On File Dictionary of Health Care Management.* New York: Facts On File, 1988.

Richardson, Diane. *Women & AIDS.* New York: Methuen, 1988.

Richter, Alan. *Dictionary of Sexual Slang: Words, Phrases & Idioms from AC/DC to Zig-zig.* New York: Wiley, 1993.

Rieder, Ines and Patricia Ruppelt. *AIDS: The Women.* San Francisco: Cleis, 1988.

Rudd, Andrea and Darien Taylor, eds. *Positive Women: Voices of Women Living with AIDS.* Toronto: Second Story Press, 1992.

Rybacki, James J. and James W. Long. *The Essential Guide to Prescription Drugs 1997.* New York: HarperCollins, 1996.

Scanlon, Valerie C. and Tina Sanders. *Essentials of Anatomy and Physiology.* 2nd ed. Philadelphia: F. A. Davis, 1995.

Shernoff, Michael, ed. *Counseling Chemically Dependent People with HIV Illness.* Binghamton, N.Y.: Harrington Park, 1991.

Shilts, Randy. *And the Band Played On: Politics, People, and the AIDS Epidemic.* New York: St. Martin's, 1987.

Siegel, Bernie S. *Love, Medicine & Miracles: Lessons Learned About Self-Healing from a Surgeon's Experience with Exceptional Patients.* New York: Harper & Row, 1986.

Sontag, Susan. *AIDS and Its Metaphors.* New York: Farrar, Straus and Giroux, 1989.

———. *Illness as Metaphor.* New York: Farrar, Straus and Giroux, 1978.

Sternberg, Robert J., ed. *Encyclopedia of Human Intelligence.* New York: Macmillan, 1994.

Taber's Cyclopedic Medical Dictionary. 17th ed. Philadelphia: F. A. Davis, 1993.

Tauber, Jeffrey T. *Dictionary of AIDS Related Terminology.* New York: Neal-Schuman, 1993.

Terl, Allan H. *AIDS and the Law: A Basic Guide for the Non-lawyer.* Taylor & Francis, 1992.

Thain, Michael and Michael Hickman. *The Penguin Dictionary of Biology.* 9th ed. rev. New York: Penguin, 1995.

Tilleraas, Perry. *Living with HIV: A Spiritual Response to HIV: The Twelve Steps.* Center City, Minn.: Hazelden Educational Materials, 1990.

U.S. Department of Health and Human Services, Public Health Service, Agency for Health Care Policy and Research. *Evaluation and Management of Early HIV Infection.* Rockville, Md.: U.S. Department of Health and Human Services, 1994. AHCPR Publication No. 94–0572.

Watstein, Sarah Barbara and Robert Anthony Laurich. *AIDS and Women: A Sourcebook.* Phoenix: Oryx, 1991.

Whipple, Beverly and Gina Ogden. *Safe Encounters: How Women Can Say Yes to Pleasure and No to Unsafe Sex.* New York: Pocket Books, 1989.

White, Evelyn C., ed. *The Black Women's Health Book.* Seattle: Seal Press, 1990.

Wilson, Josleen. *Woman: Your Body, Your Health: The Essential Guide for Well-Being.* New York: Harcourt Brace Jovanovich, 1990.

Wood, Gary James and Robert Marks, with James W. Dilley. *AIDS Law for Mental Health Professionals: A Handbook for Judicious Practice.* San Francisco: The AIDS Health Project, University of California–San Francisco, 1992.

INDEX

INDEX

This index contains important terms and names found within the dictionary entries. For definitions and primary discussions of terms, consult the A–Z section of the dictionary.

BRMs *See* biological response
modifiers
Broviac, Dr.   45
bubonic plague   213
bureaucracy   234–35, 280
burning   95
buyers' clubs   7, 240

C

CAF (cell antiviral factor)   50
California   85
Callen, Michael   215
camphor   254
cancer
  brain   37
  breast   38, 171–72
  cervical   49, 205
  chemotherapy   51, 67,
    101, 178, 263, 271
  colorectal   162
  laser therapy   159
  liver   164
  metastasis   177–78
  oral   198
  ovarian   201
  skin   30
candidiasis   3, 56, 94, 101,
  158, 198–99
carbon dioxide   134
carcinoma   42, 185
caregiver
  buddy   39–40
  burnout   40
carotene   31
Carrisyn   2
case definition   7–8, 262
cat   99
CAT scan   60, 73
catheter   122, 144
cattle   37
CC chemokine receptor 5
  (CCR5)   165
CD4 cells   139, 165, 197
  and antiretrovirals   21
  baseline count   30
  Concorde study   60
  and Cytolin   68
  and diagnosis   75
  and dinitrochlorobenzene
    77
  and glutathione   112
  and gp   120, 125, 222
  and HIV measurement   126
  and interleukin   147–48
  in pregnancy   218
  Pro 2000   222
  soluble   254
  and T cells   265
  and therapeutic vaccine
    268
CD8 cells   48, 50, 68, 69, 77,
  219–20, 264, 265
CDC *See* Centers for Disease
  Control and Prevention
Ceftin   48
celibacy   1
cells   22, 24, 69, 134, 257, 291

cellular latency   160
Centers for Disease Control
  and Prevention (CDC)   7,
  57, 142, 203, 239, 262, 283,
  285–86
central nervous system   189,
  219
central venous catheter   45
cerebrospinal fluid   256
Cerubidine   71
cervical cap   255
cervical intraepithelial neoplasia (CIN)   204, 205
cervix   24, 57, 90, 95, 122,
  166, 182, 204, 205
chemotaxis   59
chemotherapy   67, 101, 154,
  163, 178, 193, 263, 271
"chi" points   3, 4
childbirth   149, 276
children
  AIDS in   208
  and drug use   82
  emergency assistance pro-
    gram   89
  failure to thrive   97
  foster care   104
  Individuals with Disabili-
    ties Education Act   143
  orphans   10, 200
  Reye's syndrome   238
  testing of   280
  treatment of   279
Chinese medicine   3, 4
chlamydia   101
Chlor-Trimeton   52
chlorhexidine   276
chlorine bleach   33
Chloromyecitin   52
chloroquine   171
Chow, Yang-kung   63
chromosomes   117
CICs *See* circulating immune
  complexes
CIN *See* cervical intraepithelial neoplasia
circulating immune complexes
  (CICs)   134
citrovorum factor   162
civil rights   158
clinical latency   160
clinical trials   95, 142, 147,
  220, 233–34, 280
Clinton, Bill   80, 137, 291
Clostridium difficile   54
clotting   214, 226
clotting factor,   35, 119–20, 273
CMV *See* cytomegalovirus
cocaine   64, 81, 104
coenzyme Q   285
coinsurance   63
colitis   69
collagen   101
colony-stimulating factor drugs
  154
colorectal cancer   162
colostrum   38
combination therapy   63, 191,
  269, 281–82

compound Q *See* GLQ223
computer bulletin board   40
Comtrex   52
condoms   99–100, 188, 216,
  243, 244, 271
confidentiality   221–22
consent   144
Consumer Product Safety Act
  150
Contact Allergy Formula   266
contraception   98, 100, 102,
  108, 149, 185, 199, 223,
  255–56
contrast agent   107
control   90
convulsions   19, 246
corpus luteum   166
corticosteroids   258
Cotrimoxale   281
counseling   78–79, 125, 192,
  218, 227, 235–36
Cranston, Alan   155
Cranston-Gonzalez National
  Affordable Housing Act
  129
Creutzfeldt-Jakob virus   223
cross-species transplant   37
cryotherapy   153
Cryptosporidium   65
cryptosporidosis   206
cunnilingus   199
cyclophilin A   224
cystitis   94, 156, 226, 287
cytokines   2, 154, 260, 284
cytomegalovirus (CMV)   52,
  57, 99, 106, 107, 189
cytosine arabinoside   223
cytotoxic T cells   119, 219–20,
  265, 291
Cytovene   106

D

DDAVP   74
ddC *See* dideoxycytidine
ddI *See* didanosine
DDS *See* Disability Determination Service
DEA *See* Drug Enforcement
  Agency
delavirdine   89, 193
DeMarco, Chuck   135
dementia   9
dendritic cell   77, 102
Denenberg, Risa   205
denial   226–27
dental dam   244
Department of Veterans Affairs
  (VA)   7
dependency   227
dependent variable   292
depression   19, 102, 181, 206
dermatitis   245
descending neuropathy   190
desert fever   56
diabetes insipidus   74
diagnosis   71, 77, 218
dialysis   211

Diamond, Aaron   125
diaphragm   99–100, 255
diarrhea   19, 54, 55, 111, 165,
  170–71, 179, 196, 197
diastolic blood pressure   34,
  135
didanosine (ddI)   21, 26, 63,
  70, 138
dideoxycytidine (ddC)   21,
  138, 269
diet
  macrobiotic   169
  malnutrition   171
  nutritional supplementa-
    tion   13, 76–77, 99, 195
Diflucan   101
dignity   71
Dirline   70
Disability Determination Service (DDS)   78
disabled   7, 89, 141, 142, 143,
  218, 254, 297
discourse   9, 11, 58
discrimination   14, 54, 64, 78,
  90, 97–98, 128–29, 228
disseminated Kaposi's sarcoma
  154
diuretic   268
DNA (deoxyribonucleic acid)
  95, 125, 130, 150, 194, 255
  antisense   21
  branched assay   38
  facilitated inoculation   97
  and famciclovir   98
  and immune system   139
  in Kaposi's sarcoma   155
  mutation   84
  polymerase chain reaction
    test   215
  recombinant   234
  thymidine   270
  topoisomerase   271
  triple helix   281
  vidarabine   293
  zinc finger   306
domestic relations law   98
donovanosis   113
Dornan, Robert K.   80
douche   291
Drug Enforcement Agency
  (DEA)   88
drug(s)
  accelerated approval   1–2
  activity   3
  addiction   5, 235
  adjuvant   6
  anti-infective   20
  approval process   95
  assistance programs   9–10
  blind test   33
  buyers' clubs   7, 41, 240
  chemotherapy   51
  clinical endpoint   55
  clinical trials   55, 63, 95,
    233–34, 280
  colony-stimulating factor
    154
  combination therapy   58,
    63, 191, 269, 281–82